Hematopoietic Cell Transplantation for Malignant Conditions

Hematopoietic Cell Transplantation for Malignant Conditions

EDITED BY

QAISER BASHIR, MD
Stem Cell Transplantation & Cellular Therapy
UT MD Anderson Cancer Center
Houston, TX, United States

MEHDI HAMADANI, MD
Professor of Medicine
Director
BMT and Cellular Therapy Program CIBMTR
Medical College of Wisconsin
Milwaukee, WI, United States

ELSEVIER

Publisher: Dolores Meloni
Acquisition Editor: Robin Carter
Editorial Project Manager: Karen Miller
Project Manager: Kiruthika Govindaraju
Designer: Alan Studholme

**Working together
to grow libraries in
developing countries**

3251 Riverport Lane
St. Louis, Missouri 63043

www.elsevier.com • www.bookaid.org

List of Contributors

Mufti Naeem Ahmad, MD
Fellow, Hematology and Oncology
Levine Cancer Institute
Atrium Health
Charlotte, NC, United States

Sairah Ahmed, MD
Assistant Professor
Department of Stem Cell Transplant and Cellular
    Therapy
University of Texas, MD Anderson Cancer Center
Houston, TX, United States

Shukaib Arslan, MD
Doctor
Hematology/Oncology
Michigan State University, Providence-Providence
    Park Hospital
Southfield, MI, United States

Farrukh T. Awan, MD
Associate Professor of Medicine
Hematology
The Ohio State University
Columbus, OH, United States

Qaiser Bashir, MD
Stem Cell Transplantation & Cellular Therapy
UT MD Anderson Cancer Center
Houston, TX, United States

Didier Blaise, DB, MD
Transplantation and Cellular Immunotherapy Unit
Department of Hematology
Institut Paoli Calmettes
Marseille, France

Centre de Recherche en Cancérologie de Marseille
    (CRCM) Inserm UMR1068
CNRS UMR7258
(3) Aix Marseille Université U105
Marseille, France

Hematology Department
Institut Paoli Calmettes
Marseille, France

Megan Bodge, PharmD, BCOP
Clinical Pharmacy Specialist
Pharmacy
WVU Medicine
Morgantown, WV, United States

Stefania Bramanti, SB, MD
Department of Hematology
BMT Unit
Humanitas Clinical and Research Hospital
Milan, Italy

Luca Castagna, LC, MD
Department of Hematology
BMT Unit
Humanitas Clinical and Research Hospital
Milan, Italy

Luciano J. Costa, MD, PhD
Associate Professor of Medicine
Division of Hematology and Oncology
University of Alabama at Birmingham
Birmingham, AL, United States

Aaron Cumpston, PharmD, BCOP
Clinical Pharmacy Specialist
Department of Pharmacy
West Virginia University Medicine
Morgantown, WV, United States

Anita D'Souza, MD, MS
Assistant Professor of Medicine
Medicine
Medical College of Wisconsin
Milwaukee, WI, United States

Marcos de Lima, MD
Professor of Medicine
Department of Medicine
University Hospitals and Case Western Reserve
    University
Clevelan, OH, United States

Raynier Devillier, RD, MP, PhD
Transplantation and Cellular Immunotherapy Unit
Department of Hematology
Institut Paoli Calmettes, Marseille, France

Centre de Recherche en Cancérologie de Marseille
  (CRCM) Inserm UMR1068
CNRS UMR7258
(3) Aix Marseille Université U105
Marseille, France

Hematology Department
Institut Paoli Calmettes
Marseille, France

Rebecca Devlin, PhD
Scientific Associate
Department of Medical Oncology and Hematology
Princess Margaret Cancer Centre
Toronto, ON, Canada

Fiona L. Dignan, MBChB, FRCP, FRCPath, MD
Doctor
Clinical Haematology
Manchester University Foundation Trust
Manchester, United Kingdom

Sabine Furst, SF, MD
Transplantation and Cellular Immunotherapy Unit
Department of Hematology
Institut Paoli Calmettes
Marseille, France

Ragisha Gopalakrishnan, MD
Hematology Oncology Fellow
Vanderbilt Ingram Cancer Center (Hematology
  Oncology)
Vanderbilt University Medical Center
Nashville, TN, United States

Alison Gulbis, PharmD, BCOP
Manager, Clinical Pharmacy Services
Division of Pharmacy
MD Anderson Cancer Center
Houston, TX, United States

Vikas Gupta, MD, FRCP, FRCPath
Associate Professor
Department of Medicine
University of Toronto
Toronto, ON, Canada

Ali Haider, MD
Assistant Professor
Palliative, Rehabilitation, and Integrative Medicine
Houston, TX, United States

Parameswaran Hari, MD, MS
Director
Adult Blood and Marrow Transplant Program
Division of Hematology Oncology
Medical College of Wisconsin
Milwaukee, WI, United States

Professor
Hematology Oncology
Milwaukee, WI, United States

Chitra Hosing, MD
Professor
Stem Cell Transplantation and Cellular Therapy
MD Anderson Cancer Center
Houston, TX, United States

Mohammed Junaid Hussain, MD
Plasma Cell Disorders Section
Department of Hematologic Oncology & Blood
  Disorders
Levine Cancer Institute/Carolinas Healthcare System
Charlotte, NC, United States

Racquel Innis-Shelton, MD
Assistant Professor of Medicine
Division of Hematology and Oncology
Department of Medicine
University of Alabama at Birmingham
Birmingham, AL, United States

Madan Jagasia, MBBS
Professor of Medicine
Medicine/Division of Hematology Oncology
Vanderbilt University Medical Center
Nashville, TN, United States

Abraham S. Kanate, MD
Assistant Professor
Osborn Hematological Malignancy and
  Transplantation Program
Dept of Internal Medicine
West Virginia University
Morgantown, WV, United States

Partow Kebriaei, MD
Professor
Stem Cell Transplant and Cellular Therapy
MDACC
Houston, TX, United States

Maliha Khan, MD
Leukemia Department
University of Texas
MD Anderson Cancer Center
Houston, TX, United States

Shakila P. Khan, MD
Associate Professor
Pediatrics
Mayo Clinic
Rochester, MN, United States

Mohamed A. Kharfan-Dabaja, MD, MBA
Professor of Medicine
Division of Hematology-Oncology
Blood and Marrow Transplantation Program
Mayo Clinic
Jacksonville, FL, United States

Sola Kim, MD
Department of Palliative, Rehabilitation, and
    Integrative Medicine
University of Texas
MD Anderson Cancer Center
Houston, TX, United States

Mira A. Kohorst, MD
Assistant Professor of Pediatrics
College of Medicine
Division of Pediatric Hematology-Oncology
Department of Pediatric and Adolescent Medicine
Mayo Clinic
Rochester, MN, United States

Amrita Krishnan, MD
The Judy and Bernard Briskin for Multiple Myeloma
    Research
City of Hope Medical Center
Duarte, CA, United States

Rohtesh S. Mehta, MD, MPH, MS
Assistant Professor
Stem Cell Transplantation and Cellular Therapies
The University of Texas
MD Anderson Cancer Center
Houston, TX, United States

Muhammad Ayaz Mir, MBBS, FACP
Chief
Hematology & Oncology
Shifa International Hospital
Islamabad, Pakistan

Ravi Kishore Narra, MD
Assistant Professor
Medicine, Division of Hematology/Oncology
Medical College of Wisconsin
Brookfield, WI, United States

Nhu-Nhu Nguyen, MD
Physician
Palliative, Rehabilitation and Integrative Medicine
MD Anderson Cancer Center
Houston, TX, United States

Yago Nieto, MD, PhD
Professor of Medicine
Stem Cell Transplantation and Cellular Therapy
The University of Texas
MD Anderson Cancer Center
Houston, TX, United States

Liana Nikolaenko, MD
Assistant Clinical Professor
Hematology/Bone Marrow Transplant
City of Hope
Duarte, CA, United States

Amanda Olson, MD
Assistant Professor
Stem Cell Transplantation and Cellular Therapy
MD Anderson Cancer Center
Houston, TX, United States

Kelly E. Pillinger, PharmD
University of Rochester Medical Center
Strong Memorial Hospital
Rochester, NY, United States

Chelsea C. Pinnix, MD, PhD
Assistant Professor
Radiation Oncology
University of Texas
MD Anderson Cancer Center
Houston, TX, United States

L.M. Poon
Senior Consultant
Hematology Oncology
National University Cancer Institute, Singapore
Singapore, Singapore

Kelly G. Ross, MD
Assistant Professor of Medicine
Hematology/Oncology
West Virginia University
Morgantown, WV, United States

Muhammad A. Saif, MBBS, MRCP, FRCPath, MD
Consultant Haematologist
Clinical Haematology
Central Manchester University Hospital
Manchester, United Kingdom

Nirav N. Shah, MD, MS
Assistant Professor of Medicine
Internal Medicine
Medical College of Wisconsin
Milwuakee, WI, United States

Zainab Shahid, MD, FACP
Medical Direction Bone Marrow Transplant Infectious
    Diseases
Levine Cancer Institute
Carolians Healthcare System
Charlotte, NC, United States

Bronwen E. Shaw, MBChB, PhD
Professor of Medicine
Hem-Onc
Medical College of Wisconsin/CIBMTR
Milwaukee, WI, United States

Elizabeth J. Shpall, MD
Stem Cell Transplantation and Cellular Therapy
The University of Texas MD Anderson Cancer Center
Houston, TX, United States

Rabbia Siddiqi, MBBS
Department of Internal Medicine
Dow University of Health Sciences
Karachi, Pakistan

Roni Tamari, MD
Assistant Attending
Bone Marrow Transplant, Department of Medicine
Memorial Sloan Kettering Cancer Center
New York, NY, United States

Benjamin Tomlinson, MD
Assistant Professor
Internal Medicine, Division of Hematology and
    Oncology
University Hospitals Seidman Cancer Center
Cleveland, OH, United States

Saad Zafar Usmani, MD, FACP
Chief
Plasma Cell Disorders Section
Hematologic Oncology & Blood Disorders
Levine Cancer Institute/Carolinas Healthcare System
Charlotte, NC, United States

Lauren Veltri, MD
Assistant Professor
Hematology/Oncology
West Virginia University School of Medicine
Morgantown, WV, United States

Daniel Weisdorf, MD
Professor
Medicine
University of Minnesota
Minneapolis, MN, United States

Ibrahim Yakoub-Agha, MD, PhD
Professor
Hematology
University Hospital CHRU
Lille, France

Lily Yan, PharmD, BCOP
Pharmacy Clinical Specialist
Stem Cell Transplant
University of Texas
MD Anderson Cancer Center
Houston, TX, United States

Contents

CHAPTER 1

History and Current Status of Hematopoietic Cell Transplantation

ROHTESH S. MEHTA, MD, MPH, MS • DANIEL WEISDORF, MD

INTRODUCTION

In an atomic age, with reactor accidents, not to mention stupidities with bombs, somebody is going to get more radiation than is good for him. If infusion of marrow can induce recovery in a mouse or monkey after lethal radiation, one had best be prepared with this form of treatment in man.[1]

E. DONNALL THOMAS.

Research in the field of bone marrow transplantation (BMT) accelerated with the disaster caused by atomic bombs which ended World War II in August 1945. Within a few months, the US government, in coordination with Japanese scientists, formed a joint commission to investigate biological effects of the bomb, especially bone marrow (BM) failure. Comprehensive epidemiological, clinical, and genetic studies were started under the auspices of the Atomic Bomb Casualty Commission that was formed in 1947.[2,3]

BMT Developments in 1950s to Early 1960s

In 1950, Jacobson noticed "ectopic blood formation" and rapid recovery of hematopoietic tissues in rabbits treated with total body irradiation (TBI) if their spleens were shielded with lead.[4] In subsequent experiments, they witnessed increased survival of lethally irradiated mice that were infused intraperitoneally with freshly removed allogeneic spleens as compared to mice who did not receive splenic implants.[5] It was proposed that if the mechanism of this enhanced hematopoietic recovery after splenic shielding was "seeding of hematopoietic elements to various organs," then "seeding with the cellular constituents of bone marrow, as by intravenous injection, should also be effective in hastening recovery."[6] Soon, multiple studies investigated the role of BM infusion in mice, dogs, and monkeys with leukemia treated with lethal doses of TBI.[7–16]

In 1957 E.D. Thomas reported 6 attempted cases of allogeneic BMT in patients with refractory chronic myelogenous leukemia (CML), multiple myeloma, chronic lymphocytic leukemia, metastatic tumor of unknown primary, metastatic ovarian tumor, and a comatose patient with massive cerebral haemorrhage.[1] Patients received conditioning with TBI, nitrogen mustard, or triethylene melamine, followed by infusion of BM from either fetal or adult cadavers. Engraftment was assessed based on the appearance of donor-type red blood cells (RBCs) in the recipient's circulation. Although none of the patients had sustained engraftment and only 2 patients had even temporary engraftment, several noteworthy findings emerged from this series which laid the foundation of modern hematopoietic cell transplantation (HCT). First, these cases demonstrated safety of intravenous infusion of BM without concerns of pulmonary emboli. Then it was hypothesized that prolonged engraftment could occur if the dose of TBI was increased to a degree sufficient to cause marrow aplasia. It was also realized that engraftment of allogeneic BM would fail in an individual with an intact immune system necessitating immune ablation before HCT as well. Finally, the remarkable finding was that BM could be collected and stored safely for future infusions.

Two years later, E.D. Thomas reported the first cases of syngeneic BMT in two children with refractory acute leukemia from their twins presumed to be identical, based on their appearance and blood types.[17] Both of these transplants led to successful marrow recovery within 2 weeks after lethal dose of TBI. Posttransplant BM biopsy showed complete remission of their leukemia, though leukemia relapsed in both children within 2–3 months. From these cases, it was learned that more intense conditioning was needed in addition to TBI

Hematopoietic Cell Transplantation for Malignant Conditions. https://doi.org/10.1016/B978-0-323-56802-9.00001-8

1

to prevent malignant disease relapse in patients who receive immunologically identical grafts.

In 1965 Mathe et al. summarized results of 14 allogeneic BMTs after lethal-dose TBI.[18] This series provided detailed description of the "secondary syndrome" after transplant, an entity later recognized as graft-versus-host disease (GVHD) and its treatment with steroids. In addition, the clinical use of donor lymphocyte infusion (DLI) and its incitement of GVHD was described for the first time. Some of these patients died of aplasia without engraftment; some had temporary engraftment with no "secondary syndrome"; some patients had persistent engraftment for up to 3 months, whereas others had complete engraftment, but died of "secondary syndrome." One long-term survivor after transplant was a 26-year-old physician with refractory acute lymphoblastic leukemia (ALL). He was conditioned with 6-mercaptopurine and TBI, followed a week later by infusion of pooled BM obtained from 6 related donors (father, mother, 3 brothers, and 1 sister). Recovery of neutrophils and platelets occurred around day 15 and day 28, respectively. About a week after transplant, he developed "secondary syndrome" manifesting as severe diarrhea, vomiting, 15-kg weight loss, generalized skin desquamation, hepatosplenomegaly, and transaminitis. He was treated with steroids, which led to improvement after 2 months. He was noted to have engrafted from one of his brothers, based on the RBC phenotype. In addition, he received skin grafts from all six donors, which he rejected except for the graft from the same brother whose RBCs were circulating in the recipient. About 6 months after transplantation, he was given four-weekly DLIs from the same donor, after which the "secondary syndrome" reappeared which was again successfully treated with steroids. He was alive in remission at 1 year after transplantation.[18]

Although there were occasional success stories and vigorous interest in BMT until early 1960s, the enthusiasm withered due to extremely poor outcomes.[19] This was elegantly summarized by Bortin in a compendium of 203 allogeneic transplants performed between 1939 and 1969,[19] of which 75% were performed before 1962. No engraftment was observed in 62% (125/203), and the overall mortality was about 75% (152/203). The indications for BMT were acute leukemia (42%), aplastic anemia (36%), other malignant disorder (15%), or immune deficiency (7%). Many of these transplants were performed without any conditioning; some used steroids alone, others used TBI, and some received chemotherapy with 6–MP or cyclophosphamide ± other agents. In the absence of any understanding of GVHD, no prophylaxis was used. Donor sources included cadavers, twins, siblings, other family members, or some other random donor. Some cases received BMs from multiple donors. Also, with no knowledge of human leukocyte antigen (HLA) typing, procedures for most of these cases were carried out without any matching; in some cases ABO-matched donors were used, and only 3 of 203 transplants performed in the later period used an "HLA-matched" donor when the awareness of HLA began to surface.

The Significance of HLA Matching in Transplant

Some of the pioneers in the discovery of Major Human Histocompatibility Complex were Jean Dausset and J.J. van Rood who described the existence of leukocyte antibodies in late 1950s.[20,21] Dausset detected alloreactive antibodies in the serum of a leukopenic patient who had received multiple blood transfusions, which were able to bind leukocytes of another individual. This led him to believe that human leukocyte groups similar to the ABO group existed, but antibodies against them appeared only after immunization in contrast to the naturally existing ABO antibodies. In subsequent experiments, he realized that alloimmune antibodies reacted against almost half of the volunteer donors, suggesting that the same leukocyte groups were present in those individuals, which he called "MAC" (acronym of initials of the first three donors whose serum did not react). He then tested sera from 50 different individuals and established the existence of at least 8 leukocyte groups presumably related to a single genetic system, which he named as Hu-1 ("Hu" for human and "1" for the first system). This was shown to correlate with the fate of skin and kidney grafts. The Hu-1 was later renamed as Human Leukocyte Antigen. Jean Dausset was awarded the Nobel Prize of Medicine in 1980 for his discovery. Further experiments by J.J van Rood[22] and Rose Payne[23] established the presence of distinct antigenic and allelic groups in the population. Experiments by Bach and Amos in 1967[24] suggested that major histocompatibility antigens in humans were controlled by single genetic locus (HLA) at which multiple alleles may operate.

The significance of HLA matching in animal models of BMT was identified in the early 1950s. In 1953 Snell demonstrated the role of mouse histocompatibility genes, especially H-2, in transplantation.[25] In 1957 Uphoff showed that transplantation of either parental or allogeneic marrow that differed at the H2 locus caused death of F1 hybrid mice due to the *"reactions caused by graft against the host"* and noticed that this syndrome could be evaded if the donor and the recipient were H-2 identical.[26] Later, similar findings were noted by others in dogs.[27-29] Soon, a series of experiments conducted by E.D. Thomas' group in late 1960s through early 1970s revealed that lethally irradiated dogs that received marrow from dog leukocyte antigen–matched dogs, especially those who received methotrexate, had long-term survival as compared with those who received graft from DLA-mismatched dogs who died of graft rejection or GVHD.[27,30,31] Thereafter, BMTs using HLA-matched donors began in humans.

Late 1960s: The First Successful HLA-Matched Sibling BMTs

HLA testing in that era was performed using serological methods which detected antibodies in human serum that were capable of agglutinating human peripheral blood (PB) T cells (HLA class I) or B cells (HLA class II), using techniques such as the mixed leukocyte reaction (MLR) and lymphocyte typing,[24,32,33] lymphocytotoxic approach,[34] or the complement fixation technique.[35] Using these methods, the first cases of successful HLA-matched sibling BMTs in pediatric patients with nonmalignant disorders were reported in 1968 in the same issue of *Lancet*. One of these, performed at the University of Minnesota[36] involved a 5-month-old male who had sex-linked lymphopenic immunological deficiency, who received PB buffy coat and BM from HLA-matched sibling, which restored cellular and humoral immunity. The other one[37] performed at the University Hospitals, Madison, involved a 2-year-old boy with Wiskott-Aldrich syndrome, who received azathioprine and prednisone before BMT, which was unsuccessful. Thereafter, he received an infusion of PB leukocytes from the same donor, followed by administration of high-dose cyclophosphamide and then BMT from the same donor. The patient became transfusion independent, and his spleen size normalized. This case highlighted the importance of eliminating recipient's alloreactive immune cells (incited by donor PB cells and then eradicated with cyclophosphamide) to allow engraftment.

Interest in BMT Re-Emerged in 1970s and Transplants Were Tested in Earlier Stage Malignant Disease

As it was becoming clear that treating animals with methotrexate not only improved engraftment but also survival by limiting their "secondary syndrome,"[27,30,31,38-43] the concept of GVHD prophylaxis was clinically introduced in the 1970s. This, along with increasing knowledge of HLA matching, reignited the interest and clinical activity in BMT.

In 1977, E.D. Thomas reported a series of 100 consecutive patients with acute leukemia (acute myelogenous leukemia [AML], n = 54, and ALL, n = 46) who underwent BMT between 1971 and 1975 from their HLA identical siblings.[44] After treating first 10 patients with TBI alone, it was recognized that further intensive conditioning was needed to reduce the risk of recurrent leukemia. Subsequently, chemotherapies such as cyclophosphamide, 1,3-bis(2-chloroethyl)-1-nitrosourea (BCNU), and/or others were added to TBI. All patients received methotrexate for prevention of GVHD, at a dose of 15 mg/m^2 on day 1, followed by 10 mg/m^2 on days 3, 6, and 11 and weekly thereafter for first 100 days (known as long-course methotrexate). About 75% of the patients developed GVHD, which was often treated with antithymocyte globulin (ATG). Only 1 patient rejected the graft; six patients died before engraftment while all others (94 of 100) engrafted. Overall, 55 patients died before day 100 due to GVHD, interstitial pneumonia, recurrent leukemia, or other medical complications. Long-term survival of up to 9 years[45] seen in some of these refractory end-stage leukemia patients suggested that BMT should be considered early during their disease trajectory.

Subsequently, Thomas and his collaborators started performing transplants in patients with AML in first remission. In 1979 they reported outcomes of 19 such patients who underwent HLA-matched sibling BMT after a preparative regimen of intrathecal methotrexate, cyclophosphamide, and high-dose TBI.[45] All patients received GVHD prophylaxis with the long course of methotrexate as described. Only 1 patient relapsed, and 12 of the 19 (63%) patients survived. In the same year the group from City of Hope Medical Center reported significantly improved survival after HLA-matched sibling BMT in "good-risk" AML patients in first remission (n = 26) as compared to a control group (n = 21) who did not undergo BMT because they had no donor.[46] Soon several reports described cure of diseases with BMT that were considered incurable with traditional therapies, including chronic leukemia,[47-51] thalassemia,[52,53] and sickle cell anemia.[54]

Late 1970s to Mid-1980s: Use of Unrelated Donors

With the success with HLA-matched sibling BMT, the donor selection was expanded to HLA-matched unrelated donors (MUDs) for those who lacked sibling donors. The first successful MUD HCT was performed in 1973 at the Westminster Hospital, London, on a boy named Simon Bostic who was born with X-linked chronic granulomatous disorder (CGD).[55,56] He had no HLA-matched family donor, and prior cases of

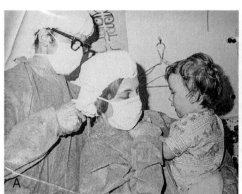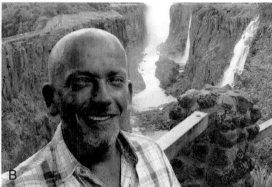

FIG. 1.1 **(A)** Simon Bostic with parents Elizabeth and Roger. **(B)** Simon Bostic at Victoria Falls in Zambia during a Comic Relief 2013 celebrity Zambezi challenge. ((A and B) *Courtesy of the Daily Mirror.*)

MUD transplant in other diseases had been unsuccessful.[57] However, as his elder brother, who also had CGD, died at the age of 2 years, his family agreed to pursue MUD HCT. Simon's mother commenced determined campaigning to look for unrelated donors, starting with getting her friends tested. The story got published in local and national press and soon numerous people from several continents got their blood tested. Eventually, a 29-year-old female was found to be a match at HLA-A, HLA-B, and HLA-D loci. At the age of almost 2 years, Simon received MUD BMT after conditioning with cyclophosphamide (60 mg/kg). He had mixed chimerism after transplant but later completely lost donor cells by the age of 7 years. They refused the idea of second transplant, and he struggled with recurrent infections while on chronic antibiotics but was reported alive for over 40 years (Fig. 1.1).[58]

The first HLA-MUD BMT for a malignant condition was performed at the Fred Hutchinson Cancer Research Center on September 4, 1979, in a 10-year-old girl with ALL in second remission who had no HLA-identical sibling. However, based on the published population HLA analysis,[59] she was noted to have inherited two relatively common HLA haplotypes. Therefore five normal donors were randomly screened, and one of them was noted to be ABO, HLA-A, HLA-B, HLA-D (MLR typing), and DR matched with the patient. She received BMT after conditioning with methotrexate, cyclophosphamide, and TBI, followed by long-course methotrexate for GVHD prophylaxis. She was reported to be well at least until 10 months after transplantation without GVHD.[60]

Shortly afterward, two successful cases of MUD BMTs were reported in 1982 in patients with aplastic anemia,[61] a disease which offers challenges for engraftment due to multiple prior blood transfusions and potential alloimmunizations. Since then, with the establishment of the National Marrow Donor Program (NMDP) in the United States and the Anthony Nolan Donor Registry in the UK and progressively easier access to search for donors, the numbers of MUD HCTs increased rapidly and surpassed the numbers of HLA-matched sibling HCTs after mid-late 2000s, both in the United States (Fig. 1.2) and in Europe. In Europe, MUD HCT constituted 53% of all allogeneic HCTs in 2014 and represented an 80% increase over the past 15 years.[62,63]

1980–90: Use of PB as Autograft

The recognition of hematopoietic progenitor cells in PB of mice, dogs, and nonhuman primates has been recognized since the 1960s,[7,64,65] followed by attempts to harvest these from circulation in man. One of the ground-breaking steps toward this goal was the development of closed system continuous-flow apheresis technology, which was first developed in 1960s by a collaborative effort of the National Cancer Institute and the International Business Machines Corporation (NCI-IBM).[66,67] A decade later, this was put to clinical testing at the M.D. Anderson Cancer Center.[68] Another decade passed before the feasibility of collecting large quantities of PB progenitor cells (PBPCs) from adult volunteers was demonstrated by Körbling M et al.[69]

The finding that autologous PB could be used for successful marrow recovery in man was first shown by Goldman et al. in 1979 in a patient with chronic phase CML by using cryopreserved buffy coat cells[70,71] and again by Korbling et al.[72] in 1981 using cryopreserved PBPCs obtained by leukaphereses. The follow-up

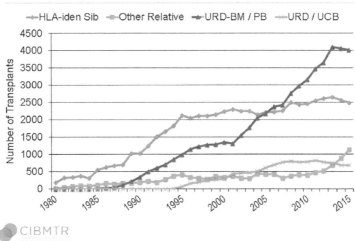

FIG. 1.2 Numbers of allogeneic HCTs performed in the United States by donor type since 1980s. *HCT,* hematopoietic cell transplantation; URD-BM/PB, Unrelated donor bone marrow/peripheral blood; UCB, Umbilical cord blood.

period in these studies was too short to draw any clinical conclusions about its use. It took another 5 years before long-term safety and efficacy of PB HCT could be established. In 1986 Korbling et al.[73] demonstrated sustained engraftment and marrow cellularity for >7 months after autologous PB HCT in a patient with Burkitt's lymphoma. Leukaphereses and collection of PBPCs were done after COMP (cyclophosphamide, vincristine, methotrexate, and prednisone) chemotherapy. The patient was reportedly alive and well 25 years after transplantation.[74]

The use of granulocyte colony–stimulating factor (G-CSF) or granulocyte macrophage colony–stimulating factor for collection was introduced in late 1980s and early 1990s, with several reports of successful autologous PB HCT.[73,75–79] Since then, the number of autologous HCTs has been constantly increasing, especially in older patients, including those over the age of 70 years (Fig. 1.3).[62,63]

Early 1990s: Rapid Increase in Allogeneic Transplantation Using PB Grafts

The notion of using PBPC in the allogeneic setting was initially faced with resistance in the 1970s-1980s due to concerns about their lower self-renewal potential,[80] which was emphasized after 2 reports of failed syngeneic donor PB HCTs.[81,82] In 1979, Hershko et al.[81] reported a case of paroxysmal nocturnal hemoglobinuria, who

received PBPC (7.1×10^{10} total nucleated cells [TNCs] containing 3.4×10^4 myeloid progenitors colony-forming unit cell (CFU–C)/kg) obtained by leukapheresis from an identical-twin. After no marrow recovery by 2 months, he received a BM graft from the same donor that contained significantly fewer cells (1.3×10^{10} TNCs) but almost double the numbers of myeloid progenitors (6.4×10^4 CFU-C/kg), which resulted in prompt marrow recovery.[81] Then in 1980 Abrams et al.[82] described a case of a patient with Ewing's sarcoma who received PBPCs from identical twin by leukapheresis (9.8×10^{10} TNCs containing 40×10^4 CFU-C), which did not support either neutrophil or platelet engraftment. Subsequent infusion of autologous BM restored blood counts.

It took another decade before PBPCs were reintroduced in the allogeneic setting. In 1989 Kessinger et al.[83] from the University of Nebraska reported a case of HLA-matched sibling donor PB HCT in an 18-year-old male with ALL whose sibling preferred to donate PB than BM. Although the patient engrafted neutrophils on day 11 and achieved 100% engraftment from donor cells, he unfortunately died on day 32 after transplant from disseminated aspergillosis, likely due to T cell depletion from the graft which was performed to reduce the risk of GVHD. The first successful G-CSF–mobilized PB HCT was reported in 1993 by Dreger et al.[84] from the University of Kiel, in a 47-year-old

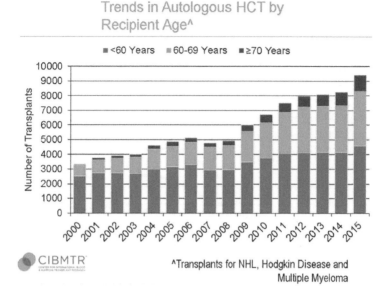

FIG. 1.3 Trend of autologous HCT performed in the United States since 2000 by age. *HCT*, hematopoietic cell transplantation.

female with AML using HLA-matched sibling after two prior failed BMTs from the same donor. A few months later, Russell et al.[85] reported a PB HCT in 45-year-old male with ALL using an HLA-matched sibling donor.

In the early 1990s there was steep growth in allogeneic G-CSF (filgrastim) mobilized PB HCT, after trials led by M.D. Anderson Cancer Center,[86] University of Kiel, Germany,[87] and the Fred Hutchinson Cancer Research Center[88] established the safety and efficacy of PB HCT in patients with relapsed/refractory hematologic malignancies. However, concerns also began to emerge about potentially higher risks of GVHD than BMT.[88] This was resolved more than a decade and a half later in numerous randomized trials comparing BM versus PB grafts, most of which showed significantly higher risks of chronic GVHD with PB HCT.[89] Despite this, PB remains the most commonly used graft source (75%–80%) for adult patients undergoing either HLA-sibling (Fig. 1.4A) or unrelated donor (Fig. 1.4B) HCT, in the United States and in Europe.[62,63] No clear data suggest the scientific rationale for this dependence on PBPC grafts for adults. In contrast, PB is the not preferred as a graft source (about 20%) for pediatric recipients of either HLA sibling (Fig. 1.4C) or unrelated donor (Fig. 1.4D) HCT.[62]

Haploidentical Stem Cell Transplantation

The possibility of using related donors other than HLA identical siblings was explored in the late 1970s,[90–92] but the results were discouraging due to high rates of GVHD, graft failure, and excessive risk of toxicities including pulmonary injury and multiorgan failure.[93,94] For instance, in a study reported in 1985 by Beatty et al.,[93] the risk of graft rejection and grade II-IV acute GVHD was significantly higher (70% vs. 42%, $P < .001$) after myeloablative haploidentical HCT (n = 105) than HLA-matched sibling BMT (n = 728).

As the role of T cells in the pathogenesis of GVHD became apparent,[95–99] several cases of T cell–depleted haploidentical transplant were reported in early 1980s,[100–102] with $<5 \times 10^4$ CD3 cells/kg recognized as the safe threshold for preventing GVHD.[103] Although T cell depletion seemed effective in patients with severe combined immunodeficiency, it did not prevent disease relapse or graft failure/rejection in patients with acute leukemia.[104,105] The risk of graft failure/rejection was noted to be 50% in recipients of T cell–depleted HLA-mismatched grafts in contrast to only 10% in recipients of T cell–depleted HLA identical graft and 1% or less in recipients of unmodified BM grafts from HLA identical donors.[100] Graft failure occurred due to the emergence of host-derived T cells even after patients had received conditioning with myeloablative TBI, cyclophosphamide, and in some cases, ATG.[106,107]

The concept of infusing massive doses of progenitor cells, which in preclinical studies was shown to overcome the HLA barrier,[108,109] was explored by the Perugia group

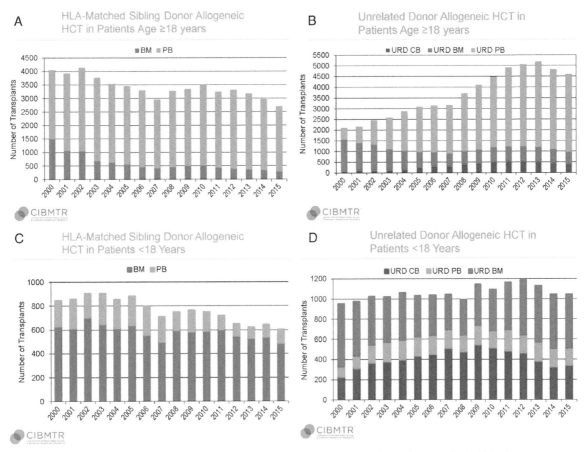

FIG. 1.4 **(A)** Trend of sibling donor HCT in patients older than 18 years by graft source in the United States. **(B)** Trend of MUD HCT in patients older than 18 years by graft source in the United States. **(C)** Trend of sibling donor HCT in patients younger than 18 years by graft source in the United States. **(D)** Trend of MUD HCT in patients younger than 18 years by graft source in the United States. *BM*, bone marrow; *HCT*, hematopoietic cell transplantation; *PB*, peripheral blood.

in the 1990s. They performed T cell–depleted transplants with grafts containing "mega doses" of hematopoietic cells obtained from BM plus G-CSF–mobilized PB.[110] The final graft contained $>10.8 \times 10^6$ CD34 cells/kg and a median of 2×10^5 CD3 cells/kg. Intensive conditioning with TBI, cyclophosphamide, thiotepa, and ATG provided both immunosuppression and myeloablation. With no further GVHD prophylaxis, only 18% of the patients developed acute GVHD. In their subsequent study,[111] even more intense T cell depletion was performed, resulting in one-tenth the dose of CD3+ cells as compared to the prior study, and cyclophosphamide was replaced with fludarabine. This completely abrogated the risk of graft failure and prevented both acute and chronic GVHD, but almost half of the patients with ALL relapsed.

Other strategies attempted to balance the risk of GVHD and disease relapse after haploidentical HCT included partial T cell depletion using combination of in vivo and ex vivo monoclonal antibodies or immunotoxin,[112,113] in vivo T cell depletion with the anti-CD52 monoclonal antibody alemtuzumab,[114,115] or ATG.[116] More recently, the field has reverted back to using T-cell replete grafts using novel GVHD prophylaxis regimens such as posttransplant cyclophosphamide[117] or selective $\alpha\beta + T$ cell–depleted grafts.[118,119] With these novel strategies, the outcomes of haploidentical HCT have improved remarkably and now approach those of MUD HCT.[120,121] As a result, the numbers of haploidentical HCT are increasing steadily both in the

United States (Fig. 1.2) and in Europe,[62,63] with PB grafts being used more frequently than BM (Fig. 1.5).

History of Umbilical Cord Blood Transplant

Among all donor/graft sources, the field of umbilical cord blood transplant (UCBT) is the most juvenile, although the notion is ancient. The potential of using fetal or newborn progenitor cells as a graft source was first observed in the 1950s when studies in lethally irradiated mice showed that liver/spleen hematopoietic cells from newborns provided longer term survival than adult marrow cells.[122] Fetal liver as a graft source was investigated in animals in late 1950s[123,124] and shortly thereafter in humans by Scott et al.,[125] but the outcomes were disappointing.[125] Logistical difficulties in obtaining the graft and success of HCTs with BM or PB grafts further limited interest in the cord blood approach.

In early 1980s it was shown that samples from newborn umbilical cord blood (UCB) contained hemopoietic colony-forming cells which could be grown in liquid suspension culture for over 3 months and provided the best enrichment of immature myeloid cells in vitro as compared to adult BM or PB.[126,127] These findings ignited the interest in using UCB as a graft source. The clinical translation of these findings rooted from research in Fanconi anemia (FA) and was a result of multi-institutional collaborative effort between investigators at the Rockefeller University (A.D. Auerbach), Indiana University (H.E. Broxmeyer), Memorial Sloan Kettering Cancer Center (E.A. Boyse), Duke University Medical Center (J. Kurtzberg), and Hôpital Saint Louis, Paris (E. Gluckman). Auerbach et al. developed a method of prenatal diagnosis of FA by chorionic villous and amniotic fluid sampling in fetuses at risk and simultaneously performed HLA typing to determine if they would be HLA identical to the affected sibling.[128] If they tested negative, UCB was harvested at the time of birth, which was found to be a rich source of progenitor cells. Further studies by Broxmeyer et al.[129] showed that human UCB contained multipotent colony-forming units (CFU-GEMM), erythroid burst-forming units, and granulocyte-macrophage (CFU-GM) progenitor cells, in frequencies similar or greater than that in adult marrow and sufficient to allow marrow recovery[128,129] based on reported cell doses from BMTs. This was confirmed in lethally irradiated mice by Boyse in an unpublished work.[129]

This extensive preclinical work led to the first UCBT which was performed on October 6, 1988, in a 5-year-old boy with FA named Matthew Farrow.[130] This was a combined effort of the investigators mentioned previously, but the transplant was conducted at Hôpital Saint Louis under the supervision of E. Gluckman due to her expertise in managing these patients.[131] Matthew

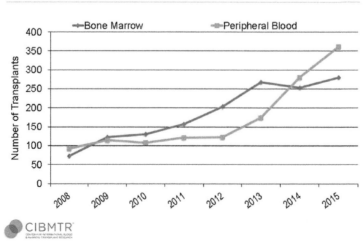

CIBMTR

FIG. 1.5 Trend of haploidentical HCT in the United States over time by graft source. *HCT*, hematopoietic cell transplantation.

was diagnosed with FA at the Duke University Medical Center at the age of 2 years. When his mother became pregnant again, prenatal testing at the Rockefeller University revealed the female fetus not only to be unaffected by FA but also 6/6-HLA match to him. Matthew's physician, Joanne Kurtzberg, proposed UCBT from his yet-to-be-born sister. Cord blood was collected and cryopreserved at birth and hand delivered from Indiana to Paris when he was admitted for transplant. He received reduced intensity conditioning (RIC) with low-dose cyclophosphamide (20 mg/kg) and 5 Gy thoraco-abdominal irradiation, a regimen previously shown by Gluckman to be effective and safe in FA patients.[132] Cord blood cells were thawed and infused without further processing at a dose of 0.4×10^8 TNCs/kg. GVHD prophylaxis constituted of cyclosporine from day 1 through 6 months after transplantation. On day 15, he developed histological grade 1 skin GVHD and hepatic GVHD, which was successfully treated with steroids. Signs of engraftment appeared on day 22. He required blood and platelet transfusions until day 54 and 43, respectively, after which he became transfusion independent. Day 120 BM analysis showed 100% cells of donor origin (46, XX), but he had mixed chimerism in the PB (64% donor) through 204 days after transplantation. He is doing well without any GVHD more than 33 years after the transplant (Fig. 1.6).[130,131]

The applicability of UCBT was soon extended to several malignant and nonmalignant disorders using matched[133–136] or partially matched[137] sibling donors and later from mismatched unrelated donors as well.[137–139] Common findings from these studies were delayed neutrophil engraftment, lower risks of GVHD, and comparable survival with UCBT compared with BMT. By early-mid 1990s, the field expanded to include adult patients.[138,140] But the cell dose in a single UCB unit was soon recognized to be inadequate for many adults. This was addressed by Barker et al. at the University of Minnesota who pioneered the use of double unit UCBT,[141] which has now become a standard in those with insufficient cell dose in a single unit. Later, multiple novel ex vivo graft manipulation techniques were introduced to increase the progenitor cell dose and accelerate engraftment, leading to improved outcomes (reviewed in the studies of Mehta et al.[142–144]).

Other major landmarks in the history of UCBT were the establishment of several UCB banks after the first unrelated UCB bank was created in 1991 by Rubinstein at the New York Blood Center.[145–147] With a large inventory of UCB banks and the establishment of several registries (see section "Origin of Donor and Transplant Registries"), the numbers of UCBT in the United States increased steadily from 2003 to 2011 but are now slowly declining as the number of haploidentical HCTs surpassed that of UCBTs in 2014.

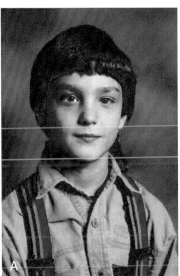
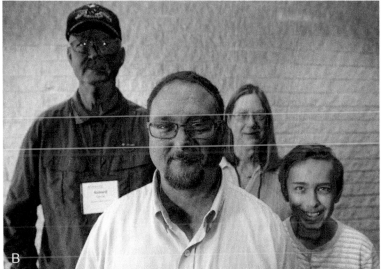

FIG. 1.6 **(A)** Matthew Farrow, age 5 years, 1988. **(B)** Recent photograph of Matthew Farrow—now a husband and a father. ((A) *Courtesy: www.bmtinfonet.org.* (B) *Courtesy: photo by fellow transplantee Rodney Curtis/RodneyCurtis.com and www.bmtinfonet.org with permission from Matthew Farrow.*)

In pediatrics, UCBT constituted about half (48%) of all unrelated donor grafts in 2009 but declined thereafter and were about one-third of all MUDs in 2015. In adults the number of UCBTs plateaued since 2010 and accounted for less than 10% of all MUDs in 2015 (Fig. 1.4B and D).[62] Similarly, in Europe, in recent years (2011–14), the number of UCBT dropped slightly as haploidentical HCT have increased by 25% annually.[63]

Late 1990s to Early 2000s: Introduction of RIC

Until the 1980s, the success of HCT relied on myeloablative conditioning with high-dose TBI (10–15 Gy) with or without cyclophosphamide (120–200 mg/kg) or other chemotherapies and later with high-dose oral busulfan (16 mg/kg)[148] as an alternative to TBI. As there is a positive dose-response correlation of most hematological malignancies to alkylating agents and radiation, it made sense to administer exceptionally high doses of chemotherapy and/or radiation to eradicate tumors before transplant.

The existence of graft-versus-tumor effect was recognized in late 1950s in murine models by Barnes et al. who noted that allogeneic, but not syngeneic, marrow infusion into irradiated mice resulted in eradication of leukemia.[12,149] But it was not until the late 1970s and early 1980s, when the graft-versus-leukemia (GVL) effect was observed in human studies that demonstrated significantly lesser risk of leukemia relapse in patients who developed GVHD than those without.[150-153] In addition, there was an increased risk of relapse with T cell depletion[150] and induction of remission after DLIs.[154] These all further provided evidence for GVL effect of HCT. Thus, it was hypothesized that the power of HCT could be harnessed without myeloablation.

One of the earliest attempts to reduce toxicities was to reduce the doses of chemotherapies.[155-157] However, it was also noted that adequate immunosuppression was critical to prevent graft rejection mediated by recipient T cells.[106,107] With preclinical data suggesting that fludarabine plus TBI yielded sufficient immunosuppression as achieved with TBI plus cyclophosphamide, but with fewer toxicities,[158] fludarabine was included in conditioning regimens in the mid-late 1990s.[111,158-162] This opened the opportunities for development of a wide variety of nonmyeloablative (NMA) and RIC regimens with various combinations of fludarabine plus reduced doses of alkylating agents such as low-dose busulfan

(8 mg/kg),[161] melphalan,[163] thiotepa,[164] and cyclophosphamide[164-166] with or without low-dose TBI (generally 200 cGy).[165-168] The risk of toxicities in these studies was noted to be significantly lower than that reported with conventional myeloablative regimens.

With the advent of NMA/RIC regimens, the number of patients aged 60–70 years or older undergoing HCT steadily increased (Fig. 1.7). In 2015, 30% of the allogeneic HCTs performed in the United Staes included patients older than 60 years.[62]

Origin of Donor and Transplant Registries

After the first successful MUD HCT was performed in 1973, this news reached Australia and to Shirley Nolan, whose 2-year-old child, Anthony Nolan, was born with Wiskott-Aldrich syndrome and had no available HLA-matched donor. She came to the UK with hopes that Simon's doctors could also save Anthony.[58] With an idea to start a BM registry to search for potential unrelated donors, she started campaigning and fundraising which led to the establishment of the world's first marrow donor registry, the Anthony Nolan Bone Marrow Registry in 1974 in Westminster Children's Hospital, where Anthony was being treated (Fig. 1.8). Although it could not help Anthony, who died in 1979, the registry continued to expand and currently includes 600,000 potential donors. In 1988 it became a founding member of Bone Marrow Donors Worldwide (BMDW), and in 2008 it established the UK's first dedicated UCB bank (https://www.anthonynolan.org/).

In the United States, Dr. Mortimer M. Bortin and several colleagues established the International Bone Marrow Transplant Registry (IBMTR) at the Medical College of Wisconsin in 1972 to gather patient data and analyze their outcomes. In 1986 a national registry of unrelated volunteer donors, the National Bone Marrow Donor Registry (later renamed as National Marrow Donor Program, NMDP) was established in St. Paul, MN, as a joint effort of the Graves' family (whose 10-year-old daughter with leukemia was saved by a MUD HCT), other patient families, doctors, US Congressional support, and funding from the US Navy (https://bethematch.org). In July 2004, the IBMTR and NMDP collaboratively formed the Center for International Blood and Marrow Transplant Research (CIBMTR) with a mission to improve transplantation access and outcomes for patients. The CIBMTR has been collecting outcomes data on nearly all allogeneic transplantations performed in the United States for over 40 years and has data on

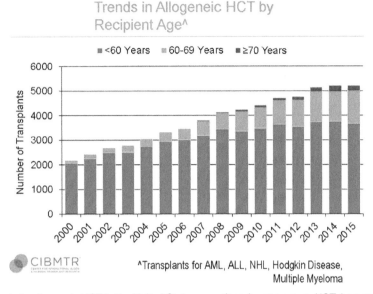

FIG. 1.7 Trends in allogeneic HCT in the United States over time, by age group. *HCT*, hematopoietic cell transplantation.

more than 465,000 patients (https://www.cibmtr.org/). It also receives voluntary data on autologous transplants and some allogeneic HCTs performed internationally. With similar goals, transplant teams from Paris, Leiden, London, and Basel started meeting since 1975, which in 1979 ultimately led to the formal establishment of the European Society for Blood and Marrow Transplantation in the Netherlands (https://www.ebmt.org/).

The idea of World Marrow Donor Association (WMDA) was initiated in 1988 to identify donors in an international collaboration by three pioneers—E. Donnall Thomas (US), John Goldman (UK), and J.J. van Rood (NL). Foundation of the WMDA was formally established in 1994, and in January 2017 BMDW joined the WMDA. Its goal is to facilitate exchange of high-quality progenitor cells for patients worldwide and to promote the interests of donors. It currently represents 75 donor registries, 158 cord blood banks, 350 donor centers, and 1615 transplant hospitals from 52 different countries (https://www.wmda.info/).

Likewise, to improve outcomes of UCBT, international registries were formed such as the Eurocord in 1995 (http://www.eurocord.org/) to collect UCBT outcome data and NetCord in 1998 (http://www.netcord.org/) to establish

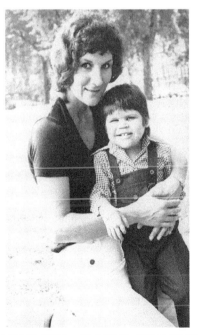

FIG. 1.8 Shirley Nolan with Anthony. (*Courtesy of the Daily Mirror.*)

good manufacturing practices for collection and storage of UCB units and to facilitate donor searching. The NMDP has a similar and internationally linked cord blood banking program (https://bethematch.org).

With the aid of these registries, it is easier than ever to identify unrelated donors from across the world. As a result, more than 8900 unrelated donor HCTs were performed in 2014 in Europe and about 4000 in the United States.[62,63]

CONCLUSION

The progress in the field of HCT since the 1950s, after a hesitant beginning, exemplifies a story of triumph over adversity. It took more than half a century and painstaking efforts from innumerable researchers to advance the field from the earliest era when transplants were performed using a random or multiple donors, without the knowledge of HLA or GVHD, to the modern era where highly sophisticated molecular techniques are used to match donor-recipient pairs at an allele level with a plethora of therapies available to prevent or treat GVHD. In earlier times, HCT was an experimental therapy reserved for patients with terminal illnesses who had exhausted all other forms of treatment, and transplant was performed as a desperation therapy. Now, it is routine to introduce the discussion of HCT in the early stages of disease as a standard consolidation therapy, especially in those with matched related donors. The fact that it has been a challenging effort to search for unrelated donors and an equally courageous attempt to perform MUD HCT may seem like an overstatement to the modern-day reader. Current computerized national and international registries, with which a donor can be identified promptly, are the result of intelligent foresight of early transplant physicians and the tireless quest of family members to save their children from fatal illnesses, a story that cannot be simply be put into words. The use of haploidentical or UCB transplants, PBPC grafts, and the introduction of RIC regimens have all opened the scope of HCT to a broader population. With advancements in supportive care, GVHD prophylaxis and treatment, refinements in conditioning regimens, and novel graft manipulation techniques, the outcomes of HCT are expected to continue to improve.

If you do not know where you come from, then you don't know where you are, and if you don't know where you are, then you don't know where you're going. And if you don't know where you're going, you're probably going wrong.

TERRY PRATCHETT.

REFERENCES

1. Thomas ED, Lochte Jr HL, Lu WC, Ferrebee JW. Intravenous infusion of bone marrow in patients receiving radiation and chemotherapy. *N Engl J Med.* 1957;257(11):491–496.
2. Putnam FW. The atomic bomb casualty commission in retrospect. *Proc Natl Acad Sci USA.* 1998;95(10):5426–5431.
3. Shigematsu I. Greetings: 50 years of atomic bomb casualty commission-radiation effects research foundation studies. *Proc Natl Acad Sci USA.* 1998;95(10):5424–5425.
4. Jacobson LO, Simmons EL, Bethard WF. Studies on hematopoietic recovery from radiation injury. *J Clin Invest.* 1950;29(6):825.
5. Jacobson LO, Simmons EL, Marks EK, Gaston EO, Robson MJ, Eldredge JH. Further studies on recovery from radiation injury. *J Lab Clin Med.* 1951;37(5):683–697.
6. Lorenz E, Congdon C, Uphoff D. Modification of acute irradiation injury in mice and Guinea-pigs by bone marrow injections. *Radiology.* 1952;58(6):863–877.
7. Cavins JA, Scheer SC, Thomas ED, Ferrebee JW. The recovery of lethally irradiated dogs given infusions of autologous leukocytes preserved at -80 C. *Blood.* 1964;23:38–42.
8. Bagdasarov AA, Sukiasian GV, Novikova MN, Raushenbakh MO. Transplantation of homologous bone marrow in acute radiation injury in dogs and monkeys. *Mem Acad Chir (Paris).* 1961;6:26–34.
9. Newsome FE, Overman RR. The effect of homologous marrow transplantation on the survival of monkeys following sublethal whole-body radiation. *Blood.* 1960;16:1762–1769.
10. Mannick JA, Lochte Jr HL, Ashley CA, Thomas ED, Ferrebee JW. Autografts of bone marrow in dogs after lethal total-body radiation. *Blood.* 1960;15:255–266.
11. Rothberg H, Blair EB, Gomez AC, Mc NW. Observations on chimpanzees after whole-body radiation and homologous bone marrow treatment. *Blood.* 1959;14:1302–1321.
12. Barnes DW, Loutit JF. Treatment of murine leukaemia with x-rays and homologous bone marrow. II. *Br J Haematol.* 1957;3(3):241–252.
13. Trentin JJ. Mortality and skin transplantability in x-irradiated mice receiving isologous, homologous or heterologous bone marrow. *Proc Soc Exp Biol Med.* 1956;92(4):688–693.
14. Ford CE, Hamerton JL, Barnes DW, Loutit JF. Cytological identification of radiation-chimaeras. *Nature.* 1956;177(4506):452–454.
15. Nowell PC, Cole LJ, Habermeyer JG, Roan PL. Growth and continued function of rat marrow cells in x-radiated mice. *Cancer Res.* 1956;16(3):258–261.
16. Main JM, Prehn RT. Successful skin homografts after the administration of high dosage X radiation and homologous bone marrow. *J Natl Cancer Inst.* 1955;15(4):1023–1029.

17. Thomas ED, Lochte Jr HL, Cannon JH, Sahler OD, Ferrebee JW. Supralethal whole body irradiation and isologous marrow transplantation in man. *J Clin Invest.* 1959;38:1709–1716.

18. Mathe G, Amiel JL, Schwarzenberg L, et al. Successful allogenic bone marrow transplantation in man: chimerism, induced specific tolerance and possible anti-leukemic effects. *Blood.* 1965;25:179–196.

19. Bortin MM. A compendium of reported human bone marrow transplants. *Transplantation.* 1970;9(6):571–587.

20. Dausset J. Iso-leuko-antibodies. *Acta Haematol.* 1958;20(1–4):156–166.

21. Van Rood JJ, Eernisse JG, Van Leeuwen A. Leucocyte antibodies in sera from pregnant women. *Nature.* 1958;181(4625):1735–1736.

22. van Rood JJ, van Leeuwen A, Schippers A, Balner H. Human histocompatibility antigens in normal and neoplastic tissues. *Cancer Res.* 1968;28(7):1415–1422.

23. Payne R, Tripp M, Weigle J, Bodmer W, Bodmer J. A new leukocyte isoantigen system in man. *Cold Spring Harb Symp Quant Biol.* 1964;29:285–295.

24. Bach FH, Amos DB. Hu-1: major histocompatibility locus in man. *Science.* 1967;156(3781):1506–1508.

25. Snell GD. The genetics of transplantation. *J Natl Cancer Inst.* 1953;14(3):691–700; discussion, 701-694.

26. Uphoff DE. Genetic factors influencing irradiation protection by bone marrow. I. The F1 hybrid effect. *J Natl Cancer Inst.* 1957;19(1):123–130.

27. Storb R, Epstein RB, Bryant J, Ragde H, Thomas ED. Marrow grafts by combined marrow and leukocyte infusions in unrelated dogs selected by histocompatibility typing. *Transplantation.* 1968;6(4):587–593.

28. Good RA, Martinez C, Gabrielsen AE. Progress toward transplantation of tissues in man. *Adv Pediatr.* 1964;13:93–127.

29. Simonsen M. Graft versus host reactions. Their natural history, and applicability as tools of research. *Prog Allergy.* 1962;6:349–467.

30. Storb R, Rudolph RH, Thomas ED. Marrow grafts between canine siblings matched by serotyping and mixed leukocyte culture. *J Clin Invest.* 1971;50(6):1272–1275.

31. Storb R, Epstein RB, Graham TC, Thomas ED. Methotrexate regimens for control of graft-versus-host disease in dogs with allogeneic marrow grafts. *Transplantation.* 1970;9(3):240–246.

32. Bach FH, Kisken WA. Predictive value of results of mixed leukocyte cultures for skin allograft survival in man. *Transplantation.* 1967;5(4):1046–1052.

33. Bach F, Hirschhorn K. Lymphocyte interaction: a potential histocompatibility test in vitro. *Science.* 1964;143(3608):813–814.

34. Terasaki PI, Bernoco D, Park MS, Ozturk G, Iwaki Y. Microdroplet testing for HLA-A, -B, -C, and -D antigens. The Phillip Levine award lecture. *Am J Clin Pathol.* 1978;69(2):103–120.

35. Mittal KK, Mickey MR, Singal DP, Terasaki PI. Serotyping for homotransplantation. 18. Refinement of microdroplet lymphocyte cytotoxicity test. *Transplantation.* 1968;6(8):913–927.

36. Gatti RA, Meuwissen HJ, Allen HD, Hong R, Good RA. Immunological reconstitution of sex-linked lymphopenic immunological deficiency. *Lancet.* 1968;2(7583):1366–1369.

37. Bach FH, Albertini RJ, Joo P, Anderson JL, Bortin MM. Bone-marrow transplantation in a patient with the Wiskott-Aldrich syndrome. *Lancet.* 1968;2(7583):1364–1366.

38. Thomas ED, Kasakura S, Cavins JA, Ferrebee JW. Marrow transplants in lethally irradiated dogs: the effect of methotrexate on survival of the host and the homograft. *Transplantation.* 1963;1:571–574.

39. Lochte Jr HL, Levy AS, Guenther DM, Thomas ED, Ferrebee JW. Prevention of delayed foreign marrow reaction in lethally irradiated mice by early administration of methotrexate. *Nature.* 1962;196:1110–1111.

40. Thomas ED, Collins JA, Herman Jr EC, Ferrebee JW. Marrow transplants in lethally irradiated dogs given methotrexate. *Blood.* 1962;19:217–228.

41. Uphoff DE. Drug-induced immunological "tolerance" for homotransplantation. *Plast Reconstr Surg.* 1961;28:12–16.

42. Hager EB, Mannick JA, Thomas ED, Ferrebee JW. Dogs that survive "lethal" exposures to radiation. *Radiat Res.* 1961;14:192–205.

43. Uphoff DE. Alteration of homograft reaction by A-methopterin in lethally irradiated mice treated with homologous marrow. *Proc Soc Exp Biol Med.* 1958;99(3):651–653.

44. Thomas ED, Buckner CD, Banaji M, et al. One hundred patients with acute leukemia treated by chemotherapy, total body irradiation, and allogeneic marrow transplantation. *Blood.* 1977;49(4):511–533.

45. Thomas ED, Buckner CD, Clift RA, et al. Marrow transplantation for acute nonlymphoblastic leukemia in first remission. *N Engl J Med.* 1979;301(11):597–599.

46. Beutler E, Blume KG, Bross KJ, et al. Bone marrow transplantation as the treatment of choice for "good risk" adult patients with acute leukemia. *Trans Assoc Am Physicians.* 1979;92:189–195.

47. Thomas ED, Clift RA, Fefer A, et al. Marrow transplantation for the treatment of chronic myelogenous leukemia. *Ann Intern Med.* 1986;104(2):155–163.

48. Goldman JM, Apperley JF, Jones L, et al. Bone marrow transplantation for patients with chronic myeloid leukemia. *N Engl J Med.* 1986;314(4):202–207.

49. Goldman JM, Baughan AS, McCarthy DM, et al. Marrow transplantation for patients in the chronic phase of chronic granulocytic leukaemia. *Lancet.* 1982;2(8299):623–625.

50. Clift RA, Buckner CD, Thomas ED, et al. Treatment of chronic granulocytic leukaemia in chronic phase by allogeneic marrow transplantation. *Lancet.* 1982;2(8299):621–623.

51. Fefer A, Cheever MA, Thomas ED, et al. Disappearance of Ph1-positive cells in four patients with chronic granulocytic leukemia after chemotherapy, irradiation and marrow transplantation from an identical twin. *N Engl J Med.* 1979;300(7):333–337.

52. Lucarelli G, Polchi P, Izzi T, et al. Allogeneic marrow transplantation for thalassemia. *Exp Hematol.* 1984;12(8):676–681.

53. Thomas ED, Buckner CD, Sanders JE, et al. Marrow transplantation for thalassaemia. *Lancet.* 1982;2(8292):227–229.

54. Johnson FL, Look AT, Gockerman J, Ruggiero MR, Dalla-Pozza L, Billings 3rd FT. Bone-marrow transplantation in a patient with sickle-cell anemia. *N Engl J Med.* 1984;311(12):780–783.

55. The-Westminster-Hospitals-Bone-Marrow-Transplant-Team. Bone-marrow transplant from an unrelated donor for chronic granulomatous disease. *Lancet.* 1977;1(8005):210–213.

56. Humble JG, Barrett AJ. Technique of bone marrow transplantation. *Proc R Soc Med.* 1975;68(9):580–582.

57. Speck B, Zwaan FE, van Rood JJ, Eernisse JG. Allogeneic bone marrow transplantation in a patient with aplastic anemia using a phenotypically HL-A-identifcal unrelated donor. *Transplantation.* 1973;16(1):24–28.

58. *Simon celebrates 40 years since his bone marrow transplant – the world's first from an unrelated donor.* ; Thursday, April 18, 2013. Available online at: https://www.anthonynolan.org/news/2013/04/18/simon-celebrates-40-years-his-bone-marrow-transplant-worlds-first-unrelated-donor. https://www.anthonynolan.org/news/2013/04/18/simon-celebrates-40-years-his-bone-marrow-transplant-worlds-first-unrelated-donor.

59. Pickbourne P, Piazza A, Bodmer W. Population analysis. In: Bodmer WF, Batchelor JR, Bodmer JG, Festenstein H, Morris PJ, eds. *Histocompatibility testing Copenhagen: Munksgaard, 1977.* 1978;259(78).

60. Hansen JA, Clift RA, Thomas ED, Buckner CD, Storb R, Giblett ER. Transplantation of marrow from an unrelated donor to a patient with acute leukemia. *N Engl J Med.* 1980;303(10):565–567.

61. Gordon-Smith EC, Fairhead SM, Chipping PM, et al. Bone-marrow transplantation for severe aplastic anaemia using histocompatible unrelated volunteer donors. *Br Med J (Clin Res Ed).* 1982;285(6345):835–837.

62. D'Souza A, Zhu X. *Current uses and outcomes of hematopoietic cell transplantation (HCT): CIBMTR summary slides;* 2016. Available at: http://www.cibmtr.org.

63. Passweg JR, Baldomero H, Bader P, et al. Hematopoietic stem cell transplantation in Europe 2014: more than 40 000 transplants annually. *Bone Marrow Transpl.* 2016;51(6):786–792.

64. Storb R, Graham TC, Epstein RB, Sale GE, Thomas ED. Demonstration of hemopoietic stem cells in the peripheral blood of baboons by cross circulation. *Blood.* 1977;50(3):537–542.

65. Goodman JW, Hodgson GS. Evidence for stem cells in the peripheral blood of mice. *Blood.* 1962;19:702–714.

66. Judson G, Jones A, Kellogg R, et al. Closed continuous-flow centrifuge. *Nature.* 1968;217(5131):816–818.

67. Freireich EJ, Judson G, Levin RH. Separation and collection of leukocytes. *Cancer Res.* 1965;25(9):1516–1520.

68. McCredie KB, Hersh EM, Freireich EJ. Cells capable of colony formation in the peripheral blood of man. *Science.* 1971;171(3968):293–294.

69. Korbling M, Fliedner TM, Pflieger H. Collection of large quantities of granulocyte/macrophage progenitor cells (CFUc) in man by means of continuous-flow leukapheresis. *Scand J Haematol.* 1980;24(1):22–28.

70. Goldman JM, Catovsky D, Goolden AW, Johnson SA, Galton DA. Buffy coat autografts for patients with chronic granulocytic leukaemia in transformation. *Blut.* 1981;42(3):149–155.

71. Goldman JM. Autografting cryopreserved buffy coat cells for chronic granulocytic leukaemia in transformation. *Exp Hematol.* 1979;7(suppl 5):389–397.

72. Korbling M, Burke P, Braine H, Elfenbein G, Santos G, Kaizer H. Successful engraftment of blood derived normal hemopoietic stem cells in chronic myelogenous leukemia. *Exp Hematol.* 1981;9(6):684–690.

73. Korbling M, Dorken B, Ho AD, Pezzutto A, Hunstein W, Fliedner TM. Autologous transplantation of blood-derived hemopoietic stem cells after myeloablative therapy in a patient with Burkitt's lymphoma. *Blood.* 1986;67(2):529–532.

74. Korbling M, Freireich EJ. Twenty-five years of peripheral blood stem cell transplantation. *Blood.* 2011;117(24):6411–6416.

75. Huan SD, Hester J, Spitzer G, et al. Influence of mobilized peripheral blood cells on the hematopoietic recovery by autologous marrow and recombinant human granulocyte-macrophage colony-stimulating factor after high-dose cyclophosphamide, etoposide, and cisplatin. *Blood.* 1992;79(12):3388–3393.

76. Elias AD, Ayash L, Anderson KC, et al. Mobilization of peripheral blood progenitor cells by chemotherapy and granulocyte-macrophage colony-stimulating factor for hematologic support after high-dose intensification for breast cancer. *Blood.* 1992;79(11):3036–3044.

77. Sheridan WP, Begley CG, Juttner CA, et al. Effect of peripheral-blood progenitor cells mobilised by filgrastim (G-CSF) on platelet recovery after high-dose chemotherapy. *Lancet.* 1992;339(8794):640–644.

78. Gianni AM, Siena S, Bregni M, et al. Granulocyte-macrophage colony-stimulating factor to harvest circulating haemopoietic stem cells for autotransplantation. *Lancet.* 1989;2(8663):580–585.

79. Juttner CA, To LB, Haylock DN, et al. Autologous blood stem cell transplantation. *Transpl Proc.* 1989;21(1 Pt 3):2929–2931.

80. Micklem HS, Anderson N, Ross E. Limited potential of circulating haemopoietic stem cells. *Nature.* 1975;256(5512):41–43.

81. Hershko C, Gale RP, Ho WG, Cline MJ. Cure of aplastic anaemia in paroxysmal nocturnal haemoglobinuria by marrow transfusion from identical twin: failure of peripheral-leucocyte transfusion to correct marrow aplasia. *Lancet.* 1979;1(8123):945–947.

82. Abrams RA, Glaubiger D, Appelbaum FR, Deisseroth AB. Result of attempted hematopoietic reconstitution using isologous, peripheral blood mononuclear cells: a case report. *Blood.* 1980;56(3):516–520.

83. Kessinger A, Smith DM, Strandjord SE, et al. Allogeneic transplantation of blood-derived, T cell-depleted hemopoietic stem cells after myeloablative treatment in a patient with acute lymphoblastic leukemia. *Bone Marrow Transpl.* 1989;4(6):643–646.

84. Dreger P, Suttorp M, Haferlach T, Loffler H, Schmitz N, Schroyens W. Allogeneic granulocyte colony-stimulating factor-mobilized peripheral blood progenitor cells for treatment of engraftment failure after bone marrow transplantation. *Blood.* 1993;81(5):1404–1407.

85. Russell NH, Hunter A, Rogers S, Hanley J, Anderson D. Peripheral blood stem cells as an alternative to marrow for allogeneic transplantation. *Lancet.* 1993;341(8858):1482.

86. Korbling M, Przepiorka D, Huh YO, et al. Allogeneic blood stem cell transplantation for refractory leukemia and lymphoma: potential advantage of blood over marrow allografts. *Blood.* 1995;85(6):1659–1665.

87. Schmitz N, Dreger P, Suttorp M, et al. Primary transplantation of allogeneic peripheral blood progenitor cells mobilized by filgrastim (granulocyte colony-stimulating factor). *Blood.* 1995;85(6):1666–1672.

88. Bensinger WI, Weaver CH, Appelbaum FR, et al. Transplantation of allogeneic peripheral blood stem cells mobilized by recombinant human granulocyte colony-stimulating factor. *Blood.* 1995;85(6):1655–1658.

89. Anasetti C, Logan BR, Lee SJ, et al. Peripheral-blood stem cells versus bone marrow from unrelated donors. *N Engl J Med.* 2012;367(16):1487–1496.

90. Clift RA, Hansen JA, Thomas ED, et al. Marrow transplantation from donors other than HLA-identical siblings. *Transplantation.* 1979;28(3):235–242.

91. Dupont B, O'Reilly RJ, Pollack MS, Good RA. Use of HLA genotypically different donors in bone marrow transplantation. *Transpl Proc.* 1979;11(1):219–224.

92. Falk PM, Herzog P, Lubens R, et al. Bone marrow transplantation between a histocompatible parent and child for acute leukemia. *Transplantation.* 1978;25(2):88–90.

93. Beatty PG, Clift RA, Mickelson EM, et al. Marrow transplantation from related donors other than HLA-identical siblings. *N Engl J Med.* 1985;313(13):765–771.

94. Powles RL, Morgenstern GR, Kay HE, et al. Mismatched family donors for bone-marrow transplantation as treatment for acute leukaemia. *Lancet.* 1983;1(8325):612–615.

95. Wagemaker G, Vriesendorp HM, van Bekkum DW. Successful bone marrow transplantation across major histocompatibility barriers in rhesus monkeys. *Transpl Proc.* 1981;13(1 Pt 2):875–880.

96. Reisner Y, Itzicovitch L, Meshorer A, Sharon N. Hemopoietic stem cell transplantation using mouse bone marrow and spleen cells fractionated by lectins. *Proc Natl Acad Sci USA.* 1978;75(6):2933–2936.

97. Boehmer H, Sprent J, Nabholz M. Tolerance to histocompatibility determinants in tetraparental bone marrow chimeras. *J Exp Med.* 1975;141(2):322–334.

98. Yunis EJ, Good RA, Smith J, Stutman O. Protection of lethally irradiated mice by spleen cells from neonatally thymectomized mice. *Proc Natl Acad Sci USA.* 1974;71(6):2544–2548.

99. Rodt H, Thierfelder S, Eulitz M. Anti-lymphocytic antibodies and marrow transplantation. 3. Effect of heterologous anti-brain antibodies on acute secondary disease in mice. *Eur J Immunol.* 1974;4(1):15–19.

100. O'Reilly RJ, Collins N, Dinsmore R, et al. Transplantation of HLA-mismatched marrow depleted of T-cells by lectin agglutination and E-rosette depletion. *Tokai J Exp Clin Med.* 1985;10(2–3):99–107.

101. O'Reilly RJ, Kirkpatrick D, Kapoor N, et al. A comparative review of the results of transplants of fully allogeneic fetal liver and HLA-haplotype mismatched, T-cell depleted marrow in the treatment of severe combined immunodeficiency. *Prog Clin Biol Res.* 1985;193:327–342.

102. Prentice HG, Blacklock HA, Janossy G, et al. Use of anti-T-cell monoclonal antibody OKT3 to prevent acute graft-versus-host disease in allogeneic bone-marrow transplantation for acute leukaemia. *Lancet.* 1982;1(8274):700–703.

103. Muller S, Schulz A, Reiss U, et al. Definition of a critical T cell threshold for prevention of GVHD after HLA nonidentical PBPC transplantation in children. *Bone Marrow Transpl.* 1999;24(6):575–581.

104. Reisner Y, Kapoor N, Kirkpatrick D, et al. Transplantation for severe combined immunodeficiency with HLA-A, B,D,DR incompatible parental marrow cells fractionated by soybean agglutinin and sheep red blood cells. *Blood.* 1983;61(2):341–348.

105. Reisner Y, Kapoor N, Kirkpatrick D, et al. Transplantation for acute leukaemia with HLA-A and B nonidentical parental marrow cells fractionated with soybean agglutinin and sheep red blood cells. *Lancet.* 1981;2(8242):327–331.

106. Kernan NA, Flomenberg N, Dupont B, O'Reilly RJ. Graft rejection in recipients of T-cell-depleted HLA-nonidentical marrow transplants for leukemia. Identification of host-derived antidonor allocytotoxic T lymphocytes. *Transplantation.* 1987;43(6):842–847.

107. Sondel PM, Hank JA, Trigg ME, et al. Transplantation of HLA-haploidentical T-cell-depleted marrow for leukemia: autologous marrow recovery with specific immune sensitization to donor antigens. *Exp Hematol.* 1986;14(4):278–286.

108. Lubin I, Segall H, Erlich P, et al. Conversion of normal rats into SCID-like animals by means of bone marrow transplantation from SCID donors allows engraftment of human peripheral blood mononuclear cells. *Transplantation.* 1995;60(7):740–747.

109. Lapidot T, Lubin I, Terenzi A, Faktorowich Y, Erlich P, Reisner Y. Enhancement of bone marrow allografts from nude mice into mismatched recipients by T cells void of graft-versus-host activity. *Proc Natl Acad Sci USA.* 1990;87(12):4595–4599.

110. Aversa F, Tabilio A, Terenzi A, et al. Successful engraftment of T-cell-depleted haploidentical "three-loci" incompatible transplants in leukemia patients by addition of recombinant human granulocyte colony-stimulating factor-mobilized peripheral blood progenitor cells to bone marrow inoculum. *Blood.* 1994;84(11):3948–3955.

111. Aversa F, Tabilio A, Velardi A, et al. Treatment of high-risk acute leukemia with T-cell-depleted stem cells from related donors with one fully mismatched HLA haplotype. *N Engl J Med.* 1998;339(17):1186–1193.

112. Henslee-Downey PJ, Abhyankar SH, Parrish RS, et al. Use of partially mismatched related donors extends access to allogeneic marrow transplant. *Blood.* 1997;89(10):3864–3872.

113. Henslee-Downey PJ, Parrish RS, MacDonald JS, et al. Combined in vitro and in vivo T lymphocyte depletion for the control of graft-versus-host disease following haploidentical marrow transplant. *Transplantation.* 1996;61(5):738–745.

114. Lee KH, Lee JH, Lee JH, et al. Reduced-intensity conditioning therapy with busulfan, fludarabine, and antithymocyte globulin for HLA-haploidentical hematopoietic cell transplantation in acute leukemia and myelodysplastic syndrome. *Blood.* 2011;118(9):2609–2617.

115. Rizzieri DA, Koh LP, Long GD, et al. Partially matched, nonmyeloablative allogeneic transplantation: clinical outcomes and immune reconstitution. *J Clin Oncol.* 2007;25(6):690–697.

116. Huang XJ, Liu DH, Liu KY, et al. Treatment of acute leukemia with unmanipulated HLA-mismatched/haploidentical blood and bone marrow transplantation. *Biol Blood Marrow Transpl.* 2009;15(2):257–265.

117. Luznik L, O'Donnell PV, Symons HJ, et al. HLA-haploidentical bone marrow transplantation for hematologic malignancies using nonmyeloablative conditioning and high-dose, posttransplantation cyclophosphamide. *Biol Blood Marrow Transpl.* 2008;14(6):641–650.

118. Lang P, Feuchtinger T, Teltschik HM, et al. Improved immune recovery after transplantation of TCRalphabeta/CD19-depleted allografts from haploidentical donors in pediatric patients. *Bone Marrow Transpl.* 2015;50(suppl 2):S6–S10.

119. Airoldi I, Bertaina A, Prigione I, et al. Gammadelta T-cell reconstitution after HLA-haploidentical hematopoietic transplantation depleted of TCR-alphabeta+/CD19+ lymphocytes. *Blood.* 2015;125(15):2349–2358.

120. Sun Y, Beohou E, Labopin M, et al. Unmanipulated haploidentical versus matched unrelated donor allogeneic stem cell transplantation in adult patients with acute myelogenous leukemia in first remission: a retrospective pair-matched comparative study of the Beijing approach with the EBMT database. *Haematologica.* 2016;101(8):e352–e354.

121. Ciurea SO, Zhang MJ, Bacigalupo AA, et al. Haploidentical transplant with posttransplant cyclophosphamide vs matched unrelated donor transplant for acute myeloid leukemia. *Blood.* 2015;126(8):1033–1040.

122. Barnes DW, Ilbery PL, Loutit JF. Avoidance of secondary disease in radiation chimaeras. *Nature.* 1958;181(4607):488.

123. Urso IS, Congdon CC, Owen RD. Effect of foreign fetal and newborn blood-forming tissues on survival of lethally irradiated mice. *Proc Soc Exp Biol Med.* 1959;100(2):395–399.

124. Uphoff DE. Perclusion of secondary phase of irradiation syndrome by inoculation of fetal hematopoietic tissue following lethal total-body x-irradiation. *J Natl Cancer Inst.* 1958;20(3):625–632.

125. Scott RB, Matthias JQ, Constandoulakism K, Lucas PF, Whiteside JD. Hypoplastic anaemia treated by tranfusion of foetal haemopoietic cells. *Br Med J.* 1961;2(5264):1385–1388.

126. Nakahata T, Ogawa M. Hemopoietic colony-forming cells in umbilical cord blood with extensive capability to generate mono- and multipotential hemopoietic progenitors. *J Clin Invest.* 1982;70(6):1324–1328.

127. Salahuddin SZ, Markham PD, Ruscetti FW, Gallo RC. Long-term suspension cultures of human cord blood myeloid cells. *Blood.* 1981;58(5):931–938.

128. Auerbach AD, Liu Q, Ghosh R, Pollack MS, Douglas GW, Broxmeyer HE. Prenatal identification of potential donors for umbilical cord blood transplantation for Fanconi anemia. *Transfus (Paris).* 1990;30(8):682–687.

129. Broxmeyer HE, Douglas GW, Hangoc G, et al. Human umbilical cord blood as a potential source of transplantable hematopoietic stem/progenitor cells. *Proc Natl Acad Sci USA.* 1989;86(10):3828–3832.

130. Gluckman E, Broxmeyer HA, Auerbach AD, et al. Hematopoietic reconstitution in a patient with Fanconi's anemia by means of umbilical-cord blood from an HLA-identical sibling. *N Engl J Med.* 1989;321(17):1174–1178.

131. Gluckman E. History of cord blood transplantation. *Bone Marrow Transpl.* 2009;44(10):621–626.

132. Gluckman E, Devergie A, Dutreix J. Radiosensitivity in Fanconi anaemia: application to the conditioning regimen for bone marrow transplantation. *Br J Haematol.* 1983;54(3):431–440.

133. Wagner JE, Kernan NA, Steinbuch M, Broxmeyer HE, Gluckman E. Allogeneic sibling umbilical-cord-blood transplantation in children with malignant and nonmalignant disease. *Lancet.* 1995;346(8969):214–219.

134. Issaragrisil S, Visuthisakchai S, Suvatte V, et al. Brief report: transplantation of cord-blood stem cells into a patient with severe thalassemia. *N Engl J Med.* 1995;332(6):367–369.

135. Bogdanic V, Nemet D, Kastelan A, et al. Umbilical cord blood transplantation in a patient with Philadelphia chromosome-positive chronic myeloid leukemia. *Transplantation.* 1993;56(2):477–479.

136. Wagner JE, Broxmeyer HE, Byrd RL, et al. Transplantation of umbilical cord blood after myeloablative therapy: analysis of engraftment. *Blood.* 1992;79(7):1874–1881.

137. Kurtzberg J, Graham M, Casey J, Olson J, Stevens CE, Rubinstein P. The use of umbilical cord blood in mismatched related and unrelated hemopoietic stem cell transplantation. *Blood Cells.* 1994;20(2–3):275–283. discussion 284.

138. Kurtzberg J, Laughlin M, Graham ML, et al. Placental blood as a source of hematopoietic stem cells for transplantation into unrelated recipients. *N Engl J Med.* 1996;335(3):157–166.

139. Vilmer E, Sterkers G, Rahimy C, et al. HLA-mismatched cord blood transplantation in a patient with advanced leukemia. *Bone Marrow Transpl.* 1991;7(suppl 2):125.

140. Laporte JP, Gorin NC, Rubinstein P, et al. Cord-blood transplantation from an unrelated donor in an adult with chronic myelogenous leukemia. *N Engl J Med.* 1996;335(3):167–170.

141. Barker JN, Weisdorf DJ, DeFor TE, et al. Transplantation of 2 partially HLA-matched umbilical cord blood units to enhance engraftment in adults with hematologic malignancy. *Blood.* 2005;105(3):1343–1347.

142. Mehta RS, Dave H, Bollard CM, Shpall EJ. Engineering cord blood to improve engraftment after cord blood transplant. *Stem Cell Investig.* 2017;4:41.

143. Mehta RS, Shpall EJ, Rezvani K. Cord blood as a source of natural killer cells. *Front Med.* 2015;2:93.

144. Mehta RS, Rezvani K, Olson A, et al. Novel techniques for ex vivo expansion of cord blood: clinical trials. *Front Med.* 2015;2:89.

145. Rubinstein P, Dobrila L, Rosenfield RE, et al. Processing and cryopreservation of placental/umbilical cord blood for unrelated bone marrow reconstitution. *Proc Natl Acad Sci USA.* 1995;92(22):10119–10122.

146. Rubinstein P, Taylor PE, Scaradavou A, et al. Unrelated placental blood for bone marrow reconstitution: organization of the placental blood program. *Blood Cells.* 1994;20(2–3):587–596; discussion 596–600.

147. Rubinstein P, Rosenfield RE, Adamson JW, Stevens CE. Stored placental blood for unrelated bone marrow reconstitution. *Blood.* 1993;81(7):1679–1690.

148. Santos GW, Tutschka PJ, Brookmeyer R, et al. Marrow transplantation for acute nonlymphocytic leukemia after treatment with busulfan and cyclophosphamide. *N Engl J Med.* 1983;309(22):1347–1353.

149. Barnes DW, Corp MJ, Loutit JF, Neal FE. Treatment of murine leukaemia with X rays and homologous bone marrow; preliminary communication. *Br Med J.* 1956;2(4993):626–627.

150. Horowitz MM, Gale RP, Sondel PM, et al. Graft-versus-leukemia reactions after bone marrow transplantation. *Blood.* 1990;75(3):555–562.

151. Weiden PL, Sullivan KM, Flournoy N, Storb R, Thomas ED. Seattle Marrow Transplant T. Antileukemic effect of chronic graft-versus-host disease: contribution to improved survival after allogeneic marrow transplantation. *N Engl J Med.* 1981;304(25):1529–1533.

152. Weiden PL, Flournoy N, Sanders JE, Sullivan KM, Thomas ED. Antileukemic effect of graft-versus-host disease contributes to improved survival after allogeneic marrow transplantation. *Transpl Proc.* 1981;13(1 Pt 1):248–251.

153. Weiden PL, Flournoy N, Thomas ED, et al. Antileukemic effect of graft-versus-host disease in human recipients of allogeneic-marrow grafts. *N Engl J Med.* 1979;300(19):1068–1073.

154. Kolb HJ, Schattenberg A, Goldman JM, et al. Graft-versus-leukemia effect of donor lymphocyte transfusions in marrow grafted patients. *Blood.* 1995;86(5):2041–2050.

155. Tutschka PJ, Copelan EA, Klein JP. Bone marrow transplantation for leukemia following a new busulfan and cyclophosphamide regimen. *Blood.* 1987;70(5):1382–1388.

156. Lucarelli G, Polchi P, Izzi T, et al. Marrow transplantation for thalassemia after treatment with busulfan and cyclophosphamide. *Ann NY Acad Sci.* 1985;445:428–431.

157. Hobbs JR, Hugh-Jones K, Barrett AJ, et al. Reversal of clinical features of Hurler's disease and biochemical improvement after treatment by bone-marrow transplantation. *Lancet.* 1981;2(8249):709–712.

158. Terenzi A, Aristei C, Aversa F, et al. Efficacy of fludarabine as an immunosuppressor for bone marrow transplantation conditioning: preliminary results. *Transpl Proc.* 1996;28(6):3101.

159. Giralt S, Thall PF, Khouri I, et al. Melphalan and purine analog-containing preparative regimens: reduced-intensity conditioning for patients with hematologic malignancies undergoing allogeneic progenitor cell transplantation. *Blood.* 2001;97(3):631–637.

160. Khouri IF, Keating M, Korbling M, et al. Transplant-lite: induction of graft-versus-malignancy using fludarabine-based nonablative chemotherapy and allogeneic blood progenitor-cell transplantation as treatment for lymphoid malignancies. *J Clin Oncol.* 1998;16(8):2817–2824.

161. Slavin S, Nagler A, Naparstek E, et al. Nonmyeloablative stem cell transplantation and cell therapy as an alternative to conventional bone marrow transplantation with lethal cytoreduction for the treatment of malignant and nonmalignant hematologic diseases. *Blood.* 1998;91(3):756–763.

162. Giralt S, Estey E, Albitar M, et al. Engraftment of allogeneic hematopoietic progenitor cells with purine analog-containing chemotherapy: harnessing graft-versus-leukemia without myeloablative therapy. *Blood.* 1997;89(12):4531–4536.

163. Tauro S, Craddock C, Peggs K, et al. Allogeneic stem-cell transplantation using a reduced-intensity conditioning regimen has the capacity to produce durable remissions and long-term disease-free survival in patients with high-risk acute myeloid leukemia and myelodysplasia. *J Clin Oncol*. 2005;23(36): 9387–9393.

164. Corradini P, Zallio F, Mariotti J, et al. Effect of age and previous autologous transplantation on nonrelapse mortality and survival in patients treated with reduced-intensity conditioning and allografting for advanced hematologic malignancies. *J Clin Oncol*. 2005;23(27):6690–6698.

165. Majhail NS, Brunstein CG, Tomblyn M, et al. Reduced-intensity allogeneic transplant in patients older than 55 years: unrelated umbilical cord blood is safe and effective for patients without a matched related donor. *Biol Blood Marrow Transpl*. 2008;14(3):282–289.

166. Schmid C, Schleuning M, Schwerdtfeger R, et al. Long-term survival in refractory acute myeloid leukemia after sequential treatment with chemotherapy and reduced-intensity conditioning for allogeneic stem cell transplantation. *Blood*. 2006;108(3):1092–1099.

167. Sandmaier BM, Mackinnon S, Childs RW. Reduced intensity conditioning for allogeneic hematopoietic cell transplantation: current perspectives. *Biol Blood Marrow Transpl*. 2007;13(1 suppl 1):87–97.

168. McSweeney PA, Niederwieser D, Shizuru JA, et al. Hematopoietic cell transplantation in older patients with hematologic malignancies: replacing high-dose cytotoxic therapy with graft-versus-tumor effects. *Blood*. 2001;97(11):3390–3400.

CHAPTER 2

Pharmacology of Drugs Used in Hematopoietic Cell Transplantation

MEGAN BODGE, PHARMD, BCOP • AARON CUMPSTON, PHARMD, BCOP

INTRODUCTION

Medication regimens used for allogeneic hematopoietic cell transplantation (allo-HCT) are often extremely complex. Core components of the medication regimen include immunosuppression for graft-versus-host disease (GVHD) prophylaxis and potentially treatment, antimicrobial prophylaxis and/or treatment, and medications for symptoms such as diarrhea or mucositis in addition to any preexisting maintenance medications for comorbid conditions. Expertise is required to successfully manage drug-drug interactions (DDIs) (Table 2.1) and balance a number of concurrent issues including the potential for medication toxicities, GVHD, infection, and disease relapse. This chapter will outline pharmacologic considerations for common medications associated with allo-HCT, as well as any relevant pearls to guide the clinician when using each medication in practice.

IMMUNOSUPPRESSANTS

Immunosuppression is a critical component of allo-HCT. Strategies used must effectively suppress the host immunity to allow engraftment, and then subsequently suppress donor immunity to prevent GVHD. This must be balanced though, to avoid risk of infection and disease relapse. Regimens for immune suppression post-allo-HCT typically contain an agent designed to prevent T cell activation (i.e., calcineurin inhibitor) and an agent to prevent T cell proliferation (i.e., a short course of methotrexate or mycophenolate). In general, these agents all work to inhibit and minimize the activity of donor T cells to reduce the risk of GVHD. Either antithymocyte globulin or alemtuzumab can be added to the conditioning regimen for in vivo T cell depletion to assist in engraftment and minimizing GVHD.

Currently, there is no standard regimen for immunosuppression used by all transplant centers. For myeloablative regimens, most centers use a combination of a calcineurin inhibitor (tacrolimus or cyclosporine) and methotrexate administered after transplantation, whereas mycophenolate mofetil is commonly substituted for methotrexate in reduced intensity and nonmyeloablative conditioning regimens as well as for use in patients undergoing a cord blood and haploidentical transplant.[1] Recently, there has been interest in alternative immunosuppressants such as sirolimus and post-transplant cyclophosphamide.

Cyclosporine

Cyclosporine is an 11-amino-acid cyclic peptide which was first extracted in the late 1960s from the fungus *Tolypocladium inflatum*. Cyclosporine is a small molecule drug which binds to cyclophilin, an intracellular protein of the immunophilin family. This complex leads to a block of calcium-dependent signal transduction downstream to the T cell receptor activation and ultimately works to inhibit production of interleukin-2 (IL-2) and T cell activation.[2]

Both cyclosporine and tacrolimus are highly lipophilic and exhibit variable absorption. Cyclosporine undergoes extensive hepatic metabolism to approximately 25 metabolites through cytochrome P450 3A4 (CYP3A4), and clearance is also influenced by the efflux pump p-glycoprotein (PgP).[1] Therefore, numerous drug-drug and drug-food interactions exist. Genetic polymorphisms of CYP3A4 enzymes may alter the pharmacokinetics of both cyclosporine and tacrolimus.

Oral bioavailability is poor with mean values around 25%, but wide interpatient variation is observed. Bioavailability is also approximately 23%–50% higher with modified cyclosporine than with nonmodified

TABLE 2.1
Common Drug Interactions to Consider in Hematopoietic Cell Transplant (HCT) Recipients

Drug-Drug Interaction	Mechanism	Effect	Recommendation
Busulfan-acetaminophen	Competition for glutathione	↑ Busulfan exposure and toxicity	Avoid acetaminophen for 72 h before and after busulfan
Busulfan-azole antifungals	↓ Busulfan clearance	↑ Busulfan exposure	Avoid when possible; monitor busulfan concentrations
Busulfan-metronidazole	↓ Busulfan clearance	↑ Busulfan exposure	Avoid metronidazole for 72 h before and after busulfan
Busulfan-phenytoin	↑ Busulfan clearance	↓ Busulfan exposure	Consider alternative agents (levetiracetam or benzodiazepines); monitor busulfan concentrations; busulfan TDM was originally validated in the context of concomitant phenytoin
Etoposide-azole antifungals	↓ Etoposide clearance	↑ Etoposide exposure	Avoid when possible
Cyclosporine-azole antifungals	↓ Cyclosporine clearance	↑ Cyclosporine exposure	Monitor serum concentrations and reduce cyclosporine dose by 20%–50% (fluconazole 400 mg), 50% (voriconazole 200 mg BID), and 25%[a] (posaconazole 200 mg suspension TID).
Tacrolimus-azole antifungals	↓ Tacrolimus clearance	↑ Tacrolimus exposure	Monitor serum concentrations and reduce tacrolimus dose by 40% (fluconazole 400 mg), 66% (voriconazole 200 mg BID), and 66%–75%[a] (posaconazole 200 mg suspension TID).
Sirolimus-azole antifungals	↓ Sirolimus clearance	↑ Sirolimus exposure	Monitor serum concentrations closely and reduce sirolimus dose by 50%–70% (fluconazole 400 mg). Voriconazole/posaconazole is contraindicated with sirolimus because of the severity of the interaction. If necessary to use concomitantly, decrease sirolimus dose by 90%.

[a]Larger dose reductions may be necessary when given with posaconazole delayed-release tablet formulation due to higher concentrations of posaconazole.
BID, twice daily; *mg*, milligram; *TID*, three times daily; *TDM*, therapeutic drug monitoring.

preparations. Absorption is significantly increased when cyclosporine is administered with a high-fat meal. Patients are therefore recommended to be consistent with administering in relation to meals. Less than 1% of the administered parent drug is excreted unchanged in the urine or feces, and approximately 95% of the metabolites are excreted in the feces. Cyclosporine appears to be the most active compound. Other major metabolites include AM1, AM9, and AM4N with AM1 having the highest immunosuppressive activity (20%–80% as active as cyclosporine).[1] The maximum plasma concentration and area under the concentration-time curve (AUC) values of both cyclosporine and tacrolimus are higher in the morning than in the afternoon.[1] Dosing for cyclosporine is typically 3 mg/kg per day intravenous (IV) or 6 mg/kg per day of cyclosporine (modified) orally (PO) divided every 12 h.

DDIs with calcineurin inhibitors are commonly managed in practice through the utilization of therapeutic drug monitoring (TDM). Dose adjustments may need to be made when initiating or discontinuing a medication with known interaction. Medications which may decrease cyclosporine concentrations include phenytoin, phenobarbital, carbamazepine, rifampin, nafcillin, octreotide, and cyclophosphamide. Medications such as azole antifungals, aprepitant, grapefruit juice, corticosteroids, diltiazem, verapamil, nicardipine, and erythromycin may increase cyclosporine concentrations. It should also be noted that certain medications such as nonsteroidal anti-inflammatory drugs (NSAIDs), amphotericin, angiotensin-converting enzyme (ACE) inhibitors, and aminoglycosides may increase the risk for nephrotoxicity and should be used with caution in patients receiving calcineurin inhibitors.

Given the narrow therapeutic index for calcineurin inhibitors and the interpatient variability in pharmacokinetic parameters, both cyclosporine and tacrolimus require TDM most commonly through obtaining trough concentrations. Several studies in solid organ transplant have found better correlation to exposure with 2-h concentration (C2) assessment, as compared to trough levels, but limited data are available in HCT recipients. Dosage adjustments are made for both cyclosporine and tacrolimus in relation to the presence/risk of GVHD, risk of disease relapse, and changes in serum creatinine or other toxicities. There are limited data to suggest a correlation between trough concentrations and clinical outcomes related to GVHD.[1] Results have been conflicting regarding the correlation of calcineurin activity with presence of acute GVHD. One study reported lower activity in patients with acute GVHD while a subsequent study reported higher activity.[3,4] There are currently no established standards for the optimal cyclosporine trough concentrations, and targets vary among centers. Recommendations from the European Group for Blood and Marrow Transplantation and the European LeukemiaNet Working Group are for a goal cyclosporine trough of 200–300 ng/mL during the first 3–4 weeks, then 100–200 ng/mL until day +90 in the absence of GVHD and toxicity.[5] At that time point, tapering often begins with planned discontinuation around day +180.

Common toxicities related to cyclosporine administration include nephrotoxicity, hypertension, neurotoxicity, electrolyte abnormalities (i.e., hypomagnesemia, hyper/hypokalemia), gingival hyperplasia, skin changes, hirsutism, and metabolic complications (i.e., posttransplant diabetes mellitus, hyperlipidemia). Acute nephrotoxicity is attributed to renal vasoconstriction and ischemia and is typically reversible. Hypertension occurs in up to 50% of patients treated and is also related to renal vasoconstriction. Fine tremor, particularly in the hands, is the most common neurotoxicity experienced. More serious complications include thrombotic microangiopathy (TMA) and posterior reversible encephalopathy syndrome. Toxicities are thought to be concentration related.

Pearls

Cyclosporine is available as a nonmodified and a modified product with several distinct formulations that are not interchangeable. The modified formulation has been reported to increase absorption by as much as 30%. The IV formulation has an IV:PO ratio of 1:2 or 1:3 when converting to a microemulsion formulation. Since CYP3A4 is located in the gastrointestinal (GI) tract, concomitant use of enzyme inducers/inhibitors may alter the conversion ratio from IV to PO.

IV cyclosporine and tacrolimus are formulated with castor oil that causes the drug to leach to tubing. Non-PVC tubing is required. When IV administration is required, constant vigilance must be undertaken to ensure that one lumen is dedicated for TDM and a separate lumen for drug administration to avoid contamination of the line and falsely elevated drug concentrations.[1]

Tacrolimus

Tacrolimus is a highly hydrophobic macrolide lactone antifungal agent derived from *Streptomyces tsukubaensis* which binds to FKBP-12 to form a pentameric complex with Ca^{2+}, calmodulin, and calcineurin. Similarly, this complex inhibits the phosphatase activity of calcineurin and leads to potent downregulation of IL-2 gene expression.[2] Calcineurin inhibition by tacrolimus directly blocks ability to dephosphorylate nuclear transcription factor of activated T cells which is required for translocation and ultimately IL-2 gene expression.[6] Tacrolimus also prevents the conversion of precursor helper T lymphocytes to activated helper T lymphocytes. Tacrolimus has been demonstrated to have immunosuppressive activity that is 50–100 times higher than cyclosporine.[7]

Tacrolimus exhibits many of the same pharmacokinetic properties as cyclosporine. One exception is that food may decrease bioavailability and slow absorption of tacrolimus. Tacrolimus undergoes extensive hepatic metabolism to approximately 15 metabolites. The metabolite present in highest concentrations is 13-O-demethyl-tacrolimus (1/10th activity of tacrolimus), and the primary minor metabolite is 31-O-demethyltacrolimus with activity similar to tacrolimus.

Tacrolimus is available as oral capsules and an IV solution. An extended-release capsule and tablet are manufactured; however, not commonly utilized for allo-HCT patients. Owing to its increased potency compared with cyclosporine, dosing for tacrolimus is approximately 100-fold lower. The initial starting dose for tacrolimus is either 0.03 mg/kg per day, based on lean body weight, as a continuous IV infusion, or 0.09–0.12 mg/kg per day PO divided every 12 h. These doses may need reduced if concomitant use of a CYP3A4 inhibitor is present, and many centers will empirically initiate therapy at lower than recommended doses because of presence of interactions. Limited data suggest that a 2-h intermittent bolus infusion administered twice daily is also feasible with comparable outcomes when compared with continuous IV infusion.[8] Some clinicians prefer the continuous infusion approach to help ensure the same lumen is used for all doses to avoid contamination. Target trough concentrations for tacrolimus are generally 5–15 ng/mL, and higher trough levels typically correlate with toxicity.

Numerous potential DDIs also exist for tacrolimus because of its extensive hepatic metabolism. Medications that interact with cyclosporine are largely the same as those that may interact with tacrolimus. The adverse effect profile of tacrolimus is also overall similar to that of cyclosporine as described previously. However, there appears to be a lower incidence of hypertension, hyperlipidemia, and skin changes. Hirsutism and gingival hyperplasia are typically not observed. A higher incidence of posttransplant diabetes mellitus and neurotoxicity is observed with tacrolimus than with cyclosporine.

Pearls

The IV:PO ratio for tacrolimus is typically either 1:4 or 1:3, although different conversion ratios may be required depending on the presence of DDIs.

Sublingual administration of tacrolimus has been reported primarily in regards to solid organ transplantation. Dose conversions are variable, but most commonly converted as 2 mg oral to 1 mg sublingual. Sublingual administration is commonly accomplished via opening oral capsules and administering the contents.[9]

Methotrexate

Methotrexate is an antimetabolite agent which is a structural analog of aminopterin, a folic acid antagonist. Folic acid is a required cofactor for the synthesis of purines and thymidine. Methotrexate exerts cytotoxic effects through inhibition of dihydrofolate reductase and thus inhibits purine and thymidylate synthesis.[1,7] Methotrexate is thought to prevent GVHD through its ability to deplete proliferating donor lymphocytes; however, the exact mechanism for methotrexate's activity to prevent GVHD is unknown.

Methotrexate primarily binds to albumin and is approximately 50% protein-bound. Methotrexate exhibits third-spacing into fluid pockets and care must be taken to ensure that no ascites or effusions are present prior to drug administration. The drug is primarily excreted through the urine as unchanged drug (80%–90%) with <10% excreted through the feces.

Methotrexate administration post-allo-HCT typically consists of four IV doses with the first dose administered approximately 24 h following the completion of the hematopoietic cell infusion. Subsequent doses are administered on days +3, +6, and +11. Dosing regimens are traditionally 15 mg/m² on day +1, followed by 10 mg/m² on days +3, +6, and +11, or may commonly be reduced to 5 mg/m² for all four doses (i.e., mini-methotrexate).[1,5]

TDM is not commonly employed for patients who receive methotrexate at low doses post-allo-HCT. However, TDM may be reasonable for patients at risk for prolonged exposure and toxicity due to third-spaced fluid (i.e., ascites, pleural effusions) or for patients with renal impairment.

DDIs have been well described for patients receiving high-dose methotrexate and include medications which may delay elimination (penicillins, NSAIDs) and medications which may increase toxicity (trimethoprim-sulfamethoxazole). Significance of DDIs with low-dose methotrexate is unknown; however, an interaction with penicillins has been described.[10]

Common toxicities of methotrexate include mucositis, nephrotoxicity, hepatotoxicity, and delayed engraftment. Renal and hepatic monitoring is required throughout methotrexate administration, and it is recommended to hold the dose in cases of total bilirubin >5 mg/dL or serum creatinine >2 mg/dL.[1,7] Owing to delay in engraftment, methotrexate use is generally avoided for recipients of cord blood transplantation.

Folinic acid (leucovorin) rescue after methotrexate is not standard among centers, but is used by some centers shortly after methotrexate administration in an attempt to reduce toxicity. The dose, timing of administration, and schedule for administration vary considerably. Dosing is typically delayed at least 12 h after methotrexate administration and often 24 h after methotrexate administration.

Mycophenolate

Mycophenolate mofetil (MMF) and mycophenolate sodium are prodrugs that are hydrolyzed by esterases in the intestines and blood to release MPA, a selective, noncompetitive inhibitor of the type 2 isoform of inosine monophosphate dehydrogenase (IMPDH) expressed in activated T- and B-lymphocytes. IMPDH is the rate-limiting step in de novo purine synthesis which lymphocytes are dependent upon.[6]

MPA is derived from penicillium molds. MPA reversibly inhibits inosine monophosphate dehydrogenase, a key enzyme required for de novo purine synthesis, and therefore inhibits T and B cell proliferation as well as antibody production.[7,11]

Wide interpatient and intrapatient variability in plasma concentrations of total MPA, unbound

MPA, and MPA 7-O-glucuronide (MPAG) have been reported. The oral bioavailability of total MPA in allo-HCT patients has been reported as a mean value of 67%.[11] MPA is extensively distributed into the tissues with a large volume of distribution (V_d). The metabolism of MMF is complex. Uridine diphosphate glucurosyltransferase (UGT) enzymes are responsible for MPA metabolism. UGT1A9 is the main enzyme involved in formation of MPAG with UGT1A8 and UGT1A10 also reported as contributing to formation of MPAG. The minor acyl glucuronide metabolite is formed by UGT2B7 and comprises approximately 5% of the total MPA metabolic pathway. MPAG may be converted back to MPA through enterohepatic recirculation in the intestines which then allows for MPA to be reabsorbed into systemic circulation. Less than half of allo-HCT patients may experience a secondary peak in MPA concentration-time profiles secondary to this phenomenon.[11]

MMF is available as an IV infusion and as an oral therapy with a 1:1 conversion between IV and PO. Oral dosage forms include an immediate-release preparation and an extended-release preparation. Data in allo-HCT patients are limited with the extended-release formulation.[12]

MMF dosing in adults is often administered at a dose of 15 mg/kg (or fixed dose of 1000 mg) administered two or three times daily.[5] No dosage adjustments are currently recommended in the setting of renal impairment, although unbound MPA concentrations may be increased in this patient population. Similarly, although pharmacokinetics are likely altered in the setting of hepatic dysfunction, due to a lack of clinical studies, there are no recommended dose adjustments currently recommended for patients with hepatic impairment. The duration for MMF prophylaxis is variable, but often 4 weeks and up to 3 months.

Cyclosporine is a common DDI which may be present for patients undergoing allo-HCT and has been associated with an approximately 34% increase in total MPA clearance when compared with patients who receive tacrolimus.[11] MMF dose adjustments may be necessary when coadministration with cyclosporine occurs, but no clear recommendations are currently available. This effect is likely mediated by inhibition of the multidrug-resistance–associated protein 2 transporter by cyclosporine which results in decreased biliary excretion and enterohepatic recycling of MPAG and therefore more rapid clearance of total MPA. Other DDIs which have been reported to decrease MMF exposure include proton pump inhibitors, metronidazole, ciprofloxacin, and amoxicillin-clavulanic acid. In general, antibiotics

may have varying effects on enterohepatic recirculation of MPA which may affect pharmacokinetic parameters. Oral magnesium salts may decrease the serum concentration of MMF and administration should be separated when taken concurrently. Mycophenolate has also been shown to increase plasma concentrations of acyclovir/valacyclovir and ganciclovir/valganciclovir.

Common toxicities of MMF include gastrointestinal symptoms, primarily diarrhea, and hematologic toxicities.[6] TDM is not commonly employed in clinical practice, although some centers will monitor trough concentrations, AUC, or Bayesian estimates of AUC. Trough targets vary based on graft source and likely correlate weakly with AUC for total and unbound MPA concentrations. It has been reported that a target total MPA $C_{SS} > 2.96 \mu g/mL$ is appropriate for patients who undergo nonmyeloablative conditioning prior to receipt of an unrelated donor graft. Correlation has been shown between total MPA AUC and acute GVHD for cord blood transplants specifically.[13,14]

Sirolimus

Sirolimus is a lipophilic macrocytic lactone derived from *S. hygroscopicus* from Easter Island which is structurally similar to tacrolimus and thought to exhibit immunosuppressive, antitumor, and antiviral properties.[11,15] Similar to tacrolimus, sirolimus also exerts its effect through binding to FKBP-12, although at a different binding site. The complex formed leads to inhibition of the mammalian target of rapamycin and IL-2-driven T cell proliferation; however, it does not lead to calcineurin inhibition.[2] Multiple cytokine-stimulated cell pathways are inhibited through a reduction in DNA transcription, DNA translation, protein synthesis, and cell signaling. Sirolimus is thought to spare CD4+ CD25+ FoxP3+ regulatory T cells, which are thought to be protective for GVHD while possibly sparing the graft-versus-leukemia effect.[7] Sirolimus also inhibits antigen presentation and dendritic cell maturation. Sirolimus exhibits poor oral bioavailability at approximately 15% for the oral suspension and 19% for the tablets. This is likely impacted by extensive intestinal and hepatic first-pass metabolism by CYP3A4 and transport by PgP. Elimination is primarily through the fecal and biliary pathways with an estimated terminal elimination half-life of approximately 62 h.

Sirolimus is available as a tablet formulation and an oral solution. There is no IV formulation currently available. Dosing is commonly a fixed dose in adults of a 6–12 mg loading dose followed by 2–4 mg once daily. There are no dose adjustments recommended for renal impairment; however, a 60% sirolimus dose reduction is recommended for patients with severe hepatic impairment. Trough concentrations are monitored for all patients. Goal trough ranges vary among transplant types with reported target trough concentrations ranging from 3 to 15 ng/mL.[16] Owing to a long half-life, trough levels should be obtained 5–7 days after initiation of therapy or dosage change.[16] Drug levels drawn before this time should be interpreted in context, considering that steady-state concentrations have probably not been reached.

DDIs for sirolimus are similar to that seen with tacrolimus and cyclosporine due to metabolism through CYP3A4. Medications that affect PgP would also be expected to alter sirolimus concentrations and clearance. An empiric sirolimus dose reduction of 90% has been reported to be necessary with concomitant administration of voriconazole, a strong CYP3A4 inhibitor.

Adverse effects attributable to sirolimus include hyperlipidemia, thrombocytopenia, impaired wound healing, mouth ulcers, pneumonitis, and interstitial lung disease.

Pearls

When sirolimus is used in combination with a calcineurin inhibitor, there is an increased incidence of TMA, nephrotoxicity, and hypertension. Combination with tacrolimus should be chosen over cyclosporine because of synergy when combined with tacrolimus and reduced toxicity compared to combination with cyclosporine. Goal tacrolimus concentrations should be kept in the lower end of the therapeutic range (3–7 or 5–10 ng/mL). Clinicians should also be aware of higher incidence of SOS in patients receiving sirolimus during myeloablative preparative regimens.

Cyclophosphamide

Posttransplant cyclophosphamide is a relatively novel approach to GVHD prophylaxis. Early clinical studies using posttransplant cyclophosphamide were conducted in patients undergoing haploidentical transplantation, and trials have sought to expand use to other donor sources. Cyclophosphamide is commonly given as an IV infusion at a dose of 50 mg/kg per day on days +3 and +4 for GVHD prophylaxis.

Cyclophosphamide is a prodrug which is extensively metabolized via hepatocytes to an active metabolite, phosphoramide mustard, and a toxic metabolite, acrolein. Phosphoramide mustard is further converted to an inactive metabolite, carboxycyclophosphamide, via the enzyme aldehyde dehydrogenase. Hematopoietic stem cells possess high amounts of this enzyme rendering the stem cells resistant to the cytotoxic effects

of cyclophosphamide and thus allowing the drug to be used post-allo-HCT without impairing engraftment.[17] In addition, cyclophosphamide is one of only a few medications able to induce T cell apoptosis and upregulate Fas (CD95) expression to trigger activation-induced cell death rapidly following activation.[17] The drug is excreted <30% as unchanged drug and 85%–90% as metabolites. The elimination half-life is 3–12 h. Dose adjustments may be indicated in the setting of severe renal impairment or hepatic impairment. Cyclophosphamide is a major substrate of CYP2B6 and therefore may exhibit DDIs with medications that also use this enzyme for metabolism.

The dose-limiting toxicity of cyclophosphamide is cardiac toxicity which may manifest as arrhythmias, cardiac tamponade, congestive heart failure, hemorrhagic myocarditis, or myocardial necrosis. In addition, cyclophosphamide has been associated with sinusoidal obstruction syndrome (SOS), especially when combined with total body irradiation or busulfan. Other toxicities of cyclophosphamide include gastrointestinal effects (nausea/vomiting, diarrhea), myelosuppression, secondary malignancies, alopecia, and hemorrhagic cystitis. The potential for hemorrhagic cystitis is mitigated by aggressive hydration and administration of mesna, a chemoprotectant which binds to and inactivates acrolein.

Antithymocyte Globulin

Antithymocyte globulin (ATG) consists of polyclonal gamma immunoglobulin (IgG) and is available as horse ATG, rabbit ATG, and rabbit ATG-Fresenius. The IgG is then harvested and toxic antibodies are absorbed out. Rabbit ATG works to block T cell membrane proteins to cause in vivo depletion of T lymphocytes which typically lasts greater than 1 year after administration.

Rabbit ATG is more potent than equine ATG and has been demonstrated to be more protective in terms of grade 2–4 acute GVHD and chronic GVHD for patients undergoing a myeloablative conditioning regimen.[7,18] For these reasons, rabbit ATG is preferred in this setting. ATG appears to have the most impact on chronic GVHD compared to acute, and possibly has more role in peripheral blood transplants compared to bone marrow product. In addition, ATG may also be used in cases of steroid-refractory acute GVHD, although results in this setting have been disappointing.

Rabbit ATG has a half-life of approximately 30 days compared with 5.7 days for equine ATG. Rabbit ATG also has higher specificity for human T lymphocytes. Rabbit ATG clearance occurs primarily through apoptosis and may be influenced by various factors including the recipient's lymphocyte count at the time of administration, the number of infused donor cells, and the development of anti-ATG antibodies. Detection of ATG in the recipient's plasma may still occur 25–60 days after allo-HCT.

The dosing and schedule for rabbit ATG is variable among centers, but is commonly administered at a total dose of 7.5 mg/kg given over 3 days between days −3 and −1 when administered as prophylaxis.[5] Lower doses may be reasonable, especially for matched related donors. Early administration of ATG (before day 5) is less potent than late administration (closer to day 0). For GVHD treatment, there is no standard dosing approach. Common doses for equine ATG include 5–40 mg/kg daily × 3–10 days, and for rabbit ATG include 2–5 mg/kg daily × 3–7 days.[19]

Common toxicities of ATG include a cytokine-release syndrome during administration (fever, chills, and hypotension), thrombocytopenia, leukopenia, increased infection risk, serum sickness, and possible allergic reactions. Serum sickness is characterized by fever, malaise, arthralgia, lymphadenopathy, and cutaneous manifestations.

Pearls

Acetaminophen and diphenhydramine are recommended pre-medications prior to ATG administration to prevent infusion reactions. Premedication with steroids may provide additional tolerability. Infusion time varies, but is typically 4–8 h. Patients should be assessed frequently and monitored closely for any signs or symptoms of reaction.

Rabbit ATG, rabbit ATG-Fresenius, and equine ATG have unique pharmacokinetic properties and should not be considered interchangeable.

Alemtuzumab

Alemtuzumab is a humanized monoclonal antibody of the IgG1 subtype which targets the human CD52 + antigen on the surface of normal and malignant B and T lymphocytes, most monocytes, macrophages, and natural kill cells.[6,7] This binding induces cytotoxicity via antibody-dependent cellular mediated lysis and ultimately leads to prolonged depletion. Owing to these effects, it is commonly used in HCT recipients for in vivo T cell depletion. Alemtuzumab also has reports of efficacy in the management of steroid-refractory GVHD.

Alemtuzumab is available for IV administration, although administration via the subcutaneous route has been used with less infusion reactions. Alemtuzumab exhibits decreased clearance with repeated dosing because of loss of CD52 receptors in the periphery which results in an increase in AUC. The half-life elimination is 11 h (range: 2–32 h). DDIs through metabolic pathways are not expected; however, due to its immunosuppressive properties, additive immunosuppression is exhibited with other agents that suppress the immune system.

Adverse effects related to alemtuzumab administration include the possibility of cytokine-release syndrome (primarily with the first dose), neutropenia, anemia, idiosyncratic pancytopenia, autoimmune thrombocytopenia, pneumonitis, and thyroid dysfunction.

Pearls

Owing to prolonged lymphopenia post-alloHCT, patients receiving T cell depletion with alemtuzumab should receive prolonged PCP and antiviral prophylaxis, and should be monitored for recovery of CD4 cells before cessation of prophylaxis.

Corticosteroids

Corticosteroids are currently used as the cornerstone of first-line treatment for GVHD, and are rarely included in the prophylaxis regimen. Commonly used medications include methylprednisolone (IV) and prednisone (oral). These agents are thought to exert their efficacy through binding to cytosolic receptors leading to translocation into the nucleus and activation of the glucocorticoid response to regulate certain messenger RNA expression. Steroids have a direct lymphocytotoxic effect and lead to down-regulation of pro-inflammatory cytokines (tumor necrosis factor-α).[6,7]

Dosing regimens vary among centers. For acute GVHD, methylprednisolone is often initiated at a dose of 1–2 mg/kg per day and subsequently converted to oral administration and tapered over several weeks once response is attained. For chronic GVHD, prednisone at 1 mg/kg per day is commonly initiated either with or without cyclosporine. Doses are also tapered gradually over time based on response to therapy.

Major side effects of corticosteroids are numerous and include typical steroid-induced complications. Toxicities observed may include hyperglycemia, hypertension, peptic ulcer disease with potential for gastrointestinal hemorrhage, cataracts, muscle atrophy, osteoporosis, and a high incidence of bacterial/fungal/viral infections.

Pearls

Consider initiation of an antacid medication when prolonged corticosteroid courses are anticipated in order to prevent or lessen gastrointestinal complications.

Anti-infective prophylaxis (PCP, viral, fungal) may be continually used for patients who remain on high-dose corticosteroid treatment for extended durations. In addition, prophylaxis against encapsulated organisms should be considered.

ANTIMICROBIAL AGENTS

Patients undergoing allo-HCT will require an antimicrobial regimen for prophylaxis against infection. An initial regimen is comprised of an antibacterial, antiviral, and antifungal agent with an agent for *Pneumocystis* prophylaxis typically added after engraftment. This regimen may need to be altered in the presence of confirmed infection, viral reactivation, or with the addition of GVHD treatment. See Table 2.2 for recommended duration of antimicrobial agents in HCT recipients.

Antibacterial
Quinolones (ciprofloxacin, levofloxacin, and moxifloxacin)

Quinolone antibiotics have become a mainstay of hematopoietic cell transplantation, specifically in the prophylactic setting. Attractive characteristics of these agents include their broad antimicrobial spectrum (increased activity against Gram-negative bacteria, including *P. aeruginosa* in particular), excellent oral absorption, preservation of the anaerobic flora of the alimentary tract (selective decontamination), systemic bactericidal activity, good tolerability, and lack of myelosuppression. Quinolones have a novel

mechanism of action, targeting bacterial topoisomerases. They specifically target bacterial DNA gyrase (topoisomerase II) and topoisomerase IV, leading to cessation of DNA replication. The first-generation quinolone, nalidixic acid, was enhanced with the addition of a fluorine at position 6, to create the fluoroquinolone class. The most commonly used fluoroquinolone agents are the second-generation agent, ciprofloxacin, and the third-generation agents: levofloxacin and moxifloxacin.

The absorption of oral formulations of fluoroquinolones yields concentrations similar to intravenous routes, allowing early conversion to oral therapies, even in severe infections. Absorption may be blocked by oral intake of sucralfate, aluminum, magnesium, zinc, iron, or calcium; and coadministration with these products should be avoided for at least 2 h. The fluoroquinolones penetrate most tissues well, specifically lung and urine, with the exception of moxifloxacin which does not get significantly excreted into the urine. The spectrum of antibacterial coverage is similar between the three agents, with the exception of improved streptococcal coverage with levofloxacin and moxifloxacin. Moxifloxacin does have a benefit of additional anaerobic bacterial coverage. Fluoroquinolones are bactericidal against susceptible organisms, and commonly exhibit a post-antibiotic effect, continuing to inhibit bacterial growth even after serum concentrations are below the minimal inhibitory concentration (MIC). The fluoroquinolone agents are well tolerated with some gastrointestinal (GI) upset, headache, mild QTc interval prolongation,

TABLE 2.2
Duration of Prophylactic Antimicrobials for Hematopoietic Cell Transplant (HCT) Recipients

Antimicrobial Agent	Autologous HCT	Allogeneic HCT	Comments
Fluoroquinolone	Continue until neutrophil engraftment	Continue until neutrophil engraftment	
Fluconazole	Continue until neutrophil engraftment	Continue until day +75–100	Consider change to posaconazole in patients with GVHD on high-dose steroids
Acyclovir/Valacyclovir	Continue for 1 year after transplantation	Continue for a minimum of 1 year after transplantation and until discontinuation of all immunosuppressants	Consider adding letermovir in CMV seropositive patients undergoing allogeneic HCT
Pneumocystis prophylaxis	High-risk patients to receive from engraftment until day +100–180	From engraftment for at least 6 months and until discontinuation of all immunosuppressants	

CMV, cytomegalovirus; *GVHD*, graft-versus-host disease; *HCT*, hematopoietic stem cell transplant.

rash, photosensitivity, and tendinitis/rupture. Ciprofloxacin has more drug interactions than the other quinolones. Of note, ciprofloxacin substantially increases the concentrations of ibrutinib, methotrexate, bendamustine, and pomalidomide.

Pearl

Quinolones have in vitro activity against BK virus, and are commonly used for prophylaxis and treatment. Limited data are available supporting clinical outcomes.[20]

Trimethoprim/Sulfamethoxazole

Trimethoprim (TMP) and sulfamethoxazole (SMX) inhibit different steps in the folic acid synthesis pathway. SMX competitively inhibits bacterial dihydropteroate synthase, blocking incorporation of p-aminobenzoic acid into dihydrofolic acid. TMP works by competitively binding dihydrofolate reductase, inhibiting the conversion of dihydrofolic acid to tetrahydrofolic acid. TMP/SMX has antimicrobial activity for a variety of pathogens, including common organisms such as *Staphylococcus aureus*, *Streptococcus pneumoniae*, *Haemophilus influenzae*, *Moraxella catarrhalis*, *Escherichia coli*, *Morganella morganii*, *Proteus mirabilis*, *Klebsiella pneumoniae*, and *Enterobacter* species. TMP/SMX also covers many less commonly seen pathogens, but very important organisms in the HCT patient, such as *Pneumocystis jiroveci* (formerly *Pneumocysitis carinii*), *Toxoplasma gondii*, *Burkholderia cepacia*, *Stenotrophomonas maltophilia*, *Nocardia* species, and *Listeria monocytogenes*. The most common indication in HCT recipients is for *Pneumocystis* prophylaxis with standard dosing being one TMP/SMX double strength tablet every Monday, Wednesday, and Friday; or a single strength tablet daily.

TMP and SMX both have excellent oral absorption, obtaining similar concentrations as intravenous administration. Both agents have substantial renal elimination, requiring dose adjustments in renal dysfunction. TMP/SMX is generally well tolerated, but can cause GI side effects, rash, fever, and hyperkalemia. Serum creatinine concentrations can be slightly elevated because of competitive inhibition of excretion by TMP. Rare, but serious adverse effects include Stevens-Johnson syndrome, toxic epidermal necrolysis (TEN), aplastic anemia, agranulocytosis, immune-mediated thrombocytopenia, and hepatic necrosis. Allergic cross-reactivity with nonantibiotic sulfonamides is very low (and possibly nonexistent),[21,22] excluding the agent sulfasalazine which may cross-react because of arylamine component of this medication.[23] Competition with methotrexate and warfarin for plasma protein binding may increase levels of these agents, when coadministered with TMP/SMX. TMP/SMX may also increase concentrations of phenytoin, sulfonylureas, and digoxin.

Piperacillin/Tazobactam

Piperacillin (Pip) is a semisynthetic penicillin derived from the ampicillin molecule with acyl side-chain adaptations. Like other penicillins, Pip inhibits cell wall synthesis by binding to one or more of the penicillin-binding proteins. Tazobactam (Tazo) is a β-lactamase inhibitor that is combined with Pip, to enhance efficacy. Pip/Tazo is active against *Staphylococcus aureus* (excluding methicillin-resistant strains), *Streptococcus* species, *Enterococcus* species (except vancomycin-resistant strains), many gram-negative bacteria (including *Pseudomonas*), and most anaerobic bacteria. Pip/Tazo is a commonly used agent for treatment of febrile neutropenia and a variety of the major infections that occur in the immunocompromised patient. Standard dosing is Pip/Tazo 3.375 g IV every 6 h, with higher doses (4.5 g every 6 h) in cases of hospital-acquired pneumonia or more severe infections. The drug is cleared by the kidneys and requires dose adjustments in patients with impaired renal function. Pip/Tazo is typically well tolerated with possible hypersensitivity reactions, rash, serum sickness, fever, interstitial nephritis, thrombocytopenia, and reversible neutropenia. Nephrotoxicity of vancomycin also appears to be higher, in patients receiving concomitant Pip/Tazo.[24–28]

Pearl

Lower doses of Pip/Tazo can be used if prolonged infusion (4 h) administration is used.

Cephalosporins

The most commonly used cephalosporins in HCT patients are ceftazidime and cefepime because of their broad coverage and specifically their coverage of *Pseudomonas* and other hospital-acquired gram-negative pathogens. Ceftazidime is classified as a third-generation cephalosporin because of enhanced gram-negative bacterial coverage, and cefepime is considered a fourth-generation agent due to excellent gram-negative and gram-positive activity. Cephalosporins exert their antibacterial effect by similar mechanisms as penicillins, as previously described. Ceftazidime and cefepime can both be administered either intramuscular or intravenously. Ceftazidime has limited gram-positive bacterial activity but has enhanced activity against gram-negative infections, although resistance is dramatically increasing due to β-lactamase–producing strains. Of specific importance in HCT recipients, is the unreliable activity against viridans streptococci pathogens, which can be a common and dangerous infection in patients with mucositis. Cefepime has much better gram-positive coverage (excluding methicillin-resistant staphylococcus aureus (MRSA) and enterococcus), and has increased stability from hydrolysis by plasmid and chromosomally mediated β-lactamases. Common dosing for ceftazidime and cefepime is 2 g every 8 h. Both cephalosporins are cleared renally and require dose adjustments in patients with renal failure. Adverse effects are similar to that seen with penicillins, with the addition of neurotoxicity with ceftazidime and cefepime, typically seen in patients with renal dysfunction without dose reductions.

Carbapenems

Carbapenems are β-lactams that differ from penicillins by the substitution of a carbon atom for a sulfur atom and by the addition of a double bond to the five-member ring system of the penicillin nucleus. These agents have a broader spectrum of activity than most other β-lactam antibiotics. The four carbapenem agents available in the US include imipenem, meropenem, doripenem, and ertapenem. The spectrums of activity are similar for the first three agents, with ertapenem having reduced activity (specifically of importance is the lack of *Pseudomonas* activity). Owing to this reduced coverage, ertapenem is not an acceptable agent for empiric management of febrile neutropenia, where the other three agents have excellent coverage of the necessary pathogens.

Imipenem is combined with the agent cilastatin to prevent rapid hydrolysis by dehydropeptidase I. They are combined in equal amounts (1:1 ratio), and dosing is commonly described by the imipenem component. Imipenem is very resistant to hydrolysis by most β-lactamases, making it the drug of choice for many of these resistant pathogens. It has a very broad spectrum of gram-positive and gram-negative coverage, including excellent activity against most anaerobic pathogens. The standard dosing strategy for this agent is 500 mg every 6 h. Imipenem is eliminated renally, and requires dose reduction in patients with reduced renal function. Adverse effects include nausea/vomiting, diarrhea, rash, fever, and seizures (1.5%).[29] Cross-reactivity with penicillin-allergic patients is very low (<1%),[30,31] even though structure is similar.

Meropenem has similar therapeutic activity as imipenem, without the need for cilastatin since it is resistant to renal dipeptidase hydrolysis. Meropenem dosing is typically 500 mg every 6 h, but the dose should be increased to 2 g every 8 h for meningitis. It is also cleared renally, and the toxicity profile is similar to imipenem, with the exception of possibly less

seizure risk (0.5%), although this benefit is debatable.[32] The spectrum of activity for doripenem is also similar to meropenem and imipenem, with possibly improved activity against some resistant *Pseudomonas* isolates. Standard doripenem dosing is 500 mg every 8 h.

Vancomycin

Vancomycin is a complex glycopeptide that exerts its antibacterial effect by inhibiting the biosynthesis of peptidoglycan, the major structural polymer of the bacterial cell wall. Vancomycin has broad coverage of gram-positive infections, with bactericidal activity against most pathogens, except having bacteriostatic killing of enterococcus. Vancomycin has no useful activity against gram-negative bacteria. Vancomycin is poorly absorbed from the gastrointestinal tract, making it an attractive agent for local treatment of *Clostridium difficile* colitis when administered orally. Resistance to vancomycin in gram-positive infections is fairly uncommon, although vancomycin-resistant enterococcus is becoming a more common pathogen, especially in the HCT population due to high vancomycin utilization.

Vancomycin displays a concentration-independent killing, making the time above the minimal inhibitory concentration (MIC) more important than the peak levels. Higher concentrations are still important for tissue penetration into difficult-to-penetrate sites (i.e., central nervous system [CNS], lungs, and so forth). Serum concentration monitoring is commonly performed for this agent because of high interpatient variability. Goal trough levels are typically 10–15 μg/mL, but may be escalated to 15–20 μg/mL in patients with infections in locations with poor tissue penetration. Vancomycin is primarily cleared by the kidneys and needs dose adjustments in patients with altered renal function. Common adverse effects include infusion-related flushing ("red man syndrome"), nephrotoxicity, ototoxicity, thrombocytopenia, and neutropenia. Nephrotoxicity was previously considered low with this agent, but more aggressive dosing used in the current era has increased the incidence and requires close monitoring.[33] As discussed previously, the incidence of nephrotoxicity also appears higher with concomitant use of piperacillin/tazobactam.[24–28]

Pearl

Oral vancomycin is available as a capsule or oral solution. The oral solution may be a more cost effective strategy, but is limited by poor oral tolerability. Compounding recipes incorporating cherry syrup or other additives are available to improve this aspect.

Metronidazole

Metronidazole was first discovered in the 1950s as a synthetically made agent to treat protozoal infections (*Trichomonas, Giardia*, etc.). It was later recognized as a highly effective agent for treatment of anaerobic bacteria, but lacks any additional bacterial coverage outside of these pathogens. It has become a standard therapy for serious anaerobic infections, specifically for intraabdominal infections (neutropenic colitis) and *Clostridium difficile* colitis in HCT patients. Metronidazole acts by diffusing into the organism, damaging DNA and causing cell death. This process occurs regardless of the growth phase of the organism, which allows the drug to work even in nondividing organisms.

Metronidazole is almost completely absorbed through oral administration, resulting in similar serum concentrations when administered orally or intravenously. The common dose is 500 mg every 8 h. The drug is primarily metabolized by the liver, with the majority of the metabolites excreted in the urine. Dose reductions are typically not necessary in mild/moderate renal or hepatic impairment, but if severe impairment exists, some dose reductions could be considered (e.g., 500 mg every 12 h). Adverse effects that can be seen with high doses or prolonged therapy include CNS toxicities and peripheral neuropathy. A disulfiram-like reaction may occur with concomitant alcohol ingestion. Drug interactions include increased exposure of busulfan and warfarin.

Antivirals

Acyclovir/valacyclovir. Acyclovir is a nucleoside analog that possesses activity against the herpes family of viruses, including herpes simplex virus type 1 and 2 (HSV-1 and HSV-2) and varicella-zoster virus (VZV). Acyclovir has low activity against Epstein–Barr virus (EBV), cytomegalovirus (CMV), and human herpesvirus 6 (HHV-6). Acyclovir dosing for HSV/VZV prophylaxis is typically 400–800 mg PO twice daily or 250 mg/m2 IV twice daily. Prophylaxis is typically continued for a minimum of 1 year after HCT, and continued for as long as patients continue to require immunosuppressive medications. Acyclovir is primarily excreted by the kidneys, requiring dose reductions in patients with renal dysfunction. High-dose acyclovir can cause neurotoxicity and renal toxicity.

Valacyclovir is a prodrug for acyclovir, being rapidly and almost completely converted to acyclovir by hepatic and intestinal metabolism. Valacyclovir has substantially improved bioavailability with approximately 55%–70% absorption compared to only about 10%–20% absorption with the traditional acyclovir formulation. The recommended dose of valacyclovir for HSV/VZV prophylaxis is 500 mg PO once to twice daily.

Ganciclovir/valganciclovir. Ganciclovir is similar in structure to acyclovir, with the addition of a hydroxymethyl group. Ganciclovir maintains activity against HSV and VZV, with enhanced activity against CMV, EBV and HHV-6. Ganciclovir has become the standard of care for treatment of CMV, with documented clinical use in these infections. Clinical efficacy in the management of EBV and HHV-6 infections is low. Oral ganciclovir has poor oral absorption, with less than 10% being absorbed. Valganciclovir is an oral prodrug that is rapidly converted to ganciclovir, which substantially improves oral absorption. When taken with food, oral valganciclovir will achieve similar concentrations as intravenous ganciclovir at therapeutic doses. Ganciclovir dosing for CMV treatment is 5 mg/kg IV every 12 h for 2 weeks and then reduced to 5 mg/kg IV q24 for an additional 2 weeks of therapy. Valganciclovir dosing is 900 mg PO twice daily for 2 weeks, and then reduced to 900 mg PO daily for an additional 2 weeks. Ganciclovir is primarily excreted by the kidneys and needs dose adjustment in renal dysfunction. The primary adverse effect of ganciclovir is myelosuppression, with many patients requiring granulocyte colony–stimulating factor support to maintain white blood cell counts. Valganciclovir has similar myelosuppression, with some additional gastrointestinal toxicities.

Foscarnet. Foscarnet is a pyrophosphate analog with inhibitory activity against all the herpesviruses. It is effective for treatment of ganciclovir-resistant CMV infections, and also acyclovir-resistant HSV and VZV infections. Oral bioavailability is low, requiring IV administration. Vitreous concentrations are similar to plasma, and CNS concentrations are approximately two-thirds of plasma concentrations. Foscarnet dosing for CMV management is 60 mg/kg IV every 12 h for 2 weeks and then 90 mg/kg every 24 h for maintenance therapy. Foscarnet is cleared renally and requires dose adjustments if renal function is compromised. Primary toxicities include nephrotoxicity and severe electrolyte wasting. Electrolytes most commonly affected include calcium, phosphorus, potassium, and magnesium. Caution should be taken with IV calcium administration because of significant incompatibility with foscarnet.

Cidofovir. Cidofovir is a cytidine nucleotide analog with inhibitory activity against human herpes, papilloma, polyoma, pox, and adenoviruses. Oral bioavailability and CNS penetration are both low with this antiviral agent. The active metabolites of cidofovir have a very long intracellular half-life, allowing infrequent dosing even though the serum concentrations may clear much faster. Cidofovir dosing for CMV management is typically 5 mg/kg IV weekly × 2 weeks, and then every other week for maintenance duration. Cidofovir is almost exclusively cleared by the kidney by glomerular filtration and renal tubular secretion. High-dose probenecid is typically given to compete for tubular secretion, prolonging the exposure to cidofovir and also decreasing nephrotoxicities. Lower doses of cidofovir have been given safely given in transplant recipients without probenecid for treatment of BK virus nephropathy. Most common adverse events include a high incidence of nephrotoxicity and neutropenia.

Letermovir. Letermovir inhibits the CMV DNA terminase complex (UL56) which is required for viral DNA processing and packaging. This mechanism of action is different than previously available agents, and does not exhibit cross resistance, making it an attractive agent for CMV prophylaxis or multidrug-resistant cases. The drug is well tolerated, without side effects previously seen with anti-CMV agents, such as myelosuppression and nephrotoxicities. Side effects include nausea/vomiting, edema, dyspnea, hepatotoxicity and atrial fibrillation/flutter. Dosing of letermovir for CMV prophylaxis is 480 mg PO or IV once a day. Concomitant use of cyclosporine increases letermovir exposure, and the dose should be reduced to 240 mg once daily in these patients. Letermovir does not have activity against HSV/VZV and prophylaxis for these infections is still required in addition to letermovir.

Antifungals

Amphotericin B. Amphotericin B is a polyene antifungal that exerts its activity by binding to ergosterol in fungal cell membranes, developing holes in the membrane and allowing cell components to leak out, causing cell death. Amphotericin B is the broadest spectrum antifungal available, with activity against a variety of yeasts and molds. It has activity against *Candida* (excluding *C. lusitaniea*), *Aspergillus* (excluding *A. terreus*), *Cryptococcus neoformans*, *Coccidioides* species, *Blastomyces*, *Histoplasma*, *Fusarium* (variable coverage), *Scedosporium* (variable coverage), and Zygomycetes (variable coverage). The most common adverse effects include nephrotoxicity, electrolyte wasting, and infusion reactions (fevers, chills, rigors, nausea/vomiting). Nephrotoxicity may be reduced by saline loading and aggressive electrolyte replace-

ment. Infusion reactions may be reduced by premedication with acetaminophen and diphenhydramine.[34] Corticosteroids may also decrease infusion reactions, but may not be ideal in the setting of treating a fungal infection.

The conventional formulation of amphotericin B contains deoxycholate for stabilization, adding significant toxicity to the drug. Dosing of amphotericin B is in the range of 0.5–1.5 mg/kg IV daily. There are three lipid-based formulations developed to decrease toxicities associated with the conventional formulation: liposomal amphotericin B (L-AMB), amphotericin B lipid complex (ABLC), and amphotericin B colloidal dispersion (ABCD). Standard dosing for these agents is 3–6 mg/kg IV daily. These formulations have all shown a decrease in nephrotoxicity compared to conventional amphotericin B. L-AMB and ABLC have also shown decreased infusion reactions, but ABCD has several reports of higher rate and more life-threatening infusion reactions than conventional amphotericin B. Because of this, ABCD is a rarely used option, and has been removed from the market in the United States. Only one prospective comparison has been completed comparing the remaining two lipid formulations. In the setting of empiric treatment of febrile neutropenia, L-AMB was found to have significantly lower rates of nephrotoxicity and infusion reactions compared to ABLC.[35] L-AMB also has improved CNS penetration compared to other formulations.

Triazoles. Availability of the triazole antifungal agents made a substantial impact on antifungal treatment approaches because of their safety, efficacy, and excellent oral bioavailability. The triazoles exert their antifungal effects by inhibiting ergosterol synthesis in the fungal cell membrane. Three of the most commonly used triazoles in HCT are fluconazole, voriconazole, and posaconazole. All of these medications have significant drug interactions, many of which are specifically important in the HCT patient. See Table 2.3 for a listing of some of the medications commonly used in HCT that will have significant increases in exposure when coadministered with a triazole antifungal agent. Fluconazole and voriconazole are inhibitors of cytochrome P450 enzymes 3A4, 2C9, and 2C19. Posaconazole is an inhibitor of 3A4 only.

- **Fluconazole**
  Fluconazole is almost completely absorbed through oral dosing, and is not affected by food consumption or gastric pH. Fluconazole has good tissue and site penetration with high levels in the CNS, lungs, urine, peritoneal fluid, eyes, and skin. It has

TABLE 2.3
Common Medications in Hematopoietic Stem Cell Transplant Recipients That Will Have Increased Exposure With Concomitant Triazole Antifungal Administration

Apixiban	Digoxin	Rivaroxaban
Aprepitant	Fentanyl	Ruxolitinib
Atorvastatin	Ibrutinib	Sirolimus
Bortezomib	Idelalisib	Sorafenib
Brentuximab vedotin	Methadone	Tacrolimus
Budesonide	Midostaurin	Venetoclax
Busulfan	Oxycodone	Vinca alkaloids
Calcium channel blockers	Phenytoin	Warfarin
Corticosteroids	Philadelphia chromosome agents	
Cyclosporine		

excellent activity against most *Candida* species, excluding *C. krusei* and *C. glabrata*. *C. krusei* exhibits inherent fluconazole resistance, where *C. glabrata* has an acquired resistance and can still be treated in many cases with higher fluconazole dosing. Fluconazole also has good activity against *Cryptococcus neoformans* and *Coccidioides* species. This agent is well tolerated with low risk of gastrointestinal toxicities, hepatotoxicities, and QTc prolongation.

- **Voriconazole**
Similar to fluconazole, voriconazole has excellent oral absorption, but with an extended spectrum of activity. Voriconazole improves coverage of *C. krusei* and *C. glabrata*, and is the drug of choice for *Aspergillus* species. It has modest activity against *Scedosporium* and *Fusarium* species. Minimal amounts of active voriconazole are excreted in the urine. Voriconazole exhibits a saturable metabolism, so increases in the dose may result in nonlinear increases in concentrations. Polymorphisms in CYP2C19 can result in fourfold increases in exposure, with 15%–20% of Asians being homozygous poor metabolizers. IV voriconazole contains cyclodextrin, which is primarily excreted renally. Toxicities of cyclodextrin are unclear, so oral dosing in renal dysfunction is preferred. Voriconazole is well tolerated, with adverse effects including hepatoxicity, reversible visual disturbances, and QTc prolongation.

- **Posaconazole**
Posaconazole is a synthetic analog of itraconazole, with similar yeast and *Aspergillus* species activity in vitro as voriconazole. Posaconazole adds enhanced activity against zygomycosis. Posaconazole is available as an IV product and orally as a suspension or delayed-release tablet formulation, with the tablets having a significant improvement in absorption and attainment of goal serum concentrations.[36,37] Absorption of the suspension is decreased by acid suppressing drugs, and increased by high-fat foods. The tablet formulation does not seem to be affected by these factors. Most efficacy data are in the prophylactic setting, although some reports of treatment efficacy have been reported.

Echinocandins. Caspofungin, micafungin, and anidulafungin are the three echinocandins available for use. These agents target 1,3-β-D-glucans in the fungal cell wall. They are fungicidal against *Candida* species and have fungistatic activity against *Aspergillus* species. All 3 drugs have poor oral absorption and require IV administration, poor CNS and urine concentrations, are not eliminated by the kidneys, and only have modest increase in exposure with hepatic impairment. Their novel mechanism of action make them an attractive option for combination antifungal therapy since they do not display antagonism with the triazoles or amphotericin B. Caspofungin concentrations are increased by concomitant cyclosporine administration. Caspofungin appears to increase tacrolimus exposure by 16%. Micafungin has been reported to increase sirolimus concentrations. This minimal drug interaction profile makes echinocandins a good option when triazole interactions are of concern. The echinocandins are well-tolerated agents, with the most common adverse events being hepatotoxicity, fever, and phlebitis at the infusion site. Caspofungin has some rare cases of histamine-related symptoms during infusion.

ANTIDIARRHEAL AGENTS
Loperamide
Loperamide is a selective antidiarrheal opioid which works directly on circular and longitudinal intestinal muscles, through the opioid receptor, to inhibit peristalsis and prolong transit time. The medication also reduces fecal volume, increases viscosity, and diminishes fluid and electrolyte loss. In addition, loperamide increases anal sphincter tone.

Loperamide is absorbed poorly and undergoes extensive hepatic metabolism through oxidative N-demethylation. It is a major substrate of CYP3A4 and also undergoes metabolism through CYP2C8, CYP2B6, and CYP2D6. Half-life elimination is 9.1–14.4 h and excretion is primarily through the feces.

Loperamide is available as a capsule and a liquid formulation. Dosing for acute diarrhea is 4 mg initially followed by 2 mg after each loose stool, up to 16 mg/day. Prior to initiation, alternative causes for diarrhea should be excluded, specifically *Clostridium difficile* infection.

Owing to its extensive CYP metabolism, numerous potential DDIs exist with loperamide. Loperamide is also a substrate of PgP which also increases the potential for DDIs. Loperamide contains a boxed warning for torsades de pointes and sudden death, therefore QTc-prolonging medications should be avoided when possible.

Adverse reactions attributable to loperamide may include dizziness, abdominal cramps, constipation, and nausea. More rarely, loperamide may cause anaphylactic reactions, ileus, or more severe skin reactions such as Stevens-Johnson syndrome and TEN.

Diphenoxylate and Atropine

Diphenoxylate is an analog of meperidine which inhibits excessive GI motility and propulsion by stimulation of mu and delta opiate receptors in the bowel. Diphenoxylate is formulated with atropine in subtherapeutic amounts to decrease abuse potential. This combination agent is approved for use for adjunctive management of diarrhea.

The onset of action for diphenoxylate is within 45–60 min with peak serum concentrations reached in approximately 2 h. It is well absorbed and extensively metabolized through the liver via ester hydrolysis to the active metabolite, diphenoxylic acid. The half-life elimination for diphenoxylate is 2.5 and 12–14 h for diphenoxylic acid. Excretion is primarily through the feces.

DDIs exist primarily in regards to agents which may also cause CNS depression or anticholinergic effects as additive toxicity may occur. Adverse reactions observed with diphenoxylate may include CNS depression, flushing, tachycardia, pruritis, urinary retention, and gastrointestinal symptoms such as abdominal distention. More rarely, effects such as ileus or anaphylaxis may be seen. Patients should be cautious with performing tasks such as driving or operating machinery while taking this medication.

Octreotide

Octreotide is a somatostatin analog which may be used as an antidiarrheal agent in refractory cases. This agent works as a mimic of natural somatostatin to block serotonin release; additionally, gastrin, VIP, insulin, glucagon, secretin, motilin, and pancreatic polypeptide are also inhibited. In healthy subjects, the antidiarrheal properties diminished over a 1 week administration period, thought to be related to adaption of the somatostatin receptors.[38]

Ocreotide is available for subcutaneous injection or IV infusion. A long-acting depot formulation is also available for intramuscular administration. The subcutaneous formulation has a rapid onset of action with peak plasma concentrations reached within 0.4 h. The duration of action for the subcutaneous formulation is 6–12 h. Octreotide is metabolized extensively through the liver and has a half-life elimination of 1.7–1.9 h, although half-life elimination may be prolonged in certain disease states such as cirrhosis as well as in elderly patients. Octreotide is excreted through the urine with 32% excretion as unchanged drug. Usual dosage for HCT patients with uncontrolled diarrhea is 100–500 mcg every 8 h, with close monitoring for toxicity and ileus.

When using octreotide, caution should be taken to avoid other QTc-prolonging medications when possible. Additive toxicity may be observed when octreotide is used concomitantly with other medications that may affect glucose levels or cardiovascular function. Octreotide should be used cautiously in patients with a history of cardiovascular disease as bradycardia, conduction abnormalities, and arrhythmias have been observed in some patients treated with the agent. Other adverse effects may include local injection site reactions, cholelithiasis, impaired glucose regulation, hypothyroidism, and pancreatitis.

MISCELLANEOUS
Defibrotide

Defibrotide is a single-stranded oligonucleotide drug derived from porcine intestinal tissue which has been approved for the treatment of adult and pediatric patients with hepatic SOS with concurrent renal and/or pulmonary dysfunction following HCT. Defibrotide has been shown to exhibit antithrombotic, anti-ischemic, and anti-inflammatory properties.[39,40] Activity of the drug is primarily through augmentation of plasmin enzymatic activity to hydrolyze fibrin clots. This activity leads to reduced endothelial cell (EC) activation and increased EC-mediated fibrinolysis via plasminogen activator and thrombomodulin expression. The mechanism for defibrotide for treatment of VOD has not been fully elucidated.

Defibrotide is not thought to undergo appreciable hepatic metabolism and is likely metabolized via nucleotidases, nucleosidases, deaminases and phosphorylases. Half-life elimination is <2 h and 5%–15% of the total dose is excreted in the urine as defibrotide sodium.

Dosing for defibrotide is 6.25 mg/kg IV every 6 h for a minimum of 21 days, or until signs and symptoms of VOD have resolved (maximum 60 days of therapy). Dosing should be based on pre-transplant body weight. The agent is administered as a 2 h infusion.

Concomitant systemic anticoagulation or fibrinolytic therapy should be avoided with defibrotide as antithrombotic or antifibrinolytic effects may be enhanced. No other major DDIs are known at this time.

Patients treated with defibrotide may be at an increased risk of bleeding and the medication is not recommended in patients with active bleeding. Other adverse reactions associated with defibrotide include hypotension, diarrhea, vomiting, nausea, and epistaxis.

Ursodiol

Ursodeoxycholic acid (ursodiol) is a naturally occurring hydrophilic bile acid which has been demonstrated to decrease cholestasis. Ursodiol has been postulated to reduce the hydrophobic bile acids in the hepatobiliary system to lessen the potential for hepatotoxicity. It has been extensively evaluated in prophylaxis of SOS, with modest benefits. Ursodiol has also been postulated to exhibit immunomodulatory and antiapoptotic properties and may be used as an adjunctive therapy for patients with acute or chronic GVHD of the liver.[40,41]

Ursodiol is available for oral administration as a tablet, suspension, or capsule. Dosing is commonly 600–900 mg/day in divided doses started with initiation of the preparative chemotherapy regimen for allo-HCT. Ursodiol is ~70% protein-bound and undergoes extensive enterohepatic recycling following hepatic conjugation and biliary secretion. Excretion is primarily through the feces with <1% excreted renally. DDIs with ursodiol include aluminum hydroxide and bile acid sequestrants which may both decrease the serum concentrations of ursodiol.

Deferasirox

Deferasirox is an iron chelating agent used for treatment of iron overload. The agent works to selectively bind iron leading to complexes which are then excreted primarily through the feces.[42] Deferasirox is available as an oral soluble tablet, an oral tablet, and as an oral packet. Dosing varies based on formulation and may be titrated every 3–6 months based on serum ferritin trends.

The agent is primarily metabolized through glucuronidation, mainly by UGT1A1. Excretion is largely through the feces with approximately 8% excreted renally. The elimination half-life ranges from 8 to 16 h. DDIs may exist since it is a modest CYP3A4/5 inducer, a moderate CYP2C8 inhibitor, and a moderate CYP1A2 inhibitor. In addition, UGT inducers (phenytoin, phenobarbital, rifampin, etc.) and bile acid sequestrants should be avoided when possible because of decreased exposure of deferasirox.

The most common adverse effects attributed to deferasirox include skin rash, nephrotoxicity, hepatotoxicity, cytopenias, hearing loss, and GI toxicities (nausea, vomiting, diarrhea, and abdominal pain).

Intravenous Immune Globulin

Intravenous immunoglobulin (IVIG) is a plasma-derived product which contains immune globulins, or antibodies.[6] IVIG is manufactured from pooled plasma donated from >1000 donors and prepared in such a way to fractionate plasma into immune globulin fractions. Products are stabilized with additives such as glucose, maltose, glycine, sucrose, sorbitol, or albumin. IVIG is primarily used to passively replace antibodies in patients with impaired immunity in conjunction with antimicrobial therapy.

IVIG is available for parenteral administration only. The most common route for administration is via IV infusion, although other studied routes of administration include intramuscular (IM) and subcutaneous injection. Several products are commercially available and may vary in terms of antibody content or additives. Certain preparations contain very high antibody titers to specific infectious organisms, such as cytomegalovirus, when compared to standard IVIG. In addition, preparations vary in terms of IgA content and patients with known IgA deficiency who receive IVIG should receive a product with the lowest IgA content available.

The half-life in hematopoietic stem cell transplantation patients has been demonstrated to be approximately 6 days which is shorter than what has been reported in healthy subjects (22 days).[43]

Patients who receive IVIG may be at risk for infusion reactions and can be premedicated with acetaminophen and diphenhydramine. Infusion reactions may include fever, chills, nausea, vomiting, and headache.

These reactions are typically transient and related to the infusion rate. Rates of infusion reactions have been reported at 1%–15% with <5% of patients experiencing clinically significant reactions. Acute renal failure has been reported with IVIG, but is commonly thought to be attributed to sucrose exposure. Sucrose-containing preparations should be avoided in patients with baseline renal dysfunction. Other adverse reactions may include thromboembolic events, pulmonary or dermatologic toxicity, hyperviscosity, aseptic meningitis, arthritis, cerebral infarction, and hemolysis.

Palifermin

Palifermin is a recombinate keratinocyte growth factor (KGF) which is used as a chemoprotective agent to reduce mucositis. KGF is produced endogenously in response to epithelial tissue injury.[44] The onset of action for palifermin is approximately 48 h, but varies based on dose. Half-life elimination has been reported at 4.5 h but may range from 3.3 to 5.7 h. Palifermin is generally well tolerated, but may cause taste changes, tongue thickening, tongue erythema, sensation of burning in the skin, rash, pruritis, and amylase/lipase elevations which are usually transient.

REFERENCES

1. McCune JS, Bemer MJ. Pharmacokinetics, pharmacodynamics and pharmacogenomics of immunosuppressants in allogeneic haematopoietic cell transplantation: part 1. *Clin Pharmacokinet.* 2016;55(5):525–550.
2. Halloran PF. Immunosuppressive drugs for kidney transplantation. *N Engl J Med.* 2004;351(26):2715–2729.
3. Sanquer S, Schwarzinger M, Maury S, et al. Calcineurin activity as a functional index of immunosuppression after allogeneic stem-cell transplantation. *Transplantation.* 2004;77:854–858.
4. Pai SY, Fruman DA, Leong T, et al. Inhibition of calcineurin phosphatase activity in adult bone marrow transplant patients treated with cyclosporine A. *Blood.* 1994;84:3974–3979.
5. Ruutu T, Gratwohl A, de Witte T, et al. Prophylaxis and treatment of GVHD: EBMT-ELN working group recommendations for a standardized practice. *Bone Marrow Transpl.* 2014;49:168–173.
6. Wiseman AC. Immunosuppressive medications. *Clin J Am Soc Nephrol.* 2016;11(2):332–343.
7. Ram R, Storb R. Pharmacologic prophylaxis regimens for acute graft-versus-host disease: past, present, and future. *Leukemia Lymphoma.* 2013;54(8):1591–1601.
8. Skeens M, Pai V, Garee A, et al. Twice daily i.v. bolus tacrolimus infusion for GVHD prophylaxis in children undergoing stem cell transplantation. *Bone Marrow Transpl.* 2012;47(11):1415–1418.
9. Doligalski CT, Liu EC, Sammons CM, et al. Sublingual administration of tacrolimus: current trends and available evidence. *Pharmacotherapy.* 2014;34(11):1209–1219.
10. Kim IW, Yun HY, Choi B, et al. ABCB1 C3435T genetic polymorphism on population pharmacokinetics of methotrexate after hematopoietic stem cell transplantation in Korean patients: a prospective analysis. *Clin Ther.* 2012;34(8):1816–1826.
11. McCune JS, Bemer MJ, Long-Boyle J. Pharmacokinetics, pharmacodynamics and pharmacogenomics of immunosuppressants in allogeneic haematopoietic cell transplantation: part 2. *Clin Pharmacokinet.* 2016;55(5):551–593.
12. Weber T, Niestadtkötter J, Wienke A, et al. Enteric-coated mycophenolate sodium containing GvHD prophylaxis reduces GvHD rate after allogeneic HSCT. *Eur J Haematol.* 2016;97(3):232–238.
13. Jacobson P, Rogosheske J, Barker JN, et al. Relationship of mycophenolic acid exposure to clinical outcome after hematopoietic cell transplantation. *Clin Pharmacol Ther.* 2005;78:486–500.
14. Harnicar S, Ponce DM, Hilden P, et al. Intensified mycophenolate mofetil dosing and higher mycophenolic acid trough levels reduce severe acute graft-versus-host disease after double-unit cord blood transplantation. *Biol Blood Marrow Transpl.* 2015;21:920–925.
15. Abouelnasr A, Roy J, Cohen S, et al. Defining the role of sirolimus in the management of graft-versus-host disease: from prophylaxis to treatment. *Biol Blood Marrow Tranpslant.* 2013;19(1):12–21.
16. Stenton SB, Partovi N, Ensom MH. Sirolimus: the evidence for clinical pharmacokinetic monitoring. *Clin Pharmacokinet.* 2005;44(8):769–786.
17. Al-Homsi AS, Roy TS, Cole K, et al. Post-transplant high-dose cyclophosphamide for the prevention of graft-versus-host disease. *Biol Blood Marrow Transpl.* 2015;21(4):604–611.
18. Storek J, Mohty M, Boelens JJ. Rabbit Anti-T cell globulin in allogeneic hematopoietic cell transplantation. *Biol Blood Marrow Transpl.* 2015;21:959–970.
19. Hsu B, May R, Carrum G, et al. Use of antithymocyte globulin for treatment of steroid-refractory acute graft-versus-host disease: an international practice survey. *Bone Marrow Transpl.* 2001;28(10):945–950.
20. Miller AN, Glode A, Hogan KR, et al. Efficacy and safety of ciprofloxacin for prophylaxis of polyomavirus BK virus-associated hemorrhagic cystitis in allogeneic hematopoietic stem cell transplantation recipients. *Biol Blood Marrow Transpl.* 2011;17(8):1176–1181.
21. Brackett CC, Singh H, Block JH. Likelihood and mechanisms of cross-allergenicity between sulfonamide antibiotics and other drugs containing a sulfonamide functional group. *Pharmacotherapy.* 2004;24(7):856–870.
22. Johnson KK, Green DL, Rife JP, Limon L. Sulfonamide cross-reactivity: fact or fiction?. [published correction appears in Ann Pharmacother. 2005;39(7-8):1373] *Ann Pharmacother.* 2005;39(2):290–301.

23. Zawodniak A, Lochmatter P, Beeler A, et al. Cross-reactivity in drug hypersensitivity reactions to sulfasalazine and sulfamethoxazole. *Int Arch Allergy Immunol.* 2010;153(2):152–156.

24. Cotner SE, Rutter WC, Burgess DR, et al. Influence of beta-lactam infusion strategy on acute kidney injury. *Antimicrob Agents Chemother.* 2017. [Epub ahead of print].

25. LeCleir LK, Pettit RS. Piperacillin-tazobactam versus cefepime incidence of acute kidney injury in combination with vancomycin and tobramycin in pediatric cystic fibrosis patients. *Pediatr Pulmonol.* 2017;52(8):1000–1005.

26. Rutter WC, Cox JN, Martin CA, et al. Nephrotoxicity during vancomycin therapy in combination with piperacillin-tazobactam or cefepime. *Antimicrob Agents Chemother.* 2017;61(2).e02089–e16.

27. Navalkele B, Pogue JM, Karino S, et al. Risk of acute kidney injury in patients on concomitant vancomycin and piperacillin-tazobactam compared to those on vancomycin and cefepime. *Clin Infect Dis.* 2017;64(2):116–123.

28. Hammond DA, Smith MN, Li C, et al. Systematic review and meta-analysis of acute kidney injury associated with concomitant vancomycin and piperacillin/tazobactam. *Clin Infect Dis.* 2017;64(5):666–674.

29. Calandra GB, Brown KR, Grad LC, et al. Review of adverse experiences and tolerability in the first 2,516 patients treated with imipenem/cilastatin. *Am J Med.* 1985;78(suppl 6A):73–78.

30. Kula B, Djordjevic G, Robinson JL. A systematic review: can one prescribe carbapenems to patients with IgE-mediated allergy to penicillins or cephalosporins? *Clin Infect Dis.* 2014;59:1113–1122.

31. Romano A, Viola M, Guéant-Rodriguez RM, et al. Imipenem in patients with immediate hypersensitivity to penicillins. *N Engl J Med.* 2006;354:2835–2837.

32. Cannon JP, Lee TA, Clark NM, et al. The risk of seizures among the carbapenems: a meta-analysis. *J Antimicrob Chemother.* 2014;69(8):2043–2055.

33. Lodise TP, Patel N, Lomaestro BM, et al. Relationship between initial vancomycin concentration-time profile and nephrotoxicity in hospitalized patients. *Clin Infect Dis.* 2009;49:507–514.

34. Goodwin SD, Cleary JD, Walawander CA, et al. Pretreatment regimens for adverse events related to infusion of amphotericin B. *Clin Infect Dis.* 1995;20:755–761.

35. Wingard JR, White MH, Anaissie E, et al. A randomized, double-blind comparative trial evaluating the safety of liposomal amphotericin B versus amphotericin B lipid complex in the empirical treatment of febrile neutropenia. L Amph/ABLC collaborative study group. *Clin Infect Dis.* 2000;31:1155–1163.

36. Cumpston A, Caddell R, Shillingburg A, et al. Superior serum concentrations with posaconazole delayed-release tablets compared to suspension formulation in hematological malignancies. *Antimicrob Agents Chemother.* 2015;59(8):4424–4428.

37. Pham AN, Bubalo JS, Lewis 2nd JS. Comparison of posaconazole serum concentrations from haematological cancer patients on posaconazole tablet and oral suspension for treatment and prevention of invasive fungal infections. *Mycoses.* 2016;59(4):226–233.

38. Londong W, Angerer M, Kutz K, et al. Diminishing efficacy of octreotide (SMS 201-995) on gastric functions of healthy subjects during one-week administration. *Gastroenterology.* 1989;96:713–722.

39. Ho VT, Revta C, Richardson PG. Hepatic veno-occlusive disease after hematopoietic stem cell transplantation: update on defibrotie and other current investigational therapies. *Bone Marrow Transpl.* 2008;41:229–237.

40. Strasser SI, McDonald GB. Gastrointestinal and hepatic complications. In: Blume KG, Forman SJ, Appelbaum FR, eds. *Thomas' Hematopoietic Cell Transplantation.* 3rd ed. Blackwell Publishing Ltd; 2007:1–42(Print).

41. Johnson DB, Savani BN. How can we reduce hepatic veno-occlusive disease-related deaths after allogeneic stem cell transplantation? *Exp Hematol.* 2012;40(7):513–517.

42. Tanaka C. Clinical pharmacology of deferasirox. *Clin Pharmacokinet.* 2014;53(8):679–694.

43. Sokos DR, Berger M, Lazarus HM. Intravenous immunoglobulin: appropriate indications and uses in hematopoietic stem cell transplantation. *Biol Blood Marrow Transpl.* 2002;8:117–130.

44. Vadhan-Raj S, Goldberg JD, Perales MA, et al. Clinical applications of palifermin: amelioration of oral mucositis and other potential indications. *J Cell Mol Med.* 2013;17(11):1371–1384.

CHAPTER 3

High-Dose Chemotherapy Regimens

LILY YAN, PHARMD, BCOP • ALISON GULBIS, PHARMD, BCOP

GOALS OF CONDITIONING REGIMENS

The majority of autologous and allogeneic hematopoietic stem cell transplants (HCTs) are used primarily for the treatment of malignant diseases. However, HCTs can also be used to treat nonmalignant diseases including acquired or congenital bone marrow failure disorders, hemoglobinopathies, inherited metabolic disorders, or primary immunodeficiencies.[1] High-dose chemotherapy/conditioning (HDC) regimens are given directly before the HCT with the following goals, which may vary depending on the patient's disease state and type of transplant[2]:

- Provide sufficient tumor reduction
- Create space in bone marrow
- Provide adequate immunosuppression
- Avoid overlapping toxicity profiles

When HCTs are used to treat malignancies, HDC regimens should reduce the tumor burden and eradicate disease if possible. Furthermore, the conditioning treatment should make space in the bone marrow for the newly transplanted cells to proliferate. In the setting of allogeneic HCT for malignant or nonmalignant diseases, HDC regimens should provide sufficient immunosuppression to allow stem cell engraftment and prevent graft-versus-host disease (GVHD). Ideally, these HDC regimens should avoid overlapping toxicities but provide synergistic cytotoxicity.[2]

TYPES OF CONDITIONING REGIMENS

Conditioning regimens for individual patients are based on several factors[3]:

- Age
- Performance status
- Comorbidities
- Type of disease
- Disease stage at transplant
- Graft-versus-tumor (GVT) effect in disease
- Graft source

Ideally, HDC regimens should optimize dose intensity to reduce the risk of relapse. Furthermore, these regimens should not increase the risk of nonrelapse mortality through toxicities such as GVHD as this would outweigh any survival benefit gained by better disease control. The intensity of conditioning regimens can be defined in 3 categories: (1) myeloablative (MA), (2) nonmyeloablative (NMA), and (3) reduced-intensity conditioning (RIC).[3,4]

Historically, MA conditioning refers to total-body irradiation (TBI), which is given with alkylating agents such as cyclophosphamide (Cy). Recently, busulfan (Bu) has replaced the role of TBI as a primary myeloablative agent in treating various hematologic malignancies. The goal of MA regimens is to eradicate disease and lead to rapid engraftment. Within 7–21 days after administration, MA regimens induce profound cytopenia and myeloablation, which is usually irreversible and fatal unless given stem cell support. The higher dose intensity of MA regimens has also been associated with higher rates of GVHD and increased treatment-related mortality (TRM) but a lower risk of relapse than RIC or NMA regimens.[3,5,6] Examples of MA regimens can be found in Table 3.1.

Treatment-related toxicities associated with MA conditioning have limited the use of HCT in elderly patients and in those with comorbidities. In the last 20 years, the introduction of fludarabine (Flu) and lower doses of alkylating agents has allowed for a reduction in dose intensity of conditioning regimens with the goal of decreasing TRM. These newer regimens are categorized as NMA or RIC regimens.[3] Rather than maximizing tumor reduction, the goal of these NMA or RIC conditioning regimens is to exploit a graft-versus-tumor (GVT) effect to eradicate malignancy and minimize TRM.[3,7,8] Over the years, donor lymphocyte infusions have demonstrated efficacy in treating relapse after allogeneic HCTs. This highlights the significance of the immune-mediated GVT effect of alloreactive T cells instead of focusing on the elimination of malignant cells with HDC to treat the disease.[7]

Unlike MA regimens, NMA regimens do not require stem cell support but still provide sufficient immunosuppression to allow engraftment of newly

Hematopoietic Cell Transplantation for Malignant Conditions. https://doi.org/10.1016/B978-0-323-56802-9.00003-1

TABLE 3.1
Definitions of MA, RIC, and NMA Regimens[3,4,8,10]

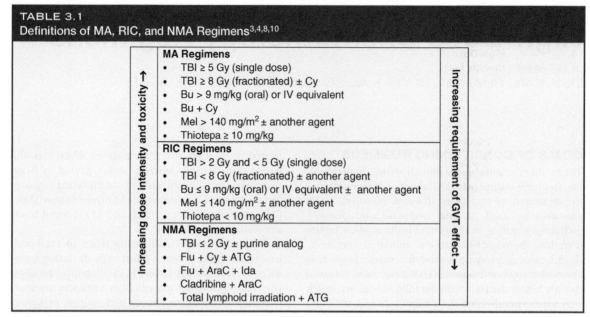

Increasing dose intensity and toxicity ↑	**MA Regimens** • TBI ≥ 5 Gy (single dose) • TBI ≥ 8 Gy (fractionated) ± Cy • Bu > 9 mg/kg (oral) or IV equivalent • Bu + Cy • Mel > 140 mg/m² ± another agent • Thiotepa ≥ 10 mg/kg **RIC Regimens** • TBI > 2 Gy and < 5 Gy (single dose) • TBI < 8 Gy (fractionated) ± another agent • Bu ≤ 9 mg/kg (oral) or IV equivalent ± another agent • Mel ≤ 140 mg/m² ± another agent • Thiotepa < 10 mg/kg **NMA Regimens** • TBI ≤ 2 Gy ± purine analog • Flu + Cy ± ATG • Flu + AraC + Ida • Cladribine + AraC • Total lymphoid irradiation + ATG	Increasing requirement of GVT effect →

AraC, cytarabine; *ATG*, antithymocyte globulin; *Bu*, busulfan; *Cy*, cyclophosphamide; *Flu*, fludarabine; *GVT*, graft-versus-tumor; *Gy*, Gray; *Ida*, idarubicin; *IV*, intravenous; *MA*, myeloablative; *Mel*, melphalan; *NMA*, nonmyeloablative; *RIC*, reduced-intensity conditioning; *TBI*, total-body irradiation.

transplanted cells. This conditioning differs from MA regimens in several ways[9]:
- Less inflammatory cytokine release
- Establishment of immune tolerance due to mixed chimerism
- Different type and duration of immunosuppression
- Higher number of recipient antigen-presenting cells after the conditioning

All these factors may contribute to the lower rates of acute and chronic GVHD associated with NMA regimens than MA conditioning.[5] Furthermore, GVHD is usually delayed with NMA regimens and may occur after day 100, which is best defined as late-onset acute GVHD. Nonrelapse mortality is much lower with NMA regimens than with MA regimens, and this conditioning is more tolerable for older patients and those with comorbidities.[3,9] Examples of NMA regimens can be found in Table 3.1.

RIC refers to regimens that do not fit the MA or NMA definitions. The Center for International Blood and Marrow Transplant Research agreed on 3 of the 5 "Champlin Criteria" in defining RIC regimens[4]:
- Results in reversible myelosuppression (usually within 4 weeks) if given without stem cell rescue
- Results in initial mixed chimerism in a proportion of patients
- Associated with low rates of nonhematologic toxicities

RIC differs from MA conditioning in that the dose of the alkylating agents and/or TBI is decreased by 30%, and it is also associated with higher risk of relapse.[4,8,10] Unlike NMA regimens, RIC regimens cause cytopenia, which can be prolonged and require rescue with stem cells.[4,8] Examples of these regimens can be found in Table 3.1.

NONCHEMOTHERAPY AGENTS IN CONDITIONING REGIMENS

Ideal characteristics of HDC regimens include a steep dose-response curve and myelosuppression as the dose-limiting toxicity. Thus, TBI has been the traditional myeloablative agent used as part of conditioning regimens. The majority of drugs used are alkylating agents, which also exhibit these desirable characteristics. Other agents include the antimetabolites, topoisomerase II inhibitors, anti–T lymphocyte antibody therapies, and more recently, rituximab. Examples and characteristics of these chemotherapy drugs can be found in Table 3.3. Examples of commonly used MA, RIC, and NMA regimens can be found in Table 3.4.

Total-Body Irradiation

Total-body irradiation is often a key component of the conditioning regimen for HCT and can provide both the myeloablative and immune-ablative components required for a successful HCT. TBI, when combined with

TABLE 3.2
Regimens With RIT Plus Chemotherapy[20]

RIT Agent	High-Dose Chemo-therapy Regimen	Transplant Type
90Y-IT	• BEAM • Bu/VP-16/Cy • Cy/VP-16	Autologous
131I–T[a]	• BEAM • Cy/VP-16	Autologous
90Y-IT	• Flu/Cy • Flu/Bu • Flu/Mel • Thiotepa/Flu/Mel	Allogeneic

131I-T, I,131I-Tositumumab; 90Y-IT, 90Y-Ibritumomab tiuxetan; BEAM, carmustine, etoposide, cytarabine, melphalan regimen; Bu, busulfan; Cy, cyclophosphamide; Flu, fludarabine; Mel, melphalan; RIT, radioimmunotherapy; VP-16, etoposide.
[a]No longer produced or sold.

chemotherapy, is effective at eradicating residual malignant disease and provides sufficient immunosuppression before HCT. It will be discussed in more detail in Chapter 5.

Radioisotopes and Radioimmunotherapy

The ability of radioisotopes to be "bone seeking" and cause less systemic toxicity generated interest in the use of radiopharmaceuticals in the HCT setting. Strontium-89, Samarium-153-ethylenediamene-tetramethylenephosphoric, and Holmium-166 1,4,7,10 tetraazcyclododecane-1,4,7,10 tetramethylenephosphonate acid were investigated in the early 1990s to treat bone metastases and osteosarcoma and later studied in the multiple myeloma (MM) population coupled with HCT as a means of marrow ablation.[11-19] Holmium-166 was coupled with melphalan (Mel) in one study, and engraftment and acute toxicity profiles were similar to giving Mel alone. However, some late toxicities not traditionally seen with Mel were observed, including hemorrhagic cystitis, thrombotic microangiopathy of the kidney, and late renal dysfunction.[14] In a later study, continuous bladder irrigation was effectively used to avoid hemorrhagic cystitis. However, late renal dysfunction was still observed in a small fraction of patients. Though Holmium-166 demonstrated trends toward higher complete response rate and higher but nonsignificant overall survival at 5 years, it has not been studied further.[15]

Because lymphomas are radiation-sensitive, radioimmunotherapy (RIT) was introduced for CD20-positive B-cell malignancies, non-Hodgkin's lymphoma (NHL), and follicular lymphoma (FL). However, adding TBI to conditioning regimens was too toxic. Given the success of 90 Y-Ibritumomab tiuxetan (90Y-IT) and I,131I-Tositumumab

(131I-T) for consolidation in NHL and FL, investigators explored their use in HCT conditioning. Both 90Y-IT and 131I-T are capable of targeted radiation to the CD20-positive cells, and myelosuppression is the major adverse effect, which can be overcome with an HCT. Standard and high-dose RIT studied with and without HDC have shown promising disease control without increased toxicity. In the autologous setting, studies have combined RIT with high-dose chemotherapy using either high-dose BEAM (carmustine [BCNU], etoposide [VP-16], cytarabine [AraC], and Mel) or high-dose Cy, VP-16 with or without Bu. In the allogeneic setting, RIT has been combined with RIC (Bu plus Flu) or NMA (Flu plus Cy) regimens (Table 3.2).[20] When RIT is combined with chemotherapy, it is given 7–14 days before the initiation of the conditioning regimen. Though data exist for 131I-T in HCT, it is no longer being produced or sold as of 2014.

90Y-Ibritumomab Tiuxetan

Ibritumomab tiuxetan binds specifically to the CD20 antigen and is the result of a stable thiourea covalent bond between ibritumomab and a linker-chelator, tiuxetan. The tiuxetan provides the chelation site for Yttrium-90, which is a beta emitter with a half-life of approximately 2.67 days. The beta emission from Y-90 induces cellular damage via free radical formation. Zirconium-90 is the radiation decay product and is nonradioactive.

When compared to historical controls, RIT combined with high-dose chemotherapy for autologous HCT appeared to be feasible and improved clinical outcomes in phase I and phase II studies.

Few randomized studies exist comparing RIT versus rituximab added to the chemotherapy-conditioning regimen. The BMT Clinical Trials Network phase III trial randomized chemotherapy-sensitive diffuse large B-cell lymphoma patients to receive either 131I-T–BEAM or rituximab-BEAM, followed by an autologous HCT. The primary endpoint was 2-year progression-free survival, and no added benefit was seen in the 131I-T–BEAM group compared with the rituximab-BEAM group (47.9% vs. 48.6%; P = .94). Engraftment and toxicities were similar between groups except for mucositis, which was higher in the 131I-T–BEAM group.[21]

CHEMOTHERAPY AGENTS IN CONDITIONING REGIMENS

Chemotherapy is classified as cell cycle specific or nonspecific. Cell cycle–specific agents are only able to kill cells during a certain phase, whereas cell cycle–nonspecific agents can kill in any phase of the cell cycle. A large majority of HCT conditioning regimens include at least one cell cycle–nonspecific agent.

TABLE 3.3
Commonly Used Chemotherapy Drugs and Dosing in HDC Regimens

Class	Drug	Dose Range	Nonhematologic Toxicities	Drug Interactions	Pharmacokinetics	Other Considerations
Alkylating agents	Busulfan (Bu)[2,22,23,27–30,77,78]	IV: 130 mg/m² IV daily for 2–4 days OR 3.2 mg/kg IV daily for 2–4 days OR Target AUC: 4000–6000 micromol* min/day for 2–4 days PO: 4 mg/kg per day in 4 divided doses for 2–4 days	• Hepatotoxicity (VOD/SOS)[a] • Lowers seizure threshold • GI toxicity[a] • Radiation recall phenomenon[a] • Pulmonary fibrosis[a] • Gonadal toxicity • Hyperpigmentation	• Phenytoin increases clearance (CYP3A4) • Acetaminophen (GSH), azoles (CYP3A4), metronidazole (CYP3A4, GSH) decrease clearance • Increases Cy toxicity (CYP450) - give before or 24h after Bu	• Highly lipophilic • Hepatic metabolism • Conjugated by glutathione S-transferase • Crosses BBB • Partially cleared via dialysis	• Dosing based on TDM • Requires antiseizure prophylaxis, starting evening prior and then daily until the morning after last dose given • Avoid acetaminophen and metronidazole • 0.8 mg IV equals 1 mg PO
	Cyclophosphamide (Cy)[2,29–32,36,79]	MA: 50–60 mg/kg IV daily for 2–4 days RIC: 50 mg/kg IV daily for 4 days NMA: 750–1000 mg/m² IV daily for 2–3 days	• Cardiotoxicity including hemorrhagic myocarditis[a] • Nephrotoxicity[a] • Hemorrhagic cystitis (due to acrolein)[a] • Pulmonary toxicity • Hepatotoxicity (VOD/SOS) • SIADH	• Azoles affect metabolism (CYP3A4, 2C9) • Thiotepa decreases activation (CYP2B6) • Bu or phenytoin affects clearance (CYP450) – give before or 24h after Bu	• Prodrug (activated by CYP450) & predominantly hepatically metabolized • Parent drug & metabolites renally eliminated & cleared via dialysis	• Give with aggressive hydration to decrease cystitis • Give mesna (for high doses)
	Ifosfamide (Ifos)[35,36]	Up to 10 g/m² (course maximum)	• Nephrotoxicity[a] • Hemorrhagic cystitis (due to acrolein)[a] • Neurotoxicity (lethargy, confusion, seizures)[a]	• Azoles affect metabolism (CYP3A4)	• Prodrug (activated by CYP450) & predominantly hepatically metabolized • Parent drug & metabolites renally eliminated & cleared via dialysis	• Give with aggressive hydration to decrease cystitis • Give mesna (for high doses)

Class	Drug	Dose	Drug interactions	Toxicities	Pharmacology	Considerations
	Melphalan (Mel)[2,36,39–41, 43–45,80,81]	ALKERAN®: Single agent: 140–200 mg/m² IV × 1; Combination: 100–140 mg/m² IV × 1 or 70–90 mg/m² IV daily for 2 days; EVOMELA®: Single agent: 100 mg/m² IV daily for 2 days; Combination: 140 mg/m² IV × 1	N/A	• GI toxicity/mucositis[a] • Hepatotoxicity (VOD/SOS)[a] • Pulmonary toxicity • SIADH	• 90% protein bound • Rapidly hydrolyzed to inactive metabolites in plasma • Hepatic metabolism • Partial renal elimination	• Limited stability with ALKERAN formulation – must be reconstituted in propylene glycol & administered within 60 min of reconstitution • Use cryotherapy to prevent mucositis
	Thiotepa[2,36,46–50]	Usual dose: 5–10 mg/kg total; 5 mg/kg/dose IV daily or BID for 1–2 days (max 20 mg/kg total) OR 250 mg/m² IV daily for 3 days	• Decreases Cy activation (CYP2B6) – give after Cy	• Neurotoxicity[a] • GI toxicity/mucositis[a] • Skin toxicity[a] • Hepatotoxicity (VOD/SOS)[a] • Interstitial pneumonitis • Cardiotoxicity	• Highly lipophilic • Extensive hepatic metabolism • Active metabolite (TEPA) has longer half-life (4.9–17.6 h)	• Partially excreted through skin via sweat – bathe at least 2×/day for up to 48 h after last dose
	Carmustine (BCNU)[2,41,46,80,82–84]	300–400 mg/m² IV × 1	• Impaired clearance & increased myelosuppression with cimetidine	• Pulmonary fibrosis[a] • Hepatotoxicity (VOD/SOS)[a] • Hypotension • Myocardial ischemia • Mucositis	• Highly lipophilic • Crosses blood brain barrier • Spontaneously hydrolyzed & rapidly hepatically metabolized • Mostly renal elimination & partially via lungs	• Contains 3.3 mg of drug in ethanol 10%. Diluent may cause hypotension, headaches and flushing • Recommended max infusion rate is 3 mg/m²/min
	Bendamustine[36,51,53]	130 mg/m² IV daily for 3 days	N/A	• GI toxicity[a] • Hepatotoxicity • Infusion reactions	• Extensive hepatic metabolism • Partial renal elimination	• Considered NMA, typically given with Flu • Consider pre-meds (acetaminophen, diphenhydramine, hydrocortisone) to avoid infusion reactions
Antimetabolites	Fludarabine (Flu)[26,27,49,51,55]	25–40 mg/m² IV daily for 3–5 days (course max of 200 mg/m²)	N/A	• Neurotoxicity • Hemolytic anemia	• Active metabolite: 2-fluoro-ara-A • Renal elimination	• Typically given with Bu, Mel, or Cy-containing regimens

Continued

Class	Drug	Dose Range	Nonhematologic Toxicities	Drug Interactions	Pharmacokinetics	Other Considerations
	Clofarabine (Clo)[61,62,85,86]	30–40 mg/m² IV daily (course max of 160 mg/m²)	• Hepatotoxicity • Nephrotoxicity • CLS/SIRS	• Limited hepatic metabolism • Substrate of OAT1, OAT2, OCT3	• Active metabolite: clofarabine 5'-triphosphate • Renal elimination	• Has been combined with Bu-based regimens for ALL • Consider prophylactic hydrocortisone pre-medication to prevent CLS/SIRS
	Cytarabine (AraC)[41,80]	400 mg/m²/day IV divided q12 h for 4 days	• Cerebellar dysfunction • GI toxicity/mucositis • Cytarabine syndrome • Conjunctivitis/keratitis • Biliary stasis	N/A	• Active metabolite: aracytidine triphosphate • Hepatic metabolism and partially detoxified in liver • Renal elimination	• Corticosteroids can be used to prevent or treat cytarabine syndrome • At doses higher than in BEAM, an ocular corticosteroid may prevent or minimize conjunctivitis
	Gemcitabine (Gem)[63,64]	800 mg/m² IV × 1 OR Single dose max: 2775 mg/m² IV daily (course max: 5500 mg/m² IV in divided doses)	• Hepatotoxicity • Hemolytic uremic syndrome • Pulmonary toxicity • Erythematous rash	N/A	• Metabolized by nucleoside kinases to active diphosphate and triphosphate metabolites • Renal elimination	• Infuse at 10 mg/m²/min
Plant alkaloid	Etoposide (VP-16)[41,67,80]	200–400 mg/m² per day IV divided q12 h for up to 4 days OR 60 mg/kg IV × 1	• GI toxicity/mucositis[a] • Infusion reaction (usually hypotension) • Risk of secondary AML • Elevated LFTs • Peripheral neuropathy • Sialoadenitis	• CYP3A4 (major) • CYP2E1 and 1A2 (minor) • P-glycoprotein	• Extensive hepatic metabolism • Renal elimination	• Monitor for hypotension during infusion • For 60 mg/kg dose: given as undiluted IV piggyback over 4 h into freely flowing normal saline running at 300 mL/h
Platinum agent	Carboplatin[65,66,87,88]	300–700 mg/m² IV daily for 3 days	• Ototoxicity (irreversible) • Nephrotoxicity • Hepatotoxicity[a] • GI toxicity/mucositis[a] • Peripheral neuropathy[a]	• Increased risk of nephrotoxicity when combined with other nephrotoxins	• Renal elimination	• Maintain adequate hydration • Monitor for hyponatremia

Anti-T lymphocyte antibody therapies	Alemtuzumab[72–74]	20 mg (flat dose) IV daily for 4–5 days	• Autoimmune effects • Infusion reactions • Severe immunosuppression	N/A	N/A	• Give with pre-meds (acetaminophen, diphenhydramine, hydrocortisone) to avoid infusion reactions. • Only available through Campath® Distribution Program on a patient-specific basis
	Lymphocyte immune globulin (equine)[70]	15–30 mg/kg dose over 3–5 days	• Fatal allergic reactions • Hemolysis • Hepatic dysfunction • Serum sickness	N/A	N/A	• A skin test is recommended prior to initial dose • Give with pre-meds (acetaminophen, diphenhydramine, hydrocortisone) to avoid infusion reactions. • Have emergency medications on hand (hydrocortisone, epinephrine, diphenhydramine)
	Antithymocyte globulin (rabbit ATG)[68–70]	No established consensus for dosing or timing relative to HCT. Total dose varies from 4 to 32 mg/kg (median 7.5 mg/kg) split over 2–4 days.	• Anaphylaxis • Flu-like symptoms	N/A	N/A	• Give with pre-meds (acetaminophen, diphenhydramine, hydrocortisone) to avoid infusion reactions. • Have emergency medications on hand (hydrocortisone, epinephrine, diphenhydramine)
CD20 antibody	Rituximab[21,31,51,56,75,89]	375 mg/m² IV daily for 2–4 doses	• Infusion reactions • Hepatitis B reactivation • Increased risk of opportunistic infections • PML	N/A	N/A	• Give with pre-meds (acetaminophen, diphenhydramine, hydrocortisone) to avoid infusion reactions

ALL, acute lymphoblastic leukemia; *AML*, acute myeloid leukemia; *AUC*, area under the curve; *BBB*, blood brain barrier; *BID*, twice daily; max, maximum; *CLS*, capillary leak syndrome; *CYP*, cytochrome; *GI*, gastrointestinal; *GSH*, glutathione; *HDC*, high-dose chemotherapy/conditioning; *IV*, intravenous; *LFT*, liver function test; *MA*, myeloablative; *N/A*, not available; *NMA*, nonmyeloablative; *OAT*, ornithine aminotransferase; *OCT*, ornithine transcarbamylase; *PO*, oral; *RIC*, reduced-intensity conditioning; *SIADH*, syndrome of inappropriate antidiuretic hormone secretion; *SIRS*, systemic inflammatory response syndrome; *SOS*; sinusoidal obstruction syndrome; *TDM*, therapeutic drug monitoring; *VOD*, veno-occlusive disease.

[a]Dose-limiting toxicity.

TABLE 3.4
Common HDC Regimens

Regimen Intensity	Name	Regimen Details	Transplant Type	Disease
MA	Cy/TBI[90]	Cy 60 mg/kg IV daily × 2 days Fractionated TBI 10–12 Gy	Allogeneic	Heme
	TBI/Etoposide[91]	Fractionated TBI 10–16 Gy Etoposide 60 mg/kg IV × 1 day	Allogeneic	ALL, AML
	Bu/Cy4[92]	Bu 1 mg/kg PO every 6 h[a] × 4 days Cy 50 mg/kg IV daily × 4 days	Allogeneic Autologous	Heme
	Bu/Cy2[93]	Bu 1 mg/kg PO every 6 h[a] × 4 days Cy 60 mg/kg IV daily × 2 days	Allogeneic Autologous	Heme
	Flu/Bu[57]	Bu 130 mg/m² IV daily × 4 days (target AUC 5000–6000 micromol* min/day) Flu 40 mg/m² IV daily × 4 days	Allogeneic	Heme
	BEAM[41,80] or BEAM/R[21]	BCNU 300 mg/m² IV × 1 day Etoposide 100–200 mg/m² IV q12 h × 4 days AraC 200 mg/m² IV q12 h × 4 days Mel 140 mg/m² IV × 1 day ±Rituximab 375 mg/m² IV weekly × 2–3 doses (pre- and post-HCT) for CD20 + malignancy	Autologous Allogeneic	Lymphoid
	CBV[94]	Cy 1500–1800 mg/m² IV daily × 4 days BCNU 300–600 mg/m² IV daily × 1 day Etoposide 600–2400 mg/m² per total IV over 4 days	Autologous	Lymphoid
	Mel[39, 40]	140–200 mg/m² IV × 1 day	Autologous	MM Amyloid
RIC	FM[45] or FMR[95]	Flu 25 mg/m² IV daily × 5 days OR 30 mg/m² IV daily × 4 days Mel 50–70 mg/m² IV daily × 2 days OR 100–140 mg/m² × 1 day ±Rituximab 375 mg/m² IV weekly × 3 doses (pre- and post-HCT) for CD20 + malignancy	Allogeneic	Lymphoid Myeloid MM
	Flu/Bu[7]	Bu 1 mg/kg PO every 6 h[a] × 2 days OR 130 mg/m² IV daily × 2 days (target AUC 4000 micromol* min/day) Flu 30 mg/m² IV daily × 6 days ATG (rabbit) 10 mg/kg IV daily × 4 days	Allogeneic	AML MDS CML
	Flu/Cy/Thio[96]	Thio 5–15 mg/kg/day IV × 1 day Cy 30 mg/kg IV daily × 2 days Flu 30 mg/m² IV daily × 2 days	Allogeneic	Lymphoid
	Cy/ATG[32]	Cy 50 mg/kg IV daily × 4 days ATG (equine) 30 mg/kg IV daily × 3 days	Allogeneic	SAA (<40 years old)
NMA	FC[97] or FCR[31, 56]	Flu 30 mg/m² IV daily × 3 days Cy 750–1000 mg/m² IV daily × 3 days ±Rituximab 375 mg/m² IV weekly × 3 doses (pre- and post-HCT) for CD20 + malignancy	Allogeneic	CLL Lymphoid
	Flu/TBI[98]	Flu 30 mg/m² IV daily × 3 days TBI 2 Gy	Allogeneic	Lymphoid Myeloid MM

ALL, acute lymphoblastic leukemia; *AML*, acute myeloid leukemia; *AraC*, cytarabine; *ATG*, antithymocyte globulin; *AUC*, area under the curve; *BCNU*, carmustine; *Bu*, busulfan; *CLL*, chronic lymphocytic leukemia; *CML*, chronic myeloid leukemia; *Cy*, cyclophosphamide; *Flu*, fludarabine; *Gy*, Gray; *HCT*, hematopoietic stem cell transplant; *HDC*, high-dose chemotherapy/conditioning; *Heme*, hematologic malignancies; *IV*, intravenous; *Lymphoid*, lymphoid malignancies; *MA*, myeloablative; *MDS*, myelodysplastic syndrome; *Mel*, melphalan; *MM*, multiple myeloma; NMA, nonmyeloablative; *PO*, oral; *RIC*, reduced-intensity conditioning; *SAA*, severe aplastic anemia; *TBI*, total-body irradiation; *Thio*, thiotepa.
[a]Total daily oral dose of busulfan equivalent to 3.2 mg/kg per day IV.

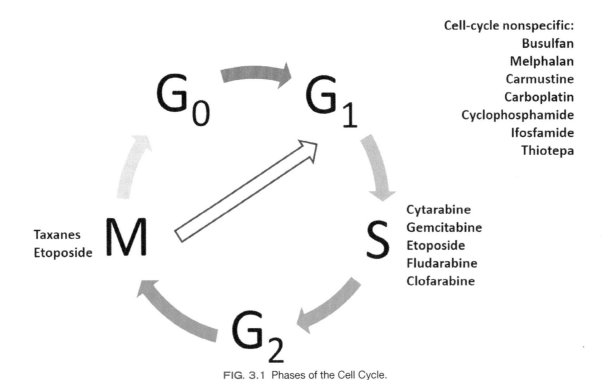

Cell-cycle nonspecific:
Busulfan
Melphalan
Carmustine
Carboplatin
Cyclophosphamide
Ifosfamide
Thiotepa

Cytarabine
Gemcitabine
Etoposide
Fludarabine
Clofarabine

Taxanes
Etoposide

FIG. 3.1 Phases of the Cell Cycle.

The different phases of the cell cycle can be found in Fig. 3.1 and include:

- G0: resting phase
- G1: gap 1 or growth phase
- S: synthesis phase, where DNA replication occurs
- G2: gap 2 or second growth phase
- M: mitosis phase, where cell division occurs

ALKYLATING AGENTS

Alkylating agents were the first chemotherapy drugs to be used in HDC regimens. These agents are cell cycle nonspecific, targeting malignant cells at any point in the cell cycle. Furthermore, they do not exhibit cross-resistance. The primary mechanism of alkylating agents is via binding of the alkyl groups to electrophilic sites on DNA to inhibit replication.[2]

Busulfan

Among the alkylating agents, Bu has shown activity against various malignancies such as acute lymphoblastic leukemia (ALL), acute myeloid leukemia (AML), lymphoma, MM, myeloid metaplasia, testicular cancers, Ewing's sarcoma, and breast cancer.[2] As an alternative to TBI, Bu continues to be a primary myeloablative

agent and has been given successfully in combination with a variety of chemotherapy agents in MA and RIC regimens for hematologic malignancies.[22]

A limitation in optimizing Bu use in conditioning regimens is due to significant interindividual variability in Bu absorption with the oral formulation, which has been attributed to factors such as age, weight, disease, hepatic function, circadian rhythm, drug interactions, and bioavailability.[23] Studies have shown that plasma Bu concentration, expressed as area under the curve (AUC), plays an important role in determining risk of graft failure and subsequent relapse versus transplant-related toxicities such as veno-occlusive disease (VOD) or sinusoidal obstruction syndrome (SOS). This pharmacokinetic variability in systemic exposure of Bu resulted in major differences in clinical response and toxicities in patients receiving the same dose of the drug.[24,25]

The availability of an intravenous (IV) preparation of Bu has greatly reduced the interindividual variability in AUC values compared with the oral formulation. Intravenous Bu bypasses the hepatic first pass effect of oral Bu, resulting in decreased drug concentrations in the hepatic sinusoids and thereby reduces VOD/SOS risk.[2] Studies have also shown that the distribution of the more convenient once daily IV Bu dosing is similar to that of the conventional 4 times daily oral Bu, easing administration and further optimizing the use of Bu in conditioning regimens.[26,27] In addition, at HCT centers, therapeutic drug monitoring (TDM) has become the standard of practice in guiding Bu dosing to maximize clinical outcomes and minimize toxicities.[2]

Aside from VOD/SOS, the other dose-limiting toxicities of Bu include neurotoxicity, which requires the use of an antiseizure medication for prophylaxis, mucositis, and pulmonary fibrosis. Bu undergoes extensive hepatic metabolism and has many significant drug interactions. The azole antifungals and phenytoin affect its clearance via CYP450 metabolism, and acetaminophen should be avoided in combination with Bu due to competition for glutathione. Metronidazole should also not be used concurrently as it can lead to decreased Bu clearance and increased VOD/SOS risk.[28]

Cyclophosphamide

High-dose Cy is used traditionally with TBI or an alkylating agent before HCT as MA conditioning for a variety of malignancies.[29,30] Although Cy provides sufficient immunosuppression for stem cell engraftment, it is not myeloablative and has also been incorporated into many RIC and NMA regimens.[31] For example, Cy with or without antithymocyte globulin (ATG) is a common RIC regimen for severe aplastic anemia.[2,32] Recent studies have shown Cy to be safe and effective in reducing GVHD when given posttransplant as GVHD prophylaxis in combination with HDC.[33,34] Its primary dose-limiting toxicity is cardiotoxicity such as hemorrhagic myocarditis, which is more frequent at doses greater than 150 mg/kg. At high doses, Cy can cause hemorrhagic cystitis and should be given with mesna.[2]

Ifosfamide

Ifosfamide (Ifos) is given before autologous HCTs in combination with carboplatin and VP-16 (ifosfamide, carboplatin, and etoposide regimen) for relapsed or refractory lymphomas.[35] As an analog of Cy, Ifos has a comparable toxicity profile but with increased risk of nephrotoxicity, hemorrhagic cystitis, and neurotoxicity. Similarly to high-dose Cy, it should be administered with mesna to decrease bladder toxicity.[2,36] Patients with low serum albumin (indicator of impaired hepatic function), high serum creatinine, and pelvic disease are at higher risk for developing ifos-induced metabolic encephalopathy. Thus, albumin and renal function should be closely monitored in patients receiving Ifos.[37] Furthermore, methylene blue has been effectively used to treat ifosfamide-induced encephalopathy and can also be used for prophylaxis.[38]

Melphalan

As a treatment of choice for HCT in MM, high-dose Mel has been widely used as a single agent or with other agents.[39,40] It is also frequently combined with BCNU, VP-16, and AraC (BEAM regimen) for relapsed or refractory lymphomas before autologous HCTs.[41] The lyophilized Mel formulation (ALKERAN®) must be reconstituted in propylene glycol and administered within 60 min of reconstitution.[42] A newer propylene glycol-free Mel formulation (EVOMELA®) overcomes these limitations. EVOMELA® has shown comparable safety and efficacy when substituted for Mel before autologous HCTs for MM and also in BEAM for lymphomas.[43,44] In the allogeneic setting, Mel has been studied with Flu as RIC for hematologic malignancies.[45] Mucositis and VOD/SOS are the primary dose-limiting toxicities.[2]

Thiotepa

Thiotepa is effective in combination with carmustine or added to Bu/Cy before autologous HCT for primary CNS (central nervous system) lymphoma (PCNSL), obviating the use of whole brain radiation therapy and reducing the risk for neurotoxicity.[46,47] It has also been studied with Flu plus Mel before haploidentical and cord blood transplants for hematologic malignancies.[48,49] Thiotepa is converted to the active metabolite TEPA, which has a much longer plasma half-life than the parent drug and is responsible for most of the central nervous system, gastrointestinal, liver and skin toxicities.[2] It is partially excreted through the skin by sweat, and patients should be advised to bathe at least twice daily for up to 48 h after the last dose of thiotepa.[50]

Carmustine

Carmustine is active against a variety of malignancies and is commonly given with VP-16, AraC and Mel (BEAM regimen) for relapsed or refractory lymphomas before autologous HCTs.[41] It is also used with high-dose thiotepa for PCNSL.[46] Its dose-limiting toxicities are pulmonary fibrosis and hepatotoxicity.[2]

Bendamustine

Bendamustine is a newer alkylating agent that has been studied with Flu and is considered NMA conditioning.[51] Bendamustine has also been promising as a substitution to BCNU in a modified BEAM combination with VP-16, AraC and Mel (BeEAM regimen) before autologous HCTs for relapsed or refractory lymphomas.[52] Dose-limiting toxicities are similar to that of other alkylating agents including GI toxicity.[36] Premedications should be given before bendamustine to avoid infusion reactions.[53]

ANTIMETABOLITES

Antimetabolites include the purine and pyrimidine analogs, which are cell cycle specific to the S-phase. The purine analogs inhibit purine synthesis, which in turn interferes with DNA and RNA function. Purine analogs typically used in HDC regimens include Flu and/or clofarabine, and they are traditionally given with an alkylating agent. Based on preclinical data, cladribine has comparable synergistic cytotoxicity when added to Flu/Bu regimen but is not well studied in a clinical HCT setting.[54] Pyrimidine analogs inhibit DNA polymerase, which interferes with DNA synthesis and RNA function. Pyrimidine analogs that are used in HCT conditioning regimens include AraC and gemcitabine (Gem).

Fludarabine

Fludarabine is commonly combined with an alkylating agent, most notably Bu or Mel, and possesses similar immunosuppressive activity to Cy.[55] Flu has been successfully incorporated into NMA, RIC, and MA regimens.[45,56,57] The Flu/Bu regimen has been compared to Bu/Cy2 and displayed similar engraftment kinetics, relapse, and nonrelapse mortality. Both regimens appear to have similar efficacy; however, the Flu/Bu regimen has a better safety profile.[27,58]

Clofarabine

Clofarabine (Clo) is a later generation purine analog that has improved antileukemic efficacy compared to Flu. When Clo was studied in human cell lines combined with Flu and Bu, it demonstrated a high level of synergy compared with Flu/Bu or Clo/Bu alone.[59,60] Clofarabine has been combined with Bu or added to the Flu/Bu regimen with successful outcomes and a favorable safety profile.[61,62]

Cytarabine

Cytarabine has been used in both the allogeneic and autologous setting for many years. It is part of the BEAM conditioning regimen as mentioned previously.[41]

Gemcitabine

Though Gem has been used in solid tumors for many years, it is starting to emerge as an effective agent for conditioning before HCT mostly in the autologous setting. In vitro data suggest that Gem has synergistic cytotoxicity when given in combination with an alkylating agent. It has been studied with docetaxel, Mel, and carboplatin (Gem-DMC) in germ cell tumors and with Bu and Mel with or without a histone deacetylase inhibitor (Gem-Bu-Mel ± vorinostat) in refractory lymphoid malignancies with promising results. In most HCT studies, Gem has been given using a fixed dose rate of $10 \, mg/m^2$ per minute.[63] In the allogeneic setting, it has been added to Mel and Flu for Hodgkin's Disease.[64]

PLATINUM AGENTS

Active in solid tumors such as ovarian and testicular cancers, platinum agents are ideal options for HCT in these malignancies. Of the platinum agents, carboplatin is the agent used in HCT.

Carboplatin

Carboplatin is typically added to another alkylating agent and/or a plant alkaloid for autologous HCT in germ cell tumors. In the setting of HCT, carboplatin is dosed using an mg/m^2 approach instead of an AUC-based dose which is traditionally used in non-HCT patients.[35,65,66]

PLANT ALKALOIDS

Plant alkaloids are used in HDC regimens and coupled with either other agents or TBI. Etoposide is the most common agent in this class that can be used in HCT conditioning although others have been studied.

Etoposide

The podophyllotoxin, VP-16, is commonly used in HCT conditioning regimens for hematologic malignancies and germ cell cancer. It is part of the BEAM regimen for autologous HCT and has been incorporated into the MA regimen, VP-16/TBI, for ALL.[67]

ANTI-T CELL ANTIBODIES

The anti-T-cell globulins are polyclonal and are most commonly of rabbit or horse origin. The anti-T cell globulins provide an in vivo form of T-cell depletion. Rabbit antithymocyte globulin (rATG) or equine lymphocyte immune globulin (ATGAM®) can be added to conditioning regimens for GVHD prevention and/or to prevent rejection. Rabbit ATG is more extensively studied in the context of HCT and use has increased over the years. Some data have looked at lower versus higher doses of rATG in the setting of GVHD prevention. However, optimal dose and schedule is yet to be determined.[68–70] In vitro data suggested that rATG is approximately 10 times more potent than the horse formulation.[71] All anti-T-cell globulins can cause infusion reactions and serum-sickness reactions and carry an increased risk of infection.

Alemtuzumab (Campath®), a humanized anti–CD-52 monoclonal antibody, is another T-cell antibody used to provide in vivo T-cell depletion. It has been studied most with RIC regimens for allogeneic HCT in nonmalignant diseases. Like anti-T cell globulins, alemtuzumab can help prevent GVHD. However, limitations to its use include profound immunosuppression, delayed immune recovery, and delayed time to full donor chimerism or persistent mixed chimerism.[72,73] As of 2012, alemtuzumab can only be obtained through a restricted distribution program.[74]

MONOCLONAL ANTIBODIES
Rituximab

As a CD20 targeting monoclonal antibody, rituximab has been more recently incorporated in combination with HDC before HCTs in lymphoid malignancies.[75] It has demonstrated efficacy in increasing overall survival when combined with BEAM before autologous HCTs for CD20-positive lymphomas.[21] Furthermore, studies have shown rituximab may induce a stronger GVT effect after allogeneic HCTs and has beneficial effects

on chronic GVHD.[76] It has been successfully combined with a variety of agents in RIC and NMA conditioning regimens before allogeneic HCTs for CD20-positive lymphomas.[31,51,56,75] Premedications should be given before rituximab to avoid infusion reactions.

DOSING CONSIDERATIONS
Organ Dysfunction

HCT candidates may present with varying degrees of renal and hepatic insufficiency. Changes in organ function can significantly impact clearance of HDC or transformation to active metabolites, which rely on hepatic metabolism. Inadequate doses of chemotherapy may lead to graft failure, whereas supratherapeutic concentrations may result in treatment-related toxicities. There is a paucity of published data for conditioning regimens in these situations, but a compilation of case reports in consensus guidelines and dosing suggestions in patients with renal and hepatic insufficiency can be found in Tables 3.5 and 3.6. Dose adjustments for these drugs should be based on the patient's level of renal

TABLE 3.5
Dosing Considerations for HDC Regimens in Renal Insufficiency

Drug	Dosing Adjustments	Extent of Renal Elimination	Other Comments
Alemtuzumab[99–101]	No change[a]	None	
Lymphocyte immune globulin (equine)[99,102]	No change[a]	None	
Antithymocyte Globulin (rabbit ATG)[99,103]	No change[a]	None	
Bendamustine[53,104]	CrCl < 40 mL/min: avoid use[b]	Partial (metabolites)	• Increased thrombocytopenia seen with renal insufficiency (CrCl < 40 mL/min) in NHL patients.
Busulfan[99,105,106]	No change	Partial (metabolites)	• Efficiently removed via HD
Carboplatin[88,107]	CrCl < 60 mL/min: reduce dose[b] OR GFR 10–50 mL/min: reduce by 50%. GFR < 10 mL/min: reduce by 75%. HD: reduce by 50%.[b,c]	Primary (parent drug)	• Increased toxicities seen with CrCl < 60 mL/min.
Carmustine[82,108]	CrCl 46–60 mL/min: reduce by 20%. CrCl 31–45 mL/min: reduce by 25%. CrCl ≤ 30 mL/min: consider alternative drug.[b]	Primary (parent drug and metabolites)	

TABLE 3.5
Dosing Considerations for HDC Regimens in Renal Insufficiency—cont'd

Drug	Dosing Adjustments	Extent of Renal Elimination	Other Comments
Clofarabine[85,86,99,109,110]	CrCl 30–60 mL/min: reduce by 50%. CrCl < 30 mL/min: insufficient information for dosing recommendation.[b]	Partial (parent drug)	• May be administered if on HD. • Significant risk of AKI, especially in renal insufficiency and/or elderly.
Cyclophosphamide[99,101,105,107]	Mild impairment: no change. Moderate to severe impairment: consider dose reduction. HD: administer after HD. OR CrCl < 10 mL/min: reduce by 25%.[b] HD: reduce by 50%. Administer after HD.[b]	Partial (parent drug and metabolites)	• May be administered if on HD (20%–50% dialyzed). • Decreased clearance seen with renal insufficiency. • CKD patients may have increased myocardial toxicity and prolonged myelosuppression.
Etoposide[105,107,111]	CrCl 15–50 mL/min: reduce by 25%. CrCl < 15 mL/min: data N/A. Consider further dose reductions.[b] OR CrCl 10–50 mL/min: reduce by 25%. CrCl < 10 mL/min or HD: Reduce by 50%. Supplemental HD dose not necessary.[b]	Partial (parent drug)	• May be administered if on HD.
Fludarabine[99,101,107,112,113]	Mild to moderate impairment: reduce by 20%–25%. Severe impairment or HD: reduce by 50%. OR CrCl 10–50 mL/min: reduce by 25%. CrCl < 10 mL/min: reduce by 50%. HD: reduce by 50%. Administer after HD.[b,c]	Primary (metabolites)	• Dialyzable. • May be administered if on HD with dose reduction.
Gemcitabine[114,115]	Mild to severe impairment: No change.[b]	Primary (inactive metabolite)	• Begin HD 6–12 h after infusion.
Melphalan[99,100,116,117]	Renal impairment or HD: 100–140 mg/m². OR CrCl 15–59 mL/min or HD: reduce to 100–140 mg/m².	Minimal (parent drug—oral)	• Not dialyzable but short half-life in water may lead to poor detection in dialysate. • CKD patients may have prolonged mucositis.
Rituximab[99,118]	No change[d]	None	• Not dialyzable.
Thiotepa[50,99,119]	Mild to moderate impairment: no change. Severe impairment: may be contraindicated. OR moderate or severe impairment: monitor for toxicity.[b]	Minimal (parent drug and active metabolite)	• Extensive hepatic metabolism • However, renal impairment may lead to decreased renal excretion. • Dialyzable.

AKI, acute kidney injury; *ATG*, antithymocyte globulin; *CKD*, chronic kidney disease; *CrCl*, creatinine clearance; *GFR*, glomerular filtration rate; *HCT*, hematopoietic stem cell transplant; *HD*, hemodialysis; *HDC*, high-dose chemotherapy/conditioning; *N/A*, not available; *NHL*, non-Hodgkin's Lymphoma.

[a]This drug has not been studied in renal insufficiency. Per case reports in renally impaired and/or dialysis-dependent HCT patients, no dose adjustment used.

[b]Dosing suggestion is based on package insert or other case reports, which may not apply to HCT patients.

[c]Dosing suggestion is for adults only.

[d]This drug has not been studied in renal insufficiency. Per case reports in renally impaired and/or dialysis-dependent non-HCT patients, no dose adjustment used.

TABLE 3.6
Dosing Considerations for HDC Regimens in Hepatic Insufficiency

DRUG REGIMENS		Dosing Adjustments	Other Comments

MA[a]	Cy/TBI[b]	• Total Cy dose: 90–110 mg/kg
		• Max TBI dose: ≤12 Gy[77,121]
			• To reduce risk of VOD/SOS:
			  • Recommend VOD/SOS prophylaxis with ursodiol starting 14 days before initiation of all MA regimens.
			  • Consider antifungal prophylaxis with echinocandins instead of azoles until engraftment.
			  • Consider switching phenytoin to levetiracetam or benzodiazepines for seizure prophylaxis if receiving Bu.
			  • Discontinue all other hepatotoxic meds if possible.
			  • Diurese aggressively to prevent fluid overload.[77,122]
			• Cy/TBI: Synergistic in causing sinusoidal injury.[2,77,123]
			• Bu: Extensive hepatic metabolism. Avoid medications that decrease Bu clearance such as azoles and metronidazole.[2,77,77a]

	Cy-based regimens[b]	• When available, recommend dosing Cy using TDM.[77] • If TDM not available, empirically reduce Cy by 10%–20%.[2,77]	
	Bu/Cy[b]	• When available, recommend dosing Bu and Cy using TDM.[77] • If TDM not available, empirically reduce Cy by 10%–20%.[2,77] Administer Cy before Bu or delay Cy by 1–2 days after Bu administration.[77,124]	
RIC[a] or NMA	Bu-based regimens	• If available, recommend dosing Bu using TDM.[77]	• Bu: Extensive hepatic metabolism. Avoid medications that decrease Bu clearance such as azoles and metronidazole.[2,77,77a] • Flu: Potentially associated with hyperbilirubinemia.[120] Recommend drain pleural fluid or ascites before Flu administration and monitor closely for toxicities.[77,125,126] • Mel: Not hepatotoxic at standard doses but mild, transient transaminitis and elevated bilirubin reported with 140 mg/m². Associated with lower risk of VOD/SOS than Bu/Cy.[77,127]
	Flu-based regimens	• Mild to moderate impairment: may be acceptable with no adjustment.[77,128,129]	
	Mel-based regimens	• No adjustment reported.	

Bu, busulfan; *Cy*, cyclophosphamide; *Flu*, fludarabine; *Gy*, gray; *HDC*, high-dose chemotherapy/conditioning; *MA*, myeloablative; *Max*, maximum; *Mel*, melphalan; *NMA*, nonmyeloablative; *RIC*, reduced-intensity conditioning; *SOS*, sinusoidal obstruction syndrome; *TBI*, total-body irradiation; *TDM*, therapeutic drug monitoring; *VOD*, veno-occlusive disease.
[a]These regimens are contraindicated in minimally compensated cirrhosis. If inflammatory hepatitis or well-compensated cirrhosis, recommend reduce dose of Cy or TBI, substitute less hepatotoxic drug for Cy or select NMA regimen.[2,77]
[b]MA regimens associated with higher incidence of VOD/SOS, which is more frequent and severe if inflammatory hepatitis.[2,77,121,123]

and hepatic insufficiency and specific pharmacokinetic properties of each drug.[77,99]

Renal
Patients with chronic kidney disease (CKD) are frequently excluded from HCT. However, select HDC regimens have been safely and effectively given to patients with renal insufficiency and/or dialysis dependency.

Hepatic
In all patients before HCT, hepatic function should be evaluated with the help of the following: (1) comprehensive liver panel (including serum aspartate aminotransferase, alanine aminotransferase, bilirubin, albumin and prothrombin time), (2) hepatitis workup, and (3) if hepatic dysfunction present, liver imaging and biopsy if possible to assess for fibrosis or cirrhosis.[77,120,121]

Dosing Principles
Chemotherapy used in HCT conditioning regimens sometimes uses weight-based (mg/kg) dosing versus body surface area (BSA)-based (mg/m²) dosing. Given the prevalence of obese patients, some instances occur

---

TABLE 3.7
Weight and Dosing Calculations

Type of Weight	Comment
Total body weight (TBW)	Also considered actual weight
Ideal body weight (IBW)	
Adjusted body weight (ABW or AIBW)	ABW25 represents 25% of the difference between TBW and IBW ABW40 represents 40% of the difference between TBW and IBW

CALCULATING IDEAL BODY WEIGHT

$$IBW\ (men) = 50 + 2.3 * (Ht\ [inches] - 60)$$
$$IBW\ (women) = 45.5 + 2.3 * (Ht\ [inches] - 60)$$

CALCULATING ADJUSTED BODY WEIGHT

$$ABW25 = IBW + (0.25 * [TBW - IBW])$$
$$ABW40 = IBW + (0.40 * [TBW - IBW])$$

CALCULATING BODY SURFACE AREA (BSA)

Formula	Calculation to Obtain BSA in m^2
Mosteller[130]	$\sqrt{\dfrac{Ht\ [cm] * \quad Wt\ [kg]}{3600}}$
DuBois and DuBois, 1916[131]	$0.20247 * (Ht\ [m])^{0.725} * (Wt\ [kg])^{0.425}$
Gehan and George[132]	$0.0235 * (Ht\ [cm])^{0.42246} * (Wt\ [kg])^{0.5145}$
Haycock et al.[133]	$0.024265 * (Ht\ [cm])^{0.3964} * (Wt\ [kg])^{0.5378}$

---

when an adjusted weight might be considered instead of actual weight for dosing of cytotoxic agents. The equations for these calculations can be found in (Table 3.7).

Dosing in Obese Patients

Obesity in the United States has increased over the past 20 years. In the approximately 40-year span from the 1960s to 2002, both men and women gained more than 10 kg on average and only gained about 2.5 cm in height in the same time period.[134] Increased obesity rates complicates health care by bringing with it not only increased comorbidities, but also increased complexity of dosing medications, such as high-dose chemotherapy.[135]

The American Society of Clinical Oncology released clinical practice guidelines in 2012 regarding conventional chemotherapy dosing in adult cancer patients. Owing to a lack of evidence that short- or long-term toxicity is higher for obese patients receiving full doses, the guidelines recommended use of full weight-based doses for obese patients receiving conventional doses of chemotherapy.[136] Unfortunately, HCT and pediatric patients were excluded from these recommendations. In 2014 the American Society of Blood and Marrow Transplant (ASBMT) sought to address the dosing of HCT conditioning regimens in obese patients. The review was unable to provide level I or II evidence-based conclusions for HCT chemotherapy dosing in obese patients but did summarize the data that did exist into a consensus guideline.[135] The recommendations from this consensus guideline are summarized in Table 3.8.

TABLE 3.8
Dosing Considerations for HDC Regimens in Obesity

Antineoplastic Agent	Package Insert	ASBMT 2014 Consensus[135]
Antithymocyte globulin (rabbit) or lymphocyte immune globulin (equine)	Not addressed	TBW
Busulfan[78]	Adult: mg/kg dosing based on the lesser of IBW or TBW In obese or severely obese: clearance best predicted when dosed on adjusted body weight using ABW25	Adult: ABW25 for mg/kg dosing and TBW for BSA-based dosing • Recommend PK targeting for regimens using >12 mg/kg PO equivalent Pediatric: TBW using similar guidelines for PK targeting
Carboplatin[88]	Not addressed	Adult: TBW for BSA-based dosing Pediatric: TBW
Carmustine[80]	Not addressed	Adult: TBW for BSA-based dosing unless >120% IBW, then use ABW25
Clofarabine[86]	Actual height and weight for BSA-based dosing	Adult and Pediatric: TBW for BSA-based dosing
Cyclophosphamide	Not addressed	Cy200: lesser of TBW or IBW Cy120 (Adult): IBW (preferred) or TBW unless >120% IBW, then use ABW25 Cy120 (Pediatric): TBW unless >120% IBW, then use ABW25
Cytarabine	Not addressed	Adult and Pediatric: TBW for BSA-based dosing
Etoposide	Not addressed	Adult: ABW25 for mg/kg dosing and TBW for BSA-based dosing
Fludarabine	Not addressed	Adult: TBW for BSA-based dosing
Melphalan (ALKERAN®)[42]	Not addressed	Adult: TBW for BSA-based dosing
Melphalan (EVOMELA®)[81]	Adult: TBW unless >130% IBW, then use ABW	N/A
Thiotepa[50]	Not addressed	Adult: TBW for BSA-based dosing unless >120% IBW, then use ABW40

ABW25, adjusted body weight = IBW + 0.25 (TBW-IBW); *ABW40*, adjusted body weight = IBW + 0.4 (TBW-IBW); *ASBMT*, American Society of Blood and Marrow Transplant; *BSA*, body surface area; *Cy120*, cyclophosphamide 120 mg/kg; *Cy200*, cyclophosphamide 200 mg/kg; *HDC*, high-dose chemotherapy/conditioning; *IBW*, ideal body weight; *PK*, pharmacokinetics; *PO*, oral; *TBW*, total body weight or actual body weight.

REFERENCES

1. Majhail NS, Farnia SH, Carpenter PA, et al. Indications for autologous and allogeneic hematopoietic cell transplantation: guidelines from the American Society for blood and marrow transplantation. *Biol Blood Marrow Transpl.* 2015;21(11):1863–1869.
2. Thomas ED, Blume KG, Forman SJ, et al. *Thomas' Hematopoietic Cell Transplantation.* 3rd ed. Malden, Mass: Blackwell Pub.; 2004.
3. Bacigalupo A, Ballen K, Rizzo D, et al. Defining the intensity of conditioning regimens: working definitions. *Biol Blood Marrow Transpl.* 2009;15(12):1628–1633.
4. Giralt S, Ballen K, Rizzo D, et al. Reduced-intensity conditioning regimen workshop: defining the dose spectrum. Report of a workshop convened by the center for international blood and marrow transplant research. *Biol Blood Marrow Transpl.* 2009;15(3):367–369.
5. Couriel DR, Saliba RM, Giralt S, et al. Acute and chronic graft-versus-host disease after ablative and nonmyeloablative conditioning for allogeneic hematopoietic transplantation. *Biol Blood Marrow Transpl.* 2004;10(3):178–185.

6. Clift RA, Buckner CD, Appelbaum FR, et al. Long-term follow-up of a randomized trial of two irradiation regimens for patients receiving allogeneic marrow transplants during first remission of acute myeloid leukemia. *Blood.* 1998;92(4):1455–1456.

7. Slavin S, Nagler A, Naparstek E, et al. Nonmyeloablative stem cell transplantation and cell therapy as an alternative to conventional bone marrow transplantation with lethal cytoreduction for the treatment of malignant and nonmalignant hematologic diseases. *Blood.* 1998;91(3):756–763.

8. Gyurkocza B, Sandmaier BM. Conditioning regimens for hematopoietic cell transplantation: one size does not fit all. *Blood.* 2014;124(3):344–353.

9. Mielcarek M, Martin PJ, Leisenring W, et al. Graft-versus-host disease after nonmyeloablative versus conventional hematopoietic stem cell transplantation. *Blood.* 2003;102(2):756–762.

10. Champlin R. Reduced intensity allogeneic hematopoietic transplantation is an established standard of care for treatment of older patients with acute myeloid leukemia. *Best Pract Res Clin Haematol.* 2013;26(3):297–300.

11. Durrant S, Irving I, Morton J, et al. Sm-153 lexidronam, limb irradiation and stem cell transplant for the treatment of multiple myeloma [abstract]. *Blood.* 2001;98:778a.

12. Bayouth JE, Macey DJ, Boyer AL, et al. Radiation dose distribution within the bone marrow of patients receiving holmium-166-labeled-phosphonate for marrow ablation. *Med Phys.* 1995;22(6):743–753.

13. Bayouth JE, Macey DJ, Kasi LP, et al. Pharmacokinetics, dosimetry and toxicity of holmium-166-DOTMP for bone marrow ablation in multiple myeloma. *J Nucl Med.* 1995;36(5):730–737.

14. Giralt S, Bensinger W, Goodman M, et al. 166Ho-DOTMP plus melphalan followed by peripheral blood stem cell transplantation in patients with multiple myeloma: results of two phase 1/2 trials. *Blood.* 2003;102(7):2684–2691.

15. Christoforidou AV, Saliba RM, Williams P, et al. Results of a retrospective single institution analysis of targeted skeletal radiotherapy with (166)Holmium-DOTMP as conditioning regimen for autologous stem cell transplant for patients with multiple myeloma. Impact on transplant outcomes. *Biol Blood Marrow Transplant.* 2007;13(5):543–549.

16. Spiers FW, Vaughan J. The toxicity of the bone seeking radionucleotides. *Leuk Res.* 1989;13:347–350.

17. Porter AT, Davis LP. Systemic radionuclide therapy of bone metastases with strontium-89. *Oncol (Willist Park).* 1994;8(2):93–96; discussion 96, 99–101.

18. Collins C, Eary JF, Donaldson G, et al. Samarium-153-EDTMP in bone metastases of hormone refractory prostate carcinoma: a phase I/II trial. *J Nucl Med.* 1993;34(11):1839–1844.

19. Bruland OS, Skretting A, Solheim OP, et al. Targeted radiotherapy of osteosarcoma using 153 Sm-EDTMP. A new promising approach. *Acta Oncol.* 1996;35(3):381–384.

20. Gisselbrecht C, Vose J, Nademanee A, et al. Radioimmunotherapy for stem cell transplantation in non-Hodgkin's lymphoma: in pursuit of a complete response. *Oncologist.* 2009;14(suppl 2):41–51.

21. Vose JM, Carter S, Burns LJ, et al. Phase III randomized study of rituximab/carmustine, etoposide, cytarabine, and melphalan (BEAM) compared with iodine-131 tositumomab/BEAM with autologous hematopoietic cell transplantation for relapsed diffuse large B-cell lymphoma: results from the BMT CTN 0401 trial. *J Clin Oncol.* 2013;31(13):1662–1668.

22. Ciurea SO, Andersson BS. Busulfan in hematopoietic stem cell transplantation. *Biol Blood Marrow Transpl.* 2009;15(5):523–536.

23. Hassan M. The role of busulfan in bone marrow transplantation. *Med Oncol.* 1999;16(3):166–176.

24. Grochow LB, Jones RJ, Brundrett RB, et al. Pharmacokinetics of busulfan: correlation with veno-occlusive disease in patients undergoing bone marrow transplantation. *Cancer Chemother Pharmacol.* 1989;25(1):55–61.

25. Slattery JT, Sanders JE, Buckner CD, et al. Graft-rejection and toxicity following bone marrow transplantation in relation to busulfan pharmacokinetics. *Bone Marrow Transpl.* 1995;16(1):31–42.

26. Russell JA, Tran HT, Quinlan D, et al. Once-daily intravenous busulfan given with fludarabine as conditioning for allogeneic stem cell transplantation: study of pharmacokinetics and early clinical outcomes. *Biol Blood Marrow Transpl.* 2002;8(9):468–476.

27. Andersson BS, de Lima M, Thall PF, et al. Once daily i.v. busulfan and fludarabine (i.v. Bu-Flu) compares favorably with i.v. busulfan and cyclophosphamide (i.v. BuCy2) as pretransplant conditioning therapy in AML/MDS. *Biol Blood Marrow Transpl.* 2008;14(6):672–684.

28. Glotzbecker B, Duncan C, Alyea E, et al. Important drug interactions in hematopoietic stem cell transplantation: what every physician should know. *Biol Blood Marrow Transpl.* 2012;18(7):989–1006.

29. Socié G, Clift RA, Blaise D, et al. Busulfan plus cyclophosphamide compared with total-body irradiation plus cyclophosphamide before marrow transplantation for myeloid leukemia: long-term follow-up of 4 randomized studies. *Blood.* 2001;98(13):3569–3574.

30. Hartman AR, Williams SF, Dillon JJ. Survival, disease-free survival and adverse effects of conditioning for allogeneic bone marrow transplantation with busulfan/cyclophosphamide vs total body irradiation: a meta-analysis. *Bone Marrow Transpl.* 1998;22(5):439–443.

31. Khouri IF, Saliba RM, Giralt SA, et al. Nonablative allogeneic hematopoietic transplantation as adoptive immunotherapy for indolent lymphoma: low incidence of toxicity, acute graft-versus-host disease, and treatment-related mortality. *Blood.* 2001;98(13):3595–3599.

32. Storb R, Blume KG, O'Donnell MR, et al. Cyclophosphamide and antithymocyte globulin to condition patients with aplastic anemia for allogeneic marrow transplantations: the experience in four centers. *Biol Blood Marrow Transpl.* 2001;7(1):39–44.

33. Mielcarek M, Furlong T, O'Donnell PV, et al. Posttransplantation cyclophosphamide for prevention of graft-versus-host disease after HLA-matched mobilized blood cell transplantation. *Blood*. 2016;127(11):1502–1508.

34. Gaballa S, Ge I, El Fakih R, et al. Results of a 2-arm, phase 2 clinical trial using post-transplantation cyclophosphamide for the prevention of graft-versus-host disease in haploidentical donor and mismatched unrelated donor hematopoietic stem cell transplantation. *Cancer*. 2016;122(21):3316–3326.

35. Kleiner S, Kirsch A, Schwaner I, et al. High-dose chemotherapy with carboplatin, etoposide and ifosfamide followed by autologous stem cell rescue in patients with relapsed or refractory malignant lymphomas: a phase I/II study. *Bone Marrow Transpl*. 1997;20(11):953–959.

36. Goodman LS, Brunton LL, Chabner B, et al. *Goodman & Gilman's the Pharmacological Basis of Therapeutics*. 12th ed. New York: McGraw-Hill; 2011.

37. Meanwell CA, Blake AE, Kelly KA, et al. Prediction of ifosfamide/mesna associated encephalopathy. *Eur J Cancer Clin Oncol*. 1986;22(7):815–819.

38. Pelgrims J, De Vos F, Van den Brande J, et al. Methylene blue in the treatment and prevention of ifosfamide-induced encephalopathy: report of 12 cases and a review of the literature. *Br J Cancer*. 2000;82(2):291–294.

39. Cunningham D, Paz-Ares L, Gore ME, et al. High-dose melphalan for multiple myeloma: long-term follow-up data. *J Clin Oncol*. 1994;12(4):764–768.

40. Child JA, Morgan GJ, Davies FE, et al. High-dose chemotherapy with hematopoietic stem-cell rescue for multiple myeloma. *N Engl J Med*. 2003;348(19):1875–1883.

41. Mills W, Chopra R, McMillan A, et al. BEAM chemotherapy and autologous bone marrow transplantation for patients with relapsed or refractory non-Hodgkin's lymphoma. *J Clin Oncol*. 1995;13(3):588–595.

42. [package insert]. *Alkeran(R) (Melphalan)*. Research Triangle Park, NJ: GlaxoSmithKline; June 2011. https://www.accessdata.fda_docs/label/2011/020207s016lbl.pdf.

43. Hari P, Aljitawi OS, Arce-Lara C, et al. A phase IIb, multicenter, open-label, safety, and efficacy study of high-dose, propylene glycol-free melphalan hydrochloride for injection (EVOMELA) for myeloablative conditioning in multiple myeloma patients undergoing autologous transplantation. *Biol Blood Marrow Transpl*. 2015;21(12):2100–2105.

44. Cashen AF, Fletcher T, Ceriotti C, et al. Phase II study of propylene glycol-free melphalan combined with carmustine, etoposide, and cytarabine for myeloablative conditioning in lymphoma patients undergoing autologous stem cell transplantation. *Biol Blood Marrow Transpl*. 2016;22(12):2155–2158.

45. Giralt S, Thall PF, Khouri I, et al. Melphalan and purine analog-containing preparative regimens: reduced-intensity conditioning for patients with hematologic malignancies undergoing allogeneic progenitor cell transplantation. *Blood*. 2001;97(3):631–637.

46. Kasenda B, Schorb E, Fritsch K, et al. Prognosis after high-dose chemotherapy followed by autologous stem-cell transplantation as first-line treatment in primary CNS lymphoma–a long-term follow-up study. *Ann Oncol*. 2012;23(10):2670–2675.

47. DeFilipp Z, Li S, El-Jawahri A, et al. High-dose chemotherapy with thiotepa, busulfan, and cyclophosphamide and autologous stem cell transplantation for patients with primary central nervous system lymphoma in first complete remission. *Cancer*. 2017;123(16):3073–3079.

48. Ciurea SO, Saliba R, Rondon G, et al. Reduced-intensity conditioning using fludarabine, melphalan and thiotepa for adult patients undergoing haploidentical SCT. *Bone Marrow Transpl*. 2010;45(3):429–436.

49. Ciurea SO, Saliba RM, Hamerschlak N, et al. Fludarabine, melphalan, thiotepa and anti-thymocyte globulin conditioning for unrelated cord blood transplant. *Leuk Lymphoma*. 2012;53(5):901–906.

50. [package insert]. *Tepadina(R) (Thiotepa)*. SA, Switzerland: Adienne; January 2017. September 19, 2017. https://www.accessdata.fda.gov/drugsatfda_docs/label/2017/208264s000lbl.pdf.

51. Khouri IF, Wei W, Korbling M, et al. BFR (bendamustine, fludarabine, and rituximab) allogeneic conditioning for chronic lymphocytic leukemia/lymphoma: reduced myelosuppression and GVHD. *Blood*. 2014;124(14):2306–2312.

52. Visani G, Malerba L, Stefani PM, et al. BeEAM (bendamustine, etoposide, cytarabine, melphalan) before autologous stem cell transplantation is safe and effective for resistant/relapsed lymphoma patients. *Blood*. 2011;118(12):3419–3425.

53. [package insert]. *Treanda(R) (Bendamustine)*. North Wales, PA: Teva Pharmaceuticals USA, Inc.; October 2016. https://www.accessdata.fda.gov/drugsatfda_docs/label/2016/022249s022lbl.pdf.

54. Valdez BC, Li Y, Murray D, et al. Comparison of the cytotoxicity of cladribine and clofarabine when combined with fludarabine and busulfan in AML cells: enhancement of cytotoxicity with epigenetic modulators. *Exp Hematol*. 2015;43(6):448–461.e442.

55. Terenzi A, Aristei C, Aversa F, et al. Efficacy of fludarabine as an immunosuppressor for bone marrow transplantation conditioning: preliminary results. *Transpl Proc*. 1996;28(6):3101.

56. Khouri IF, McLaughlin P, Saliba RM, et al. Eight-year experience with allogeneic stem cell transplantation for relapsed follicular lymphoma after nonmyeloablative conditioning with fludarabine, cyclophosphamide, and rituximab. *Blood*. 2008;111(12):5530–5536.

57. de Lima M, Couriel D, Thall PF, et al. Once-daily intravenous busulfan and fludarabine: clinical and pharmacokinetic results of a myeloablative, reduced-toxicity conditioning regimen for allogeneic stem cell transplantation in AML and MDS. *Blood*. 2004;104(3):857–864.

58. Ben-Barouch S, Cohen O, Vidal L, et al. Busulfan fludarabine vs busulfan cyclophosphamide as a preparative regimen before allogeneic hematopoietic cell transplantation: systematic review and meta-analysis. *Bone Marrow Transpl.* 2016;51(2):232–240.

59. Valdez BC, Andersson BS. Interstrand crosslink inducing agents in pretransplant conditioning therapy for hematologic malignancies. *Environ Mol Mutagen.* 2010;51(6):659–668.

60. Valdez BC, Li Y, Murray D, et al. The synergistic cytotoxicity of clofarabine, fludarabine and busulfan in AML cells involves ATM pathway activation and chromatin remodeling. *Biochem Pharmacol.* 2011;81(2):222–232.

61. Kebriaei P, Basset R, Ledesma C, et al. Clofarabine combined with busulfan provides excellent disease control in adult patients with acute lymphoblastic leukemia undergoing allogeneic hematopoietic stem cell transplantation. *Biol Blood Marrow Transpl.* 2012;18(12):1819–1826.

62. Andersson BS, Valdez BC, de Lima M, et al. Clofarabine +/- fludarabine with once daily i.v. busulfan as pretransplant conditioning therapy for advanced myeloid leukemia and MDS. *Biol Blood Marrow Transpl.* 2011;17(6):893–900.

63. Wang E, Gulbis A, Hart JW, et al. The emerging role of gemcitabine in conditioning regimens for hematopoietic stem cell transplantation. *Biol Blood Marrow Transpl.* 2014;20(9):1382–1389.

64. Anderlini P, Saliba RM, Ledesma C, et al. Gemcitabine, fludarabine and melphalan as a reduced-intensity conditioning regimen for allogeneic stem cell transplant in relapsed and refractory Hodgkin lymphoma: preliminary results. *Leuk Lymphoma.* 2012;53(3):499–502.

65. Nieto Y, Tu SM, Bassett R, et al. Bevacizumab/high-dose chemotherapy with autologous stem-cell transplant for poor-risk relapsed or refractory germ-cell tumors. *Ann Oncol.* 2015;26(10):2125–2132.

66. Suleiman Y, Siddiqui BK, Brames MJ, et al. Salvage therapy with high-dose chemotherapy and peripheral blood stem cell transplant in patients with primary mediastinal nonseminomatous germ cell tumors. *Biol Blood Marrow Transpl.* 2013;19(1):161–163.

67. Bruserud O, Reikvam H, Kittang AO, et al. High-dose etoposide in allogeneic stem cell transplantation. *Cancer Chemother Pharmacol.* 2012;70(6):765–782.

68. Bashir Q, Munsell MF, Giralt S, et al. Randomized phase II trial comparing two dose levels of thymoglobulin in patients undergoing unrelated donor hematopoietic cell transplant. *Leuk Lymphoma.* 2012;53(5):915–919.

69. Bryant A, Mallick R, Huebsch L, et al. Low-dose antithymocyte globulin for graft-versus-host disease prophylaxis in matched unrelated allogeneic hematopoietic stem cell transplantation. *Biol Blood Marrow Transpl.* 2017;23(12):2096–2101.

70. Ruutu T, van Biezen A, Hertenstein B, et al. Prophylaxis and treatment of GVHD after allogeneic haematopoietic SCT: a survey of centre strategies by the European Group for Blood and Marrow Transplantation. *Bone Marrow Transpl.* 2012;47(11):1459–1464.

71. Chen G, Kook H, Zeng W, et al. Is there a direct effect of antithymocyte globulin on hematopoiesis? *Hematol J.* 2004;5(3):255–261.

72. Sauter CS, Chou JF, Papadopoulos EB, et al. A prospective study of an alemtuzumab containing reduced-intensity allogeneic stem cell transplant program in patients with poor-risk and advanced lymphoid malignancies. *Leuk Lymphoma.* 2014;55(12):2739–2747.

73. Gandhi S, Kulasekararaj AG, Mufti GJ, et al. Allogeneic stem cell transplantation using alemtuzumab-containingregimens in severe aplastic anemia. *Int J Hematol.* 2013;97(5):573–580.

74. Genzyme S. *US Campath Distribution Program*; 2013. https://www.campathproviderportal.com/Home.aspx?ReturnUrl=%2fSecure%2fWelcome.aspx.

75. Kharfan-Dabaja MA, Nishihori T, Otrock ZK, et al. Monoclonal antibodies in conditioning regimens for hematopoietic cell transplantation. *Biol Blood Marrow Transpl.* 2013;19(9):1288–1300.

76. Khouri IF. Reduced-intensity regimens in allogeneic stem-cell transplantation for non-hodgkin lymphoma and chronic lymphocytic leukemia. *Hematol Am Soc Hematol Educ Prog.* 2006:390–397.

77. Bodge MN, Culos KA, Haider SN, et al. Preparative regimen dosing for hematopoietic stem cell transplantation in patients with chronic hepatic impairment: analysis of the literature and recommendations. *Biol Blood Marrow Transpl.* 2014;20(5):622–629.

77a. Nilsson G, Aschan J, Hentschke P, et al. The effect of metronidazole on busulfan pharmacokinetics in patients undergoing hematopoietic stem cell transplantation. *Bone Marrow Transplant.* 2003;31(6):429–435.

78. [package insert]. *Busulfex(R) (Busulfan)*. Tokyo, 101–8535 Japan: Otsuka Pharmaceutical Co., Ltd.; January 2016.

79. Marr KA, Leisenring W, Crippa F, et al. Cyclophosphamide metabolism is affected by azole antifungals. *Blood.* 2004;103(4):1557–1559.

80. Przepiorka D, van Besien K, Khouri I, et al. Carmustine, etoposide, cytarabine and melphalan as a preparative regimen for allogeneic transplantation for high-risk malignant lymphoma. *Ann Oncol.* 1999;10(5):527–532.

81. [package insert]. *Evomela(R) (Melphalan)*. Irvine, CA: Spectrum Pharmaceuticals, Inc.; March 2016. http://www.evomela.com/web/download/Evomela-Prescribing-Information.pdf.

82. [package insert]. *BiCNU(R) (Carmustine)*. Eatontown, NJ: Heritage Pharmaceuticals, Inc.; March 2017. https://www.accessdata.fda.gov/drugsatfda_docs/label/2017/017422s055lbl.pdf.

83. Dorr RT, Soble MJ. H2-antagonists and carmustine. *J Cancer Res Clin Oncol.* 1989;115(1):41–46.

84. Woo MH, Ippoliti C, Bruton J, et al. Headache, circumoral paresthesia, and facial flushing associated with high-dose carmustine infusion. *Bone Marrow Transpl.* 1997;19(8):845–847.

85. van Besien K, Stock W, Rich E, et al. Phase I-II study of clofarabine-melphalan-alemtuzumab conditioning for allogeneic hematopoietic cell transplantation. *Biol Blood Marrow Transpl.* 2012;18(6):913–921.

86. [package insert]. *Clolar(R) (Clofarabine).* Cambridge, MA: Genzyme Corporation; October 2016. https://www.accessdata.fda.gov/drugsatfda_docs/label/2016/021673s025lbl.pdf.

87. Adra N, Abonour R, Althouse SK, et al. High-dose chemotherapy and autologous peripheral-blood stem-cell transplantation for relapsed metastatic germ cell tumors: the Indiana university experience. *J Clin Oncol.* 2017;35(10):1096–1102.

88. [package insert]. *Paraplatin(R) (Carboplatin).* Princeton, NJ: Bristol-Myers Squibb Company; July 2010. https://www.accessdata.fda.gov/drugsatfda_docs/label/2010/020452s005lbl.pdf.

89. Srour SA, Li S, Popat UR, et al. A randomized phase II study of standard-dose versus high-dose rituximab with BEAM in autologous stem cell transplantation for relapsed aggressive B-cell non-hodgkin lymphomas: long term results. *Br J Haematol.* 2017;178(4):561–570.

90. Thomas ED, Buckner CD, Banaji M, et al. One hundred patients with acute leukemia treated by chemotherapy, total body irradiation, and allogeneic marrow transplantation. *Blood.* 1977;49(4):511–533.

91. Snyder DS, Chao NJ, Amylon MD, et al. Fractionated total body irradiation and high-dose etoposide as a preparatory regimen for bone marrow transplantation for 99 patients with acute leukemia in first complete remission. *Blood.* 1993;82(9):2920–2928.

92. Santos GW, Tutschka PJ, Brookmeyer R, et al. Marrow transplantation for acute nonlymphocytic leukemia after treatment with busulfan and cyclophosphamide. *N Engl J Med.* 1983;309(22):1347–1353.

93. Tutschka PJ, Copelan EA, Klein JP. Bone marrow transplantation for leukemia following a new busulfan and cyclophosphamide regimen. *Blood.* 1987;70(5):1382–1388.

94. Ahmed T, Ciavarella D, Feldman E, et al. High-dose, potentially myeloablative chemotherapy and autologous bone marrow transplantation for patients with advanced Hodgkin's disease. *Leukemia.* 1989;3(1):19–22.

95. Bashir Q, Khan H, Thall PF, et al. A randomized phase II trial of fludarabine/melphalan 100 versus fludarabine/melphalan 140 followed by allogeneic hematopoietic stem cell transplantation for patients with multiple myeloma. *Biol Blood Marrow Transpl.* 2013;19(10):1453–1458.

96. Corradini P, Tarella C, Olivieri A, et al. Reduced-intensity conditioning followed by allografting of hematopoietic cells can produce clinical and molecular remissions in patients with poor-risk hematologic malignancies. *Blood.* 2002;99(1):75–82.

97. Khouri IF, Keating M, Körbling M, et al. Transplant-lite: induction of graft-versus-malignancy using fludarabine-based nonablative chemotherapy and allogeneic blood progenitor-cell transplantation as treatment for lymphoid malignancies. *J Clin Oncol.* 1998;16(8):2817–2824.

98. Maris MB, Niederwieser D, Sandmaier BM, et al. HLA-matched unrelated donor hematopoietic cell transplantation after nonmyeloablative conditioning for patients with hematologic malignancies. *Blood.* 2003;102(6):2021–2030.

99. Bodge MN, Reddy S, Thompson MS, et al. Preparative regimen dosing for hematopoietic stem cell transplantation in patients with chronic kidney disease: analysis of the literature and recommendations. *Biol Blood Marrow Transpl.* 2014;20(7):908–919.

100. van Besien K, Schouten V, Parsad S, et al. Allogeneic stem cell transplant in renal failure: engraftment and prolonged survival, but high incidence of neurologic toxicity. *Leuk Lymphoma.* 2012;53(1):158–159.

101. Gerrie A, Marsh J, Lipton JH, et al. Marrow transplantation for severe aplastic anemia with significant renal impairment. *Bone Marrow Transpl.* 2007;39(5):311–313.

102. Hamaki T, Katori H, Kami M, et al. Successful allogeneic blood stem cell transplantation for aplastic anemia in a patient with renal insufficiency requiring dialysis. *Bone Marrow Transpl.* 2002;30(3):195–198.

103. Kersting S, Verdonck LF. Successful outcome after non-myeloablative allogeneic hematopoietic stem cell transplantation in patients with renal dysfunction. *Biol Blood Marrow Transpl.* 2008;14(11):1312–1316.

104. Nordstrom BL, Knopf KB, Teltsch DY, et al. The safety of bendamustine in patients with chronic lymphocytic leukemia or non-Hodgkin lymphoma and concomitant renal impairment: a retrospective electronic medical record database analysis. *Leuk Lymphoma.* 2014;55(6):1266–1273.

105. Ballester OF, Tummala R, Janssen WE, et al. High-dose chemotherapy and autologous peripheral blood stem cell transplantation in patients with multiple myeloma and renal insufficiency. *Bone Marrow Transpl.* 1997;20(8):653–656.

106. Ullery LL, Gibbs JP, Ames GW, et al. Busulfan clearance in renal failure and hemodialysis. *Bone Marrow Transpl.* 2000;25(2):201–203.

107. Aronoff GR, American College of Physicians. *Drug Prescribing in Renal Failure: Dosing Guidelines for Adults and Children.* 5th ed. Philadelphia: American College of Physicians; 2007.

108. Kintzel PE, Dorr RT. Anticancer drug renal toxicity and elimination: dosing guidelines for altered renal function. *Cancer Treat Rev.* 1995;21(1):33–64.

109. Bonate PL, Cunningham CC, Gaynon P, et al. Population pharmacokinetics of clofarabine and its metabolite 6-ketoclofarabine in adult and pediatric patients with cancer. *Cancer Chemother Pharmacol.* 2011;67(4):875–890.

110. Sudour H, Kimmoun A, Contet A, et al. Successful management with clofarabine for refractory leukaemia in a young adult with chronic renal failure. *Am J Hematol.* 2011;86(3):321–323.

111. [package insert]. *Toposar(TM) (Etoposide)*. Irvine, CA: Teva Parenteral Medicines, Inc; November 2009. https://dailymed.nlm.nih.gov/dailymed/archives/fdaDrugInfo.cfm?archiveid=14388.

112. Lichtman SM, Etcubanas E, Budman DR, et al. The pharmacokinetics and pharmacodynamics of fludarabine phosphate in patients with renal impairment: a prospective dose adjustment study. *Cancer Investig*. 2002;20(7–8): 904–913.

113. Kielstein JT, Stadler M, Czock D, et al. Dialysate concentration and pharmacokinetics of 2F-Ara-A in a patient with acute renal failure. *Eur J Haematol*. 2005;74(6):533–534.

114. Janus N, Thariat J, Boulanger H, et al. Proposal for dosage adjustment and timing of chemotherapy in hemodialyzed patients. *Ann Oncol*. 2010;21(7):1395–1403.

115. Li YF, Fu S, Hu W, et al. Systemic anticancer therapy in gynecological cancer patients with renal dysfunction. *Int J Gynecol Cancer*. 2007;17(4):739–763.

116. Choi HS, Kim SY, Lee JH, et al. Successful allogeneic stem-cell transplantation in a patient with myelodysplastic syndrome with hemodialysis-dependent endstage renal disease. *Transplantation*. 2011;92(6):e28–e29.

117. Dimopoulos MA, Sonneveld P, Leung N, et al. International myeloma working group recommendations for the diagnosis and management of myeloma-related renal impairment. *J Clin Oncol*. 2016;34(13):1544–1557.

118. Jillella AP, Dainer PM, Kallab AM, et al. Treatment of a patient with end-stage renal disease with Rituximab: pharmacokinetic evaluation suggests Rituximab is not eliminated by hemodialysis. *Am J Hematol*. 2002;71(3):219–222.

119. Termuhlen AM, Grovas A, Klopfenstein K, et al. Autologous hematopoietic stem cell transplant with melphalan and thiotepa is safe and feasible in pediatric patients with low normalized glomerular filtration rate. *Pediatr Transpl*. 2006;10(7):830–834.

120. Hogan WJ, Maris M, Storer B, et al. Hepatic injury after nonmyeloablative conditioning followed by allogeneic hematopoietic cell transplantation: a study of 193 patients. *Blood*. 2004;103(1):78–84.

121. McDonald GB. Hepatobiliary complications of hematopoietic cell transplantation, 40 years on. *Hepatology*. 2010;51(4):1450–1460.

122. Johnson DB, Savani BN. How can we reduce hepatic venoocclusive disease-related deaths after allogeneic stem cell transplantation? *Exp Hematol*. 2012;40(7):513–517.

123. McDonald GB, Slattery JT, Bouvier ME, et al. Cyclophosphamide metabolism, liver toxicity, and mortality following hematopoietic stem cell transplantation. *Blood*. 2003;101(5):2043–2048.

124. Rezvani AR, McCune JS, Storer BE, et al. Cyclophosphamide followed by intravenous targeted busulfan for allogeneic hematopoietic cell transplantation: pharmacokinetics and clinical outcomes. *Biol Blood Marrow Transpl*. 2013;19(7):1033–1039.

125. Mahadevan A, Kanegaonkar R, Hoskin PJ. Third space sequestration increases toxicity of fludarabine–a case report. *Acta Oncol*. 1997;36(4):441.

126. McDonald GB, Frieze D. A problem-oriented approach to liver disease in oncology patients. *Gut*. 2008;57(7): 987–1003.

127. Ayash LJ, Elias A, Wheeler C, et al. Double dose-intensive chemotherapy with autologous marrow and peripheral-blood progenitor-cell support for metastatic breast cancer: a feasibility study. *J Clin Oncol*. 1994;12(1):37–44.

128. Hamaki T, Kami M, Igarashi M, et al. Non-myeloablative hematopoietic stem cell transplantation for the treatment of adult T-cell lymphoma in a patient with advanced hepatic impairment. *Leuk Lymphoma*. 2003;44(4):703–708.

129. Jacobsohn DA, Emerick KM, Scholl P, et al. Nonmyeloablative hematopoietic stem cell transplant for X-linked hyper-immunoglobulin m syndrome with cholangiopathy. *Pediatrics*. 2004;113(2):e122–e127.

130. Mosteller RD. Simplified calculation of body-surface area. *N Engl J Med*. 1987;317(17):1098.

131. DuBois D, DuBois EF. A formula to estimate the approximate surface area if height and weight be known. 1916. *Nutrition*. 1989;5(5):303–311; discussion 312–303.

132. Gehan EA, George SL. Estimation of human body surface area from height and weight. *Cancer Chemother Rep*. 1970;54(4):225–235.

133. Haycock GB, Schwartz GJ, Wisotsky DH. Geometric method for measuring body surface area: a height-weight formula validated in infants, children, and adults. *J Pediatr*. 1978;93(1):62–66.

134. Ogden CL, Fryar CD, Carroll MD, et al. Mean body weight, height, and body mass index, United States 1960-2002. *Adv Data*. 2004;(347):1–17.

135. Bubalo J, Carpenter PA, Majhail N, et al. Conditioning chemotherapy dose adjustment in obese patients: a review and position statement by the American Society for Blood and Marrow Transplantation practice guideline committee. *Biol Blood Marrow Transpl*. 2014;20(5): 600–616.

136. Griggs JJ, Mangu PB, Anderson H, et al. Appropriate chemotherapy dosing for obese adult patients with cancer: American Society of Clinical Oncology clinical practice guideline. *J Clin Oncol*. 2012;30(13):1553–1561.

CHAPTER 4

The Role of Radiation Therapy in Hematopoietic Stem Cell Transplantation

CHELSEA C. PINNIX, MD, PHD

TOTAL-BODY IRRADIATION THERAPY

Total-body irradiation (TBI) is commonly used as a component of preparative conditioning regimens before allogeneic hematopoietic stem cell transplantation (HSCT). In this setting the potential goals of TBI are numerous. TBI can irradiate residual malignant cells and therefore has the potential to decrease tumor burden and improve disease-related outcomes. Another objective of TBI is to offer physical space for donor cells to engraft within the bone marrow compartment.[1] An additional well-recognized effect of TBI is to provide immunosuppression of the HSCT recipient which may allow improved engraftment of donor cells, potentially facilitating increased graft versus tumor effect.

The potential advantages imparted by TBI-based preparative regimens are distinct from systemic therapy.[2] First, external beam radiation therapy (RT) dose delivery is not dependent on blood supply. Thus TBI is not affected by metabolism, absorption, or clearance, in the manner that conventional drug agents are. Based on this advantage, TBI can deliver a therapeutic dose to sites that may have barriers to achieving tumoricidal concentrations of systemic therapy, so-called "sanctuary sites", such as the central nervous system (CNS) and testis. Finally, tumor cells that exhibit resistance to chemotherapy are not necessarily refractory to RT.

Myeloablative Conditioning Regimens

Myeloablative conditioning (MAC) regimens are those in which TBI and/or chemotherapeutic drugs (usually alkylating agents) are given at doses that do not allow autologous reconstitution and therefore can be fatal to patients without the administration of hematopoietic cells. This approach is often used as conditioning before allogeneic HSCT. The goal of this approach is to eliminate residual disease while offering adequate immunosuppression to mitigate

rejection of the graft. Although increased intensity of MAC regimens do confer a lower risk of relapse, this disease control benefit may be offset by increased treatment-related mortality (TRM) due to toxicity associated with treatment.[3,4]

In 1977 Thomas et al. at the University of Washington School of Medicine and the Fred Hutchinson Cancer Research Center in Seattle reported early outcomes of 100 patients with acute myeloid leukemia (AML) and acute lymphoblastic leukemia (ALL) treated with HSCT from a human leukocyte antigen (HLA)–identical sibling and established the role of TBI as a preparative regimen in this setting.[5] TBI was administered with a total dose of 10 Gy in one fraction using cobalt-60 sources with or without additional systemic therapy. In a follow-up publication, long-term remission was sustained in the majority of patients.[6] The radiation dose was incriminated with causing death in some patients, so in an effort to reduce transplant-related mortality, a randomized trial of 53 leukemia patients was conducted to compare two TBI regimens, 10 Gy in one fraction versus 12 Gy in six daily fractions.[7] Disease-free survival was superior with the fractionated regimen. Owing to small numbers and relatively short follow-up, there was not a clear difference in TRM; however, 12 Gy TBI in 2 Gy fractions administered with cyclophosphamide became a common myeloablative regimen for patients with acute leukemia.

Once fractionated regimens became the standard of care, the optimal fractionated TBI dose was debated. Doses above 12 Gy were thought to have increased tumoricidal effects; however, the question of whether this potential increase in disease control would be offset by added toxicity was unclear. Researchers in Seattle conducted a subsequent randomized trial comparing TBI to a dose of 12 Gy versus 15.75 Gy among 71 AML patients undergoing allogeneic HSCT with 120 mg/kg

59

of cyclophosphamide.[8] The increased TBI dose was associated with a lower risk of relapse (3-year probability of relapse was 35% for the 12 Gy group and 12% for the 15.75 Gy group, P=.06); however, the 3-year probability of transplant-related mortality was higher in the 15.75 Gy arm (32%) than in the 12 Gy arm (12%, P=.04). Similar results were demonstrated by a similar randomized trial conducted by this group for 57 patients with chronic myeloid leukemia (CML) comparing 12 Gy to15.75 Gy. In this study the higher dose of TBI reduced the probability of relapse but did not impact overall survival due to increased TRM.[9] In both of these randomized trials, the increased mortality in the higher dose TBI arm was due to increased death from venoocclusive disease (VOD) of the liver, cytomegalovirus (CMV) pneumonia, and acute graft versus host disease (GVHD). It is interesting that in both the studies, the higher 15.75 Gy TBI arm had increased rates of GVHD, which in many cases were fatal. In both the studies the patients in the 15.75 Gy TBI arms received less of the prescribed post-transplant GVHD prophylaxis regimen that contained methotrexate and cyclosporine, presumably due to augmented toxicity from the higher dose TBI regimen that limited patient ability to complete the GVHD prophylactic course. Therefore it was hypothesized that the increase in GVHD associated with the higher TBI dose schedule could have been due to insufficient prophylaxis and not necessarily the elevated RT dose.

With longer follow-up in several studies, however, concerns regarding toxicity which were largely attributed to RT prompted trials evaluating potential alternatives to TBI-containing preparative regimens. Given the known activity of cyclophosphamide against lymphoid tissue but modest activity against hematopoietic stem cells and myeloid tissues, coupling cyclophosphamide with an agent that possessed an enhanced anti-myeloid and hematopoietic stem cell activity was desired.[10] Santos et al. at Johns Hopkins hospital reported on the outcomes of 51 patients with acute non-lymphocytic leukemia who were administered oral busulfan and cyclophosphamide before HSCT with an HLA-identical sibling.[11] An actuarial 2-year overall survival (OS) rate of 44% was reported. The major causes of mortality were GVHD and viral infections (mainly CMV-associated interstitial pneumonia). These outcomes were stated to be on par with previous reports of TBI-based regimens, and therefore high-dose oral busulfan and cyclophosphamide were considered a worthwhile option for MAC for HSCT.

A randomized trial was conducted by the Group d'Etudes de la Greffe de Moelle Osseuse to compare disease- and treatment-related outcomes after MAC with intravenous (IV) cyclophosphamide and TBI (CyTBI) as compared to oral busulfan and IV cyclophosphamide (BuCy).[12] One hundred and one patients with AML were randomized to either preparative regimen in the first remission. At 2 years, the patients who received CyTBI had superior disease-free survival (72% vs. 47%, P < .01) and OS (75% vs. 51%, P<.02). Relapse rates at 2 years were lower among the CyTBI arm (14% vs. 34%, P<.04). Transplant mortality was also lower among the CyTBI group than among the BuCy group (8% vs. 27%, P<.06). The superiority of the CyTBI arm was maintained with extended follow-up.[13] At a median follow-up of 10.8 years, the 10-year actuarial OS rate was 59% in the CyTBI arm compared with 43% (P=.04) in the BuCy arm. The 10-year leukemia-free survival rate was 55% for CyTBI and 35% for BuCy (P=.02). On multivariate analysis, BuCy was independently associated with increased risk of failure. In a study of long-term follow-up of four randomized trials comparing CyTBI with BuCy conditioning regimens (with busulfan administered orally), similarly among AML patients, Cy-TBI was associated with superior survival.[14]

Oral busulfan has been criticized for wide variability in plasma levels that could result in excessive toxicity or reduced efficacy based on patient bioavailability levels.[12] This undesirable characteristic of orally administered busulfan prompted many investigators to compare TBI-based myeloablative regimens with IV busulfan. In a large retrospective study of 1230 AML patients undergoing HSCT with an HLA-matched sibling or unrelated donor, the Center for International Bone Marrow Transplant Research compared the outcomes of oral busulfan, IV busulfan, and TBI-based conditioning regimens.[15] Nonrelapse mortality (NRM) was lower for patients who received IV busulfan compared with TBI (relative risk, RR=0.58, P=.0066). IV busulfan and cyclophosphamide were also associated with improved leukemia-free survival and OS. The authors also retrospectively compared high-dose TBI (>12.5 Gy) with standard-dose TBI (≤12.5 Gy) and observed elevated rates of NRM with the high-dose TBI (RR = 1.46, P=.032). In a similar non-randomized cohort study of 1483 leukemia patients, IV busulfan was compared with TBI-based myeloablative regimens. Among the AML patients, 2-year OS was superior in the IV busulfan cohort (58% vs. 46%, P=.003). There were no reported differences in GVHD, although there was a higher incidence of VOD in the busulfan-treated patients (5% vs. 1%). As randomized data are not available, taken together these studies are regarded as data to support the use of IV busulfan as a standard of care regimen for HSCT of AML patients.[16]

While advances in chemotherapy delivery have been implemented over several decades to improve outcomes with chemotherapy-based conditioning regimens, similarly, RT techniques for the delivery of TBI have also evolved. These modern RT approaches however were not used in the aforementioned studies, and therefore it is feasible that outcomes with TBI may be improved with these contemporary RT approaches. Many older studies used historic cobalt-60 units which are severely outdated and have less desirable dose distribution profiles than the high-energy photons used today. Furthermore, lung shielding is often used at many tertiary transplant and RT centers to limit lung dose and minimize TBI-related pulmonary toxicity.[17] Dose escalation of TBI is limited due to the limitation of normal tissues to tolerate increased RT doses. In an effort to increase doses of RT to the marrow while limiting doses to normal organs and tissues, novel techniques in TBI targeting have been developed, including total marrow irradiation as well as total marrow and lymphoid irradiation. Additional studies with extended follow-up are required to determine if treatment-related toxicity can be limited via the use of modern TBI delivery.

Reduced-Intensity Conditioning Regimens

MAC regimens, while associated with enhanced leukemia control, also portend the potential for increased risk from toxicity. Therefore candidacy for MAC regimens is often limited to younger patients (aged less than 60 years) with optimal performance status. Regimens designed to permit donor engraftment while limiting the risk of TRM have emerged for older patients and those with perceived decreased ability to tolerate aggressive conditioning therapy. With reduced-intensity conditioning (RIC) approaches, the conditioning regimens are designed to mainly provide immunosuppression to allow engraftment with reliance on the donor graft for the antileukemia effect.[18]

The first study evaluating low-dose TBI to a dose of 2 Gy in one fraction was reported by McSweeney et al. at Fred Hutchinson Cancer Research Center.[19] In preclinical canine studies the combination of post-grafting pharmacologic immunosuppression with T-cell activation inhibitor cyclosporine (CSP) coupled with the anti–metabolite mycophenolate mofetil (MMF) reduced GVHD and allowed a decrease in the TBI dose (from 9.2 to 2 Gy) required for successful, durable engraftment.[20,21] Based on these observations the authors conducted a study of 45 patients with hematologic malignancies who underwent HSCT with an HLA-identical donor using 2 Gy TBI, CSP, and MMF.[19] Astoundingly, more than half of patients (53%) had HSCT performed in the outpatient

setting. Acute GVHD (grade 2–3) occurred in 47% of patients who maintained their graft. Graft rejection that was not fatal occurred in 20% of patients. More than half of patients with durable engraftment were in complete remission with a median follow-up of 417 days. This innovative strategy utilizing post-HSCT immunosuppression to minimize GVHD changed the landscape of HSCT, permitting administration of this potentially curative strategy to older and higher risk patients who were previously ineligible for this therapy.

In a study of patients who underwent HSCT for Philadelphia chromosome–negative ALL at University Hospitals Bristol NHS Trust in the United Kingdom, the outcome of 93 patients who received RIC was compared with that of 1428 patients who received full-intensity MAC.[22] The reduced-intensity group received busulfan (9 mg/kg or less, n = 27), melphalan (150 mg/m^2, or less, n = 23), or low-dose TBI (n = 36). The TBI regimens included 8 Gy fractionated or 5 Gy or less in a single fraction (n = 18), 2 Gy TBI with fludarabine (n = 12) or other TBI-containing regimens (n = 6). The reduced-intensity group had similar transplantation-related mortality but slightly increased rates of relapse that did not reach statistical significance (25% vs. 26%, $P = .08$). Age-adjusted survival was not significantly different. On multivariate analysis, several factors were associated with improved OS (including the use of TBI conditioning); however, conditioning intensity was not. Based on these data and other studies, reduced-intensity conditioning regimens are regarded as an effective option for patients who are unable to tolerate aggressive myeloablative programs and are being increasingly used in the older and frailer patient population.[23]

Recent data have called into question whether reduced-intensity regimens truly result in increased disease relapse compared with myeloablative regimens. Indeed, long-term follow-up of a multi-institutional randomized trial conducted in Germany of AML patients aged 18–60 years undergoing allogeneic HSCT with an HLA-matched sibling donor or 9/10 matched unrelated donor revealed no evidence of increased late relapse among patients who received reduced-intensity conditioning compared with those who received MAC.[24] The trial randomized 195 patients to reduced-intensity conditioning with 120 mg/m^2 of fludarabine with TBI to a dose of 8 Gy in four fractions administered over the course of 2 days with lung shielding or MAC with TBI to a dose of 12 Gy in six fractions given over 3 days with lung shielding administered with 120 mg/kg of cyclophosphamide. With a median follow-up of just under 10 years for survivors, the cumulative incidence of relapse was identical in both the arms (30%, $P = .99$).

Rates of 10-year NRM were 16% in the reduced-intensity conditioning arm compared with 26% in the myeloablative arm ($P = .10$). Rates of secondary malignancy were 6% in both the cohorts ($P = 1.0$). The original publication of this trial reported lower rates of early toxicity with the reduced-intensity regimen;[25] therefore based on the results of the long-term follow-up, the authors concluded that reduced-intensity conditioning with moderately reduced TBI doses should be considered as a standard of care regimen for AML patients aged 60 years or less who are undergoing allogeneic stem cell transplantation in the first remission. There are a few criticisms of this study however, the most important being that the reduced-intensity regimen used is more aggressive and potentially more toxic than more commonly used reduced-intensity programs. Some may argue that the TBI regimen of 8 Gy in 2 Gy fractions administered twice daily should not be considered low intensity. In addition, there was a smaller fraction of patients with high-risk features in this study than what would typically be expected in this patient population.[26] Nonetheless, studies such as this one challenge the notion that reduced-intensity regimens should be reserved for older patients with poor performance status and open the door to explore the potential to deescalate conditioning programs for all patients. The optimal RT dose to be used in this setting is yet to be defined.

CNS Leukemic Involvement

Patients with a history of CNS involvement either at diagnosis or at relapse who undergo allogeneic HSCT pose a unique therapeutic challenge. The blood–brain barrier may hamper penetration of cytotoxic chemotherapy in the CNS, potentially limiting the efficacy of chemotherapy-based myeloablative regimens. Furthermore, it is debated whether the graft versus leukemia effect is less prominent in the CNS.[27-29] Patients with a history of CNS involvement before allogeneic HSCT are at higher risk for post-allogeneic CNS relapse.[30] Finally CNS relapses are often difficult to salvage and can be fatal.[31] For these reasons, CNS-directed RT may be considered before allogeneic HSCT to improve local control in the brain, spine, and cerebrospinal fluid. Inclusion of RT before SCT is considered with trepidation, however, given the risk of neurotoxicity among an often vulnerable patient population with a history of extensive pretreatment with CNS-directed chemotherapy (often intrathecal or IV methotrexate and/or cytarabine).

In a study from the University of Washington of School of Medicine, 648 AML patients undergoing allogeneic HSCT with MAC between 1995 and 2005 were evaluated.[31] The majority of patients had no history of CNS leukemia (n = 577); however, 71 patients had a prior diagnosis of CNS positivity (CNS+). Of these 71 patients, 52 received intrathecal chemotherapy alone as treatment and 19 received intrathecal chemotherapy with a CNS RT boost. Among the patients with CNS positivity, those who received RT had a significantly improved relapse-free survival (RFS) and OS. The 5-year RFS was 32% for the RT group and 6% for the intrathecal-alone group ($P < .001$). Furthermore, the 5-year OS of the RT group was significantly better (42%) than that of the intrathecal chemotherapy–alone group (6%, $P = .004$). The outcomes of the CNS+ patients who received RT were comparable with those of the 577 patients who had no prior history of CNS leukemia.

In acute lymphoblastic leukemia, the addition of a cranial boost may also reduce post allogeneic stem cell relapse. In a study from the University of Minnesota, with the addition of a cranial boost to myeloablative TBI-based regimens, the 2-year risk of CNS relapse was 0% among patients with a history of CNS disease who received a boost and 21% among those with prior CNS involvement who did not ($P = .03$).[32] There are conflicting studies however that suggest that CNS RT may not impact outcome for patients with CNS involvement before allogeneic SCT. In a study conducted at the Tehran University of Medical Sciences of 161 pediatric ALL patients undergoing TBI-free allogeneic HSCT, disease-free survival and OS were not significantly different among patients with or without a history of CNS disease.[33] It is important to note however that the outcome of pediatric patients with ALL is superior to that of adult patients;[34] therefore CNS relapses may have a more devastating impact among adult patients, and treatment intensification may be necessary.

For patients with a history of CNS leukemia undergoing allogeneic HSCT with a TBI-based myeloablative regimen, a cranial or craniospinal boost is often administered to provide therapeutic doses of RT to the CNS.[35] For patients who receive a non–TBI-based conditioning regimen, craniospinal irradiation (CSI) may be considered before HSCT. CSI may be administered with proton or photon RT. Proton treatment has the distinct advantage of dramatically reducing the dose to structures anterior to the vertebral body, which may have implications for toxicity. In a study from MD Anderson Cancer Center (MDACC), 37 consecutive patients were treated with CSI between 2011 and 2015, before allogeneic HSCT.[36] CSI was administered with protons in 14 patients to a median dose of 21.8 Gy and photons in 23 patients to a median dose of 24 Gy. Proton CSI was associated with lower rates of radiation therapy oncology group (RTOG) grade 1–3 mucositis during CSI (7% vs. 44%, $P = .03$);

however, toxicities during the HSCT admission and 100 days after SCT did not differ according to technique. Only one relapse occurred in the entire cohort. Although this study did not demonstrate a dramatic difference in acute toxicity with protons compared with photons, long-term toxicity may be reduced with the strategy. Additional follow-up is required to determine the impact of proton CSI on delayed treatment-related morbidity.

Toxicity after HSCT: contributions from TBI

Acute toxicity may arise after TBI and can include nausea, vomiting, fatigue, mucositis, diarrhea, and parotitis; these side effects are often mild.[37] The greatest concern regarding morbidity related to TBI, however, is the risk of subacute and long-term toxicity. Potential risk factors from TBI-containing conditioning regimens vary based on the TBI total dose and fractionation, age of the patient at the time of transplantation, and other patient-related factors; therefore it is critical that patients are counseled regarding potential posttherapy sequelae.[38]

GVHD. GVHD is a process in which infused donor lymphocytes target host tissue, a process if not put under control with the adequate therapy might lead to end-organ damage. The donor cells are thought to be stimulated by the foreign donor environment in addition to a cytokine-rich inflammatory environment.[39] The conditioning regimen administered before allogeneic HSCT can cause host tissue injury and a resultant inflammatory state that is thought to contribute to GHVD.[40] Based on this rationale, reduced-intensity conditioning regimens that minimize host tissue damage may decrease GVHD incidence and severity. Many studies have evaluated factors associated with increased rates of GVHD and have identified factors such as utilization of myeloablative conditioning (as compared to RIC),[41,42] use of tacrolimus-based GVHD prophylaxis (as compared to cyclosporine based), female donor to male recipient,[41,43] and greater degree of HLA mismatch for unrelated donor HSCT.[41,44] Utilization of TBI has also been shown to increase risk of GVHD. In a registry study of 6848 patients from the Japan Society for Hematopoietic Cell Transplantation, MAC regimens that contained TBI were significantly associated with elevated risks of acute grade 2–4 GVHD.[45] The adverse effect on GVHD risk was especially evident among older patients (>45 years) and HLA-matched donors (as compared to HLA-mismatched donor). Given that the risks for GVHD are multifactorial, utilization of TBI, intensity of conditioning regimen, and source of graft must all be considered on an individualized patient bases when choosing the optimal HSCT strategy.

Pulmonary toxicity. Pulmonary complications of allogeneic HSCT are common and can be severe, accounting for up to roughly 25% of transplant-related deaths in some studies.[46,47] Both infectious and non-infectious causes of pulmonary toxicity can occur in this at-risk population. Numerous factors associated with an increased risk of pulmonary toxicity have been identified, including older age, the development of GVHD, lower performance status before HSCT, utilization of methotrexate as GVHD prophylaxis, and lower pre-HSCT pulmonary function.[46,47]

Although several TBI-related factors have been recognized, severe pulmonary injury can be seen among HSCT patients treated with chemotherapy-only preparative regimens.[48–50] In a French randomized trial of 120 patients with CML randomized to Cy-TBI or BuCy, interstitial pneumonitis developed in 11 patients randomized to BuCy and in 12 patients who received Cy-TBI. This unfortunate toxicity was the only cause of death in eight patients, and it contributed to the death of seven patients in this study.[48] The Nordic Bone Marrow Transplantation Group reported long-term outcomes of 167 leukemia patients randomized to BuCy versus CyTBI.[50] As expected, the busulfan-treated patients had an increased risk of VOD of the liver (12% vs. 1%, $P = .01$) as well as hemorrhagic cystitis (32% vs. 10%, $P = .003$); however, obstructive bronchiolitis was also more frequent in the busulfan group (26% vs. 5%, $P < .01$). Interstitial pneumonitis was the cause of death in six patients in the busulfan arm and five patients treated with TBI.

Radiation delivery factors associated with increased risk of post-HSCT pulmonary toxicity have been identified including the use of large single fraction sizes, higher rate of radiation delivery (dose rate) and higher RT doses.[50a] The utilization of lung heterogeneity corrections can also impact dose delivery to the lungs. In a study by Kelsey et al., TBI plans administered without correcting for lung heterogeneity increased lung dose by 6%–43% higher than the intended prescribed dose.[51] In an effort to reduce RT lung exposure many advocate using lung blocks to restrict the lung dose to 8–10 Gy.[38,52,53] The potential benefits of blocking the lungs and other organs however must be weighed against the risk of shielding disease and marrow from irradiation.[54] When lung blocks are placed, care is taken to minimize shielding of bone in the chest wall and vertebral bodies (Fig. 4.1).

Secondary malignancies. As the outcomes after allogeneic HSCT improve, a larger population of transplant recipients will become long-term survivors. The use of a TBI-containing conditioning regimen has been

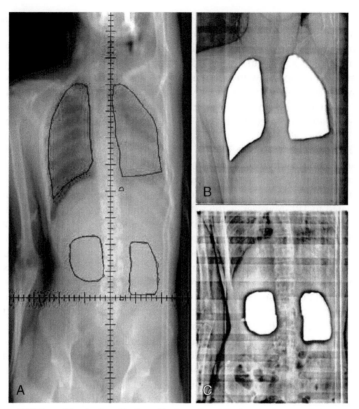

FIG. 4.1 Lung and Kidney Blocks in a Patient Undergoing Myeloablative Total-Body Irradiation for Acute Lymphoblastic Leukemia. (A) Digitally reconstructed radiograph created from a computed tomography (CT) simulation data set of a patient with Philadelphia chromosome–negative acute lymphoblastic leukemia who underwent matched unrelated donor allogeneic stem cell transplantation with a myeloablative regimen of 12 Gy total-body irradiation (delivered over 4 consecutive days in 3 Gy fractions), etoposide, and Anti-thymocyte globulin (ATG). The lung blocks and kidney blocks were delineated by the radiation oncologist with attention paid to minimizing shielding of the chest wall and vertebral bodies. The lung and kidney blocks were used for one of four fractions. Port films were acquired on the day of treatment to verify accurate positioning of the **(B)** lung and **(C)** kidney blocks before treatment delivery.

identified as an important risk factor for the development of secondary solid tumors. To date, the largest study to evaluate long-term secondary solid malignancy risk among allogeneic HSCT recipients reported the outcomes of a multi-institutional cohort of 28,874 patients with 189 solid tumors.[55] This large group of survivors had a median age of 27 years at the time of HSCT; 74% received HSCT for leukemia; and TBI was a component of conditioning for 67% of patients. Using a competing risk analysis approach, the cumulative incidence of developing a solid tumor was 1% at 10 years, 2.2% at 15 years, and 3.5% at 20 years. When a Kaplan–Meier method was used, the cumulative incidence was 2.5%, 5.8%, and 8.8% at 10, 15, and 20 years, respectively. These observations correlated with twice the risk

of the general population. The most notable risk factors identified in this large cohort study were the age at the time of allogeneic HSCT as well as RT exposure. Pediatric patients who received TBI at age 10 years or younger had a 55-fold increased risk of non–squamous cell carcinoma (SCC) second solid cancer development. Patients aged 10–19 and 20–29 years had four- to six-fold increased risk; however, for adult patients who received TBI at the age of 30 years or more, no excess risk was observed. This is an important consideration in regards to long-term risk when adult patients above the age of 30 years are considered for a TBI containing conditioning regimen prior to allogeneic HSCT. In this study the risk of SCC was linked to chronic GVHD and male gender, regardless of the age at the time of transplantation.

Interestingly in this large study, mainly myeloablative RT doses were used, either as a single fraction or fractionated, with 12–13 Gy fractionated TBI administered most commonly. Therefore in this report the impact of lower RT doses for TBI that are often used in RIC regimens is unclear. A previous study of more than 19,000 patients who underwent allogeneic HSCT between 1964 and 1992 found that lower doses of TBI (<12 Gy) were associated with lower risk of secondary cancers; however, only 11.45% of patients who received TBI were given single doses of less than 10 Gy, and it was not reported how many patients received very low TBI doses of 2–5 Gy.[56] Given data on atomic bomb survivors who have demonstrated an increased risk of secondary cancers despite lower total-body RT doses, clarification on the impact of low-dose TBI (especially 2 Gy) on secondary malignancy development is needed.[57–59]

While TBI is an important risk factor for the development of secondary solid cancers after allogeneic HSCT, chemotherapy-only conditioning regimens do confer an increased risk of secondary cancers over the general population. In a study of 4318 allogeneic HSCT recipients the risk of invasive solid cancers was 1.4 times higher than the expected rate.[60] In particular, cancers of the oral cavity, lung, brain, and esophagus were observed. Chronic GVHD was also found to be an independent risk factor for the development of solid tumors, especially those of the oral cavity. Therefore the aforementioned results suggest that second malignancies might be related to the immune suppression status.

Other toxicities. Additional toxicity concerns exist after allogeneic HSCT with MAC regimens with or without TBI, including hypothyroidism,[61] cataracts,[62] kidney dysfunction,[63] decreased bone density,[64] neurocognitive effects,[65] and sterility.[66] The magnitude of these risks vary based on the patient's age, preexisting therapies, and the conditioning regimen chosen. Therefore it is critical that the conditioning regimen chosen is individualized to optimize the regimen with the maximized therapeutic ration for each patient. In addition, for long-term survivors, follow-up is crucial to optimally manage toxicity from therapy.

THE ROLE OF RT AMONG PATIENTS WITH HODGKIN LYMPHOMA AND NON-HODGKIN LYMPHOMA UNDERGOING HSCT

Hodgkin Lymphoma

Hodgkin lymphoma (HL) is often cured with doxorubicin-based chemotherapy with or without consolidative RT.[67,68] However, a proportion of patients will relapse after initial therapy or will have disease that is refractory to frontline treatment. For this patient population, high-dose systemic therapy with autologous stem cell rescue offers improved outcomes over conventional chemotherapy.[69] After autologous SCT, sites of disease involvement at relapse are the most frequent sites of failure after intensive chemotherapy and autologous stem cell rescue.[70–72] In a study of 69 HL patients who received high-dose chemotherapy and autologous SCT, 91% of relapses were at initial sites of disease among early-stage HL patients; moreover, 71% were solely in previously involved sites.[71] In another study of patients with relapsed or refractory HL who underwent autologous SCT, 92.3% of relapses involved a site of previous disease after treatment with high-dose chemotherapy and autologous SCT alone.[72]

While no randomized studies have been conducted to evaluate the potential benefit of peritransplant RT in reducing treatment failure, numerous single and multiinstitutional studies have been performed to address this question.[70,73–77] Although the timing and indications for RT varied between studies, factors across studies that suggest a potential benefit for RT include the presence of bulky disease, limited-stage disease at the time of relapse, and the presence of positron emission tomography (PET)–positive disease just before autologous SCT (Table 4.1).

Outcomes for relapsed and refractory HL patients continue to improve with the introduction of targeted therapies. The phase III study of Brentuximab Vedotin in patients at high risk of residual HL following SCT (the AETHERA trial), randomized 329 primary refractory or unfavorable HL patients to postautologous SCT brentuximab vedotin or placebo between 2010 and 2012. To be considered for the study, patients had to have one risk factor: relapse within 12 months from initial disease remission, extranodal HL at the time of relapse before salvage chemotherapy, or primary refractory disease. Patients who received brentuximab had significantly improved progression-free survival (PFS) (HR 0.57, $P = .0013$), with a median PFS of 42.9 months (compared to 24.1 months in the placebo arm). In the study, 7% of patients in the brentuximab arm had some form of RT as a component of SCT conditioning. The proportion of patients who received consolidative RT are not reported; however, 13% of patients received RT as a subsequent form of treatment after SCT and brentuximab. There is some controversy regarding which patients should receive brentuximab after autologous SCT. The role of RT in this new era of targeted consolidative therapy remains elusive.

TABLE 4.1
Retrospective Studies Among Hodgkin Lymphoma Patients Treated with and Without Peritransplant Radiation Therapy

Study	Year	Patient#	Conditioning	Patients Receiving RT	RT Technique	Timing in Relation to HSCT	Median RT Dose (Range)	Outcome	Subsets of Patients Benefiting From RT
Biswal (East Carolina University, Duke and University of Rochester)[73]	1993–2003	62	BEAC	32	IFRT	After	30.6 Gy (6–44.2)	3-year OS, 69.6 versus 40 ($P=.05$); DSS, 82.1 versus 57.6% ($P=0.08$); and LC ($P=0.03$)	Bulky disease for DFS ($P=.032$)
Kahn (Emory)[74]	1995–2008	92	BuCyE	46	IFRT	83% before	30 Gy (21–45)	DFS not significant ($P=0.204$)	
Eroglu (Turkey)[75]	1995–2012	45	BEAM or ICE	21	IFRT	76% before	30 Gy (25–44)	5-year OS, 81% IFRT versus 48% no RT, $P=.045$ for early-stage patients	1–2 nodal regions at relapse, early-stage patients
Levis (Italy)[76]	2003–14	73	BEAM or FEAM	21	IFRT	Before or within 3 weeks	30 Gy (25.2–43.2)	Overall no difference with IFRT but worse prognostic factors in IFRT group	Limited-stage disease at relapse and PET positive had trend to improved PFS
Wilke (University of Minnesota Transplant Database)[77]	2005–14	80	Cyclophosphamide, carmustine, and etoposide	32	"localized fields limited to areas of disease involvement before transplantation or radiographically suspicious"	After	30.6 Gy (16–44)	Improved PFS with RT (67% vs. 42%, $P=.01$)	Bulky disease ($P=0.02$), B symptoms ($P=0.05$), primary refractory HL ($P=0.02$), partial response on pretransplant imaging ($P=0.02$)
Milgrom (University of Penn and MDACC)[70]	2006–15	189	BCNU, BEAM, or CBV	22	Varied	After in 95%	36 Gy (25.2–41.4)	No difference in LC, PFS, or OS	Local control benefit among primary refractory disease and FDG avid at the time of SCT ($P=0.02$)

BEAC, BCNU, etoposide, cytarabine, cyclophosphamide; *BEAM*, BCNU, etoposide, Ara–C, and melphalan; *BuCyE*, Busulfan, cyclophosphamide, and etoposide; *CBV*, cyclophosphamide, BCNU, and VP-16; *DFS*, disease-free survival; *DSS*, disease-specific survival; *IFRT*, involved field radiation therapy; *LC*, local control; *PFS*, progression-free survival.

Non-Hodgkin Lymphoma

Diffuse large B cell lymphoma (DLBCL) is the most common subtype of non-Hodgkin lymphoma (NHL), representing roughly one-third of all newly diagnosed NHL cases.[78] Chemoimmunotherapy, usually with rituximab, cyclophosphamide, vincristine, doxorubicin, and prednisone, (R–CHOP) is successful as frontline therapy in most cases; however, roughly one-third of patients will have refractory disease or relapse after a complete response to upfront treatment.[78,79] Patients who develop relapsed or refractory disease often have a poor prognosis. The PARMA trial established high-dose chemotherapy followed by autologous bone marrow transplantation as the standard of care for patients with chemotherapy-sensitive relapsed NHL over conventional salvage chemotherapy alone.[80] Patients who did not undergo autologous SCT had a 5-year event-free survival rate of only 12% and 5-year OS rate of 32%.

The rationale for the use of RT in the peritransplant setting for patients with NHL, particularly DLBCL, is similar to that of HL: Relapses at sites of previous disease involvement dominate the pattern of failure.[81–83] In a retrospective study of 100 patients with DLBCL who underwent high-dose chemotherapy and HSCT at the University of Rochester between 1992 and 2014, 40% of early-stage patients and 76% of advanced-stage patients relapsed at sites of initial disease. Furthermore, 69% of early-stage patients and 75% of advanced-stage patients relapsed in sites of initial disease only. Patterns of relapse studies such as this one highlight a potential role for RT in improving local control and PFS.

Positron emission tomography–computed tomography (PET-CT) imaging can be a useful prognostic tool, especially for patients with relapsed and refractory DLBCL. PET-CT response to salvage chemotherapy can predict outcomes after autologous SCT in this patient population. In a retrospective study from Memorial Sloan-Kettering Cancer Center of 129 adult patients with relapsed and refractory DLBCL who were undergoing autologous SCT, the only pretransplant risk factor that impacted PFS and OS was PET-CT response to salvage chemotherapy.[84] Patients with a Deauville response of 1–3 had a 3-year PFS and OS of 77% and 86%, whereas those with Deauville 4 response had inferior rates of 49% and 54%, respectively.

In the absence of randomized data, many clinicians as well as the International Lymphoma Radiation Oncology Group advocate peritransplant RT for patients with limited-stage NHL, bulky disease, as well as for those with persistent fluorodeoxyglucose (FDG) avid disease before transplantation. In each case the potential risks and benefits of RT are considered, including the anticipated toxicity profile of a given RT field, response to salvage chemotherapy, and the risk of relapse at a particular site.[85]

Toxicity Among HL and NHL Patients

As most patients who receive consolidative RT after autologous SCT have treatment fields that include the mediastinum, the most concerning acute toxicity is pneumonitis. Although most modern series have demonstrated that RT is well tolerated, some studies have reported higher TRM after involved field RT to the thorax due to radiation pneumonitis that in certain cases was fatal. Tsang et al. reported on the outcome of 50 patients with relapsed and refractory HL who underwent autologous SCT.[86] Increased toxic deaths were observed among patients who were treated with RT.

The administration of high-dose therapy and autologous SCT have been shown to the increase the risk of radiation pneumonitis. Investigators at the Dana-Farber Cancer Institute evaluated risk factors for radiation pneumonitis among 92 patients with HL treated with three-dimensional conformal mediastinal RT.[87] Among the patients treated in the peritransplant setting, 35% of patients experienced radiation pneumonitis compared with 10% of patients who were treated with mediastinal RT as a component of upfront combined modality therapy. The grade of radiation pneumonitis was also more severe in the peritransplant group. The timing of RT in reference to transplant seemed to impact risk as well, with patients who received pretransplant RT at greater risk for grade 3 radiation pneumonitis (57%) compared with those treated after transplantation (0%, $P = .015$). Dosimetric factors were also identified which increased the risk of this toxicity.

In a study evaluating risk factors for radiation pneumonitis among lymphoma patients treated with contemporary radiation via intensity-modulated radiation therapy (IMRT) to the mediastinum at MDACC, patients who received RT in the setting of high-dose chemotherapy and autologous SCT also experienced higher rates of symptomatic radiation pneumonitis (25%) than those who received RT as a component of initial combined modality therapy (10%, $P = .019$).[88] Several dosimetric factors were identified which correlated with the risk of pneumonitis, including the mean lung dose and volume of lung that received a dose of 5 Gy (V5).

Radiation oncologists can decrease the risk of radiation pneumonitis in this patient population through the utilization of advanced technology, including IMRT and deep inspiration breath hold. Deep inspiration breath hold can result in reduced RT lung doses via (1) minimization of respiratory motion, thereby permitting smaller field sizes and (2) increase in lung volume

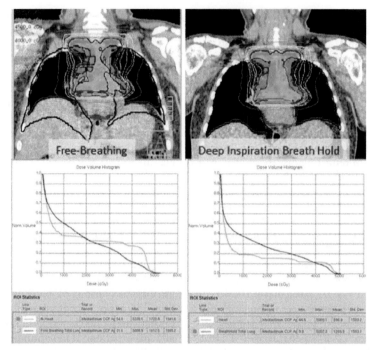

FIG. 4.2 Consolidative Mediastinal Radiation Therapy Administered After Autologous Stem Cell Transplantation. Radiation planning without motion management (free-breathing, left panel) was compared with deep inspiration breath hold planning (right panel). Deep inspiration breath hold resulted in enhanced expansion of the lung with resulting larger lung volumes. In the left panel the free-breathing lung volume is delineated in purple. The deep inspiration breath hold lung volume is superimposed on the free-breathing scan (blue). Deep inspiration breath hold planning resulted in lower mean heart dose (8.9 Gy) as compared with free breathing (17.2 Gy). The mean total lung dose was also significantly reduced with deep inspiration breath hold planning (12.6 vs. 16.1 Gy). A dose–volume histogram illustrates the differences in the volume of heart (teal) and lung (purple) exposed to various radiation doses with free-breathing planning (left) as compared with deep inspiration breath hold planning (right).

during RT delivery which results in reduced lung doses (Fig. 4.2). This technology can result in improved ability to meet lung dose constraints that are associated with decreased risk of radiation pneumonitis, including mean lung dose of less than 13.5 Gy and V5<55%.[89]

CONCLUSIONS

The outcomes of patients undergoing HSCT for hematologic malignancies are improving. TBI is a specialized RT technique that may be used in conjunction with chemotherapy as a preparative regimen before allogeneic HSCT with the goal of ablating the recipient's hematopoietic stem cell system and in some cases eradicating residual disease. As the utilization of RIC regimens increases, additional studies are required to determine the potential benefit of low-dose TBI-containing regimens over chemotherapy-alone conditioning approaches. For patients with HL and NHL undergoing autologous stem cell transplantation, RT can provide local control to sites of chemorefractory and/or bulky disease. Modern RT delivery techniques, including proton beam RT, IMRT, and breath hold are currently used with the goal of reducing normal tissue RT exposure and long-term RT morbidity. With these approaches the therapeutic ratio may be altered such that RT-related long-term toxicity is limited. With this in mind, more clinicians may opt to include RT in the peritransplant setting to improve disease control.

ACKNOWLEDGMENTS

The author would like to thank Drs. Sarah Milgrom, Jillian Gunther, and Bouthaina Dabaja for their critical feedback and meticulous proofreading of the chapter.

DISCLOSURE STATEMENT

Dr. Pinnix receives research support from Merck & Co and an honorarium from the Internation Journal of Radiation Oncology, Biology and Physics.

REFERENCES

1. Gale RP, Butturini A, Bortin MM. What does total body irradiation do in bone marrow transplants for leukemia? *Int J Radiat Oncol Biol Phys.* 1991;20:631–634.
2. Wolden SL, Rabinovitch RA, Bittner NH, et al. American College of Radiology (ACR) and American Society for radiation oncology (ASTRO) practice guideline for the performance of total body irradiation (TBI). *Am J Clin Oncol.* 2013;36:97–101.
3. Perez-Simon JA, Diez-Campelo M, Martino R, et al. Influence of the intensity of the conditioning regimen on the characteristics of acute and chronic graft-versus-host disease after allogeneic transplantation. *Br J Haematol.* 2005;130:394–403.
4. Tanaka J, Kanamori H, Nishiwaki S, et al. Reduced-intensity vs myeloablative conditioning allogeneic hematopoietic SCT for patients aged over 45 years with ALL in remission: a study from the Adult ALL Working Group of the Japan Society for Hematopoietic Cell Transplantation (JSHCT). *Bone Marrow Transpl.* 2013;48:1389–1394.
5. Thomas ED, Buckner CD, Banaji M, et al. One hundred patients with acute leukemia treated by chemotherapy, total body irradiation, and allogeneic marrow transplantation. *Blood.* 1977;49:511–533.
6. Thomas ED, Buckner CD, Clift RA, et al. Marrow transplantation for acute nonlymphoblastic leukemia in first remission. *N Engl J Med.* 1979;301:597–599.
7. Thomas ED, Clift RA, Hersman J, et al. Marrow transplantation for acute nonlymphoblastic leukemic in first remission using fractionated or single-dose irradiation. *Int J Radiat Oncol Biol Phys.* 1982;8:817–821.
8. Clift RA, Buckner CD, Appelbaum FR, et al. Allogeneic marrow transplantation in patients with acute myeloid leukemia in first remission: a randomized trial of two irradiation regimens. *Blood.* 1990;76:1867–1871.
9. Clift RA, Buckner CD, Appelbaum FR, et al. Allogeneic marrow transplantation in patients with chronic myeloid leukemia in the chronic phase: a randomized trial of two irradiation regimens. *Blood.* 1991;77:1660–1665.
10. Santos GW, Kaizer H. Bone marrow transplantation in acute leukemia. *Semin Hematol.* 1982;19:227–239.
11. Santos GW, Tutschka PJ, Brookmeyer R, et al. Marrow transplantation for acute nonlymphocytic leukemia after treatment with busulfan and cyclophosphamide. *N Engl J Med.* 1983;309:1347–1353.
12. Blaise D, Maraninchi D, Archimbaud E, et al. Allogeneic bone marrow transplantation for acute myeloid leukemia in first remission: a randomized trial of a busulfan-Cytoxan versus Cytoxan-total body irradiation as preparative regimen: a report from the Group d'Etudes de la Greffe de Moelle Osseuse. *Blood.* 1992;79:2578–2582.
13. Blaise D, Maraninchi D, Michallet M, et al. Long-term follow-up of a randomized trial comparing the combination of cyclophosphamide with total body irradiation or busulfan as conditioning regimen for patients receiving HLA-identical marrow grafts for acute myeloblastic leukemia in first complete remission. *Blood.* 2001;97:3669–3671.
14. Socie G, Clift RA, Blaise D, et al. Busulfan plus cyclophosphamide compared with total-body irradiation plus cyclophosphamide before marrow transplantation for myeloid leukemia: long-term follow-up of 4 randomized studies. *Blood.* 2001;98:3569–3574.
15. Copelan EA, Hamilton BK, Avalos B, et al. Better leukemia-free and overall survival in AML in first remission following cyclophosphamide in combination with busulfan compared with TBI. *Blood.* 2013;122:3863–3870.
16. Champlin RE. Busulfan or TBI: answer to an age-old question. *Blood.* 2013;122:3856–3857.
17. Savani BN, Montero A, Wu C, et al. Prediction and prevention of transplant-related mortality from pulmonary causes after total body irradiation and allogeneic stem cell transplantation. *Biol Blood Marrow Transpl.* 2005;11:223–230.
18. Giralt S, Estey E, Albitar M, et al. Engraftment of allogeneic hematopoietic progenitor cells with purine analog-containing chemotherapy: harnessing graft-versus-leukemia without myeloablative therapy. *Blood.* 1997;89:4531–4536.
19. McSweeney PA, Niederwieser D, Shizuru JA, et al. Hematopoietic cell transplantation in older patients with hematologic malignancies: replacing high-dose cytotoxic therapy with graft-versus-tumor effects. *Blood.* 2001;97:3390–3400. PMID: 11369628.
20. Storb R, Yu C, Wagner JL, et al. Stable mixed hematopoietic chimerism in DLA-identical littermate dogs given sublethal total body irradiation before and pharmacological immunosuppression after marrow transplantation. *Blood.* 1997;89:3048–3054.
21. Storb R, Raff RF, Appelbaum FR, et al. What radiation dose for DLA-identical canine marrow grafts? *Blood.* 1988;72:1300–1304.
22. Marks DI, Wang T, Perez WS, et al. The outcome of full-intensity and reduced-intensity conditioning matched sibling or unrelated donor transplantation in adults with Philadelphia chromosome-negative acute lymphoblastic leukemia in first and second complete remission. *Blood.* 2010;116:366–374.
23. Sorror ML, Sandmaier BM, Storer BE, et al. Long-term outcomes among older patients following nonmyeloablative conditioning and allogeneic hematopoietic cell transplantation for advanced hematologic malignancies. *JAMA.* 2011;306:1874–1883.

24. Fasslrinner F, Schetelig J, Burchert A, et al. Long-term efficacy of reduced-intensity versus myeloablative conditioning before allogeneic haemopoietic cell transplantation in patients with acute myeloid leukaemia in first complete remission: retrospective follow-up of an open-label, randomised phase 3 trial. *Lancet Haematol.* 2018;5:e161–e169.

25. Bornhauser M, Kienast J, Trenschel R, et al. Reduced-intensity conditioning versus standard conditioning before allogeneic haemopoietic cell transplantation in patients with acute myeloid leukaemia in first complete remission: a prospective, open-label randomised phase 3 trial. *Lancet Oncol.* 2012;13:1035–1044.

26. Craddock C. Conditioning intensity in HCT for AML: the jury is still out. *Lancet Haematol.* 2018;5:e132–e133.

27. Davies JK, Taussig DC, Oakervee H, et al. Long-term follow-up after reduced-intensity conditioning allogeneic transplantation for acute myeloid leukemia/myelodysplastic syndrome: late CNS relapses despite graft-versus-host disease. *J Clin Oncol.* 2006;24:e23–e25.

28. Ostronoff M, Domingues MC, Ostronoff F, et al. Reduced intensity conditioning allogeneic bone marrow transplantation following central nervous system (CNS) relapse of acute promyelocytic leukemia: evidence for a graft-versus-leukemia effect in the CNS. *Am J Hematol.* 2006;81:387–388.

29. Aoki J, Ishiyama K, Taniguchi S, et al. Outcome of allogeneic hematopoietic stem cell transplantation for acute myeloid leukemia patients with central nervous system involvement. *Biol Blood Marrow Transpl.* 2014;20:2029–2033.

30. Hamdi A, Mawad R, Bassett R, et al. Central nervous system relapse in adults with acute lymphoblastic leukemia after allogeneic hematopoietic stem cell transplantation. *Biol Blood Marrow Transpl.* 2014;20:1767–1771.

31. Mayadev JS, Douglas JG, Storer BE, et al. Impact of cranial irradiation added to intrathecal conditioning in hematopoietic cell transplantation in adult acute myeloid leukemia with central nervous system involvement. *Int J Radiat Oncol Biol Phys.* 2011;80:193–198.

32. Gao RW, Dusenbery KE, Cao Q, et al. Augmenting total body irradiation with a cranial boost before stem cell transplantation protects against post-transplant central nervous system relapse in acute lymphoblastic leukemia. *Biol Blood Marrow Transpl.* 2018;24:501–506.

33. Hamidieh AA, Monzavi SM, Kaboutari M, et al. Outcome analysis of pediatric patients with acute lymphoblastic leukemia treated with total body irradiation-free allogeneic hematopoietic stem cell transplantation: comparison of patients with and without central nervous system involvement. *Biol Blood Marrow Transpl.* 2017;23:2110–2117.

34. Muffly L, Lichtensztajn D, Shiraz P, et al. Adoption of pediatric-inspired acute lymphoblastic leukemia regimens by adult oncologists treating adolescents and young adults: a population-based study. *Cancer.* 2017;123:122–130.

35. Su W, Thompson M, Sheu RD, et al. Low-dose cranial boost in high-risk adult acute lymphoblastic leukemia patients undergoing bone marrow transplant. *Pract Radiat Oncol.* 2017;7:103–108.

36. Gunther JR, Rahman AR, Dong W, et al. Craniospinal irradiation prior to stem cell transplant for hematologic malignancies with CNS involvement: effectiveness and toxicity after photon or proton treatment. *Pract Radiat Oncol.* 2017;7:e401–e408.

37. Buchali A, Feyer P, Groll J, et al. Immediate toxicity during fractionated total body irradiation as conditioning for bone marrow transplantation. *Radiother Oncol.* 2000;54:157–162.

38. Radiology ACo. *ACR–ASTRO Practice Parameter for the Performance of Total Body Irradiation;* 2017.

39. Harris AC, Ferrara JL, Levine JE. Advances in predicting acute GVHD. *Br J Haematol.* 2013;160:288–302.

40. Ferrara JL, Levine JE, Reddy P, Holler E. Graft-versus-host disease. *Lancet.* 2009;373:1550–1561.

41. Jagasia M, Arora M, Flowers ME, et al. Risk factors for acute GVHD and survival after hematopoietic cell transplantation. *Blood.* 2012;119:296–307.

42. Mielcarek M, Martin PJ, Leisenring W, et al. Graft-versus-host disease after nonmyeloablative versus conventional hematopoietic stem cell transplantation. *Blood.* 2003;102:756–762.

43. Gale RP, Bortin MM, van Bekkum DW, et al. Risk factors for acute graft-versus-host disease. *Br J Haematol.* 1987;67:397–406.

44. Arora M, Weisdorf DJ, Spellman SR, et al. HLA-identical sibling compared with 8/8 matched and mismatched unrelated donor bone marrow transplant for chronic phase chronic myeloid leukemia. *J Clin Oncol.* 2009;27:1644–1652.

45. Nakasone H, Fukuda T, Kanda J, et al. Impact of conditioning intensity and TBI on acute GVHD after hematopoietic cell transplantation. *Bone Marrow Transpl.* 2015;50:559–565.

46. Weiner RS, Bortin MM, Gale RP, et al. Interstitial pneumonitis after bone marrow transplantation. Assessment of risk factors. *Ann Intern Med.* 1986;104:168–175.

47. Ho VT, Weller E, Lee SJ, et al. Prognostic factors for early severe pulmonary complications after hematopoietic stem cell transplantation. *Biol Blood Marrow Transpl.* 2001;7:223–229.

48. Devergie A, Blaise D, Attal M, et al. Allogeneic bone marrow transplantation for chronic myeloid leukemia in first chronic phase: a randomized trial of busulfan-cytoxan versus cytoxan-total body irradiation as preparative regimen: a report from the French Society of Bone Marrow Graft (SFGM). *Blood.* 1995;85:2263–2268.

49. Kroger N, Zabelina T, Kruger W, et al. Comparison of total body irradiation vs busulfan in combination with cyclophosphamide as conditioning for unrelated stem cell transplantation in CML patients. *Bone Marrow Transpl.* 2001;27:349–354.

50. Ringden O, Remberger M, Ruutu T, et al. Increased risk of chronic graft-versus-host disease, obstructive bronchiolitis, and alopecia with busulfan versus total body irradiation: long-term results of a randomized trial in allogeneic marrow recipients with leukemia. Nordic Bone Marrow Transplantation Group. *Blood.* 1999;93:2196–2201.

50a. Wong JYC1, Filippi AR2, Dabaja BS3. Total Body Irradiation: Guidelines from the International Lymphoma Radiation Oncology Group (ILROG). PMID: 29893272.

51. Kelsey CR, Horwitz ME, Chino JP, et al. Severe pulmonary toxicity after myeloablative conditioning using total body irradiation: an assessment of risk factors. *Int J Radiat Oncol Biol Phys.* 2011;81:812–818.

52. Della Volpe A, Ferreri AJ, Annaloro C, et al. Lethal pulmonary complications significantly correlate with individually assessed mean lung dose in patients with hematologic malignancies treated with total body irradiation. *Int J Radiat Oncol Biol Phys.* 2002;52:483–488.

53. Soule BP, Simone NL, Savani BN, et al. Pulmonary function following total body irradiation (with or without lung shielding) and allogeneic peripheral blood stem cell transplant. *Bone Marrow Transpl.* 2007;40:573–578.

54. Anderson JE, Appelbaum FR, Schoch G, et al. Relapse after allogeneic bone marrow transplantation for refractory anemia is increased by shielding lungs and liver during total body irradiation. *Biol Blood Marrow Transpl.* 2001;7:163–170.

55. Rizzo JD, Curtis RE, Socie G, et al. Solid cancers after allogeneic hematopoietic cell transplantation. *Blood.* 2009;113:1175–1183.

56. Curtis RE, Rowlings PA, Deeg HJ, et al. Solid cancers after bone marrow transplantation. *N Engl J Med.* 1997;336:897–904.

57. Hsieh MM, Fitzhugh CD, Tisdale JF. Incidence of second cancers after allogeneic hematopoietic stem cell transplantation using reduced-dose radiation. *Blood.* 2009;114: 225; author reply 225–226.

58. Preston DL, Shimizu Y, Pierce DA, et al. Studies of mortality of atomic bomb survivors. Report 13: solid cancer and noncancer disease mortality: 1950-1997. *Radiat Res.* 2003;160:381–407.

59. Preston DL, Pierce DA, Shimizu Y, et al. Dose response and temporal patterns of radiation-associated solid cancer risks. *Health Phys.* 2003;85:43–46.

60. Majhail NS, Brazauskas R, Rizzo JD, et al. Secondary solid cancers after allogeneic hematopoietic cell transplantation using busulfan-cyclophosphamide conditioning. *Blood.* 2011;117:316–322.

61. Al-Hazzouri A, Cao Q, Burns LJ, et al. Similar risks for hypothyroidism after allogeneic hematopoietic cell transplantation using TBI-based myeloablative and reduced-intensity conditioning regimens. *Bone Marrow Transpl.* 2009;43:949–951.

62. Ozsahin M, Belkacemi Y, Pene F, et al. Total-body irradiation and cataract incidence: a randomized comparison of two instantaneous dose rates. *Int J Radiat Oncol Biol Phys.* 1994;28:343–347.

63. Hingorani S. Chronic kidney disease in long-term survivors of hematopoietic cell transplantation: epidemiology, pathogenesis, and treatment. *J Am Soc Nephrol.* 2006;17:1995–2005.

64. Stern JM, Sullivan KM, Ott SM, et al. Bone density loss after allogeneic hematopoietic stem cell transplantation: a prospective study. *Biol Blood Marrow Transpl.* 2001;7:257–264.

65. Hiniker SM, Agarwal R, Modlin LA, et al. Survival and neurocognitive outcomes after cranial or craniospinal irradiation plus total-body irradiation before stem cell transplantation in pediatric leukemia patients with central nervous system involvement. *Int J Radiat Oncol Biol Phys.* 2014;89:67–74.

66. Mertens AC, Ramsay NK, Kouris S, Neglia JP. Patterns of gonadal dysfunction following bone marrow transplantation. *Bone Marrow Transpl.* 1998;22:345–350.

67. Eich HT, Diehl V, Gorgen H, et al. Intensified chemotherapy and dose-reduced involved-field radiotherapy in patients with early unfavorable Hodgkin's lymphoma: final analysis of the German Hodgkin Study Group HD11 trial. *J Clin Oncol.* 2010;28:4199–4206.

68. Engert A, Plutschow A, Eich HT, et al. Reduced treatment intensity in patients with early-stage Hodgkin's lymphoma. *N Engl J Med.* 2010;363:640–652.

69. Linch DC, Winfield D, Goldstone AH, et al. Dose intensification with autologous bone-marrow transplantation in relapsed and resistant Hodgkin's disease: results of a BNLI randomised trial. *Lancet.* 1993;341:1051–1054.

70. Milgrom SA, Jauhari S, Plastaras JP, et al. A multi-institutional analysis of peritransplantation radiotherapy in patients with relapsed/refractory Hodgkin lymphoma undergoing autologous stem cell transplantation. *Cancer.* 2017;123:1363–1371.

71. Dhakal S, Biswas T, Liesveld JL, et al. Patterns and timing of initial relapse in patients subsequently undergoing transplantation for Hodgkin's lymphoma. *Int J Radiat Oncol Biol Phys.* 2009;75:188–192.

72. Mundt AJ, Sibley G, Williams S, et al. Patterns of failure following high-dose chemotherapy and autologous bone marrow transplantation with involved field radiotherapy for relapsed/refractory Hodgkin's disease. *Int J Radiat Oncol Biol Phys.* 1995;33:261–270.

73. Biswas T, Culakova E, Friedberg JW, et al. Involved field radiation therapy following high dose chemotherapy and autologous stem cell transplant benefits local control and survival in refractory or recurrent Hodgkin lymphoma. *Radiother Oncol.* 2012;103:367–372.

74. Kahn S, Flowers C, Xu Z, Esiashvili N. Does the addition of involved field radiotherapy to high-dose chemotherapy and stem cell transplantation improve outcomes for patients with relapsed/refractory Hodgkin lymphoma? *Int J Radiat Oncol Biol Phys.* 2011;81:175–180.

75. Eroglu C, Kaynar L, Orhan O, et al. Contribution of involved-field radiotherapy to survival in patients with relapsed or refractory Hodgkin lymphoma undergoing autologous stem cell transplantation. *Am J Clin Oncol.* 2015;38:68–73.

76. Levis M, Piva C, Filippi AR, et al. Potential benefit of involved-field radiotherapy for patients with relapsed-refractory Hodgkin's lymphoma with incomplete response before autologous stem cell transplantation. *Clin Lymphoma Myeloma Leuk.* 2017;17:14–22.

77. Wilke C, Cao Q, Dusenbery KE, et al. Role of consolidative radiation therapy after autologous hematopoietic cell transplantation for the treatment of relapsed or refractory Hodgkin lymphoma. *Int J Radiat Oncol Biol Phys.* 2017;99:94–102.

78. Roschewski M, Staudt LM, Wilson WH. Diffuse large B-cell lymphoma-treatment approaches in the molecular era. *Nat Rev Clin Oncol.* 2014;11:12–23.

79. Fisher RI, Gaynor ER, Dahlberg S, et al. Comparison of a standard regimen (CHOP) with three intensive chemotherapy regimens for advanced non-Hodgkin's lymphoma. *N Engl J Med.* 1993;328:1002–1006.

80. Philip T, Guglielmi C, Hagenbeek A, et al. Autologous bone marrow transplantation as compared with salvage chemotherapy in relapses of chemotherapy-sensitive non-Hodgkin's lymphoma. *N Engl J Med.* 1995;333:1540–1545.

81. Takvorian T, Canellos GP, Ritz J, et al. Prolonged disease-free survival after autologous bone marrow transplantation in patients with non-Hodgkin's lymphoma with a poor prognosis. *N Engl J Med.* 1987;316:1499–1505.

82. Philip T, Armitage JO, Spitzer G, et al. High-dose therapy and autologous bone marrow transplantation after failure of conventional chemotherapy in adults with intermediate-grade or high-grade non-Hodgkin's lymphoma. *N Engl J Med.* 1987;316:1493–1498.

83. Dhakal S, Bates JE, Casulo C, et al. Patterns and timing of failure for diffuse large B-Cell lymphoma after initial therapy in a cohort who underwent autologous bone marrow transplantation for relapse. *Int J Radiat Oncol Biol Phys.* 2016;96:372–378.

84. Sauter CS, Matasar MJ, Meikle J, et al. Prognostic value of FDG-PET prior to autologous stem cell transplantation for relapsed and refractory diffuse large B-cell lymphoma. *Blood.* 2015;125:2579–2581.

85. Ng AK, Yahalom J, Goda JS, et al. Role of radiation therapy in patients with relapsed/refractory diffuse large B-Cell lymphoma: guidelines from the international lymphoma radiation oncology group. *Int J Radiat Oncol Biol Phys.* 2018;100:652–669.

86. Tsang RW, Gospodarowicz MK, Sutcliffe SB, et al. Thoracic radiation therapy before autologous bone marrow transplantation in relapsed or refractory Hodgkin's disease. PMH Lymphoma Group, and the Toronto Autologous BMT Group. *Eur J Cancer.* 1999;35:73–78.

87. Fox AM, Dosoretz AP, Mauch PM, et al. Predictive factors for radiation pneumonitis in Hodgkin lymphoma patients receiving combined-modality therapy. *Int J Radiat Oncol Biol Phys.* 2012;83:277–283.

88. Pinnix CC, Smith GL, Milgrom S, et al. Predictors of radiation pneumonitis in patients receiving intensity modulated radiation therapy for Hodgkin and non-Hodgkin lymphoma. *Int J Radiat Oncol Biol Phys.* 2015;92:175–182.

89. Pinnix CC1, Huo J2, Milgrom SA1, et al. Using benchmarked lung radiation dose constraints to predict pneumonitis risk: Developing a nomogram for patients with mediastinal lymphoma. *Adv Radiat Oncol.* 2018;3(3):372–381. https://doi.org/10.1016/j.adro.2018.03.005. eCollection 2018 Jul-Sep. PMID: 30202805.

CHAPTER 5

Sources of Cells for Hematopoietic Cell Transplantation: Practical Aspects of Hematopoietic Cell Collection

RACQUEL INNIS-SHELTON, MD • LUCIANO J. COSTA, MD, PHD

INTRODUCTION

Hematopoietic cell transplantation is based on the administration of a graft containing hematopoietic progenitor cells (HPCs) with the objective of restoring hematopoiesis after myeloablative chemotherapy and/or radiation, expediting hematologic recovery after intense, but not myeloablative therapy and/or replacing the patient hematopoietic (and consequently immunologic) system to provide immune surveillance and prevent recurrence of a hematologic malignancy.

A hematopoietic graft can be obtained by many different approaches depending primarily on the type of transplant being performed (allogeneic or autologous), the type of donor available, the underlying disease being treated, and some practical and financial aspects.

SOURCES OF CELLS FOR ALLOGENEIC TRANSPLANTATION

Bone Marrow

The first and most traditional source of HPCs for transplant is bone marrow obtained by multiple aspirations of the iliac crest with the donor typically under general anesthesia. The graft obtained is infused into the recipient either unprocessed or after red cell depletion (if major ABO incompatibility) and/or plasma depletion (if minor ABO incompatibility). The graft composition resembles the marrow content with relative abundance of red cells, more differentiated myeloid precursors, and paucity of true stem cells, early precursors, and mature lymphocytes when compared to a peripheral blood graft.

Traditionally the total number of nucleated white cells per kg of recipient is used as surrogate of the hematopoietic potential for the graft obtained. A total nucleated cell dose of $>2 \times 10^8$ nucleated cells/kg of recipient is considered minimal necessary for safe engraftment. Higher doses are associated with faster engraftment.[1]

From the donor perspective, bone marrow donation negates the need for mobilization using growth factors (described in the following) but carries the discomfort and risk associated with anesthesia and multiple aspirations of the iliac crest. Serious complications are extremely rare. More frequent and less serious complications are postprocedure pain and anemia.[2-4]

Peripheral Blood

The administration of filgrastim (or other similar growth factor) will cause expansion of the granulocytic population in the bone marrow and the release of proteases in the marrow environment which will disrupt several "anchors" that keep HPC within the marrow compartment, including the binding of CXCR4 in the HPC to Stromal cell-derived factor 1(SDF-1) in the marrow stroma and lead to enrichment of the otherwise very small pool of circulating HPC, characterized by expression of CD34.[5]

Typically after 4 days of growth factor administration there is substantial increase in the pool of circulating CD34+ cells. HPCs are then obtained by one or more sessions of leukapheresis optimized to capture mononuclear cells. In most cases a single session of leukapheresis is sufficient to yield an adequate graft.

The graft obtained from mobilized peripheral blood will typically contain an abundance of CD34+ and also other mononuclear cells including mature lymphocytes.[3] Because the product is obtained by leukapheresis optimized for mononuclear cells, there is minimal presence of red cells and granulocytes. The hematopoietic potential of the graft has been extensively correlated to its CD34+ dose per kg of recipient.

There is far less variation in strategies for allogeneic mobilization of HPC than there is for autologous mobilization. Long-term safety of filgrastim administration to volunteer normal donors has been established.[6] Filgrastim, typically at doses of 10 µg/kg per day, is the near-ubiquitous mobilizing agent, and mobilization failures are rare. Cell doses <1.5 × 10^6 CD34+/kg are considered inadequate and may cause engraftment failure or delayed neutrophil and platelet recovery. Higher doses are associated with faster engraftment and, in some studies, reduced risk of relapse of the underlying hematologic malignance and increase in risk of graft versus host disease (GVHD).[7] Therefore cell doses of 4–5 × 10^6 CD34+/kg are considered optimal although such determination may be influenced by the risk of recurrence of the underlying disease and baseline risk of GVHD.[8]

The CXCR4 antagonist plerixafor (further discussed under autologous mobilization) is not an approved agent for allogeneic mobilization. However, it has been tested as an alternative to filgrastim as a potentially more convenient and less toxic agent.[9] Grafts obtained with filgrastim and plerixafor mobilization have different cellular composition and lymphocyte cytokine profile, and the effects of plerixafor mobilization on GVHD and risk of disease recurrence need to be better understood.

Comparisons of Bone Marrow Versus Peripheral Blood

Although in many circumstances either a bone marrow or a peripheral blood graft can be used for allogeneic transplantation, the type of graft used has substantial implications on the outcome of the transplant. When compared with bone marrow, peripheral blood grafts have a higher content of CD34+ cells, a higher content of mature lymphocytes, and smaller volume and minimal amount of red blood cells. Owing to greater convenience, faster engraftment (REF) and peripheral blood HPCs (PB-HPCs) have become the preferred graft source accounting for approximately 65% of allogeneic transplants. Owing to its higher lymphocyte content, peripheral blood grafts are also linked to higher risk of GVHD and also potentially lower risk of relapse of the underlying malignancy due to more robust graft versus tumor (GVT) effect.

It is therefore expected that comparisons between bone marrow and peripheral blood grafts are influences by underlying risk of GVHD, risk of disease recurrence, and hematologic disease being treated. While transplants with low risk of GVHD and high risk of relapse (e.g., matched related donor transplantation for relapsed acute leukemia) would favor peripheral blood graft, transplantations for conditions that would not benefit from GVT (such as aplastic anemia) or with a baseline higher risk of GVHD (unrelated donor) would be best performed using a bone marrow graft.

Multiple studies compared bone marrow and peripheral blood grafts from matched related donors used in the treatment of malignant conditions. Findings were often conflicting or inconclusive until a large individual patient data metaanalysis was performed compiling data from 1111 adult patients enrolled in nine randomized trials.[10] This analysis confirmed higher risk of serious acute and chronic GVHD and lower risk of recurrence with peripheral blood graft and similar nonrelapse mortality translating into improved survival for patients with late-stage disease.

Only more recently bone marrow and PB-HPC as grafts for myeloablative matched unrelated donor transplant were directly compared on a large randomized trial with 551 patients.[11] There was no significant difference in survival, but with higher risk of graft failure and lower risk of chronic GVHD in the bone marrow arm.[11] Long-term follow-up of patient-reported outcomes favored bone marrow.[12] Therefore it is currently not recommended that centers performing myeloablative unrelated donor transplantation routinely use peripheral blood as their preferred graft source.[13] For reduced-intensity conditioning unrelated donor transplantation, outcomes of bone marrow and peripheral blood graft seem similar.[14]

More recently, the use of posttransplantation cyclophosphamide to abrogate alloreactivity and minimize rejection and GVHD has gained popularity and made possible the use of grafts from haploidentical related donors. Although this strategy was initially developed in the setting of bone marrow transplantation,[15] it has also been used with peripheral blood grafts without overwhelming increment in GVHD. Existing comparative data suggest higher risk of GVHD, but lower risk of graft failure, lower risk of leukemia relapse, and similar survival with peripheral blood grafts.[16,17] More data and longer follow-up will be necessary to define the optimal source of graft for haploidentical transplantation with posttransplantation cyclophosphamide.

Umbilical Cord Blood

Umbilical cord blood (UCB) is a source of HPC with no risk for the donor. Because of the immature immune status of the newborn, UCB transplantation can be performed with much greater tolerance for human leukocyte antigen (HLA) disparities, greatly extending the option of allogeneic HPC transplantation to minority patients.[18] The greatest caveats of UCB grafts consist in the relatively low number of total nucleated cells when compared with adult bone marrow grafts translating into up to 20% risk

TABLE 5.1
Implications of Different CD34+ Cell Dose in Autologous Transplantation

Cell Dose	Implications	Recommendation
$<1.5 \times 10^6$ CD34+/kg	Delayed neutrophil and platelet recovery, increased transfusion requirement, and higher risk of engraftment failure	Contraindicated
$1.5–3.0 \times 10^6$ CD34+/kg	Delayed platelet recovery	Discouraged
$3.0–5.0 \times 10^6$ CD34+/kg	Adequate neutrophil and platelet recovery	Adequate cell dose
$>5.0 \times 10^6$ CD34+/kg	Possible minimal gain in platelet and neutrophil engraftment, possible improvement in long-term platelet recovery, and fewer transfusions	Uncertain benefit

of engraftment failure and delayed and often incomplete recovery of neutrophil and platelet count.[19] In fact, outcomes are heavily influenced by cell dose, and great HLA compatibility partially negates the detrimental effect of low cell dose. Therefore selection of UCB units for transplantation is complex and requires specific expertise.[20] Strategies to increase efficacy of UCB particularly by providing a higher number of HPC include the use of two UCB units[21] and in vitro expansion[22] but with limited applicability.

SOURCES OF CELLS FOR AUTOLOGOUS TRANSPLANTATION

Since the 1990s the use of mobilized autologous PB-HPCs to support hematopoietic recovery after high-dose chemotherapy has revolutionized the treatment of several malignancies including lymphomas, plasma cell neoplasms, germ cell tumors, and other solid tumors. PB-HPCs have, for the most part, replaced marrow source grafts in the majority of the 10,000 autologous hematopoietic stem cell transplants (AHSCTs) performed yearly in the United States.

Similar to allogeneic grafts, the number of CD34+ cells/kg correlates closely with the likelihood and speed of hematopoietic recovery. Table 5.1 summarizes consensus recommendations and implications of different cell doses.[8]

It is common, particularly for patients with plasma cell neoplasms and germ cell tumors, to collect enough cells to support more than one transplant procedure. Such intention evidently needs to be taken in account the number of cells to be collected when planning.

Historically there have been two basic modalities to mobilize HPC in autologous donors: growth factor (GF) alone or chemotherapy followed by growth factor (C+GF). Most recently the advent of CXCR4 inhibitor plerixafor in combination with GF (GF+P) has

provided a third approach for HPC mobilization and generated new questions.

Regardless of the method of mobilization, most transplant centers will assess one or more objective parameters before initiation of HPC collection. Monitoring of CD34+ in peripheral blood is preferable, and most centers will not initiate leukapheresis unless CD34+> $10/\mu L$ (with variations ranging from 5 to $20/\mu L$). This approach is based on the close relationship between CD34+ in peripheral blood and yield of CD34+ in the apheresis product.[23]

There is no consensus on the volume of blood to be processed during a leukapheresis session. Most transplant centers will process at least 3 blood volumes. Large-volume leukapheresis may improve collection yields but also lead to more side effects.[24]

Growth Factor Mobilization

Growth factor administration and daily leukapheresis can continue until the desired number of CD34+ cells is obtained, but typically for not longer than 4 days. Three different GFs, filgrastim Granulocyte-colony stimulating factor (G-CSF), sargramostim granulocyte monocyte-colony stimulating factor (GM-CSF), and pegfilgrastim have been used to mobilize HPC. Their doses and characteristics are displayed on Table 5.2. Most recently, TBO-filgrastim has been shown to have near-identical performance than filgrastim yet with lower cost.[25,26] Most GFs require daily injections for 4 days before collection plus daily doses during collection. The only exception is pegfilgrastim, a pegylated modification of filgrastim[27] with longer half-life which is given as a single dose 3–4 days before planned first day of collection. In a retrospective analysis, pegfilgrastim has been shown to have at least equivalent mobilization potential to filgrastim with comparable cost.[28,29]

The type of GF to be used will often depend on institution formulary, experience, and price. There are very

TABLE 5.2
Characteristics of Different Growth Factors Utilized for Mobilization

Growth Factor	Dose	Comments
Filgrastim	Alone: 10–16 µg/kg per day After chemotherapy: 5–10 µg/kg per day	Most established GF. Superior to sargramostim when used after chemotherapy mobilization. Cost can be high in heavier patients and/or patients requiring many days of collection.
TBO-Filgrastim	Alone: 10–16 µg/kg per day After chemotherapy: 5–10 µg/kg per day	Performance near identical to filgrastim. Lower cost
Sargramostim	8 µg/kg per day or 250 µg/m^2 per day	Inferior to filgrastim when used after chemotherapy mobilization. Limited data on use without chemotherapy. Likely more side effects than figrastim
Pegfilgrastim	Alone: 6–12 mg single dose After chemotherapy: 6-mg single dose	No proper prospective comparison with filgrastim. Superior to filgrastim in retrospective analysis. More convenient to patients since single injection. Cost is high, particularly if 12 mg used.

little data indicating that combination of different GFs will yield better results than a single GF used at optimal doses and schedule.

When compared to other methods for autologous HPC mobilization, the use of GF without chemotherapy and without plerixafor is the strategy with the lowest cost. Another advantage is the predictability, allowing convenient scheduling for apheresis, and patient safety. The main limitation of this approach however is its low success rate. Mobilization failures and suboptimal mobilizations are common. In fact, approximately 30% of patients with lymphoma and 15% of patients with plasma cell neoplasm will fail to collect sufficient cells for transplantation after mobilization with GF alone.[30] Consensus guidelines discourage the use of GF alone in patients with plasma cell neoplasms and multiple prior lines of therapy and patients with lymphoma, particularly if the option of adding plerixafor based on low CD34+ in peripheral blood (as discussed in the following) is not available.[31]

Several clinical factors have been identified as associated with poor mobilization with GF, including age, premobilization platelet count, and prior therapy with certain agents (melphalan, lenalidomide, and fludarabine). However, clinical factors alone are insufficient to accurately predict the success of mobilization with GF.[32] Stratification of patients per risk factors for mobilization failure and assignment of patients to different mobilization strategies according to perceived risk are discouraged. Instead, a strategy that monitors CD34+ in peripheral blood and adds plerixafor in the event of suboptimal mobilization is preferred.

Chemotherapy Plus GF Mobilization

Many chemotherapy agents will cause significant bone marrow suppression. It has long been recognized that during the recovery from marrow suppression, there is a substantial increase in the number of circulating CD34+ cells, an effect that can be magnified by the administration of GFs. This approach will lead to a sharp increase in circulating CD34+ cells, typically 9–11 days from the administration of chemotherapy, ideal time to proceed with leukapheresis. This strategy is frequently used as patient candidates for autologous transplantations are often already on chemotherapy (particularly patients with lymphoma), and collection of HPC can occur on the "rebound" of the last intended chemotherapy cycle. Regimens such as Ifosfamide, carboplatin, etoposide(ICE), Dexamethasone, high-dose cytarabine, cisplatin(DHAP), Etoposide, metilprednisolone, high dose cytarabine, cisplatin(ESHAP), Dexamethasone, thalidomide, cisplatine, adriamycin, cyclophosphamide, etoposide(DT-PACE), and Carmustine, etoposide, cytarabine, melphalan(mini-BEAM) are routinely used as platforms for HPC mobilization.

Many centers will routinely use one cycle of single-agent chemotherapy for the purpose of HPC mobilization. The agent most routinely used is cyclophosphamide[33] in doses of 1.5–7 g/m^2. The optimal dose of cyclophosphamide is unknown, but higher doses are associated with more toxicity without any obvious gain in mobilization, so doses higher than $4\,g/m^2$ are discouraged.[31]

Although cyclophosphamide + GF will typically yield high content of CD34+ cells, collection failures occur in approximately 15% of patients depending on other characteristics.[34] The greatest limitation of this approach is however the pronounced neutropenia increasing the risk of infections. In most series 10%–20% of patients undergoing mobilization with cyclophosphamide develop fever and neutropenia requiring hospitalization and use of intravenous antibiotics.[34,35]

There is also robust literature supporting the use of etoposide in doses of 750–$2000\,mg/m^2$, but there are no prospective studies showing superiority of one mobilizing chemotherapy agent over another. Prior reports indicate success in collecting the minimal number of cells to proceed to transplant the vast majority patients with a large proportion of patients reaching the mobilization target in 1 day of collection.[36–38] High-dose etoposide is however a relatively toxic mobilizing regimen, and approximately a quarter of the patients will require transfusion of blood products and hospital admissions for fever and neutropenia.[36–38]

Vinorelbine at the dose of $35\,mg/m^2$ in combination with GF mobilizes sufficient number of HPC in near all patients.[39–41] Contrary to the experience with cyclophosphamide and etoposide, chemotherapy mobilization with vinorelbine is associated with very low risk of fever with neutropenia and need for transfusion support. Cytarabine is yet another chemotherapeutic agent used for mobilization of autologous HPC with excellent success rate including in patients with prior mobilization failure.[42]

One theoretical advantage of chemotherapy mobilization is that the chemotherapy used for mobilization would have an additional therapeutic effect on the underlying disease. In fact, some programs will routinely assign patients with suboptimal disease control before transplantation to chemotherapy mobilization. Such advantage has never been properly demonstrated. In multiple myeloma, recent evidence indicates that the use of chemotherapy mobilization does not contribute meaningfully to disease control.[43,44] Conversely, disease burden before mobilization should not be used to assign patients to a specific mobilization strategy.

Growth Factor Plus CXCR4 Antagonist

Plerixafor is a reversible partial antagonist of CXCR4 that competes with SDF-1 disrupting its interaction with CXCR4 in progenitor cells. Unattached HPCs are then released to enter the peripheral blood stream. In patients receiving GFs

for HPC mobilization, the subcutaneous administration of plerixafor leads to a sharp, threefold to fivefold increase in circulating CD34+ cells that peaks at approximately 10 h allowing for a more effective collection (REF).

The demonstration of superiority of GF + plerixafor (GF + P) over GF came from two randomized trials performed in multiple myeloma (MM) and non-Hodgkin lymphoma (NHL) patients. In the MM trial, 302 patients were randomized to receive placebo or plerixafor of $240\,\mu g/kg$ on the evening of the fourth day of filgrastim administration, continuing daily until completion of collection. The primary efficacy endpoint, the collection of 6×10^6 CD34+/kg in ≤2 leukapheresis sessions, was achieved in 71.6% of patients mobilizing with GF + plerixafor versus 34.4% of patients with GF + placebo. The median number of days required to collect 6×10^6 CD34+/kg was 1 in patients receiving plerixafor versus 4 in the control group.[45]

The NHL trial had near-identical design and included 298 patients. Fifty-nine percent of patients receiving plerixafor and only 20% of the patients receiving placebo met the primary efficacy endpoint of collecting 5×10^6 CD34+/kg in up to 4 apheresis sessions resulting in 90% of the patients in the plerixafor group versus 55% in the control group being able to undergo transplantation[46] without remobilization.

Plerixafor has a favorable side effect profile with the main toxicity being mild-to-moderate diarrhea. The greatest caveat to broader adoption of plerixafor has been cost. In fact, many patients will successfully collect an adequate number of HPC in few apheresis sessions with GF alone. Some centers have adopted the practice of using plerixafor for patients who are at perceived high risk of mobilization failure. However, this approach has important limitations due to the lack of reliable tools to precisely predict poor mobilization.[32] We believe that "just in time" is a more effective strategy to use plerixafor. With this approach, plerixafor is added to an ongoing mobilization cycle according to the number of CD34+ in the peripheral blood after 4 days of GF administration. Therefore only patients who are actual (as opposed to predicted) poor mobilizers do receive plerixafor. This approach has reduced the risk of mobilization failure to <5% while preventing "unnecessary" use of plerixafor in 40%–60% of patients.[8,23,47,48] Fig. 5.1 display the example of one algorithm for "just in time" use of plerixafor.

Comparison of Mobilization Strategies

There is no large randomized trial comparing GF with C + GF. However, there are several recognized advantages and disadvantages of each approach (Tables 5.3 and 5.4). Importantly, even though more CD34+ cells

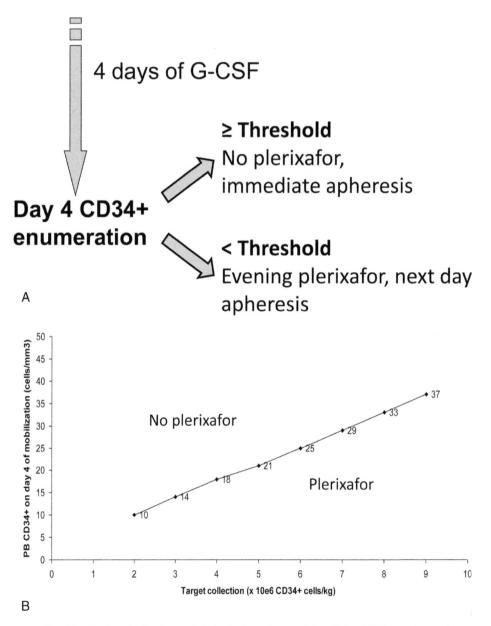

FIG. 5.1 Algorithm for "just in time" use of plerixafor based on peripheral blood CD34+ enumeration on fourth day of mobilization (panel **A**) with thresholds defined by pharmacoeconomic analysis and influenced by mobilization target (panel **B**). (Adapted from the study by Costa LJ, Alexander ET, Hogan KR, Schaub C, Fouts TV, Stuart RK. Development and validation of a decision-making algorithm to guide the use of plerixafor for autologous hematopoietic stem cell mobilization. *Bone Marrow Transpl.* 2011;46(1):64–69 with permission.)

TABLE 5.3
Selected Literature Comparing Different Mobilization Strategies

Author	N total Disease	Trial Setting	Mobilization Regimen	Mean CD34+/kg Yield	P value	Mobilization Success of Meeting CD34+/kg Target	Comments & Practice Implications
COMPARISONS BETWEEN GROWTH FACTORS							
Tuchman[33]	167 MM	Single-center retrospective analysis	Cy 3–4 g/m² + G-CSF 10 μg/kg per d vs. G-CSF 10 μg/kg per d	12×10^6 vs. 5.8×10^6	<0.01	NS	Higher yield of CD34+ cells offset by cost of toxicities to patient
Herbert[53]	52 Lymphoma, MM	Single-center retrospective analysis	Pegfilgrastim 12 or 6 mg vs. G-CSF 10 μg/kg per d	4.78×10^6 vs. 3.70×10^6	NS	91% vs. 80%	Similarity in yield deserves further exploration
Costa[28]	131 Lymphoma, MM	Single-center retrospective analysis	Pegfilgrastim 12 mg ± plerixafor (240 μg/kg) vs. G-CSF 10 μg/kg ± plerixafor (240 μg/kg)	$1.43 \pm 0.63 \times 10^6$ CFU-GMs/kg vs. $1.46 \pm 0.9 \times 10^6$ CFU-GMs/kg	NS	52/57 vs. 68/74	Similarity in yield deserves further exploration. Less need for plerixafor with pegfilgrastim
Simona[54]	64 Lymphoma, MM	Single-center retrospective	ESHAP + G-CSF 5 μg/kg per d vs. ESHAP + Pegfilgrastim 6 mg	12.3×10^6 vs. 9.4×10^6	NS	25/26 vs. 36/38	Toxicities to be considered in chemo-mobilization strategies
GF VS. GF + CXCR4 ANTAGONIST							
DiPersio[46]	298 Lymphoma	Multicenter phase III randomized double-blind placebo controlled	G-CSF 10 μg/kg per d + placebo vs. G-CSF 10 μg/kg per d + plerixafor	Median yields 1.98×10^6 vs. 5.69×10^6	NS	Target: $\geq 2 \times 10^6$ 47.3% vs. 86.7% Target: $\geq 5 \times 10^6$ 19.6% vs. 59.3%	Pivotal trial evidences safety and efficacy of plerixafor
DiPersio[45]	302 MM	Multicenter phase III randomized double-blind placebo controlled	G-CSF 10 μg/kg per d + placebo vs. G-CSF 10 μg/kg controlled	Median yields 6.18×10^6 vs. 10.96×10^6		Target: $\geq 2 \times 10^6$ 88.3% vs. 95.3% Target: $\geq 6 \times 10^6$ 34.4% vs. 71.6%	Pivotal trial evidences safety and efficacy of plerixafor

Continued

TABLE 5.3

Selected Literature Comparing Different Mobilization Strategies—cont'd

CHEMOTHERAPY + GF VS. GF ± CXCR4 ANTAGONIST

Author	N total Disease	Trial Setting	Mobilization Regimen	Mean CD34+/kg Yield	P value	Mobilization Success of Meeting CD34+/kg Target	Comments & Practice Implications
Narayanasami[55]	47 Lymphoma MM	Single-center randomized	Cyclophosphamide 5g/m^2 + G-CSF 10 μg/kg per d vs. G-CSF 10 μg/kg per d	11.9 × 10^6 vs. 3.9 × 10^6	0.004	NS	Chemo-mobilization associated with higher yield that G only, but at the cost of more toxicity and resource utilization
Antar[56]	83 MM	Single-center retrospective	Cyclophosphamide 5g/m^2 + G-CSF (n = 56) vs. G-CSF + preemptive plerixafor 240 μg/kg (n = 27)	Median yields 15.5 × 10^6 vs. 7.5 × 10^6	0.005	100% both groups	Chemo-mobilization associated with higher yield that G only, but at the cost of more toxicity and resource utilization
Shaughnessy[35]	66 Lymphomas/MM	Multi-center retrospective	Cyclophosphamide 3–5 g/m^2 + G-CSF (n = 33) vs. G-CSF + plerixafor 240 μg/kg (n = 33)	Median yields 11.6 × 10^6 vs. 10.7 × 10^6	0.5	100% both groups	More hospital admissions and more weekend apheresis with cyclophosphamide. Similar cost.
Costa[34]	131 Lymphomas/MM	Single-center retrospective	Cyclophosphamide 2 g/m^2 + G-CSF (n = 81) vs. G-CSF ± plerixafor 240 μg/kg (n = 50)	Median yields 7.7 × 10^6 vs. 7.0 × 10^6	0.08	78% vs. 98%	More infections, more hospitalizations, higher cost with cyclophosphamide + GF.
Dhakal[49]	98 Lymphomas	Multi-center retrospective	ICE chemotherapy + G-CSF (n = 35) vs. G-CSF ± plerixafor 240 μg/kg (n = 63)	Median yields 5.4 × 10^6 vs. 3.2 × 10^6	<0.001	100% vs. 87%	Lower cost with chemotherapy + GF.

GF, growth factor; MM, multiple myeloma.

TABLE 5.4
Advantages and Disadvantages of Different Mobilization Strategies

Mobilization Strategy	Advantages	Disadvantages
Growth factor mobilization	• Short time from start of mobilization to transplant. • Fewer days of GF administration • Onset of collection is more predictable	• Fewer CD34+ collected than with C + GF • High failure rate
Growth factor + CXCR4 antagonist	• Short time from start of mobilization to transplant. • Fewer days of GF administration • Onset of collection is more predictable • High success rate	• High cost
Chemotherapy + growth factor	• More CD34+ cells collected than with GF alone • Chemotherapy already used for underlying disease	• Longer stay of intravascular catheter • Higher risk of infection • Neutropenia • Thrombocytopenia • Higher risk of complications requiring hospitalization • High cost • Ideal time of apheresis is less predictable

---

are often obtained with C + GF, there is no definitive evidence that the rate of mobilization failure is different between the two methods.

Although C + GF and GF + P are both strategies to increase yield of HPC collected (over GF alone), there has not been any prospective comparison between the two methods. Retrospective comparisons have yielded different conclusions. A multicenter retrospective comparison between cyclophosphamide $(3-5\,g/m^2)$ + GF and GF + P in 66 patients (33 patients in each group) with myeloma and lymphoma found that all patients in both the groups collected sufficient number of cells to proceed to transplantation with similar estimated cost. However, apheresis was less predictable, and more patients required hospitalization and weekend apheresis with cyclophosphamide mobilization.[35] Another single-center study retrospectively compared cyclophosphamide $2\,g/m^2$ + filgrastim (n = 81) versus filgrastim (n = 50) + "just in time" use of plerixafor in patients with lymphoma or MM. Mobilization failure rate was 22% in chemotherapy + GF versus 2% in GF ± P. There was also lower risk of infections requiring hospitalization, shorter time from onset of mobilization to transplantation, and overall lower cost with GF ± P.[34] A different conclusion was achieved on another retrospective multicenter study comparing the performance

of carboplatin, ifosfamide, and etoposide (ICE) + GF (n = 35) versus GF ± plerixafor (n = 63). In this study the chemotherapy strategy was associated with higher CD34+ yields, fewer mobilization failures, and lower cost.[49] Table 5.3 displays some of the published experience comparing different mobilization strategies. Table 5.4 summarizes advantages and disadvantages of different mobilization strategies for autologous HPC.

Mobilization Failures

Mobilization failure can be defined as the failure to obtain sufficient HPC to proceed with transplantation, but the definition varies across different reports. The lack of sufficient HPC after one cycle of mobilization will either completely preclude or delay potentially life-saving or life-extending transplantation. Remobilization is often unsuccessful and exquisitely expensive. Therefore transplant programs should develop mobilization approaches optimized to decrease the risk of failure.

Mobilization failure rates depend not only on the mobilization strategy utilized but also on the characteristics of individuals studied. Most patients who fail mobilization and are still adequate candidates for autologous transplantation will be able to proceed to transplantation after remobilization. GF alone is not considered an adequate strategy for remobilization given the very high failure rate. Chemotherapy + GF can successfully mobilize HPC in a subset of patients failing GF alone. However, a strategy containing CXCR4 antagonist is recommended in the remobilization setting given a success rate >70%, particularly when a CXCR4 antagonist was not part of the initial mobilization regimen.[31,50,51] With the CXCR4 antagonist being increasingly more frequently used as initial mobilization strategy, transplant physicians will occasionally manage patients failing mobilization with GF + P. There is limited information available to guide management of these patients. Most patients will be successfully remobilized with the same regimen after a 3–4 week interval.[52] Others have combined chemotherapy + GF + P in a single mobilization cycle, but such approach is both expensive and potentially toxic.

REFERENCES

1. Remberger M, Torlen J, Ringden O, et al. Effect of total nucleated and CD34(+) cell dose on outcome after allogeneic hematopoietic stem cell transplantation. *Biol Blood Marrow Transpl J Am Soc Blood Marrow Transpl.* 2015;21(5):889–893.
2. Miller JP, Perry EH, Price TH, et al. Recovery and safety profiles of marrow and PBSC donors: experience of the National Marrow Donor Program. *Biol Blood Marrow Transpl J Am Soc Blood Marrow Transpl.* 2008;14(suppl 9):29–36.
3. Favre G, Beksac M, Bacigalupo A, et al. Differences between graft product and donor side effects following bone marrow or stem cell donation. *Bone Marrow Transpl.* 2003;32(9):873–880.
4. Burns LJ, Logan BR, Chitphakdithai P, et al. Recovery of unrelated donors of peripheral blood stem cells versus recovery of unrelated donors of bone marrow: a prespecified analysis from the phase III blood and marrow transplant clinical trials network protocol 0201. *Biol Blood Marrow Transpl J Am Soc Blood Marrow Transpl.* 2016;22(6):1108–1116.
5. Hopman RK, DiPersio JF. Advances in stem cell mobilization. *Blood Rev.* 2014;28(1):31–40.
6. Behfar M, Faghihi-Kashani S, Hosseini AS, Ghavamzadeh A, Hamidieh AA. Long-term safety of short-term administration of filgrastim (rhG-CSF) and leukophresis procedure in healthy children: application of peripheral blood stem cell collection in pediatric donors. *Biol Blood Marrow Transpl J Am Soc Blood Marrow Transpl.* 2018;24(4):866–870.
7. Perez-Simon JA, Diez-Campelo M, Martino R, et al. Impact of CD34+ cell dose on the outcome of patients undergoing reduced-intensity-conditioning allogeneic peripheral blood stem cell transplantation. *Blood.* 2003;102(3):1108–1113.
8. Duong HK, Savani BN, Copelan E, et al. Peripheral blood progenitor cell mobilization for autologous and allogeneic hematopoietic cell transplantation: guidelines from the American Society for Blood and Marrow Transplantation. *Biol Blood Marrow Transpl J Am Soc Blood Marrow Transpl.* 2014;20(9):1262–1273.
9. Schroeder MA, Rettig MP, Lopez S, et al. Mobilization of allogeneic peripheral blood stem cell donors with intravenous plerixafor mobilizes a unique graft. *Blood.* 2017;129(19):2680–2692.
10. Stem Cell Trialists' Collaborative G. Allogeneic peripheral blood stem-cell compared with bone marrow transplantation in the management of hematologic malignancies: an individual patient data meta-analysis of nine randomized trials. *J Clinical Oncol.* 2005;23(22):5074–5087.
11. Anasetti C, Logan BR, Lee SJ, et al. Peripheral-blood stem cells versus bone marrow from unrelated donors. *N Engl J Med.* 2012;367(16):1487–1496.
12. Lee SJ, Logan B, Westervelt P, et al. Comparison of patient-reported outcomes in 5-year survivors who received bone marrow vs peripheral blood unrelated donor transplantation: long-term follow-up of a randomized clinical trial. *JAMA Oncol.* 2016;2(12):1583–1589.
13. Bhella S, Majhail NS, Betcher J, et al. Choosing wisely BMT: American Society for Blood and Marrow Transplantation and Canadian Blood and Marrow Transplant Group's list of 5 tests and treatments to question in blood and marrow transplantation. *Biol Blood Marrow Transpl J Am Soc Blood Marrow Transpl.* 2018;24(5):909–913.
14. Eapen M, Logan BR, Horowitz MM, et al. Bone marrow or peripheral blood for reduced-intensity conditioning unrelated donor transplantation. *J Clin Oncol.* 2015;33(4):364–369.
15. Luznik L, O'Donnell PV, Symons HJ, et al. HLA-haploidentical bone marrow transplantation for hematologic malignancies using nonmyeloablative conditioning and high-dose, posttransplantation cyclophosphamide. *Biol Blood Marrow Transpl J Am Soc Blood Marrow Transpl.* 2008;14(6):641–650.
16. Ruggeri A, Labopin M, Bacigalupo A, et al. Bone marrow versus mobilized peripheral blood stem cells in haploidentical transplants using posttransplantation cyclophosphamide. *Cancer.* 2018;124(7):1428–1437.
17. Bashey A, Zhang MJ, McCurdy SR, et al. Mobilized peripheral blood stem cells versus unstimulated bone marrow as a graft source for t-cell-replete haploidentical donor transplantation using post-transplant cyclophosphamide. *J Clin Oncol.* 2017;35(26):3002–3009.
18. Gragert L, Eapen M, Williams E, et al. HLA match likelihoods for hematopoietic stem-cell grafts in the U.S. registry. *N Engl J Med.* 2014;371(4):339–348.
19. Rocha V, Labopin M, Sanz G, et al. Transplants of umbilical-cord blood or bone marrow from unrelated donors in adults with acute leukemia. *N Engl J Med.* 2004;351(22):2276–2285.
20. Barker JN, Byam C, Scaradavou A. How I treat: the selection and acquisition of unrelated cord blood grafts. *Blood.* 2011;117(8):2332–2339.
21. Scaradavou A, Brunstein CG, Eapen M, et al. Double unit grafts successfully extend the application of umbilical cord blood transplantation in adults with acute leukemia. *Blood.* 2013;121(5):752–758.

22. de Lima M, McNiece I, Robinson SN, et al. Cord-blood engraftment with ex vivo mesenchymal-cell coculture. *New Engl J Med.* 2012;367(24):2305–2315.

23. Costa LJ, Alexander ET, Hogan KR, Schaub C, Fouts TV, Stuart RK. Development and validation of a decision-making algorithm to guide the use of plerixafor for autologous hematopoietic stem cell mobilization. *Bone Marrow Transpl.* 2011;46(1):64–69.

24. Fontana S, Groebli R, Leibundgut K, Pabst T, Zwicky C, Taleghani BM. Progenitor cell recruitment during individualized high-flow, very-large-volume apheresis for autologous transplantation improves collection efficiency. *Transfusion.* 2006;46(8):1408–1416.

25. Bhamidipati PK, Fiala MA, Grossman BJ, et al. Results of a prospective randomized, open-label, noninferiority study of Tbo-Filgrastim (Granix) versus Filgrastim (Neupogen) in combination with plerixafor for autologous stem cell mobilization in patients with multiple myeloma and non-hodgkin lymphoma. *Biol Blood Marrow Transpl J Am Soc Blood Marrow Transpl.* 2017;23(12):2065–2069.

26. Elayan MM, Horowitz JG, Magraner JM, Shaughnessy PJ, Bachier C. Tbo-filgrastim versus filgrastim during mobilization and neutrophil engraftment for autologous stem cell transplantation. *Biol Blood Marrow Transpl J Am Soc Blood Marrow Transpl.* 2015;21(11):1921–1925.

27. Zamboni WC. Pharmacokinetics of pegfilgrastim. *Pharmacotherapy.* 2003;23(8 Pt 2):9S–14S.

28. Costa LJ, Kramer C, Hogan KR, et al. Pegfilgrastim- versus filgrastim-based autologous hematopoietic stem cell mobilization in the setting of preemptive use of plerixafor: efficacy and cost analysis. *Transfusion.* 2012;52(11):2375–2381.

29. Costa LJ, Innis-Shelton R, Bowersock J, et al. Autologous hematopoietic progenitor cells mobilization with combination of pegfilgrastim and plerixafor: efficacy and cost assessment. *Blood.* 2017;130(suppl 1):4708.

30. Gertz MA, Wolf RC, Micallef IN, Gastineau DA. Clinical impact and resource utilization after stem cell mobilization failure in patients with multiple myeloma and lymphoma. *Bone Marrow Transpl.* 2010;45(9):1396–1403.

31. Giralt S, Costa L, Schriber J, et al. Optimizing autologous stem cell mobilization strategies to improve patient outcomes: consensus guidelines and recommendations. *Biol Blood Marrow Transpl J Am Soc Blood Marrow Transpl.* 2014;20(3):295–308.

32. Costa LJ, Nista EJ, Buadi FK, et al. Prediction of poor mobilization of autologous CD34+ cells with growth factor in multiple myeloma patients: implications for risk-stratification. *Biol Blood Marrow Transpl J Am Soc Blood Marrow Transpl.* 2014;20(2):222–228.

33. Tuchman SA, Bacon WA, Huang LW, et al. Cyclophosphamide-based hematopoietic stem cell mobilization before autologous stem cell transplantation in newly diagnosed multiple myeloma. *J Clin Apher.* 2015;30(3):176–182.

34. Costa LJ, Miller AN, Alexander ET, et al. Growth factor and patient-adapted use of plerixafor is superior to CY and growth factor for autologous hematopoietic stem cells mobilization. *Bone Marrow Transpl.* 2011;46(4):523–528.

35. Shaughnessy P, Islas-Ohlmayer M, Murphy J, et al. Cost and clinical analysis of autologous hematopoietic stem cell mobilization with G-CSF and plerixafor compared to G-CSF and cyclophosphamide. *Biol Blood Marrow Transpl J Am Soc Blood Marrow Transpl.* 2011;17(5):729–736.

36. Wood WA, Whitley J, Goyal R, et al. Effectiveness of etoposide chemomobilization in lymphoma patients undergoing auto-SCT. *Bone Marrow Transpl.* 2013;48(6):771–776.

37. Wood WA, Whitley J, Moore D, et al. Chemomobilization with etoposide is highly effective in patients with multiple myeloma and overcomes the effects of age and prior therapy. *Biol Blood Marrow Transpl J Am Soc Blood Marrow Transpl.* 2011;17(1):141–146.

38. Mahindra A, Bolwell BJ, Rybicki L, et al. Etoposide plus G-CSF priming compared with G-CSF alone in patients with lymphoma improves mobilization without an increased risk of secondary myelodysplasia and leukemia. *Bone Marrow Transpl.* 2012;47(2):231–235.

39. Samaras P, Pfrommer S, Seifert B, et al. Efficacy of vinorelbine plus granulocyte colony-stimulation factor for CD34+ hematopoietic progenitor cell mobilization in patients with multiple myeloma. *Biol Blood Marrow Transpl J Am Soc Blood Marrow Transpl.* 2015;21(1):74–80.

40. Samaras P, Rutti MF, Seifert B, et al. Mobilization of hematopoietic progenitor cells with standard- or reduced-dose filgrastim after vinorelbine in multiple myeloma patients: a randomized prospective single-center phase II study. *Biol Blood Marrow Transpl J Am Soc Blood Marrow Transpl.* 2018;24(4):694–699.

41. Heizmann M, O'Meara AC, Moosmann PR, et al. Efficient mobilization of PBSC with vinorelbine/G-CSF in patients with malignant lymphoma. *Bone Marrow Transpl.* 2009;44(2):75–79.

42. Calderon-Cabrera C, Carmona Gonzalez M, Martin J, et al. Intermediate doses of cytarabine plus granulocyte-colony-stimulating factor as an effective and safe regimen for hematopoietic stem cell collection in lymphoma patients with prior mobilization failure. *Transfusion.* 2015;55(4):875–879.

43. Uy GL, Costa LJ, Hari PN, et al. Contribution of chemotherapy mobilization to disease control in multiple myeloma treated with autologous hematopoietic cell transplantation. *Bone Marrow Transpl.* 2015;50(12):1513–1518.

44. Oyekunle A, Shumilov E, Kostrewa P, et al. Chemotherapy-based stem cell mobilization does not result in significant paraprotein reduction in myeloma patients in the era of novel induction regimens. *Biol Blood Marrow Transpl J Am Soc Blood Marrow Transpl.* 2018;24(2):276–281.

45. DiPersio JF, Stadtmauer EA, Nademanee A, et al. Plerixafor and G-CSF versus placebo and G-CSF to mobilize hematopoietic stem cells for autologous stem cell transplantation in patients with multiple myeloma. *Blood.* 2009;113(23):5720–5726.

46. DiPersio JF, Micallef IN, Stiff PJ, et al. Phase III prospective randomized double-blind placebo-controlled trial of plerixafor plus granulocyte colony-stimulating factor compared with placebo plus granulocyte colony-stimulating factor for autologous stem-cell mobilization and transplantation for patients with non-Hodgkin's lymphoma. *J Clin Oncol*. 2009;27(28):4767–4773.

47. Costa LJ, Abbas J, Hogan KR, et al. Growth factor plus preemptive ('just-in-time') plerixafor successfully mobilizes hematopoietic stem cells in multiple myeloma patients despite prior lenalidomide exposure. *Bone Marrow Transpl*. 2012;47(11):1403–1408.

48. Micallef IN, Sinha S, Gastineau DA, et al. Cost-effectiveness analysis of a risk-adapted algorithm of plerixafor use for autologous peripheral blood stem cell mobilization. *Biol Blood Marrow Transpl J Am Soc Blood Marrow Transpl*. 2013;19(1):87–93.

49. Dhakal B, Veltri LW, Fenske TS, et al. Hematopoietic progenitor cell mobilization with ifosfamide, carboplatin, and etoposide chemotherapy versus plerixafor-based strategies in patients with hodgkin and non-hodgkin lymphoma. *Biol Blood Marrow Transpl J Am Soc Blood Marrow Transpl*. 2016;22(10):1773–1780.

50. Perkins JB, Shapiro JF, Bookout RN, et al. Retrospective comparison of filgrastim plus plerixafor to other regimens for remobilization after primary mobilization failure: clinical and economic outcomes. *Am J Hematol*. 2012;87(7):673–677.

51. Duarte RF, Shaw BE, Marin P, et al. Plerixafor plus granulocyte CSF can mobilize hematopoietic stem cells from multiple myeloma and lymphoma patients failing previous mobilization attempts: EU compassionate use data. *Bone Marrow Transpl*. 2011;46(1):52–58.

52. Yuan S, Nademanee A, Krishnan A, Kogut N, Shayani S, Wang S. Second time a charm? Remobilization of peripheral blood stem cells with plerixafor in patients who previously mobilized poorly despite using plerixafor as a salvage agent. *Transfusion*. 2013;53(12):3244–3250.

53. Herbert KE, Gambell P, Link EK, et al. Pegfilgrastim compared with filgrastim for cytokine-alone mobilization of autologous haematopoietic stem and progenitor cells. *Bone Marrow Transpl*. 2013;48(3):351–356.

54. Simona B, Cristina R, Luca N, et al. A single dose of Pegfilgrastim versus daily Filgrastim to evaluate the mobilization and the engraftment of autologous peripheral hematopoietic progenitors in malignant lymphoma patients candidate for high-dose chemotherapy. *Transfus Apher Sci*. 2010;43(3):321–326.

55. Narayanasami U, Kanteti R, Morelli J, et al. Randomized trial of filgrastim versus chemotherapy and filgrastim mobilization of hematopoietic progenitor cells for rescue in autologous transplantation. *Blood*. 2001;98(7):2059–2064.

56. Antar A, Otrock ZK, Kharfan-Dabaja MA, et al. G-CSF plus preemptive plerixafor vs hyperfractionated CY plus G-CSF for autologous stem cell mobilization in multiple myeloma: effectiveness, safety and cost analysis. *Bone Marrow Transpl*. 2015;50(6):813–817.

CHAPTER 6

Patient and Donor Selection and Workup for Hematopoietic Cell Transplantation

BRONWEN E. SHAW, MBCHB, PHD

PATIENT SELECTION AND WORKUP

Hematopoietic cell transplantation (HCT) is an intense procedure associated with morbidity and mortality. It is well recognized that patient factors are critical determinants of outcome, so careful patient selection is paramount for prognostication and to carefully weigh the benefits and the risks of HCT in each individual patient. Factors that have a significant impact on the outcome and should form part of the workup include (1) disease-specific factors, (2) demographic factors, (3) comorbidities, and (4) patient-reported outcomes (PROs) and socio-economic status (SES). Several tools are available to assist with standardized assessments in each of these areas.

Disease-Specific Factors

This topic will be covered in detail, for each individual disease, in Section 4 of the book. Several transplantation societies have published evidence-based guidelines, which place diseases and their stage into broad categories for autologous or allogeneic HCT, such as generally not recommended, standard of care, or clinical option.[1,2] A thorough workup of the patient's disease should be performed before HCT. This may include assessment of the bone marrow or other disease sites with morphological, histological, immunophenotypic, cytogenetic, molecular, and imaging methodologies as appropriate. These assessments should be carried out as close to the time of commencing conditioning therapy as feasible to ensure that the most current disease status is captured. Several tools and scores can be applied to the individual patient's disease status for prognostication in the context of HCT.

Demographic Factors

The primary consideration in this category is the age of the patient. Historically, older patients were excluded from transplantation by their age alone, but with the advent of less toxic conditioning regimens, general population trends of longer lifespans with individuals remaining healthier into advanced years, the recognition of the impact of comorbidities on outcome (described in the following), and the barrier of age were lifted. In the last decade the number of patients aged above 60 years receiving both autologous and allogeneic HCT has increased significantly as seen in the Center for International Blood and Marrow Transplant Research (CIBMTR) activity reports (Fig. 6.1 and 6.2). Recent date from numerous studies do not show worse outcomes for patients based on their age alone, for multiple different disease indications, in both the autologous and the allogeneic setting.[3–6] Thus biological age is generally no longer considered a barrier to HCT. However, biological age does not always correlate well with physiological age. Physiological age has been described as "the relative age of a person, especially when comparing that individual's physical status with those of other persons of the same chronological age" (http://medical-dictionary.thefreedictionary.com/physiological+age) and includes assessment of "reserve" and "frailty".[7] Loss of reserve and increased frailty correlated with worse health, and assessment of physiological age in patients aged >50 years can allow a more accurate characterization of reserve.[8] Standardized tools to perform these assessments are available and routinely used in many centers as part of a comprehensive geriatric assessment. Limitations in functional ability reported directly by the patient or by direct testing (such as a 4-min walk test) are important prognostic indicators. Results for 203 patients transplanted at the University of Chicago showed that any limitation in the activities of daily living resulted in a higher risk of nonrelapse mortality and poorer survival. These effects were even more marked in patients aged >60 years.[9] Biomarkers

Hematopoietic Cell Transplantation for Malignant Conditions. https://doi.org/10.1016/B978-0-323-56802-9.00006-7

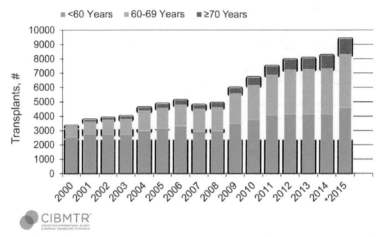

FIG. 6.1 Trends in autologous transplants by recipient age^. ^Transplants for NHL, Hodgkin Disease and Multiple Myeloma, *2015 Data incomplete. (Souza A, Zhu X. *Current Uses and Outcomes of Hematopoietic Cell Transplantation (HCT): CIBMTR Summary Slides*, 2016.)

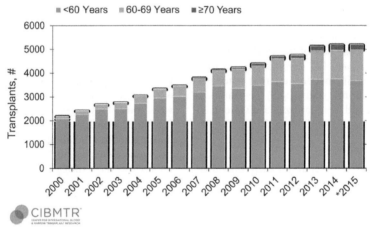

FIG. 6.2 Trends in allogeneic transplants by recipient age^. ^Transplants for AML, ALL, NHL, Hodgkin Disease, Multiple Myeloma, *2015 Data incomplete. (Souza A, Zhu X. *Current Uses and Outcomes of Hematopoietic Cell Transplantation (HCT): CIBMTR Summary Slides*, 2016.)

are being explored in this context but are not yet in routine use.[8] Centers should develop strategies for targeted assessment of their older patients, whether or not comorbidities are present.

Comorbidities

Damage or loss of function in an organ, which is not directly caused by the primary disease, can be referred to as a comorbidity. The impact of comorbidities is well studied in the allogeneic setting, and the Hematopoietic Cell Transplantation Comorbidity Index (HCT-CI) is routinely calculated before HCT in most transplant

centers for individual patient counseling and prognostication. The HCT-CI was developed by Sorror et al.[10] as an HCT-specific modification of the Charlson Comorbidity Index (CCI). The score is based on predefined abnormalities in multiple organ systems, which are assigned relative weights based on initial testing and validation studies. A patient with no comorbidities as defined by the HCT-CI will have a score of zero, and multiple abnormalities can result in scores of 5–10 or higher. An online calculator can assist with determining the score (http://www.hctci.org/Home/Calculator). Numerous studies have shown the value of the HCT-CI as a prognostic tool in determining nonrelapse mortality and survival in adults undergoing allogeneic HCT, with higher mortality and poorer survival in patients with higher scores.[11] More recently the value of the HCT-CI has been shown in children undergoing HCT[12] and in the autologous HCT setting.[12,13] Two newer variations on the HCT-CI incorporate age (the age-adjusted HCT-CI) and laboratory biomarkers (the augmented HCT-CI),[14] although these have been validated in fewer HCT settings to date.

Patient-Reported Outcomes and Socio-Economic Factors

Two recent studies in HCT have shown that pre-HCT scores, derived from measuring symptoms and function through direct patient report (using PRO measures such as the SF36 and Functional Assessment of Cancer Therapy-Bone Marrow Transplant (FACT-BMT)), are significantly associated with both survival[15] and quality of life (QOL)[16] after HCT. Minority race and lower SES[17,18] are associated with poorer transplant outcomes, the reasons for which are multifactorial and not entirely understood. Other important behavioral and social factors to consider, which are less well studied, include compliance with treatment and medication,[19] history of addictive behavior, and care-giver, social, and psychosocial support.[20]

Tools

In addition to tools for prognostication mentioned in this chapter, the CIBMTR makes available a 1-year survival calculator through their transplant center portal. This tool calculates the predicted probability of 1-year survival after allo-HCT for individual patients given their demographics, disease, and treatment characteristics, using statistical models developed for outcomes reporting. The accuracy of this tool is being tested in prospective studies. Predictive scores to determine the risk of specific post-HCT complications, including veno-occlusive disease,[21] disease relapse ,[22] and graft-versus-host disease (GVHD),[23,24] have been developed and, in some cases, validated. Use of these tools can assist with decision-making in pre-HCT family conferences.

HLA Typing and the Search Procedure

An important aspect of the (allogeneic) transplant patient's workup is determining whether a donor is available. This must be done in a timely manner, and ideally, a sample for HLA typing of the patient should be obtained as soon as possible after the diagnosis is made, particularly in the setting of a disease in which HCT is definite or highly likely to be indicated. Once the need for HCT has been confirmed, HLA typing of

siblings or other relatives should be performed. It is important to perform a brief assessment of the potential donor's health before HLA typing is done, in line with accreditation guidelines (http://www.factwebsite.org), not to perform costly and time-consuming typing for an individual who is not medically fit to donate. Reasons for deferral in this setting may include current pregnancy, malignancy, and cardiovascular or other serious health conditions. This type of screening can be carried out by phone or email. An unrelated donor (UD) search should be done as soon as possible and may include both UDs and umbilical cord blood (UCB) units as appropriate. Most recommendations[25] stress the importance of having high-resolution (allele-level) HLA typing available with which the search is performed. This can significantly reduce the time needed to test samples which are later found to be mismatched and to improve the precision of automated HLA matching algorithms.[26] Most transplant centers will work with registries or donor centers to assist with the logistics of the search and to give advice in complex cases, such as the selection of UCB units.

DONOR SELECTION AND WORKUP

Donor Selection

There are many factors that affect donor selection both in terms of the donor type and the specific donor. This includes HLA matching, relationship to the patient, donor characteristics, and donor health. Selecting between donor types takes into account clinical outcomes (explained in Chapters 8 and 9) and logistic considerations which are described in the following sections and summarized in Table 6.1. The use of cells from donors other than HLA-identical siblings has increased over the last decade, as shown by CIBMTR data (Fig. 6.3).

Donor type

HLA-identical sibling. Typically, the 'best' donor, if available, is an HLA-identical sibling. Based on Mendelian genetics, there is a 25% chance that each sibling will be matched to the recipient, and the chance of having an HLA-identical sibling will differ by family size (http://www.cancernetwork.com/cancer-management/hematopoietic-cell-transplantation). Although HLA typing for a sibling can often be rapidly obtained, it is increasingly the case that siblings live distant from the recipient and that the logistics of obtaining a blood sample can be more complex. In some cases, multiple HLA-identical siblings may be available, in which case accreditation bodies generally require that a strategy for selection is followed. The

TABLE 6.1
Relative Risks and Benefits of Different Cell Sources

	HLA-Identical Sibling	UD	MMUD	UCB[a]	Haplo[a]
Availability	25% chance each sibling is matched	75% Caucasians[b] 16%–46% other race/ethnicity	97% Caucasians[b] >66% other race/ethnicity	~100% Caucasians[b] 81% African American	Almost always
HLA match	Ideal	Restrictive	Restrictive	Less restrictive	Predictable
Speed of acquisition	Fast	Fast–medium	Fast–medium	Fast	Fast
Cell dose	Predictable	Predictable	Predictable	Low	Predictable
Quality	Predictable	Predictable	Predictable	Impacted by multiple factors	Predictable
Impact of donor-specific antibodies	Low	Recognized	Recognized	May be problematic	May be problematic
Donor complications	Increased compared to UD	Few/possible	Few/possible	Mother nil Baby unknown	Increased compared to UD
Subsequent donations	Possible	Possible	Possible	Not possible	Possible
Speed of engraftment	Fast	Fast	Slower	Slower	Slower
Graft failure	Very rare	Rare	More common	More common	More common
GVHD	Low	High without TCD	High without TCD	Lower than expected with mismatch	High without TCD
Immune reconstitution	Fast	Slow	slower	Slower	Slower
Relapse	Higher than UD	Lower than HLA-identical sibling	Lower than HLA-identical sibling	May be reduced (particularly with double UCB)	Higher in some studies
Survival	Best	Similar to HLA-identical sibling	Similar to UCB and Haplo	Similar to MMUD and Haplo	Similar to UCB and MMUD

[a]see Chapter 8 (haplo) and Chapter 9 (UCB).
[b]HLA match ≥4/6 and TNC >2.5 × 10⁷/kg of recipient body weight (from Ref. 31).
GVHD, graft-versus-host disease; *HLA*, human leukocyte antigen; *MMUD*, mismatched unrelated donor; *TCD*, T-cell depletion; *UCB*, umbilical cord blood; *UD*, unrelated donor.

health, availability, and willingness of the donor are often major considerations in making this decision; however, donor factors other than HLA, such as age, cytomegalovirus (CMV) serostatus, pregnancies, and ABO type, may be considered [although evidence for an impact of these factors is much less than when selecting an unrelated donor (UD) (described in the following)]. Stem cell collections from HLA-identical siblings are typically robust in terms of cell number and quality. Even when older donors (>60) are harvested, an acceptable minimum number of stem cells are typically obtained.[27]

Matched unrelated donor. Historically, a well-matched UD was the second choice if an HLA-identical sibling was not available. In many centers this remains the predominant practice; however, given the improvement in outcomes with alternative donor sources, as well as potential logistic benefits (e.g., availability, speed of acquisition), some centers will consider other donor types either at the same time or before a UD. The definition of a 'well-matched' UD has changed over time; however, the current gold standard is a donor matched at allele level for HLA-A, HLA-B, HLA-C, or HLA-DRB-1 (8/8).[28,29] The

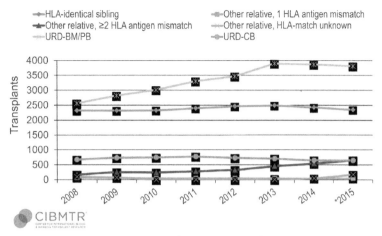

FIG. 6.3 Allogeneic transplant recipients in the US, by donor type. *2015 Data incomplete. (Souza A, Zhu X. *Current Uses and Outcomes of Hematopoietic Cell Transplantation (HCT): CIBMTR Summary Slides*, 2016.)

worldwide donor registries have continued to increase in size, and in September 2017 there are more than 30 million donors represented on the Bone Marrow Donor Worldwide (BMDW) Registry (https://www.bmdw.org/). The BMDW lists details of each donor (e.g., HLA typing), which can be variable depending on the date at which the donor joined the registry, which registry they are a member of, and whether the registry allows listing of other non-HLA characteristics. Many transplant centers will not use BMDW directly but will use the services of a national registry to assist with the donor search and selection process. Several donor registries (and the BMDW) use predictive matching algorithms based on HLA frequencies to streamline the donor search and selection process.[26] Unfortunately, not all donors listed in the BMDW will be available to donate. There are multiple reasons for this including the inability to contact the donor, temporary or permanent deferral, or change in donor willingness, which have been covered in detail in recent reviews.[30]

The most detailed analysis addressing the possibility of finding a donor, taking into account both race/ethnicity and availability, was performed by the National Marrow Donor Program/Be The Match (NMDP) in their large registry of more than 10 million adult donors.[31] They found the likelihood of there being an available 8/8 matched UD on their registry differed significantly for the 21 US racial and ethnic groups. It was high at 75% for white Europeans but lower for all other ethnicities (46% for white patients of Middle Eastern or North African descent, 16%–19% for black Americans and ranging between 27% and 52% for Hispanics, Asians, Pacific Islanders, and Native Americans).

In many cases, more than one 8/8 HLA-matched donor will be available, and 'secondary selection' characteristics can be taken into account. Several publications have addressed the impact of secondary donor characteristics on UD transplant outcomes. The age of the UD donor (younger donor age results in better recipient outcome) has been repeatedly shown to be of importance, and routine practice should be made to prioritize the youngest donor within equally HLA-matched potential donors to optimize survival.[32–37] Other characteristics that impact survival and/or other important clinical outcomes, such as GVHD and relapse, include recipient/donor ABO match status,[34,38] recipient/donor CMV match status,[35,39,40] recipient/donor race/ethnicity matching,[41] donor parity,[33,34] and gender.[42] The CIBMTR attempted to develop and validate a donor selection score that prioritizes donor characteristics associated with better survival in 8/8 HLA-matched UDs. We included >10,000 recipient/donor pairs in a series of testing and validation cohorts. Despite this very large number of recipients, we were unable to develop a donor selection score as the only donor factors consistently associated with survival was donor age. These data show that as none of the other donor factors tested were reproducibly associated with survival, flexibility in selecting UD based on these characteristics is justified (manuscript submitted). Other donor factors that may be taken into account, but have not been extensively studied in the literature, include donor weight and discrepancies between recipient/donor weight (particularly where bone marrow is the stem cell source)[43,44] and donor registry/center.[45]

Finally, although the presence and clinical impact of donor-specific antibodies (DSAs) are more commonly considered when selecting alternative donors (described in the following), it is well recognized that DSAs are frequently directed at the HLA-DP locus, which is usually mismatched in the 8/8 matched setting and commonly considered in donor selection due to its impact on outcomes.[46-48]

Several recent studies show that the survival after a matched UD HCT is not different from survival after an HLA-identical sibling donor HCT.[49,50] Given the fact that donor age has proven to be such a significant determinant of survival in the UD setting, a few studies have addressed the question of whether a younger UD may result in better outcomes than an older HLA-identical donor. The data thus far are mixed, particularly in older patients, in which one study showed that outcomes favored using the sibling donor,[51] whereas another favored the younger unrelated donor.[37] Further studies are required before a clear recommendation can be made.

The term 'alternative donor' typically includes mismatched UD (MMUD), umbilical cord blood (UCB), and haplo-identical (haplo) donors. Many studies now show that survival using any one of these donor types is similar,[52-54] although currently no data from a large randomized study are available. However, other outcomes such as graft failure and GVHD may differ depending on the source and necessitate approaches that are aimed at minimizing these issues. Importantly, the race/ethnicity of donors available on the international registries is predominantly Caucasian, and, as has been shown previously, patients from ethnic minorities frequently cannot find an 8/8 matched UD. The availability of alternative donors has significantly increased the access to transplantation for patients from ethnic minorities. One study from the United Kingdom showed no difference in the chance of undergoing HCT for patients from all race/ethnicities enrolled in a prospective study, but a significantly higher proportion of patients from ethnic minorities received an alternative donor HCT compared with Caucasians (UCB 21.3% vs. 3.8%, $P < .001$, and haplo 10.6% vs. 1.3%, $P < .001$).[55]

Mismatched unrelated donor. HLA-mismatched UD are typically used in the setting of T-cell depleting techniques to reduce the risk of GVHD, which would otherwise be prohibitively high. The degree of mismatch is usually only a single allele, and outcomes in this setting are acceptable, especially if permissive (i.e., they do not result in an increase in complications compared to an 8/8 HLA match, see Chapter 2), and a donor with

this type of mismatch, if available, should be prioritized.[56] Use of an MMUD expands the available donor pool. The NMDP found that the inclusion of 7/8 HLA-matched donors increased the likelihood of finding a UD to 97% in white Europeans and 76% for African Americans, with all race/ethnicities having a probability of finding a UD of >66%.[31] Graft failure and GVHD may be higher in this setting, and many studies have shown delayed immune reconstitution, resulting in a prolonged period at risk for infections.[57] These negative factors may be balanced against the ability to collect a large number of cells of predictable quality and the potential to obtain cells for subsequent infusions. Recently, centers have developed protocols for transplanting patients from a donor who is even more mismatched (4/8–7/8). One study has pioneered this approach in the setting of posttransplant cyclophosphamide (as in haplo transplantation, described in the following).[58] There are two large benefits to this approach: (1) Some patients do not have an available donor of any type (including related or UCB), and a multiply mismatched UD allows for the option of transplantation, and (2) Owing to the large size of the UD registries, there are multiple donors available for a patient if the restriction of HLA matching is loosened; thus other donor characteristics (such as younger age, or ABO match) can be prioritized, and certain mismatched HLA alleles can be avoided if there are DSAs in the recipient.

Haploidentical donor (see also Chapter 8). Recent advances in approaches to HCT when using a haploidentical donor have significantly changed the field, such that use of this donor type is now routine in many centers. These protocols generally incorporating T-cell depletion in some form (e.g., use of antithymocyte globulin, posttransplant cyclophosphamide, or CD34+ cell selection) have resulted in a significantly lower incidence of both acute and chronic GVHD in many studies.[59,60] Strictly speaking, an HLA-haploidentical donor is one in which a single inherited identical copy of chromosome 6 (containing the HLA loci) is shared. This donor must therefore be related to the recipient. In many situations, the second copy of chromosome 6 may be completely mismatched for the HLA loci; however, based on the frequency of particular HLA alleles in the population, it could be matched at a variable number of HLA loci. Thus there is a spectrum of mismatching possible from a 'true' haplo match (4/8) to a 6 or even 7/8 matched relative. Many publications do not clearly define the degree of HLA match in the patient/donor pairs studied; however, in studies addressing the impact of the degree of HLA mismatched on outcome, little evidence for any difference has been shown.[61] Several studies have also attempted to develop a haplo-donor selection strategy that could prioritize non-HLA donor factors, such as family relationship (sibling vs. parent vs. child), age, gender, and genetic factors such as killer immunoglobulin-like receptors (KIRs),[62,63] but thus far there is little consistent evidence for a universal algorithm which impacts outcomes. As with HLA-identical siblings, haplo donors are typically readily available, provide a robust and predictable product, and can be accessed for a subsequent donation. Conversely, DSAs can be particularly problematic in the setting of a haplo HCT, and several strategies for depleting these, with varying degrees of success, have been published.[64–66]

Umbilical cord blood (see also Chapter 9). Successful outcomes using UCB as the stem cell source for HCT in the late 1980s[67] lead to adoption of donor type, initially in children, and later, after two landmark papers describing outcomes in adults[68,69] more generally. The naivety of cells in the UCB unit allows for transplantation across a greater degree of HLA disparity (than a UD), without the expected degree of GVHD. In view of this, HLA matching algorithms for UCB selection were historically less restrictive, and matching at HLA-A, HLA-B (at a serologically level), and HLA-DRB-1 (allele level) (6/6) were the standard of care, with an acceptable match grade of ≥4/6.[70] More recently it has been shown that matching for HLA-C[71] and high-resolution matching at all loci[72,73] result in superior outcomes. A downside to the use of UCB (especially in adult patients) is the low number of stem cells [total nucleated cells (TNC) and CD34+ cells] present in the graft. Studies show both the TNC[74] and CD34+ cell count[75] to be crucial factors determining outcomes, especially graft failure and immune reconstitution. Unlike other donor types in which the HLA match is of primary importance, studies in UCB have shown that HLA match and TNC are of equal importance, making the selection of this stem cell source more complex. The large NMDP study mentioned previously[31] also addressed the question of how many UCB units are available in the registry taking into account both HLA and TNC. They found that almost all patients had an available ≥4/6 HLA-matched UCB; however, when taking the TNC into account, this differed by patient age. For children, a suitably matched UCB unit with sufficient TNC (>2.5 × 10⁷/kg of recipient body weight) could be found for almost all patients. This was similar for European adults but dropped to 81% for African American adult patients. In addition to the benefits of less restrictive HLA matching, cord blood collection facilities are frequently located in ma-

ternity units serving population with a high proportion of ethnic minorities to increase the HLA diversity of units in the bank. There are several secondary factors that should be taken into account which may impact the quality of the unit, including the age of the unit, the method of processing the unit, and the cord blood bank.[76] Strategies to overcome the restrictions due to low cell dose in a unit include (1) double UCB transplants,[77,78] (2) supplementing the UCB transplant with cells from a different source (e.g., a relative) to provide a 'bridge to engraftment,[79,80] and (3) technologies to expand the stem cells in the UCB.[81] An important benefit of UCB is that units can be rapidly available (which is a significant advantage in the setting of an urgent need for HCT) as the UCB is already stored in the bank; however, subsequent donations are not possible.

Donor Workup
All allogeneic donors need a careful workup before they can be cleared for donation. This serves two main purposes: (1) to protect the health of the patient by excluding donors (as appropriate) with conditions that can be transmitted through the product and (2) to protect the health and well-being of the donor.

Donor suitability
Donor suitability is determined by the clinical health, history (including 'high-risk' behavior, travel, and vaccinations), investigations (e.g., chest X-ray, ECG may be required), and laboratory testing [e.g., infectious disease markers (IDMs), basic chemistry and hematology panels, Hb electrophoresis] of the donor. The World Marrow Donor Association (WMDA), an organization, the goal of which is to 'foster collaboration between international registries to facilitate the exchange of hematopoietic stem cell products for the purpose of unrelated hematopoietic SCT,[82] requires all WMDA-accredited UD registries to have established guidelines to determine donor suitability. Although there is reasonable international consensus from registries about conditions and results which should lead to deferral of the donor, in general, these are recommendations rather than absolute reasons for deferral. In an attempt to harmonize and make available these criteria across all registries, the WMDA convened a working committee to develop an online resource for registries to refer to (https://wiki.wmda.info/index.php?title=Main_P age)[83] (Fig. 6.4). This wiki site has a look up function for the individual condition. The webpage is then organized to display the individual at increased risk due to the condition {recipient [e.g., transmissible disease (Fig. 6.5), donor (Fig. 6.6) or both}, the recommendations

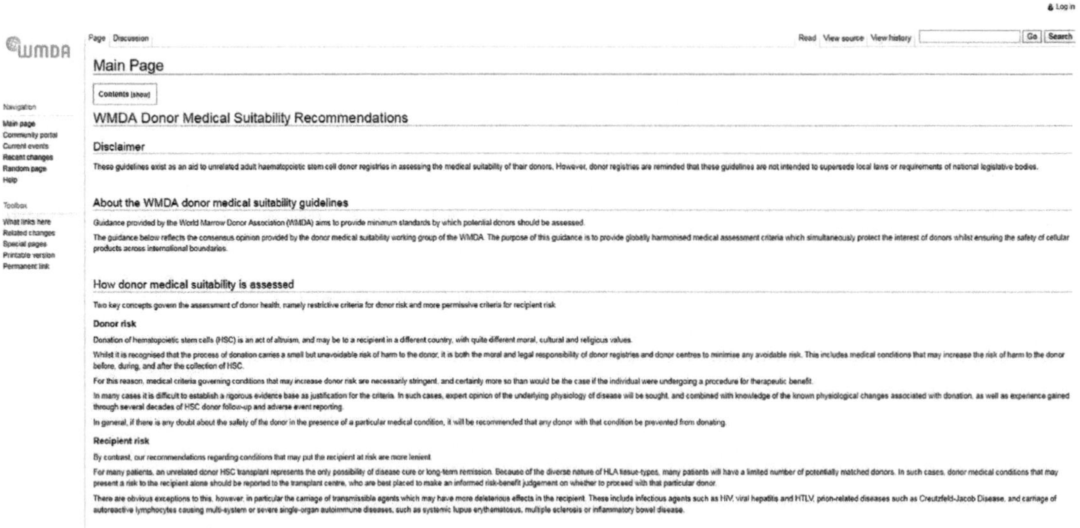

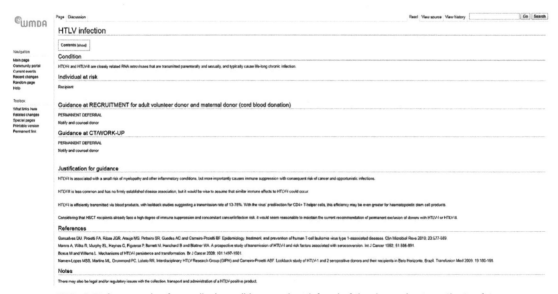

FIG. 6.4 An overview of the main page of the WMDA donor suitability tool. *WMDA*, World Marrow Donor Association.

FIG. 6.5 An example of a medical condition causing deferral of the donor due to patient safety.

for deferral, justification for the guidelines, and any available references. No similar resource exists for the assessment of related donors, although several efforts have been directed at resolving this.[84,85]

Risk to recipient

There are several categories of preexisting conditions that can be transferred through the stem cell product. These include infection (e.g., hepatitis B and C, HIV, syphilis, Chagas disease), malignancy (e.g., hematological and may be due to an unknown clonal abnormality in the donor[86]), autoimmune diseases (e.g., thyroid disease, vitiligo), and inherited diseases (e.g., hemoglobinopathies including sickle cell anemia and thalassemia). Foundation for the Accreditation of Cellular Therapy - Joint Accreditation Committee of ISCT (International Society for Cellular Therapy) (FACT-JACIE), the accreditation body for HCT centers, standards require that

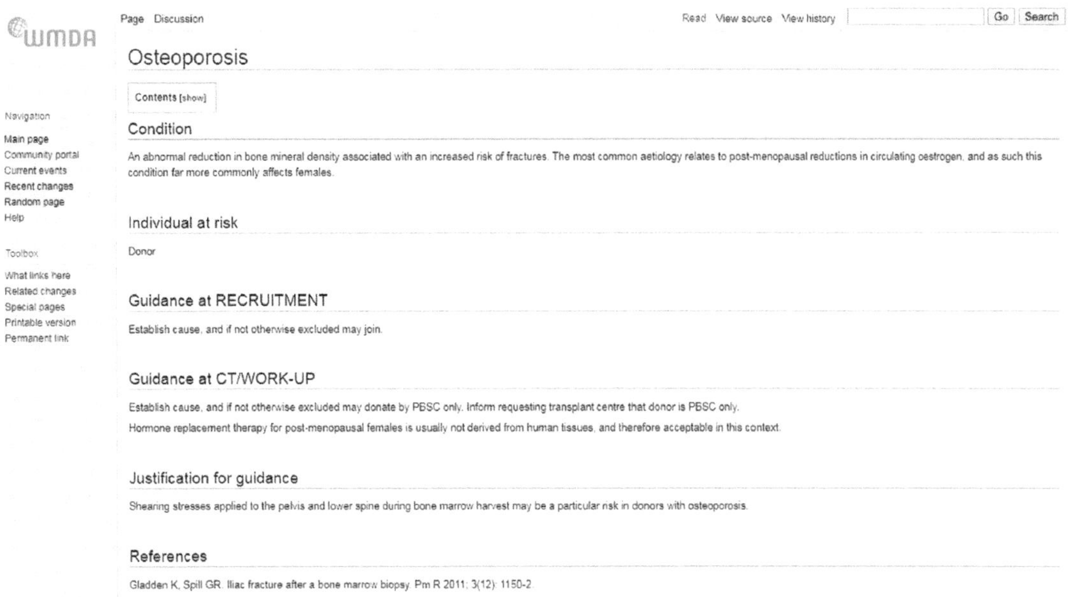
WMDA

Page Discussion

Read View source View history Go Search

Osteoporosis

Contents [show]

Navigation

Main page
Community portal
Current events
Recent changes
Random page
Help

Toolbox

What links here
Related changes
Special pages
Printable version
Permanent link

Condition

An abnormal reduction in bone mineral density associated with an increased risk of fractures. The most common aetiology relates to post-menopausal reductions in circulating oestrogen, and as such this condition far more commonly affects females.

Individual at risk

Donor

Guidance at RECRUITMENT

Establish cause, and if not otherwise excluded may join.

Guidance at CT/WORK-UP

Establish cause, and if not otherwise excluded may donate by PBSC only. Inform requesting transplant centre that donor is PBSC only.

Hormone replacement therapy for post-menopausal females is usually not derived from human tissues, and therefore acceptable in this context.

Justification for guidance

Shearing stresses applied to the pelvis and lower spine during bone marrow harvest may be a particular risk in donors with osteoporosis.

References

Gladden K, Spill GR. Iliac fracture after a bone marrow biopsy. Pm R 2011; 3(12): 1150-2.

FIG. 6.6 An example of a medical condition causing deferral of the donor due to donor safety.

testing for many of these is performed, but this may vary by geographical region (based on the prevalence of a condition) and regulatory requirements that may differ by country (https://www.fda.gov/downloads/biologicsbloodvaccines/guidancecomplianceregulatoryinformation/guidances/tissue/ucm091345.pdf). In the UD setting, donors may be deferred if one of these conditions is discovered (particularly if more than one donor is potentially available); however, deferral is more difficult with a related donor. The transplant physician needs to weigh the risk to the recipient of developing a post-HCT condition transmitted with the product versus the life-saving nature of the transplant itself. In many cases a certain level of risk is deemed to be acceptable, by both the physician and the patient.

Risk to the donor

It is important to remember that donation is a voluntary act, and every attempt should be made to minimize the risk, both physical and psychological, to the donor. Although donation of either bone marrow (BM) or peripheral blood stem cells (PBSCs) is overall a very safe procedure, serious complications (including death) have been reported.[87–89] To minimize the risk of complications, medical criteria determining suitability may appear overly 'stringent', compared to what might be an exclusion for a patient undergoing a therapeutic procedure. Although criteria are established (by registries and others), there is seldom a robust evidence base to support these, and many conditions fall into a 'grey area'. For this reason, many recommendations are based on years of experience with donors and expert and consensus opinion.[83,85] Risks to the donor may also differ based on whether PBSC or BM is donated, for example, a donor with a history of back surgery may be deferred from BM harvest but acceptable for PBSC, while a donor with a condition which may be flared by GCSF (e.g., gout or rheumatoid arthritis) may be acceptable for BM but deferred from PBSC.

Donor assessment

The timing of donor assessment differs for UD and related donors. Typically, UD will have an assessment at at least three time points: when they join the registry, when they are asked to provide a sample to confirm they are a suitable HLA match, and when they are selected for donation. Although assessments at the first two stages are less rigorous, they will nevertheless exclude donors with obvious contraindications to donation (e.g., malignancy, cardiac disease) and highlight to these donors, medical conditions to be aware of and to inform the registry about if they develop. In contrast, related donors are seldom knowledgeable about risk or procedures for stem cell donation until their relative is searching for a donor and thus may have known or unknown medical conditions which can exclude them. It is now recommended by FACT-JACIE and others[84] that all related donor have a basic medical screen before providing a sample for HLA typing.

Conflict of interest

Conflict of interest, or coercion, can occur in the donor evaluation process. This may occur in related donors as they are generally worked up and consented at the same institution where their relative is being treated. Several studies highlighted this potential conflict of interest, showing that the donor is often managed by the same physician as the patient.[90,91] This may result in nondisclosure of medical risks or conditions by the donor if they are concerned that this may lead to their deferral or become known to their family member. Conversely the physician may apply less strict deferral criteria, putting the donor at higher risk. Finally, the lack of an independent advocate for the donor may result in coercion. To address these issues, organizations such as FACT-JACIE and the WMDA[84] have made recommendation for the separation of care of the patient and donor. In some countries, particularly with vulnerable donors such as children, a donor advocate is mandated by law. This is entirely avoided in the UD setting due to the anonymous nature of the donation as set forth in the WMDA standards (https://share. wmda.info/display/ANON/WMDA+Standards?preview= /20748235/200048678/20160905-STDC-WMDA%20sta ndards%20cleared%20version.pdf).

Donor follow-up

It is recommended that a mechanism for donor follow-up is in place at a minimum to understand and resolve any serious adverse events or reactions (SAE/R) which occur.[92] UD registries comply with this requirement and report these SEA/R to the WMDA Serious Product Events and Adverse Reactions (SPEAR) registry.[93] Although, SAE/R which occur in related donors can be reported to the WMDA registry, this is not common practice as it is not mandated. Recently the European Society for Blood and Marrow Transplant (EBMT) has developed reporting through their routine patient outcome data collection system (https://www.ebmt.org/ Contents/Data-Management/Registrystructure/MED-ABdatacollectionforms/Pages/MED-AB-data-collection-forms.aspx#DonorOutcomeForms). Finally, a few studies have addressed donor QOL after donation, in general donors return to their baseline and many UD report that they are extremely satisfied with their decision to donate and the vast majority would agree to donate again.[94]

REFERENCES

1. Majhail NS, Farnia SH, Carpenter PA, et al. Indications for autologous and allogeneic hematopoietic cell transplantation: guidelines from the American Society for blood and marrow transplantation. *Biol Blood Marrow Transplant.* 2015;21:1863–1869.

2. Sureda A, Bader P, Cesaro S, et al. Indications for allo- and auto-SCT for haematological diseases, solid tumours and immune disorders: current practice in Europe, 2015. *Bone Marrow Transplant.* 2015;50:1037–1056.

3. Auner HW, Szydlo R, Hoek J, et al. Trends in autologous hematopoietic cell transplantation for multiple myeloma in Europe: increased use and improved outcomes in elderly patients in recent years. *Bone Marrow Transplant.* 2015;50:209–215.

4. Lim Z, Brand R, Martino R, et al. Allogeneic hematopoietic stem-cell transplantation for patients 50 years or older with myelodysplastic syndromes or secondary acute myeloid leukemia. *J Clin Oncol.* 2010;28:405–411.

5. McClune BL, Weisdorf DJ, Pedersen TL, et al. Effect of age on outcome of reduced-intensity hematopoietic cell transplantation for older patients with acute myeloid leukemia in first complete remission or with myelodysplastic syndrome. *J Clin Oncol.* 2010;28: 1878–1887.

6. Sorror ML, Sandmaier BM, Storer BE, et al. Long-term outcomes among older patients following nonmyeloablative conditioning and allogeneic hematopoietic cell transplantation for advanced hematologic malignancies. *JAMA.* 2011;306:1874–1883.

7. Chen X, Mao G, Leng SX. Frailty syndrome: an overview. *Clin Interv Aging.* 2014;9:433–441.

8. Artz AS. Biologic vs physiologic age in the transplant candidate. *Hematol Am Soc Hematol Ed Program.* 2016;99–105:2016.

9. Rosko A, Artz A. Reprint of: aging: treating the older patient. *Biol Blood Marrow Transplant.* 2017;23:S10–S17.

10. Sorror ML, Maris MB, Storb R, et al. Hematopoietic cell transplantation (HCT)-specific comorbidity index: a new tool for risk assessment before allogeneic HCT. *Blood.* 2005;106:2912–2919.

11. Sorror ML. Comorbidities and hematopoietic cell transplantation outcomes. *Hematol Am Soc Hematol Ed Program.* 2010;237–47:2010.

12. Sorror ML, Logan BR, Zhu X, et al. Prospective validation of the predictive power of the hematopoietic cell transplantation comorbidity index: a center for international blood and marrow transplant research study. *Biol Blood Marrow Transplant.* 2015;21:1479–1487.

13. Berro M, Arbelbide JA, Rivas MM, et al. Hematopoietic cell transplantation-specific comorbidity index predicts morbidity and mortality in autologous stem cell transplantation. *Biol Blood Marrow Transplant.* 2017;23:1646–1650.

14. Sorror ML, Estey E. Allogeneic hematopoietic cell transplantation for acute myeloid leukemia in older adults. *Hematol Am Soc Hematol Ed Program.* 2014;21–33:2014.

15. Wood WA, Le-Rademacher J, Syrjala KL, et al. Patient-reported physical functioning predicts the success of hematopoietic cell transplantation (BMT CTN 0902). *Cancer.* 2016;122:91–98.

16. Shaw BE, Brazauskas R, Millard HR, et al. Centralized patient-reported outcome data collection in transplantation is feasible and clinically meaningful. *Cancer.* 2017; 123(23):4687–4700.

17. Baker KS, Davies SM, Majhail NS, et al. Race and socio-economic status influence outcomes of unrelated donor hematopoietic cell transplantation. *Biol Blood Marrow Transplant*. 2009;15:1543–1554.
18. Knight JM, Rizzo JD, Logan BR, et al. Low socioeconomic status, adverse gene expression profiles, and clinical outcomes in hematopoietic stem cell transplant recipients. *Clin Cancer Res*. 2016;22:69–78.
19. By the American Geriatrics Society Beers Criteria Update Expert P. American geriatrics society 2015 updated beers criteria for potentially inappropriate medication use in older adults. *J Am Geriatr Soc*. 2015;63:2227–2246.
20. Goetzmann L, Ruegg L, Stamm M, et al. Psychosocial profiles after transplantation: a 24-month follow-up of heart, lung, liver, kidney and allogeneic bone-marrow patients. *Transplantation*. 2008;86:662–668.
21. Strouse C, Richardson P, Prentice G, et al. Defibrotide for treatment of severe veno-occlusive disease in pediatrics and adults: an exploratory analysis using data from the center for international blood and marrow transplant research. *Biol Blood Marrow Transplant*. 2016;22:1306–1312.
22. Shaffer BC, Ahn KW, Hu ZH, et al. Scoring system prognostic of outcome in patients undergoing allogeneic hematopoietic cell transplantation for myelodysplastic syndrome. *J Clin Oncol*. 2016;34:1864–1871.
23. Arora M, Hemmer MT, Ahn KW, et al. Center for International Blood and Marrow Transplant Research chronic graft-versus-host disease risk score predicts mortality in an independent validation cohort. *Biol Blood Marrow Transplant*. 2015;21:640–645.
24. Levine JE, Braun TM, Harris AC, et al. A prognostic score for acute graft-versus-host disease based on biomarkers: a multicentre study. *Lancet Haematol*. 2015;2:e21–e29.
25. Spellman SR, Eapen M, Logan BR, et al. A perspective on the selection of unrelated donors and cord blood units for transplantation. *Blood*. 2012;120:259–265.
26. Wadsworth K, Albrecht M, Fonstad R, et al. Unrelated donor search prognostic score to support early HLA consultation and clinical decisions. *Bone Marrow Transplant*. 2016;51:1476–1481.
27. Anderlini P. Sixty as the new forty: considerations on older related stem cell donors. *Bone Marrow Transplant*. 2017;52:15–19.
28. Lee SJ, Klein J, Haagenson M, et al. High-resolution donor-recipient HLA matching contributes to the success of unrelated donor marrow transplantation. *Blood*. 2007;110:4576–4583.
29. Pidala J, Lee SJ, Ahn KW, et al. Nonpermissive HLA-DPB1 mismatch increases mortality after myeloablative unrelated allogeneic hematopoietic cell transplantation. *Blood*. 2014;124:2596–2606.
30. Lown RN, Shaw BE. Beating the odds: factors implicated in the speed and availability of unrelated haematopoietic cell donor provision. *Bone Marrow Transplant*. 2013;48:210–219.
31. Gragert L, Eapen M, Williams E, et al. HLA match likelihoods for hematopoietic stem-cell grafts in the U.S. registry. *N Engl J Med*. 2014;371:339–348.
32. Carreras E, Jimenez M, Gomez-Garcia V, et al. Donor age and degree of HLA matching have a major impact on the outcome of unrelated donor haematopoietic cell transplantation for chronic myeloid leukaemia. *Bone Marrow Transplant*. 2006;37:33–40.
33. Kollman C, Howe CW, Anasetti C, et al. Donor characteristics as risk factors in recipients after transplantation of bone marrow from unrelated donors: the effect of donor age. *Blood*. 2001;98:2043–2051.
34. Kollman C, Spellman SR, Zhang MJ, et al. The effect of donor characteristics on survival after unrelated donor transplantation for hematologic malignancy. *Blood*. 2016;127:260–267.
35. Shaw BE, Mayor NP, Szydlo RM, et al. Recipient/donor HLA and CMV matching in recipients of T-cell-depleted unrelated donor haematopoietic cell transplants. *Bone Marrow Transplant*. 2017;52(5):717–725.
36. Ayuk F, Zabelina T, Wortmann F, et al. Donor choice according to age for allo-SCT for AML in complete remission. *Bone Marrow Transplant*. 2013;48:1028–1032.
37. Kroger N, Zabelina T, de Wreede L, et al. Allogeneic stem cell transplantation for older advanced MDS patients: improved survival with young unrelated donor in comparison with HLA-identical siblings. *Leukemia*. 2013;27:604–609.
38. Seebach JD, Stussi G, Passweg JR, et al. ABO blood group barrier in allogeneic bone marrow transplantation revisited. *Biol Blood Marrow Transplant*. 2005;11:1006–1013.
39. Ljungman P, Brand R, Einsele H, et al. Donor CMV serologic status and outcome of CMV-seropositive recipients after unrelated donor stem cell transplantation: an EBMT megafile analysis. *Blood*. 2003;102:4255–4260.
40. Ljungman P, Brand R, Hoek J, et al. Donor cytomegalovirus status influences the outcome of allogeneic stem cell transplant: a study by the European group for blood and marrow transplantation. *Clin Infect Dis*. 2014;59:473–481.
41. Morishima Y, Kawase T, Malkki M, et al. Significance of ethnicity in the risk of acute graft-versus-host disease and leukemia relapse after unrelated donor hematopoietic stem cell transplantation. *Biol Blood Marrow Transplant*. 2013;19:1197–1203.
42. Nakasone H, Remberger M, Tian L, et al. Risks and benefits of sex-mismatched hematopoietic cell transplantation differ according to conditioning strategy. *Haematologica*. 2015;100:1477–1485.
43. Anthias C, Billen A, Arkwright R, et al. Harvests from bone marrow donors who weigh less than their recipients are associated with a significantly increased probability of a suboptimal harvest yield. *Transfusion*. 2016;56:1052–1057.
44. Billen A, Madrigal JA, Szydlo RM, et al. Female donors and donors who are lighter than their recipient are less likely to meet the CD34+ cell dose requested for peripheral blood stem cell transplantation. *Transfusion*. 2014;54:2953–2960.
45. Lazarus HM, Kan F, Tarima S, et al. Rapid transport and infusion of hematopoietic cells is associated with improved outcome after myeloablative therapy and unrelated donor transplant. *Biol Blood Marrow Transplant*. 2009;15:589–596.

46. Crivello P, Zito L, Sizzano F, et al. The impact of amino acid variability on alloreactivity defines a functional distance predictive of permissive HLA-DPB1 mismatches in hematopoietic stem cell transplantation. *Biol Blood Marrow Transplant.* 2015;21:233–241.

47. Fleischhauer K, Shaw BE, Gooley T, et al. Effect of T-cell-epitope matching at HLA-DPB1 in recipients of unrelated-donor haemopoietic-cell transplantation: a retrospective study. *Lancet Oncol.* 2012;13:366–374.

48. Spellman S, Bray R, Rosen-Bronson S, et al. The detection of donor-directed, HLA-specific alloantibodies in recipients of unrelated hematopoietic cell transplantation is predictive of graft failure. *Blood.* 2010;115:2704–2708.

49. Peters C, Schrappe M, von Stackelberg A, et al. Stem-cell transplantation in children with acute lymphoblastic leukemia: a prospective international multicenter trial comparing sibling donors with matched unrelated donors-The ALL-SCT-BFM-2003 trial. *J Clin Oncol.* 2015;33:1265–1274.

50. Saber W, Opie S, Rizzo JD, et al. Outcomes after matched unrelated donor versus identical sibling hematopoietic cell transplantation in adults with acute myelogenous leukemia. *Blood.* 2012;119:3908–3916.

51. Alousi AM, Le-Rademacher J, Saliba RM, et al. Who is the better donor for older hematopoietic transplant recipients: an older-aged sibling or a young, matched unrelated volunteer? *Blood.* 2013;121:2567–2573.

52. Anasetti C, Aversa F, Brunstein CG. Back to the future: mismatched unrelated donor, haploidentical related donor, or unrelated umbilical cord blood transplantation? *Biol Blood Marrow Transplant.* 2012;18:S161–S165.

53. Raiola AM, Dominietto A, di Grazia C, et al. Unmanipulated haploidentical transplants compared with other alternative donors and matched sibling grafts. *Biol Blood Marrow Transplant.* 2014;20:1573–1579.

54. Ruggeri A, Labopin M, Sanz G, et al. Comparison of outcomes after unrelated cord blood and unmanipulated haploidentical stem cell transplantation in adults with acute leukemia. *Leukemia.* 2015;29:1891–1900.

55. Lown RN, Marsh SGE, Blake H, et al. Equality of access to transplant for ethnic minority patients through use of cord blood and haploidentical transplants. *Blood.* 2013;122:2138 (abstract).

56. Lazaryan A, Wang T, Spellman SR, et al. Human leukocyte antigen supertype matching after myeloablative hematopoietic cell transplantation with 7/8 matched unrelated donor allografts: a report from the Center for International Blood and Marrow Transplant Research. *Haematologica.* 2016;101:1267–1274.

57. de Koning C, Nierkens S, Boelens JJ. Strategies before, during, and after hematopoietic cell transplantation to improve T-cell immune reconstitution. *Blood.* 2016;128:2607–2615.

58. Kasamon YL, Ambinder RF, Fuchs EJ, et al. Prospective study of nonmyeloablative, HLA-mismatched unrelated BMT with high-dose posttransplantation cyclophosphamide. *Blood Adv.* 2016;1:288–292.

59. Chang YJ, Huang XJ. Haploidentical stem cell transplantation: anti-thymocyte globulin-based experience. *Semin Hematol.* 2016;53:82–89.

60. Robinson TM, O'Donnell PV, Fuchs EJ, et al. Haploidentical bone marrow and stem cell transplantation: experience with post-transplantation cyclophosphamide. *Semin Hematol.* 2016;53:90–97.

61. Ciurea SO, Champlin RE. Donor selection in T cell-replete haploidentical hematopoietic stem cell transplantation: knowns, unknowns, and controversies. *Biol Blood Marrow Transplant.* 2013;19:180–184.

62. Chang YJ, Luznik L, Fuchs EJ, et al. How do we choose the best donor for T-cell-replete, HLA-haploidentical transplantation? *J Hematol Oncol.* 2016;9:35.

63. McCurdy SR, Fuchs EJ. Selecting the best haploidentical donor. *Semin Hematol.* 2016;53:246–251.

64. Ciurea SO, de Lima M, Cano P, et al. High risk of graft failure in patients with anti-HLA antibodies undergoing haploidentical stem-cell transplantation. *Transplantation.* 2009;88:1019–1024.

65. Gladstone DE, Zachary AA, Fuchs EJ, et al. Partially mismatched transplantation and human leukocyte antigen donor-specific antibodies. *Biol Blood Marrow Transplant.* 2013;19:647–652.

66. Yoshihara S, Maruya E, Taniguchi K, et al. Risk and prevention of graft failure in patients with preexisting donor-specific HLA antibodies undergoing unmanipulated haploidentical SCT. *Bone Marrow Transplant.* 2012;47:508–515.

67. Gluckman E, Broxmeyer HA, Auerbach AD, et al. Hematopoietic reconstitution in a patient with Fanconi's anemia by means of umbilical-cord blood from an HLA-identical sibling. *N Engl J Med.* 1989;321:1174–1178.

68. Laughlin MJ, Eapen M, Rubinstein P, et al. Outcomes after transplantation of cord blood or bone marrow from unrelated donors in adults with leukemia. *N Engl J Med.* 2004;351:2265–2275.

69. Rocha V, Labopin M, Sanz G, et al. Transplants of umbilical-cord blood or bone marrow from unrelated donors in adults with acute leukemia. *N Engl J Med.* 2004;351:2276–2285.

70. Rocha V, Gluckman E, Eurocord-Netcord r, et al. Improving outcomes of cord blood transplantation: HLA matching, cell dose and other graft- and transplantation-related factors. *Br J Haematol.* 2009;147:262–274.

71. Eapen M, Klein JP, Sanz GF, et al. Effect of donor-recipient HLA matching at HLA A, B, C, and DRB1 on outcomes after umbilical-cord blood transplantation for leukaemia and myelodysplastic syndrome: a retrospective analysis. *Lancet Oncol.* 2011;12:1214–1221.

72. Eapen M, Wang T, Veys PA, et al. Allele-level HLA matching for umbilical cord blood transplantation for nonmalignant diseases in children: a retrospective analysis. *Lancet Haematol.* 2017;4:e325–e333.

73. Eapen M, Klein JP, Ruggeri A, et al. Impact of allele-level HLA matching on outcomes after myeloablative single unit umbilical cord blood transplantation for hematologic malignancy. *Blood.* 2014;123:133–140.

74. Barker JN, Scaradavou A, Stevens CE. Combined effect of total nucleated cell dose and HLA match on transplantation outcome in 1061 cord blood recipients with hematologic malignancies. *Blood.* 2010;115:1843–1849.

75. Sobol U, Go A, Kliethermes S, et al. A prospective investigation of cell dose in single-unit umbilical cord blood transplantation for adults with high-risk hematologic malignancies. *Bone Marrow Transplant.* 2015;50:1519–1525.

76. Querol S, Gomez SG, Pagliuca A, et al. Quality rather than quantity: the cord blood bank dilemma. *Bone Marrow Transplant.* 2010;45:970–978.

77. Cornelissen JJ, Kalin B, Lamers CHJ. Graft predominance after double umbilical cord blood transplantation: a review. *Stem Cel Investig.* 2017;4:47.

78. Scaradavou A, Brunstein CG, Eapen M, et al. Double unit grafts successfully extend the application of umbilical cord blood transplantation in adults with acute leukemia. *Blood.* 2013;121:752–758.

79. Liu H, van Besien K. Alternative donor transplantation–"mixing and matching": the role of combined cord blood and haplo-identical donor transplantation (haplo-cord SCT) as a treatment strategy for patients lacking standard donors? *Curr Hematol Malig Rep.* 2015;10:1–7.

80. Tsai SB, Liu H, Shore T, et al. Frequency and risk factors associated with cord graft failure after transplant with single-unit umbilical cord cells supplemented by haploidentical cells with reduced-intensity conditioning. *Biol Blood Marrow Transplant.* 2016;22:1065–1072.

81. Mehta RS, Dave H, Bollard CM, et al. Engineering cord blood to improve engraftment after cord blood transplant. *Stem Cel Investig.* 2017;4:41.

82. Petersdorf EW. The World Marrow Donor Association: 20 years of international collaboration for the support of unrelated donor and cord blood hematopoietic cell transplantation. *Bone Marrow Transplant.* 2010;45:807–810.

83. Lown RN, Philippe J, Navarro W, et al. Unrelated adult stem cell donor medical suitability: recommendations from the world marrow donor association clinical working group committee. *Bone Marrow Transplant.* 2014;49:880–886.

84. van Walraven SM, Nicoloso-de Faveri G, Axdorph-Nygell UA, et al. Family donor care management: principles and recommendations. *Bone Marrow Transplant.* 2010;45:1269–1273.

85. Worel N, Buser A, Greinix HT, et al. Suitability criteria for adult related donors: a consensus statement from the Worldwide network for blood and marrow transplantation standing committee on donor issues. *Biol Blood Marrow Transplant.* 2015;21:2052–2060.

86. Gondek LP, Zheng G, Ghiaur G, et al. Donor cell leukemia arising from clonal hematopoiesis after bone marrow transplantation. *Leukemia.* 2016;30:1916–1920.

87. Halter J, Kodera Y, Ispizua AU, et al. Severe events in donors after allogeneic hematopoietic stem cell donation. *Haematologica.* 2009;94:94–101.

88. Pulsipher MA, Chitphakdithai P, Logan BR, et al. Acute toxicities of unrelated bone marrow versus peripheral blood stem cell donation: results of a prospective trial from the National Marrow Donor Program. *Blood.* 2013;121:197–206.

89. Pulsipher MA, Chitphakdithai P, Miller JP, et al. Adverse events among 2408 unrelated donors of peripheral blood stem cells: results of a prospective trial from the National Marrow Donor Program. *Blood.* 2009;113:3604–3611.

90. O'Donnell PV, Pedersen TL, Confer DL, et al. Practice patterns for evaluation, consent, and care of related donors and recipients at hematopoietic cell transplantation centers in the United States. *Blood.* 2010;115:5097–5101.

91. Shaw BE. First do no harm. *Blood.* 2010;115:4978–4979.

92. Halter JP, van Walraven SM, Worel N, et al. Allogeneic hematopoietic stem cell donation-standardized assessment of donor outcome data: a consensus statement from the Worldwide Network for Blood and Marrow Transplantation (WBMT). *Bone Marrow Transplant.* 2013;48:220–225.

93. Shaw BE, Chapman J, Fechter M, et al. Towards a global system of vigilance and surveillance in unrelated donors of haematopoietic progenitor cells for transplantation. *Bone Marrow Transplant.* 2013;48:1506–1509.

94. Switzer GE, Bruce JG, Harrington D, et al. Health-related quality of life of bone marrow versus peripheral blood stem cell donors: a prespecified subgroup analysis from a phase III RCT-BMTCTN protocol 0201. *Biol Blood Marrow Transplant.* 2014;20:118–127.

CHAPTER 7

T-Cell Replete Haploidentical Transplantation

LUCA CASTAGNA, LC, MD • STEFANIA BRAMANTI, SB, MD •
RAYNIER DEVILLIER, RD, MP, PHD • SABINE FURST, SF, MD •
DIDIER BLAISE, DB, MD

The development of different transplant programs using haploidentical donors without T-cell depletion is knowing an exciting time. The feasibility and the toxic profile of T-cell replete haploidentical transplantation, very close to that obtained with conventional donors, are well demonstrated, making of these alternative donors a concrete opportunity for patients with severe disease. So far, the limit to donor availability in the right time for each patients does not exist anymore. In this chapter we revised the most important results obtained with some of the several platforms developed worldwide in patients with malignant and nonmalignant hematological diseases.

INTRODUCTION

Human leukocyte antigen (HLA)–identical stem cell transplantation is a curative option for many hematological malignancies, but the probability to have such a donor in the family is only 25%.[1] Despite the existence of a worldwide registry of HLA-typed volunteer donors (more than 20 millions), about 40% of patients do not find an HLA-identical donor. For those patients it is necessary to search for an alternative donor: partially matched unrelated donor, haploidentical relative donor, or cord blood unit.[2]

This chapter will focus on the results obtained using a haploidentical donor in the context of the now-available T-cell replete platforms.

Because any patient shares exactly one HLA haplotype with each biological parent or child and with half of siblings, a donor matched on one haplotype can be identified rapidly in nearly all cases (haploidentical donor).

While the first attempts to transplant patients with haploidentical relative donors using conventional prophylaxis translated into high toxicity and mortality because of graft failure and GVHD,[3] it appeared that deep T-cell depletion (based on CD34 negative selection) coupled with a myelo-immunoablative conditioning regimen, as developed by the Perugia group, could overcome these barriers.[4] However, the deep T-cell depletion was associated with long-lasting immunodeficiency and limited anti-leukemic effect in many situations, and results obtained in Perugia were difficult to reproduce elsewhere by other groups.

During the last decade, several groups challenged the paradigm of T-cell depletion as a sine *qua non* condition for haploidentical stem cell transplantation (haplo-SCT) and contributed developing different T-cell replete platforms.

GIAC ('G'CSF-stimulation; 'I'ntensified immunosuppression; 'A'ntithymocyte globulin; 'C'ombination of PBSC and bone-marrow) **platform**.

One of the early leading teams on T-cell replete haplo-SCT development has been the University of Beijing in China. The first attempts to perform a haplo-SCT without ex vivo T-cell depletion was made in China. Indeed, in the early 2000, because of the "one-child family" politics previously introduced and the difficulty to find an HLA-identical donor in the donor registries, the probability to identify a donor was low. For these reasons, some Chinese teams started to develop haploidentical program without ex vivo T depletion allowing to perform a transplantation from other family relatives.

In an early paper, Ji et al. reported on 15 advanced leukemia patients receiving allo-SCT from haploidentical donors. They used an adapted platform to allow a solid engraftment reducing prohibitive GVHD. The platform consisted of GCSF-primed bone marrow (BM) stimulating the donor (3–4 µg/kg for 7 days) to enhance the number of stem cells reducing the contamination by T lymphocytes, a reinforced immunosuppressive prophylaxis, in addition to cyclosporine A (CsA) and methotrexate (MTX), with antithymocyte globulin

(ATG) Fresenius, 5 mg/kg from day −4 to −1 and mycophenolate mofetil (MMF) from day +7 to +100.[5] All patients received a TBI-based myeloablative conditioning regimen (MAC). Engraftment was achieved quickly as well as full donor chimerism. The incidence of grade 2–4 acute GVHD (aGVHD) was 33%, and no patients developed severe chronic GVHD (cGVHD). The 2-year disease-free survival (DFS) at 2 years was 60%. Some years later, another team from Beijing University published on 171 patients affected by acute leukemia, myelodysplastic syndromes, and chronic myeloid leukemia, receiving a haplo-SCT with a specific protocol consisting of TBI-based MAC regimen, an intensive immunosuppressive prophylaxis with CsA, MTX, MMF, and ATG, and a combined stem cell source from GCSF-primed BM and peripheral blood stem cells (PBSCs). A full-door chimerism was achieved in all patients, and the CI of severe aGVHD (grade 3–4) was 23%, whereas the probability to relapse was 12% and 39% in standard and high-risk patients, and the leukemia-free survival was 68% and 42%, respectively.[139] The use of both primed BM and PBSC was considered of outmost importance in this platform because of the low capacity of primed BM to induce GVHD and the high number of T-cells contained in PBSC graft to reinforce the graft-versus-leukemia (GVL) effect. Indeed, in an in vitro study, they showed that the combination of primed BM and PBSC in different proportion did not affect the Th1 to Th2 polarization, and this could explain the incidence of aGVHD and cGVHD in the haplo setting similar to that observed after HLA identical transplantation.[6] The authors dissected deeply the quality of combined source of stem cells. Lv et al. reported that the high number of myeloid-derived suppressor cells (MDSCs), both the absolute number and promyelocytic and monocyte-MDSC, contained in the graft reduced the risk of aGVHD and cGVHD, independently from other factors. In this study the reconstitution of monocyte MDSC at day +15 was a predictive factor of future development of aGVHD. An important point was that the high number of MDSC did not influence the risk of relapse.[7] More recently, this team suggested that the number of regulatory B cells (B-regs) in the graft reduced the risk to develop aGVHD via T cells subsets such as Th1 and Th17.[8]

In a retrospective analysis Xu et al. showed that[9] in patients with high-risk leukemia, the OS was better using combined PBSC and G-BM than using PBSC alone, with a higher incidence of full-donor chimerism. Furthermore, the NRM and cGVHD were similar, whereas the incidence of aGVHD was higher with PBSC plus G-BM. Overall, these data confirmed that the combined stem cell source is superior to PBSC alone in this model.

The Beijing team published many papers on the safety and efficacy of their T-cell replete platform both in patients with malignant and not malignant hematological disease. Overall, in these studies including young patients (median age ranges between 23 and 28 year), the results are encouraging in terms of toxicity. As shown in Table 7.1, the median cumulative incidence of grade 2–4 and grade 3–4 aGVHD is 40% (50%–28%) and 11% (6%–23%); severe/extensive cGVHD was 21% (12%–55%) and 1–3 year nonrelapse mortality (NRM) 18% (13%–22%). In an interesting randomized study,[10] patients receiving haplo-SCT were categorized to have low or high risk to develop GVHD based on CD4/CD8 ratio[11] or number of CD56[bright12] in stem cell graft as reported in previous studies. High-risk patients were randomized to receive or not a reinforced GVHD prophylaxis with steroids (0.5 mg/kg per d IV from days +5 to +12, followed by 0.25 mg/kg per d IV for 10 days; 0.125 mg/kg per d until day +30). The CI of grade 2–4 aGVHD was reduced in the steroids arm compared to the control arm without steroids (21% vs. 48%, respectively) and not different compared to low-risk arm (26%). Similarly, the CI of moderate/severe cGVHD was lower with steroids (21% vs. 50%). Of note, infectious complications and risk of relapse were not enhanced by prophylactic steroids.

In the GIAC platform, ATG is one of the major components. However, the relationship between ATG dose and clinical results in terms of toxicity and disease control is well known.[13] To address this point in the haplo-SCT context, Wang et al. performed a randomized trial comparing the standard dose of ATG (10 mg/kg) to a lower dose (6 mg/kg). As expected, the incidence of grade 2–4 and 3–4 aGVHD was higher using lower ATG dose (41% vs. 25% and 16% vs. 5%, respectively), whereas no difference was found of moderate-to-severe cGVHD and NRM. The infectious complications were similar except for the incidence of EBV reactivation and posttransplant lymphoproliperative disease (PTLD) which were directly correlated to the ATG dose.[14] Recently this study has been updated to evaluate the impact of the ATG dose on the control of disease and long-term effects. After a median follow-up of more than 4 years, the cumulative incidence of relapse, 5-year NRM, overall survival (OS), and DFS were not statistically different in the 2 arms. However, patients receiving the higher ATG dose showed a reduced incidence of any late effect (57% vs. 71%), moderate-to-severe cGVHD (30% vs. 56%), and a better survival without severe aGVHD, severe cGVHD, and relapse (GRFS)

TABLE 7.1
Toxicity of GIAC Platform

Authors	N	Median Age	PGF	Grade 2–4 aGVHD	Grade 3–4 aGVHD	Extensive cGVHD	NRM
Huang[140]	171	23y	0	55%	23%	46.9%	19.5%
Lu[21]	135	24y	0	40%	NR	55%	22%
Huang[141]	219	25y	0	47%	NR	54%	20%
Wang[14]	1210	25y	NR	40%	12%	21%	17%
Wang[31]	231	28y	0	36%	10%	12%	13%
Wang[37]	121	26y	1 pt	28%	6%	14%	13%
Chang[10]	72	26y	/	21%	/	21%	13%
	73	30 y		48%	/	50%	10%
Chang[25]	240 MRD+ MRD–	30y	2% 1%	43% 36%	NR	70% overall 48% overall	8% 14%
Chang[25]	258 MRD+ MRD–	30y	3% 1%	32% 28%	NR	73% overall 40% overall	7% 18%

aGVHD, acute graft-versus-host disease; *cGVHD*, chronic graft-versus-host-disease; *MRD*, matched related donor; *NR*, not reported; *PGF*, primary graft failure.
Huang[139], Lu[21], Huang[140]: patients included were affected by AML, MDS, ALL, and CML.
Wang[14]: patients included were affected by AML, MDS, ALL, and CML, and not malignant diseases.
Wang[31]: patients were affected by AML in first complete remission.
Wang[37]: patients were affected by Ph-negative ALL.
Chang[10]: this is a randomized study, including patients with high-risk to develop GVHD. These patients were randomized to receive steroids[72] during the first month after haplo-SCT.
Chang[25]: this is a retrospective cohort including AML patients with positive or negative minimal residual disease (MRD).
Chang[25]: this is a prospective cohort.

(41% vs. 26%).[15] These data strongly suggest that the dose of ATG can be tuned also in GIAC platform leading to an improvement of clinical results.

Recently the same group analyzed which factors can have an impact on treatment-related mortality (TRM) after haplo-SCT in a prospective study, including patients affected by AML and ALL in first CR and using an MAC regimen. In this analysis, three clinical factors (1 point each) significantly impacted on TRM: donor age/patient age (<40 years/<30 years), gender matching (F=>M), and major ABO incompatibility. Indeed the TRM was significantly higher in patients with score 3 (31%), than score 2 (15%) and score 1 (8%). An important point is that the impact of these factors is independent from the donor (haploidentical or HLA identical sibling).[16] Yan et al. analyzed the TRM and causes of death (CODs) in 840 patients with acute leukemia or MDS after haplo-SCT and compared them with a cohort of 540 patients receiving allo-SCT from HLAid sib. The 2-y TRM in the haplo cohort was significantly higher than that in the HLAid group (27%

vs. 20%), whereas no difference was observed regarding the mortality due the relapse of disease. The COD in the haplo group were infections (49%), GVHD (6%), and others (12%). The infection-related deaths were more frequent in the haplo group (21% vs. 13%), whereas there was no difference of death from GVHD. In multivariate analysis the risk factors for TRM were high-risk disease status and to receive haplo-SCT. In the haplo group, other than characteristics of disease, diagnosis of MDS was an independent risk factor (TRM 39%).[17]

One of the major concerns using deep in vivo T-cell depletion is the high risk to develop opportunistic infections. In particular, haplo-SCT is considered a risk factor to develop invasive fungal infections (IFIs).[18] This topic was addressed by the Beijing team analyzing the incidence of IFI in 291 patients, receiving low-dose fluconazole (200 mg/day until day +75). The 1-year cumulative incidence of proven/probable IFI was 13%, and the risk factors were late platelet engraftment, severe aGVHD, and high-risk hematological disease. The diagnosis of IFI had an impact on survival compared to those patients without IFI (24% vs. 71%).[19] In a randomized trial Huang et al. compared the efficacy to prevent IFI using oral itraconazole (5 mg/kg per day) or micafungin (50 mg/day). The cumulative incidence of IFI was similar (1.4% vs. 4.4%, respectively), but the tolerance of micafungin was better, as expected.[20]

Viral infections, especially cytomegalovirus (CMV) reactivation and organ-related incidence, are a further concern. The incidence of CMV reactivation and CMV-related interstitial pneumonia in the GIAC protocol was 65% and 17%, respectively. However, most of the patients showed refractory or recurrent CMV infection (55% and 31%, respectively). In a multivariate analysis the risk to have refractory CMV (HR 2 and 1.9, respectively) and CMV disease (HR 10.5 and 2.4, respectively) was higher after haplo-SCT and aGVHD.[21] Haplo-SCT and response to the therapy were the risk factors for recurrent CMV. Finally, patients with refractory CMV had a higher NRM.[22] Based on these results, Pei et al. identified 75 patients with refractory CMV, and 44 of them were infused with CMV-specific T-cell and compared to 32 with nonrefractory CMV infection in a matched-pair analysis. Most of the patients infused (27/32) cleared the CMV within 4 weeks, whereas five patients had CMV recurrence. CMV disease was well controlled in 7 out of 10. The authors found that patients with refractory CMV had significantly less CMV-specific CD8 and CD4 T cell than patients with nonrefractory infection and that the success of cellular therapy was correlated to the expansion of infused CMV-specific T cell.[23]

Another relevant clinical point addressed in several studies was primary graft failure, including poor graft function and graft rejection. Poor graft function was defined as a hypo/aplastic BM with 2/3 factors: ANC $\leq 0.5 \times 10^9$/L; PLT $\leq 20 \times 10^9$/L; and/or hemoglobin less than 70 g/L for at least three consecutive days after day +28 after HSCT. In a prospective study the incidence of poor graft function was 5.5%. In this paper, there was a clear association between poor graft function and the presence of donor-specific antibodies (DSAs). Indeed, in a cohort of 342 patients, 25% had anti-HLA antibodies, and of them, 11% were DSAs, with a median mean fluorescence index (MFI) more than 4000. The presence in the recipient of DSA with MFI more than 2000 had a higher risk (cumulative incidence compared to patients with MFI < 2000, 27.3% vs. 1.9% in a training set and 33.3% vs. 4.5% in a validation set). In both groups of patients, the occurrence of poor graft function was associated with a higher NRM and had a strong negative impact on survival.[24] Other factors, other than presence of DSA, have been associated to

poor graft function. Shi et al. found that dysfunctional BM endothelial progenitor cells and high levels of reactive oxygen species and apoptosis were more evident in patients with poor graft function. Furthermore, they found that atorvastatin could restore the functionality of endogenous BM EPCs and stimulate their mobilization.[25] The immune system can play a role in the genesis of poor graft function as suggested by Kong et al. In this study they observed that in the BM of patients with poor graft function, there was an imbalance between Th17 and Treg cells, favoring Th17 that in BM microenvironment downregulates hematopoiesis.[26]

Regarding the primary graft rejection (defined as not achievement of ANC more than 0.5×10^9/L at day +28), the incidence was associated with the presence of the highest levels of DSA (>10 000) (20% vs. 0.3%). The NRM is higher in these patients with a significantly lower survival than in those without graft rejection.[24]

Similar to what was well known in T-cell deplete platform, donor characteristics play an important factor in the outcome of the patients. Wang et al. analyzed 1210 patients treated with the GIAC platform. In the multivariate analysis, donors younger than 30 years and male donors were associated with a reduced NRM and better survival. Mother donors were associated with a higher incidence of aGVHD, NRM, and worse survival than father. Compared with sibling, children were associated with less aGVHD, while only age impacted on NRM. For patients without children, no differences in outcome was found between father and sibling. To better ascertain the weight of donor age and sex, they performed an analysis grouping the pairs in four groups. So far, they observed that young sibling donors (less than 30 years) were associated with less aGVHD than sibling donors older than 30 years or father of any age. Sister donors aged more than 30 years, in particular when the recipient was a brother, were associated with more NRM and worse survival. Finally, the authors tested the relevance to be mismatched in noninherited maternal antigens (NIMAs). After a complex analysis, considering different donor-recipient combination, they found that NIMA mismatch played a protective against aGVHD.[27]

From the early 2000, several thousands of patients (2500 in 2016) have been treated with haplo-SCT clearly showing the efficacy and the feasibility of GIAC platform. Even if the GIAC platform is rarely used outside the Chinese boundaries, many data are accumulated allowing a great improvement of clinical results. Indeed, in China almost 99% of haplo-SCT are performed using the GIAC platform, giving a considerable reproducibility of the results.[28] Different postallogeneic

TABLE 7.2
Clinical Results Reported With GIAC Platform in AML

Authors	N	Disease Status	DFS	OS	Relapse Rate
Huang[20]	58	CR 1–3	73%	77%	12%
Wang[31] Haplo HLAid sib	231 219	CR1	74% 78%	79% 82%	15% 15%
Sun[19] GIAC MUD	68 62	CR1	73% 60%	78% 63%	12.7% 24%
Chang[15a]	339	CR1 and CR > 1	MRD+ (189) 71% MRD– (51) 73%	MRD+ 75% MRD– 75%	MRD+ 19% MRD– 15%
Chang[15b]	340	CR1 and CR > 1	MRD+ (202) 75% MRD– (56) 80%	MRD+ 83% MRD– 78%	MRD+ 13% MRD– 7%

AML, acute myeloid lymphoma; *DFS*, disease-free survival; *MRD*, matched related donor; *OS*, overall survival.
Chang[15a]: this is a retrospective cohort.
Chang[15b]: this is a prospective cohort.

complications have been addressed with possible solutions. However, the treatment-related toxicity and mortality remain quite high considering that most of the patients allografted in China are young and only 5.5% and 0.4% are aged more than 50 or 60 years.[29]

Most of the papers published by the Chinese groups included patients with acute myeloid leukemia (AML), acute lymphoblastic leukemia (ALL), and severe aplastic anemia (sAA).

Acute myeloid leukemia (AML). The clinical results in AML are illustrated in Table 7.2. Overall, most studies focused on patients transplanted in first complete remission,[30,31] while more advanced patients were included in two studies.[32,33] In the first study,[32] patients with intermediate- and high-risk AML were allocated on patient's decision to receive haplo-SCT or conventional chemotherapy. The results clearly showed that haplo-SCT was more effective with significantly higher DFS and OS and lower relapse incidence (RI). In a second randomized study, CR1 intermediate AML received transplantation from haploidentical donor or HLAid sibling. In this young population, the clinical results were undistinguishable, and no difference in any clinical endpoint was detected. This is the first randomized trial showing that the results using an alternative donor are not different compared to the conventional familiar HLAid donor.[30] In a matched-pair analysis in collaboration with the European Bone Marrow Transplantation group, Sun et al. compared the results obtained after GIAC-based haplo-SCT or transplantation from matched unrelated donor (MUD). In this population

with intermediate risk, CR1 AML receiving a busulfan-based myeloablative conditioning regimen, DFS, OS, RI, and NRM were similar between the two cohorts.[31] Finally, Chang et al. compared in a retrospective and prospective study the activity of haplo-SCT in patients with AML in CR1 or more advanced CR with positive or negative minimal residual disease (MRD, detected by cytofluorimetry). In this study the probability to relapse in MRD-positive cohort was lower after haplo-SCT than after transplantation from HLAid sibling. The positive effect on relapse and survival was confirmed in the multivariate analysis.[33]

Overall, these results confirm that haploidentical donor should be considered as a valid alternative to conventional donors. As recently reported by Xu et al., HLAid sibling remained the most preferred source of stem cells. However, haploidentical donors gained a priority place over unrelated donors in the Chinese population having a probability to find a donor in the registry of 11%.[28]

Acute lymphoblastic leukemia (ALL). The clinical results of GIAC protocol in ALL are reported in Table 7.3. In a first paper the authors analyzed standard-risk CR1 ALL receiving conventional CT or haplo-SCT. The results are impressive because the RI was 30% after haplo-SCT and 66% after CT, and as expected, the survival rate (OS and DFS) was significantly better in the haplo group.[34] In a second paper, 139 Ph1+ ALL patients were included, and of these, 101 receiving haplo-SCT were compared with 38 allo-SCT from MRD. Most of the patients were treated with tyrosin kinase inhibitor (imatinib) before

TABLE 7.3
Clinical Results Reported With GIAC Platform in ALL

Authors	N	Disease/ Status	DFS	OS	Relapse Rate
Yan[35]	79	ALL Ph-/	54%	70%	30%
Haplo	59	CR1	23%	28%	66%
CT		(standard risk)			
Chen[36]	101	ALL Ph+/	65%	74%	18%
Haplo	38	CR1	61%	68%	34%
HLAid sib					
Wang[37]	103	ALL Ph-/	61%	75%	18%
Haplo	83	CR1	60%	69%	24%
HLAid sib		(high-risk)			
Han[38]	127	ALL Ph-/	68%	70%	14%
Haplo	77	CR1	63%	69%	16%
MUD	144	(standard	67%	73%	21%
HLAid sib		risk)			

ALL, acute lymphoblastic leukemia; *DFS*, disease-free survival; *MUD*, matched unrelated donor; *OS*, overall survival.

allo-SCT and were in CR1. The conditioning regimen was myeloablative. Of note, most patients received imatinib after transplant. The clinical results were encouraging because the DFS and OS were similar in the haplo and MRD cohorts (65% vs. 61%, and 74% vs. 68%, respectively). The NRM was also not different as well as the incidence of grade 3–4 aGVHD and cGVHD. However, more patients in the haplo cohort had grade 2–4 aGVHD. In multivariate analysis the treatment with imatinib after allo-SCT improve the survival, whereas MRD positivity and resistance to imatinib were negative prognostic factors.[35] In a third paper the Chinese group randomized clinical high-risk Ph- ALL in CR1 to receive transplantation from haplo donor (n = 103) or MRD (n = 83). The clinical results in terms of survival, NRM, aGVHD, and cGVHD were not different after MRD and haplo transplantation. Of note, neither age nor conditioning regimen with total-body irradiation (TBI) nor high-risk cytogenetic affected the prognosis. In this study, preemptive, MRD-based donor lymphocyte infusion (DLI) was performed in 10 patients.[36] In the last paper published, Han et al. retrospectively compared patients with Ph-standard-risk ALL in CR1, receiving transplantation haplo (n = 127), MRD (n = 144), and MUD (n = 77). Again, the outcome was not statistically different by donor type. In multivariate analysis, the presence of MRD positivity before and after transplantation was the most important factors on survival.[37]

In ALL, haplo-SCT with GIAC platform is effective, obtaining clinical results closing to conventional donors.

Nonmalignant disease. The GIAC platform was applied to sAA failing an immunosuppressive therapy (IST) in a prospective study and compared the results in this cohort with that observed using MRD.[38] Xu et al. reported that in 101 patients receiving haplo-SCT, the OS and failure-free survival (FFS) were not different, while the cumulative incidence of grade 2–4 aGVHD and cGVHD were higher after haplo-SCT than after MRD. In this study the incidence of graft failure was low, and 94% of patients achieved a myeloid engraftment.[39] In a retrospective multicenter study, sAA patients received allo-SCT as first-line therapy: haploidentical donor was used in 89 and MRD in 88. The results were similar to the those of a previous study with more acute and chronic GVHD in the haplo-SCT cohort and same survival (OS 86% vs. 91%, FFS 85% vs. 89%, respectively).[40] More recently the authors updated the results of 57 patients treated with haplo-SCT as first-line therapy in a single center, using a busulfan-based conditioning regimen. The OS, FFS, and NRM were 83%, 83%, and 13%. The grade 2–4 and grade 3–4 aGVHD incidence was 20% and 6%, respectively, and cGVHD 25%. No case of graft failure was observed. In multivariate analysis, the comorbidity index influenced negatively the survival.[41]

DLI. The relapse rate after GIAC platform in AML is 12%–15% and 14%–30% in ALL (Tables 7.2 and 7.3). Based on this relatively high risk of relapse, several trials reported on the use of modified DLI (mDLI). mDLI consisted of donor G–CSF–mobilized peripheral blood progenitor cells. In an initial study, Huang et al. infused mDLI in 20 patients relapsing after haplo-SCT. The median time of first infusion from haplo-SCT was 177 days, and 11 patients were treated before mDLI. The 2-year probability of LFS was 40%. Because of the high incidence of aGVHD after mDLI in the first 9 patients, the successive 11 received GVHD prophylaxis, and only one developed aGVHD. The cumulative incidence of cGVHD was 64%.[42] In a retrospective study Wang et al. compared the outcome of patients with high-risk acute leukemia, receiving[61] or not[27] mDLI as prophylaxis of relapse. All patients in the mDLI cohort received GVHD prophylaxis with oral cyclosporine A or weekly low-dose methotrexate. The median number of CD3 infused was 5.7×10^7/kg. The CI of grade 2–4 and grade 3–4 aGVHD after mDLI was 41.9% and 13%, respectively. The 2-year CI of relapse was significantly lower in the mDLI cohort than that observed in the control group (37% vs. 55%, respectively), which was associated to a better OS (30% vs. 11%).[43] More recently, prophylactic mDLI was performed in patients receiving allo-SCT for relapsed/refractory acute leukemia and obtaining a CR. In this prospective multicenter study, 100 patients were included, and 62 received haplo-SCT. After mDLI, 58% obtained an MRD negativity and 3-year LFS was 50%, CI grade 2–4 aGVHD 29%, 2-year TRM 17%. These results are consistent with a major efficacy of prophylactic mDLI in a contest of patients at high risk of relapse.[38]

Other ATG-based platforms. Several other teams around the world developed ATG-based platforms to perform T-cell replete haplo-SCT.

In 2006, Ogawa et al., from Hyogo College of Medicine in Osaka, Japan, published data obtained in patients with several hematological malignancies (n = 26), using an ATG-based conditioning regimen before transplantation of PBSC from haploidentical donor. The conditioning regimen was reduced intensity, ATG dose (Fresenius) used was high (8 mg/kg), and GVHD prophylaxis was reinforced with methylprednisone (1 mg/kg/day until day +15, and then reduced in 15 days). All patients but one achieved a full-donor chimerism. The incidence of grade 2–4 aGVHD and extensive cGVHD was 20% and 25%, respectively. The NRM was 15%. This initial study proved that the platform used was quite immunoablative to achieve complete chimerism with low incidence of GVHD.[44] In a subsequent study, the same group treated advanced patients (n = 30) with a modified platform consisting of MAC, PBSC, and a GVHD prophylaxis based on tacrolimus, MTX, MMF, and methylprednisone, other than ATG in the conditioning. All patients achieved a complete chimerism, and the incidence of grade 2–3 aGVHD and extensive cGVHD was 37.9% and 29%, and the NRM was 23%. In this cohort of advanced patients, the relapse incidence was low (20%) and the 3-year OS 49%.[45] Recently, they published a multicenter phase I/II, including high-risk patients (n = 34) with busulfan-based RIC, ATG, PBSC, tacrolimus, MTX, and methylprednisone as GVHD prophylaxis. All but one patient achieved full-donor chimerism. Similar to the first study, the incidence of grade 2–4 aGVHD and extensive cGVHD was 30% and 20%, respectively. Of note, all patients with every grade aGVHD were treated with steroids. At 1 year, the NRM was 26% the OS was strongly influenced by the disease status, being 62% for those in CR and 42% in the others.[46]

Starting from the last decade, The Korean team from Asan Medical Center and the Pusan National University in Seoul published several papers on ATG-based haplo-SCT. In a first study, 31 patients with high-risk AML, ALL, and MDS (only one patient with sAA) were included (one-third of them were refractory at transplantation). All received a Busulfan-based RIC, and ATG 12 mg/kg before infusion of unmanipulated PBSC. Posttransplant GVHD prophylaxis was conventional (Cyclosporine A plus short course MTX). The OS and EFS were encouraging (63% and 47%, respectively), and the CI of grade 2–4, 3–4 aGVHD, and moderate-to-severe cGVHD was low (19%, 10%, and 20%, respectively). Finally, the NRM was only 13%.[47] In a second report including more patients (n = 83) affected by high-risk acute leukemia and MDS (half of them were refractory), the authors confirmed the same results in terms of survival and toxicity.[48] Finally, they performed a prospective phase 2 trial comparing the outcome of patients with AML in CR1-2, receiving transplantation from haploidentical donor, MUD, or MRD. The conditioning regimen was the same for haplo and MUD transplantation (Busulfan-based RIC), whereas MAC was used in the MRD cohort. ATG dose was 4.5 mg/kg in MRD cohort and 12 mg/kg in the other two cohorts. For all patients, stem cell source was PBSC. The 3-year OS, relapse-free survival, and NRM were not statistically different between haplo and MUD, or when allo-SCT from alternative donors were combined and compared to MRD group. The cumulative incidence of grade 2–4 and 3–4 aGVHD was similar, whereas the incidence of moderate-to-severe cGVHD was significantly higher in the MRD group than that observed in the other two groups (40% vs. 22%, respectively). Only the incidence of CMV and EBV reactivations were significantly lower after MSD.[49] Another Korean team from St Mary's hospital compared retrospectively the results with haplo-SCT and well matched or partially matched UD, in patients with CR1-3 AML. The platform use for haplo-SCT consisted of an MAC, ATG (total dose 6 mg/kg) followed by PBSC, and the GVHD prophylaxis was tacrolimus plus short course MTX. In this report based on a low number of AML patients, the cumulative incidence of aGVHD, cGVHD, CMV reactivation and disease, 3-year OS and DFS, NRM and relapse was not statistically different, even if the number of patients was too low to firmly conclude.[50]

An Italian group reported on haplo-SCT incorporating an original approach combining G–CSF–stimulated bone marrow alone, ATG (total dose 5 mg/kg), and four immunosuppressive drugs after stem cell infusion (MTX, Cyclosporine A, basiliximab, and MMF) to avoid GVHD. Eighty patients with several hematological diseases were included. The conditioning regimen was RIC and MAC. The 3-year OS was 45% for the whole population, better in standard-risk than high-risk diseases, the CI of relapse was 21%, and the 1-year NRM was 32%. The CI of grade 2–4 aGVHD and cGVHD was 29% and 23%, respectively. These data were considered encouraging.[51] Recently, using the same platform on 97 patients, they updated their results confirming similar results in terms of efficacy and toxicity.[52] G–CSF–primed BM was significantly different from G–CSF–primed peripheral blood because of the higher number of CD34+ cells overall and more primitive cell fraction, an enhanced number of BM mesenchymal progenitors (CFU–F) as well as T and B cells in particular of naive T cell fractions. The authors were particularly interested, for a future clinical use, to the high number of mesenchymal progenitors.[53]

POSTTRANSPLANTATION CYCLOPHOSPHAMIDE-BASED PLATFORM

In the early 2000 the Baltimore group showed in a mouse model that MHC-incompatible cells could engraft stably after nonmyeloablative conditioning with Fludarabine and low-dose TBI, avoiding immunological complications with a timely administration after stem cells infusion of high-dose Cyclophosphamide (PT-Cy).[54] The immunosuppressive activity of PT-Cy was well known since 1963, when Berenbaum et al. showed that Cy administration prolonged the survival of allogeneic skin grafts in mice, especially if the drug was given 1–3 days after placement of the skin graft.[55] In 1966, Santos and Owens found that Cy suppressed the incidence and severity of GVHD in rats given allogeneic spleen cells, especially if dosing was commenced on day 2 after the splenocyte infusion.[56] In 1989, Mayhumi et al. developed a method for inducing tolerance to major histocompatibility complex (MHC) antigens by giving mice an intravenous injection of MHC-matched, allogeneic splenocytes followed in 2–3 days by an intraperitoneal injection of high-dose Cy.[57] In 1996, Colson et al. published that the dose of TBI required for stable engraftment can be reduced from 7 Gy to 3 Gy when associated to ATG and Cy 2 days after stem cell infusion.[58] The little impact of Cy administered after stem cells infusion was explained by the high-level expression of aldehyde dehydrogenase in hematopoietic stem cells, conferring resistance to cyclophosphamide cytotoxicity.[59]

In bone marrow transplantation, donor-derived mature T cells in the marrow graft proliferate in response to alloantigens in the host. These T cells can induce GVHD. Conversely, residual T cells in the host proliferate in response to the graft and can contribute to graft failure. When cyclophosphamide is given 1–3 days after unmanipulated haploidentical stem cell infusion, it inhibits DNA replication and results in selective destruction of proliferative alloreactive T-cell clones, in both directions donor against host and host against donor. On the other hand, resting, not activated T cells in the graft were spared and can recreate the donor-derived new immune system in the patients. However, PT-Cy could reduce the alloreactivity through other mechanisms. PT-Cy creates a degree of intrathymic mixed chimerism which limits production of anti-graft immune cells through intrathymic clonal deletion and induces anergy and production of suppressor T cells which serve to protect the graft.

Starting from this background, Luznik et al. developed a murine model in which MHC-mismatched marrow cells infused into recipients conditioned with fludarabine or Cy, plus TBI (dose from 50 to 200 cGy), and Cy 200 mg/kg intraperitoneally on day 3. In this model, fludarabine and PT-Cy allowed engraftment. Additionally, fludarabine sensitized host stem cells to the toxicity of TBI because animals conditioned with both agents had higher chimerism than animals conditioned with TBI alone. Cy administered 48–72 h after the infusions of stem cells prevented GVHD by selectively eliminating T cells that have been activated by recognition of host antigens. These results indicate that PT-Cy inhibits aGVHD mediated by T cells reactive to host MHC and minor H antigens.[60]

The first phase I/II trial of PT-Cy after nonmyeloablative conditioning and transplantation of T-cell repleted, haploidentical marrow for patients with poor-risk hematologic malignancies and nonmalignant hematologic disorders was published in 2002. The conditioning regimen consisted of fludarabine (30 mg/m^2 per day from days –6 to –2) and TBI 2 Gy on day –1. All patients received Cy (50 mg/kg) on day +3, MMF from day +4 to day 35, and tacrolimus from day +4 to day ≥ 50. In a first cohort of 3 patients, 2 developed a primary graft failure. For this reason, in a second cohort (n = 10), the conditioning regimen was modified adding cyclophosphamide (14.5 mg/kg day –6 and –5). This allowed that 8 of 10 patients achieved a full-donor chimerism. The GVHD prophylaxis was also modified because of a significant incidence of aGVHD, and administration of tacrolimus was prolonged after day +100.[61] Between 1999 and 2006, 68 consecutive patients affected with high-risk hematologic malignancies or paroxysmal nocturnal hemoglobinuria were accrued in a modified protocol. Conditioning regimen consisted of Cy (14.5 mg/kg per day i.v. from day –6 and –5), fludarabine (30 mg/m2/day i.v. from day –6 to –2), and TBI (200 cGy on day –1). On day 0, patients received unmanipulated bone marrow (target collection of 4×10^8 nucleated cells/kg recipient weight). On day +3 (28 patients in Seattle) or on days +3 and +4 (40 patients in Baltimore), Cy (50 mg/kg/day) was administered. All patients received tacrolimus (dose of 1 mg i.v. daily by day +4 or +5 until day +180 and MMF until day +35, dose of 15 mg/kg orally 3 times daily). The incidence of grade 2–4 and grade 3–4 aGVHD was 33% and 6%, respectively, the 1-year NRM was 15%, and graft failure rate was 13%, even if 8 of these 9 patients had an autologous reconstitution. The OS and event-free survival (EFS) at 2 years were 36% and 26%, respectively. Relapse incidence was high (51% at 1 year), probably because of very high-risk patient population. The group from Baltimora receiving PT-Cy on day +3 and +4 had a lower incidence of cGVHD.[62]

The major histocompatibility complex encodes human leukocytes antigens (HLAs) responsible for cell surface antigen presentation. HLA molecules differences between donor and recipient are, therefore, a major determinant of the graft-versus-host response as host cell expression of HLA molecules not present in the donor elicits a strong non-self immune response by the graft within the host. This strong alloreactivity can also occur in the opposite direction, mediating a host-versus-graft response that can ultimately result in graft rejection. In haplo-SCT, only one of the two HLA haplotypes is shared, and thus the unshared haplotype encodes allogeneic HLA molecules that strongly activate the immune system. However, despite this strong background, Kasamon et al. analyzed 185 patients receiving haplo-SCT with PT-Cy founding that greater HLA disparity did not modify major outcomes. The presence of a greater number of total antigen or allele mismatches between donor and recipients was not associated with detrimental outcomes in terms of EFS, NRM, and grade II–IV aGVHD. Additionally, patients with more allele mismatches with the donor has a lower relapse risk. On univariate analysis, no statistically significant association was found between the total number of antigen or allele mismatches in the GVH direction (3 or 4 vs. fewer) and relapse, NRM, or EFS, and acute GVHD. In the HVG direction, more mismatches were associated with protective effect on relapse risk and EFS. The presence of two or more class I antigen mismatches in any direction was associated with a lower risk of relapse on univariate analysis and a lower risk for an event. Antitumor effects of this particular transplant platform seem to be not associated with acute GVHD.[63] Recently, in a retrospective single-center study, 208 consecutive donor-recipient pairs receiving PT-Cy-based haplo-SCT (both MAC and Nonmyeloablative (NMA)) were analyzed,

and the HLA disparity (≥4/10 HLA allelic mismatches [graft-versus-host direction]) resulted in relapse protection without an increase in NRM. Other HLA factors were independently associated with improved survival such as the presence of HLA-DR mismatch, HLA-DP nonpermissive mismatch, killer cell immunoglobulin-like receptor (KIR) receptor-ligand mismatch, and KIR B/x haplotype with KIR2DS2.[64] An Italian retrospective study was conducted on 318 patients receiving haplo-SCT with PTCY and MAC regimen, and the authors did not find any correlation between HLA disparity and outcomes in multivariate analysis. The data did not change even when vectorial HLA matching in both GVH or HVG directions were considered.[65]

Other non-HLA depending factors can play a role in the outcome of haplo-SCT using the Baltimore approach such as CMV serostatus, sex disparity, ABO matching, donor age.

As reported for the GIAC protocol, the availability of multiple donors for a single recipient imposed to have definite criteria to help prioritize donors. McCurdy et al.[66] in a context of NMAC haplo-SCT and bone marrow, as stem cell source, and with PT-Cy suggested a donor selection algorithm based on absence of the donor-specific antibodies, ABO matching, donor age, donor sex, and CMV serostatus match. In a previous reported study[64] donor characteristics associated with inferior survival included parental donor relationship and the use of CMV-seronegative donor for a CMV seropositive patient. Recently, the EBMT group reported, however, that donor CMV serostatus, in patients with acute leukemia and CMV positive, did not impact on main outcomes.[67] Finally, a recent study from Johns Hopkins group report the results in 33 patients undergoing Non myeloablative conditioning regimen (NMAC) regimen haplo-SCT from second- or third-degree related donors. The 1-year probability of GVHD-free, relapse-free survival was 57%. With posttransplant cyclophosphamide, haploidentical BMT from non–first-degree relatives has similar results to first-degree relatives. Non–first-degree relatives (e.g., aunts, uncles, cousins, nieces, nephews, and grandchildren) should be considered for BMT donor searches.[68]

With the use of PT-Cy, the CI of grade 2–4 aGVHD seems to be in line with results after HLA matched HSCT although the risk to develop severe aGVHD is low and most of the patients had grade 2 aGVHD. Recently, McCurdy et al. analyzed 340 adults with hematologic malignancies focusing on the impact of aGVHD on survival. The CI at 100 days of grade 2 and grades 3–4 aGVHD were 30% and 2%, respectively. The 1-year CI of cGVHD was 10%. In landmark analysis, the

4-year OS and PFS were significantly better in patients with grade 2 aGVHD compared to those with grade >2 (63% and 59% vs. 48% and 39%, respectively). In multivariable analysis, grade 2 aGVHD significantly increased the PFS as well as the higher nucleated cell graft dose in the graft. Older age and high disease risk index were associated to low PFS and OS. High hematopoietic cell transplantation-comorbidity index (HCT-CI) increased the risk of NRM, whereas this is reduced when high number of CD3+ cells was infused. Finally, grade 2 aGVHD reduced significantly the risk of relapse without an enhanced risk of NRM, contrary to those with grade 3–4 aGVHD and cGVHD. The Authors tried to identify factors associated with the development of grade 2 aGVHD founding that higher CD3+ cells in the graft and older age showed the association.[69]

Another potential clinical problem with this platform could be the primary GF. The incidence of primary GF reported in the literature, using either MAC or NMAC conditioning regimen, ranges from 0% to 30%.[70] Primary GF remains a complication associated with very poor outcome, due to increased transplant-related mortality. One of the most important factors for primary GF is the presence of DSA in the recipient, which are associated to 10-fold increased risk of primary GF in all hematopoietic cell transplantation, when transplanted with HLA mismatched donor.[71-75] In general, antibody-mediated graft rejection may occur either by antibody-dependent cell-mediated cytotoxicity or complement-mediated cytotoxicity. The largest study that take a picture of incidence of primary GF in the context of haplo-SCT with PT-Cy, was conducted at John Hopkins on 296 recipients. A total of 957 donors were evaluated, including 853 related (741 [87%] mismatched and 112 [13%] matched) and 104 unrelated donors. Detection of DSA was based on solid-phase antibody assays on the Luminex (Luminex, Austin, TX) platform and cross-match test. DSA were detected in 43 (14.5%) recipients, mostly were female. DSA with moderate-to-strong strength was more frequently encountered in the haplo-SCT than in mismatched unrelated donors. DSA were most commonly detected in female patients directed against their children. Nine patients without other available donors underwent desensitization. Eight who reduced their DSA to negative or weak levels proceeded to transplantation and achieved full donor chimerism.[156] The European Society for Blood and Marrow Transplantation (EBMT) recently published a Consensus Guidelines for the Detection and Treatment of DSA in Haploidentical setting. The panel of expert recommend to test DSA by Luminex platform and/or cell-based assays in all recipients for haploidentical donor

transplants. They stated to consider positive DSA value >1.000 MFI. In the absence of an alternative donor, it is recommended that those patients should undergo to desensitization therapy, especially with high DSA levels (>5.000 MFI). C1q testing and/or cell-based assays must be done to further assess the risk of graft failure. The choice of desensitization protocol may be based on local experience.[76]

Although many factors can influence the outcome of allogeneic transplantation, disease type and disease status at the time of transplantation are the most important predictors of survival. Armand et al. developed and later validated the Disease risk index (DRI), to stratify patients into four sub-groups based on disease type and status before HCT across conditioning regimen and histology. The refined DRI was a system for risk-stratifying heterogeneous populations of patients undergoing allo-SCT. This index applies regardless of age, conditioning regimen, donor type, and graft source.[77] McCurdy et al. retrospectively analyzed, the outcome of 372 patients with hematological malignancies treated with haplo-SCT with PT-Cy, according to the refined DRI. This analysis showed that the DRI effectively stratifies patients into low, intermediate, and high/very high risk groups with respectively 3-year PFS 65%, 37%, and 22%. The 3-year OS according DRI were 71%, 48%, and 35% in low, intermediate and high/very high risk, respectively. On multivariable analyses, the DRI was statistically significantly associated with relapse, PFS, and OS.[78]

Immunoreconstitution after haplo-SCT and PT-Cy was object of various studies. Roberto et al. demonstrated that after elimination of donor and recipient alloreactive T cell by PT-Cy, the phenotype of surviving T naive cells was that of T memory stem cell (TMSC). In the following weeks, naive-derived TSCM generate memory cells in response to exogenous antigens and, presumably, homeostatic cytokines. Adoptively transferred T cell memory, which has survived Cy, expands to detectable levels in the circulation only in the presence of the cognate antigen. Whether T-cell memory can persist in the haplo-SCT individual in the absence of the cognate antigen is currently unknown.[79] The same group performed an analysis of markers associated with B-cell differentiation showing that B cells are generated de novo after haplo-SCT. The B-cell compartment is initially characterized by the presence of transitional B cells and is progressively repopulated by mature naive B cells. Using a polychromatic flow cytometry approach, they report a new putative transitional B-cell stage, named T0, defined as CD5–CD21– cells. These cells are the first to appear during B-cell recovery. The B-cell maturation process from T0 to naive B cells takes ~6 months to complete in haplo-SCT patients.[80] PT-Cy in haplo-SCT kills also mature and proliferating NK cells infused in the recipient with the graft. Indeed, NK cells do not express aldehyde dehydrogenase, thus implying that the immature CD62L-pos/NKG2Apos/KIR- NK cells reconstituting in the recipients derive from donor stem cells. The absolute numbers of donor-derived NK cells reconstitute early after haplo-SCT with PT-Cy, but the distribution of their subset takes much longer to acquire a pattern similar to that observed in healthy donors. The transient and predominant expansion start from the second week, and it is sustained by a donor-derived unconventional subset of NKp46neg-low/CD56dim/CD16-NK cells expressing remarkable high levels of CD94/NKG2A. These immature NK cells, present at low frequency in healthy donors, are greatly expanded in the following 7 weeks after haplo-SCT and express high levels of the activating receptors NKGD. Nonetheless, these NK cells displayed a markedly defective cytotoxicity that could be reversed by blocking the inhibitory receptor CD94/NKG2A. These data opened the possibility to develop a novel immune-therapeutic approach that targets the inhibitory NKG2A check-point.[81] These results confirm and underline that long-lasting period in which most of the circulating NK cells display phenotypic features of immaturity. This immunological situation correlates with the clinical evidence of frequent viral reactivations, including those from CMV, polyomaviruses, and human herpes viruses, detected after haplo-SCT

and PT-Cy transplantation despite the relatively rapid recovery of CD8 T-cell counts .[82] Data on infections among 70 consecutive recipients of haplo-SCT affected by various hematologic malignancies showed a cumulative incidence of viral infections of 70%. At 1 year, 35 of 65 patients at risk had CMV reactivation (54%), and the rate of polyomavirus-associated cystitis was 19% (13/70). Cumulative incidence of bacterial and fungal infections at 1 year were 63% and 12%, respectively.[83] At least part of this susceptibility might be due to the ineffective protection conferred by the immature donor-derived NK cells, and future studies should verify whether the dynamics of recovery of memory.

Haplo-SCT PT-Cy in Lymphomas. Mostly of studies published with ATG-based platforms did not include patients with lymphoproliferative diseases. On the other hand, when these diseases are treated with haplo-SCT, the platform preferentially used is with PT-Cy.

As recently reported by EBMT analysis, the number of transplantations from haploidentical donors is growing steadily, even in non-Hodgkin lymphoma (NHL) and Hodgkin lymphoma (HL). The feasibility of haplo-SCT using PT-Cy platform, in terms of main toxicity, was reported in Table 7.4. The results were also encouraging because the CI of grade 2–4 and grade 3–4 aGVHD ranges from 17% to 43% and from 3% to 14%, respectively. Similarly, the CI of NRM ranges from 9% to 26%. The most remarkable finding was the low incidence of overall cGVHD ranging from 9% to 16%, which is low compared to that observed using

TABLE 7.4
Toxicity of PTCY Platform in Lymphoma Patients

Authors	HL	NHL	Grade 2–4 aGVHD	Grade 3–4 aGVHD	cGVHD	NRM
Burroughs[91]	28	0	43%	11%	35%	9%
Castagna[142]	27	22	25%	NR	5%	16%
Raiola[86]	26	0	24%		9%	4%
Garciaz[143]	0	26	NR	NR	15%	15%
Gayoso[94]	43	0	39%	14%	19%	21%
Martinez[92]	98	0	33%	9%	26%	17%
Kanate[87]	46	139	26%	8%	13%	11%
Ghosh[88]	44	136	27%	8%	12%	15%
Castagna[93]	62	0	23%	4%	16%	20%
Lacerda[144]	24	0	17%	/	24%	26%
Gauthier[95]	34	0	28%	3%	15%	9%

aGVHD, acute graft-versus-host disease; *cGVHD*, chronic graft-versus-host-disease; *NRM*, nonrelapse mortality.

TABLE 7.5
Clinical Results Reported With PTCY Platform in Lymphoma

Authors	HL	NHL	Stem Cell Source	CTX	PFS	OS	RI	GF
Burroughs[91]	28	0	BM	NMAC	51%	58%	40%	0
Castagna[116]	27	22	BM 80% PBSC 20%	RIC/NMAC	63%	71%	19%	4%
Raiola[153]	26	0	BM	NMAC	63%	77%	31%	
Garciaz[143]	0	26	BM PBSC	RIC/NMAC	65%	77%	19%	NR
Gayoso[94]	43	0	BM 28% PBSC 72%	RIC	48%	58%	24%	2%
Kanate[87]	46	139	BM 93% PBSC 7%	RIC	42%	68%	36%	NR
Ghosh[88]	44	136	BM 93% PBSC 7%	NMAC	48%	61%	37%	NR
Dietrich[a,84]	0	59	NR	MAC/RIC	55%	56%	36%	
Martinez[92]	98	0	BM 61% PBSC 39%	NMAC	43%	67%	39%	NR
Castagna[93]	62	0	BM 63% PBSC 37%	RIC/NMAC	59%	63%	21%	
Lacerda[144]	24	0	BM 54% PBSC 46%	NMAC	54%	66%	19%	
Gauthier[95]	34	0	BM 50% PBSC 50%	RIC/NMAC	66%	75%	25%	NR

BM, bone marrow; *CTX*, Conditioning regimen; *GF*, primary graft failure; *MAC*, myeloablative conditioning regimen; *NR*, not reported; *OS*, overall survival; *PBSC*, peripheral blood stem cell; *PFS*, progression free survival; *RI*, relapse incidence.
[a]In this study 13 out of 59 patients received MAC.

conventional donors with an improvement of patients' quality of life. Overall, it can be concluded that also in lymphoma patients haplo-SCT with PT-Cy was a good option from tolerability point of view.

The clinical results obtained in lymphoma patients were in Table 7.5. All the studies reported until now were retrospective single or multicenter eventually comparing results of haplo-SCT with those obtained using MRD and MUD. The results are promising using mostly RIC or NMAC conditioning regimen, only in one study,[84] 13 patients received MAC regimen. Of note, in more recently reported studies, the proportion of patients infused with PBSC was growing. The OS ranged from 56% to 75% and the PFS from 42% to 66%. The relapse incidence was between 19% and 40%. Considering that patient population was represented by advanced lymphoma patients, relapsing after autologous transplantation[85] or with active disease,[86] these results can be considered encouraging. The CIB-MTR reported the two largest retrospective comparative

studies, including both HL and NHL patients.[87,88] The first study analyzed the outcome of patients treated with haplo-SCT with PT-Cy with that obtained using MUD, with or without ATG. In the multivariate analysis, the CI of grade 2–4 aGVHD was similar while the CI of grade 3–4 was significantly lower after haplo-SCT. Similarly, the CI of cGVHD and NRM were lower in the haplo-SCT cohort. On the other hand, the OS and PFS were not statistically different.[87] In the second study, Ghosh et al. compared haplo-SCT with PT-Cy to transplantation from MRD. Again, the main outcomes were comparable between the two cohorts, except for CI of cGVHD lower in the haplo-SCT cohort.[88] The European Society for Blood and Marrow Transplantation (EBMT) compared retrospectively the outcome using haploidentical donor or MRD/MUD founding very similar results to previous studies, confirming the low incidence of cGVHD in the haplo cohort.[84]

The Baltimore group reported on the results in T-cell lymphomas, receiving allo-SCT from a haploidentical donor or HLAid sibling. The results are encouraging in a poor prognosis cohort of patients showing that the 2-year OS and PFS were 43% and 40%, respectively. The relapse incidence was 34%, and the NRM was 11% in the haplo cohort. The disease status and the timing (CR1 vs. other) were relevant for the outcome.[89] The same group performed an interesting prospective phase 2 study in B-cell lymphoma. In this study, the donor selection was based on polymorphism of gamma FC receptor of Rituximab over of HLA compatibility, using the same platform with PT-CY. Sixty-nine of 83 patients included were grafted with a haploidentical donor. In this group the CI of grade 2–4 and 3–4 aGVHD was 45% and 6%, respectively, and cGVHD 13%. The 2-year OS and PFS was 73% and 63%, while the relapse incidence was 20%. The outcomes were better when high-affinity gamma FC receptor donors were used for transplantation.[90]

Based on the suggestive results reported 10 years ago by Burroughs et al., showing that in HL patients haplo-SCT with PT-Cy seemed to induce a stronger graft versus tumor effect than conventional donors,[91] many studies were focalized on this histotype. In an EBMT study,[92] HL patients treated with haplo-SCT with PT-Cy (n = 98) were compared with those treated with MRD (n = 338) or MUD (n = 273). In the multivariate analysis, in the haplo group the NRM was similar to MTD but lower than that in the MUD group. Even if the OS and PFS were similar in the three groups, the relapse incidence was lower after haplo and MUD as well as the extensive chronic GVHD and relapse-free survival. In most of the studies in HL, several prognostic factors were identified, and in particular, a well-controlled disease before, even better if complete remission, was the most recurrent for survival, relapse and NRM.[92–95]

Finally, as expected, few patients with MM now received an allo-SCT. Regarding haplo-SCT with PT-Cy, a retrospective multicenter experience was published including 30 patients with advanced disease. The results were encouraging, and the 18-month CI of relapse and NRM were 42% and 10%, respectively. The CI of grade 2–4 aGVHD was 29%. The 18-month PFS and OS were 33% and 63%, respectively. The disease status before haplo-SCT was the most important factor for survival, as expected.[96]

Haplo-SCT with PT-Cy seemed effective and well tolerated in lymphoma patients, without any differences in terms of survival, but with a reduction on acute and chronic GVHD, compared to conventional donors. The relapse of course is a concern, and based on the tolerability of haplo-SCT, posttransplantation intervention with drugs or DLI should be tested, mainly in patients not in CR.

Haplo-SCT PT-Cy in acute Leukemia (AL). Data on toxicities after haplo-SCT with PT-Cy in AL are summarized in Table 7.6. The NRM of grade 2–4 aGVHD, cGVHD ranges respectively from 7% to 18%, 4%–35%, and 16%–40%. Graft failure was not reported in all studies, but it seemed to be not relevant.

The results with Haplo-SCT with PT-Cy in AL patients were compared with those using TCD platform, showing an improvement in outcomes. Ciurea et al. reported an improvement of 1-year NRM (16% vs. 42%, P = .02), OS (64% vs. 30%, P = .02), and PFS (50% vs. 21%, P = .02) in 32 consecutive patients treated with haplo-SCT and PT-Cy compared to a TCD with ATG followed by infusion of CD34+ selected cells. Engraftment rate and grade 2–4 aGVHD were not significantly different, whereas cGVHD was significantly lower using PT-Cy prophylaxis.[97] The place of haplo-SCT with PT-Cy, when an HLA identical donor was unavailable, was evaluated in several studies comparing haplo donor to other alternative donors. In Table 7.7, we summarized the studies comparing transplantation from a haploidentical donor to unrelated cord blood. No main differences both in terms of toxicity and clinical results were found, even if all studies are retrospective and often registry based and in some study in the haplo cohort were included different platforms.

In Table 7.8 are summarized the results obtained using haplo donor and PT-Cy and compared to other alternative donor and to MRD. Overall, the results obtained with haplo-SCT were as good as those obtained with other alternative donor. The most important study was reported by the CIBMTR comparing haplo-SCT with PT-Cy to transplantation from MUD. In this study were included patients with AML in first or second CR or with active disease (almost 30%). The CI of grade 2–4 and 3–4 aGVHD and cGVHD were significantly lower in the haplo group receiving RIC or MAC. Furthermore, in the RIC group the NRM was lower in the haplo cohort while the relapse incidence was higher. No statistically differences were observed in terms of survival.[98] Although the presumed higher antileukemic effect from haploidentical donor has been questioned,[154] in a retrospective analysis including high risk AML and myelodysplastic syndrome, we found encouraging results. Indeed, at least for CR patients, the CI of relapse was 32%, the PFS 47% and OS 62%, with an acceptable NRM (20%).[155] Of course, only prospective studies will clarify this pivotal point.

Other studies compared the results of haplo-SCT to MRD or alternative donors, in specific phase of disease. Salvatore et al. published a retrospective registry based study on AML in CR1. The Authors described results

TABLE 7.6
Toxicity in AL Patients With PTCY Haplo Platform

Authors	N	CTX	Source (Haplo)	Grade 2–4 aGVHD	cGVHD	NRM	GF
Bashey[145]	27	NMAC/MAC	BM	30%	4%	7%	NR
Haplo	55		PBSC	39%	12%	16%	
MUD	49			27%	11%	13%	
MRD							
Di Stasi[146]	32	RIC	BM	26%	17%	18%	0
Haplo	87			24%	29%	8%	
MRD	108			19%	23%	8%	
MUD							
Ciurea[97]	192	MAC/RIC	BM 82%	16%/19%a	30%/34%a	14%/9%	NR
Haplo	1245		PBSC 19%	33%/28%a	53%/52%a	20%/23%	
MUD							
Bacigalupo[113]	76	MAC	BM	18%	20%	14%	0.7%
Haplo							
Rashidi[147]	52	MAC/RIC	PBSC	40%	10%	27%	NR
Haplo	88			36%	9%	27%	
MUD							
Rubio[114]	503	MAC/RIC	BM	29%	32%		18%
Haplo			PBSC	24%	25%		
Bashey[148]	55	NMAC/RIC/	PBSC	41%	31%	17%	3%
Haplo	98	MAC	BM	48%	47%	16%	2%
MUD	79			21%	44%	14%	2%
MRD							
Raiola[149,§]	92	MAC/RIC	BM	14%a	15%	18%	1%
Haplo	43			21%	22%	33%	2%
MUD	43			42%	19%	35%	7%
mMUD	176			31%	29%	24%	0
MRD	105			19%	23%	35%	0
CB							
Rashidi[150]							
Haplo	62	MAC/RIC	PBSC	40%	6%	22%	/
MRD/MUD	21		PBSC	19%	5%	16%	/

BM, bone marrow; CB, cord blood; GF, growth factor; MRD, matched related donor; MUD, matched unrelated donor; MAC, myeloablative conditioning; mMUD, mismatched MUD; PBSC, peripheral blood stem cell; RIC, reduced-intensity conditioning.
adifferences were statistically lower in the haplo cohort.
§this study included mostly but not only leukemia patients.

TABLE 7.7
Comparative Studies of Haploidentical HCT Versus Umbilical Cord Blood Transplantation (UCB)

Authors	N	Grade 2–4 aGVHD	cGVHD	NRM	RI	OS
Brunstein[151]	50	0%	13%	7%	45%	62%
Haplo	50	21%	5%	24%	31%	54%
UCB						
El Cheikh[152]	69	5%	6%	18%	18%	69%
Haplo	81	33%	12%	23%	38%	45%
UCB						
Ruggeri[153]	360	11%	29%	27%	41%	38%
Haplo	558	12%	24%	30%	32%	42%
UCB						

aGVHD, acute graft-versus-host disease; cGVHD, chronic graft-versus-host-disease; GF, growth factor; MAC, myeloablative conditioning; MRD, matched related donor; MUD, matched unrelated donor; RIC, reduced-intensity conditioning.

TABLE 7.8
Clinical Results in AL Patients With PTCY Haplo Platform

Authors	N	CTX	Source	OS	LFS	RI
Bashey[145]	27	NMAC/MAC	PBSC/BM	64%	60%	33%
Haplo	55			67%	52%	34%
MUD	49			76%	53%	34%
MRD						
Di Stasi[146]	32	RIC	BM	56%	41%	33%
Haplo	108			66%	45%	23%
MUD	87				57%	28%
MRD						
Ciurea[97]	192	MAC/RIC	BM/PBSC	45%/46%	NR	44%/58%
Haplo	1245			50%/44%		39%/42%
MUD						
Rashidi[147]	52	MAC/RIC	PBSC	42%	NR	29%
Haplo	88			37%		43%
MUD						
Rubio[a,114]	696	MAC/RIC	BM/PBSC	38%	32%	36%
Haplo				33%	27%	40%
AML						
ALL						
Bashey[148]	55	NMAC/ MAC/	BM/PBSC	57%		39%
Haplo	98	RIC		59%		40%
MUD	79			79%		38%
MRD						
Rashidi[150]						
Haplo	62	MAC/RIC	PBSC	53%	/	31%
MRD/MUD	21		PBSC	58%	/	26%

ALL, acute lymphoblastic leukemia; *AML*, acute myeloid lymphoma; *GF*, growth factor; *MAC*, myeloablative conditioning regimen; *MRD*, matched related donor; *MUD*, matched unrelated donor; *NMAC*, nonmyeloablative conditioning regimen; *RIC*, reduced-intensity conditioning regimen.
[a]In this study, outcome was gave according to disease status and conditioning regimen.

according to cytogenetic. In multivariate analysis, for intermediate risk AML, haplo-SCT were associated with higher risk of grade 2–4 aGVHD, higher NRM ($P < .01$) lower LFS, OS and GRFS ($P < .01$), without difference in terms of cGVHD. In high risk AML, no difference was found in LFS, OS and GRFS, but higher grade 2–4 aGVHD. A trend for a lower relapse incidence was observed in haplo group both in intermediate and high-risk categories.[98] Versluis et al., on behalf the EBMT, also reported on AML in poor risk CR1, comparing haplo-SCT with MRD, UCB and mismatched UD (mMUD). In multivariable analysis, they did not found differences on OS and LFS following MRD, 10/10 MUD, or haplo-SCT, but a significantly worse OS after mMUD and UCB transplantation. The relapse rate was decreased after MUD compared to MRD and haplo-SCT, while the NRM was significantly higher for all alternative donors compared to MRD.[99] Piemontese et al. compared haplo-SCT and UD both matched and mismatched in AML patients in CR1/2. In multivariate analysis, LFS

and OS were significantly better with MUD than haplo or mMUD, while no differences were found between haplo and mMUD.[100] Canaani et al. analyzed AML patients with FLT3-ITD mutation (n=91) or without FLT3-ITD (n=201) receiving a haplo-SCT. Hal pf them were prophylaxed with PT-Cy and half with ATG. Over-all, the clinical outcomes and toxicities were not influenced by the presence of mutation, without difference between the kind of GVHD prophylaxis. Furthermore, the results observed with haploidentical donor were compared with those observed using an MRD or MUD, and again the clinical outcomes were similar, with only a lower NRM in MRD transplantation.[101] Li et al. analyzed a cohort of patients with secondary AML treated with haplo-SCT using PT-Cy (n=119) or ATG-based (n=35). The results were encouraging in particular, as expected, for CR patients. For these patients, the 2-year OS and LFS were 57% and 49%, respectively, which was better than survival observed in patients with active disease. An important point was the influence of GVHD prophylaxis used (PT-Cy vs. ATG) because in multivariate analysis, the 2-year NRM as well as the LFS, OS and GRFS were higher with ATG than PT-Cy. aGVHD and cGVHD incidence were similar in the two groups, with a higher risk using PBSC.[102] These two different approaches to prevent GVHD (PT-Cy and ATG) in CR1/CR2 AML patients have been evaluated specifically by the EBMT. In this analysis the Authors compared 193 patients with PT-Cy to 115 with ATG. As in the previous study, LFS, NRM and GRFS, but not OS, were significantly lower in the ATG group compared to PT-Cy, while no difference was observed in the relapse rate. Regarding GVHD, the risk to develop grade 2–4 aGVHD was similar, while with ATG the rate of grade 3–4 was significantly higher; the incidence of cGVHD was not different.[103]

The activity of haplo-SCT and PT-Cy has been reported also for patients affected by acute lymphoblastic leukemia (ALL). Srour et al. reported on 109 adult patients transplanted with haploidentical donor and PT-Cy. Only 33% of the patients were in CR1, and the CI of grade 2–4 and 3–4 aGVHD was 32% and 11%, the 5-year NRM 30% and the 5-year relapse rate 40%. Overall, the 3-year DFS and OS were 31% and 37%. In the multivariate analysis, only the intensity of conditioning regimen was associated with the outcome.[104] The EBMT analyzed 208 ALL patients receiving a haplo-SCT. Of these patients 28% had active disease at transplantation, 32% carried out t(9; 22), and 66% received a MAC. The GVHD prophylaxis was with PT-Cy in 57% of patients. The CI of grade 2–4 and grade 3–4 aGVHD was 30% and 11%, higher with PBSC than BM. The OS and LFS were significantly influenced by the disease status, because in CR1 group were 52% and 47% compared to 34% and 33% and 4% and 5% in CR2 and active disease groups, respectively. These results were linked to a progressively higher relapse rate in the three groups, without difference in NRM. The GVHD prophylaxis adopted did not impact on any outcome.[105] These two studies confirm the activity of haplo-SCT in ALL.

Haplo-SCT has been assayed in patients with refractory AL, with encouraging results. A trial from Germany evaluated the feasibility and efficacy of sequential therapy using clofarabine and Baltimore-based haploidentical platform with PT-Cy. They treated 18 patients (3 with ALL) with refractory or relapsed leukemia. In this series, post-transplant immunomodulation with early discontinuation of calcineurin inhibitor and donor lymphocytes infusions was not planned. The 1-year NRM was 28%, the grade 2–4 aGVHD and cGVHD incidence was 22% and 27%, respectively. The anti-leukemic effect was encouraging: relapse free survival, OS, and relapse rate were 39%, 55%, and 44%, respectively.[106] In a phase 2 prospective trial, Jaiswal et al. reported on refractory patients treated with haplo-SCT using MAC regimen, PT-Cy, early reduction of MMF, and prophylactic G–CSF–mobilized donor lymphocytes infusion (pDLI) without cyclosporine A discontinuation. The disease progression was 21% and the 18 months PFS 61.9%. When compared to those obtained with the same platform without pDLI, the disease progression and PFS was better in pDLI arm, while the incidence of cGVHD was higher after pDLI (41% vs. 11%).[107] In a single center retrospective study, How et al. analyzed a cohort of AML patients with active disease (marrow blasts > 5%), receiving transplantation from haploidentical donor (n = 24) MRD (n = 32), or MUD (n = 43). In the haplo cohort, the GVHD prophylaxis was with PT-Cy. No differences were observed in terms of engraftment, aGVHD, cGVHD, EFS, OS, TRM, and relapse rate between the three cohorts.[108] The EBMT ALWP[109] OS and LFS were 14% and 12% and RI was 61%, NRM was 23%.

Recently the acute leukemia working party of EBMT published a position paper on the use of haploidentical donor in patients with acute leukemia supporting a MUD as the best donor option in the absence of MSD, and further supports the use of a haploidentical donor or 9/10 MMUD as equally viable alternatives in the absence of a fully matched donor, or in the case of the need for an urgent transplant. Furthermore, a haplo donor could be choose, in particular situation, instead of start to search for an unrelated donor.[110]

Modifications to the Haplo-SCT PT-Cy. Although in the original protocol from Baltimore the conditioning regimen was nonmyeloablative, in several studies in leukemia patients, the conditioning regimen has been intensified, with the aim to reduce the relapse incidence. Several single-center retrospective studies reported a low risk of acute and chronic GvHD and encouraging rates of NRM and OS with MAC.[111-113] The impact of intensity of conditioning regimen was reported by the EBMT in a retrospective analysis. In this study, the Authors compared the outcome of leukemia patients conditioned by RIC (n = 271) or MAC (n = 425), but only 25% and 32%, respectively were transplanted using the Baltimore platform. The CI of aGVHD was similar after RIC and MAC, the relapse incidence was higher after RIC in AML, but no difference in terms of LFS, NRM and cGVHD. The conditioning regimens did not have any impact on OS. For PT-Cy group, the NRM was associated with a lower NRM.[114]

Another important modification of Baltimore protocol was the introduction of PBSC instead of BM. Several papers including a small number of patients reported on the use of PBSC with PT-Cy.[115-118] In a matched-pair analysis, O'Donnell et al. did not find any differences in terms of acute and chronic GVHD, NRM and survival. However, they observed a significant reduction of relapse incidence in patients infused with PBSC[119]. The CIBMTR and EBMT performed three retrospective studies on this subject. Bashey et al. compared 480 patients receiving BM to 190 PBSC graft, including all hematological diseases, and they observed that the risks of grade 2–4 aGVHD and cGVHD were lower using BM, while the survival and NRM were superimposable. The relapse risk was, however, higher with BM.[120] Ruggeri et al. compared 260 BM to 190 PBSC CR1 and CR2 leukemia patients, confirming the lower risk of grade 2–4 and grade 3–4 aGVHD using BM, while the incidence of cGVHD and relapse was similar as well as survival.[121] Finally, Savani et al. refined the previous analysis comparing only patients conditioned by and receiving either BM or PBSC. The CI of engraftment was lower in bone marrow The incidence of grade 2–4 aGVHD and cGVHD was lower in bone marrow recipients (19% vs. 24%). In multivariate analysis, the OS and LFS were higher in patients transplanted with PBSC, due to a significant reduction of relapse rate, without difference in NRM.[122]

The GVHD prophylaxis in the Baltimore protocol was based of course on PT-Cy but also on the association of tacrolimus and MMF starting from day +5. It has been published that cyclosporine A can be used instead of tacrolimus, without any change in the safety of procedure.[123] Furthermore, initially, the duration of full dose of immunosuppression was quite long (day +180).[62] Recently, the John Hopkins group reported the results of prospective trials evaluating an early stopping of tacrolimus without tapering at day +60 and day +90. All patients received NMAC regimen and BM graft. Based on strict stopping criteria, they observed that 49% and 69% of patients can stop tacrolimus at day +90 and +60 respectively, without an increased risk of acute and chronic GVHD, NRM. Interestingly, the probability of relapse and the survival seemed better in the cohort of patients sopping the immunosuppression at day +60.[124]

Haplo-SCT PT-Cy in elderly patients. The median age at diagnosis of AML is between 68 and 72 years, making the accessibility to transplantation for these patients at least difficult. A single center study and population-based data indicate that only 2%–3% of AML patients aged more than 65 years were treated with allo-HSCT.[125] Recently,

the application of haplo-HSCT in elderly patients has been reported. Kasamon et al. analyzed 271 patients, with several hematological malignancies, receiving a haplo-HSCT with PT-Cy.[126] Younger patients (50–59 years) were compared to two group of patients aged 60–69 and 70–75 years old, and overall 24% of patients were affected by AML. Conditioning regimen was NMAC. Clinical outcomes were similar, even if the incidence of grade 2–4 aGVHD was significantly higher in the oldest cohort (24% vs. 37% vs. 52%) without differences in cGVHD and NRM. Similarly, 3-year PFS, DFS, RI, and OS were not different (39% vs. 34% vs. 33%, 39% vs. 34% vs. 34%, 48% vs. 46% vs. 44%, 48% vs. 45% vs. 44%, respectively). The patients were regrouped following the disease risk index (DRI),[77] showing that in low, intermediate, and high/very high risk groups, the 3-year PFS and OS were 62% and 68%, 36% and 44%, and 15% and 31%, respectively. Blaise et al. compared the outcome of 31 patients older than 55 years (median age 62 years) receiving haplo-HSCT using Baltimore platform, with those receiving ATG-based MRD or MUD. One third of patients suffered by AML. The characteristics of three groups were similar, with statistically differences for stem cell source and conditioning regimen (more BM and NMAC regimen in the haplo group). The 2-year OS was not different in the three groups, while NRM and PFS were similar in the haplo and MRD group but statistically lower compared to MUD group (10% vs. 11% vs. 34% and 67% vs. 64% vs. 38%). Similarly, the incidence of grade 2–4 aGVHD was significantly higher in the MUD group (23% vs. 21% vs. 44%), as well as cGVHD (13% vs. 35% vs. 24%). The 2-year PFS without severe cGVHD was always higher in the haplo and MRD groups (67% vs. 51% vs. 31%). This retrospective study, for the first time, questioned the role of extra-familiar donors in aged patients.[127] The same group made the same comparison only in AML patients. Overall, 94 patients (median age 65 years) were included and 33 were transplanted with haploidentical donor, 31 with MSD, and 30 from UD. The outcome, in terms of PFS, OS, NRM, relapse, and GRFS, were similar, but the cumulative incidence of grade 3–4 aGVHD was significantly higher in the UD group.[128] Bashey et al. performed a similar study, confirming that the OS, NRM, and aGVHD were not statistically different after MRD, MUD and haplo-SCT, while the C of moderate-severe cGVHD was significantly lower fater haplo-SCT.[129] The feasibility of haplo-SCT in elderly patients has been confirmed in two other studies.[130,131]

Finally, the EBMT compared 250 AML elderly patients receiving haplo-SCT to 2589 transplanted with an MUD. The GVHD prophylaxis was performed by PT-Cy in 65% of patients. Although the patient characteristics were not well balanced in terms of disease status (more patients in advanced disease, lower performance status, longer time to transplant in the haplo cohort), in multivariate analysis the risk to develop acute and chronic GVHD was independent from the donor type. However, the risk to have extensive cGVHD was more frequent in MUD. The donor type did not influence the risk of NRM, relapse incidence, LS, OS, and GRFS. All these results were confirmed in a matched-pair analysis.[132]

Haplo-SCT PT-Cy in Nonmalignant Diseases

The results obtained with Haplo-SCT and PT-Cy to treat severe nonmalignant diseases have been now reported in several publications. The most extensive experience have been reported for sAA. The first paper was published by the Clay et al. reporting on 8 heavily pretreated patients (haplo-SCT was second allo-SCT in 4), conditioned with the Baltimore regimen with conventional PT-Cy and PSBC. The median age was 32 years.[19-57] They observed 2 DSA-related graft failure. The other patients obtained a sustained engraftment and full-donor chimerism. Only one patient had grade 2 aGVHD, and no cGVHD was observed.[133] Esteves et al. treated 16 refractory patients which included using the same protocol. All patients but one were transplanted with BM, and two patients having graft failure were retransplanted with PBSC. The median age was 17 years.[5-39] Most of the patients obtained full-donor chimerism (87%), and three patients had primary or secondary graft failure. After a median follow-up of 1 year approximately, the OS was 67%. The risk to develop aGVHD was low (2 patients) as well as cGVHD (3 patients had a limited form).[134] Finally, DeZern et al. treated 13 patients out of 16 with haplo-SCT and PT-Cy in a prospective phase 2 study. The median age was 30 years.[11-30,31-69] Fourteen patients were transplanted with BM. No primary or secondary graft failure, neither severe acute nor chronic GVHD, nor toxic-related deaths were observed. All patients with clonal karyotypic abnormalities[11] normalized after transplantation.[135] Severe hemoglobinopathies, such as sickle cell anemia (SCA) and beta-thalassemia (β-thal), can be treated by allo-SCT. Some experience has been reported with haplo-SCT and PT-Cy. The Baltimore group reported on 14 adult SCA patients (median age 30 years, range 15–46). Their classical scheme was modified adding ATG (day −9 to −7 4.5 mg/kg), sirolimus instead of tacrolimus to reduce the incidence of posterior reversible encephalopathy syndrome (PRES), and some donors were harvested after bone marrow priming with G-CSF (5 days); all received unmanipulated bone marrow. Six patients (43%) rejected their graft with an autologous reconstitution, whereas 11 patients completely reverse SCA phenotype, and they became asymptomatic. No GVHD, acute or chronic, was observed, and three patients developed PRES on tacrolimus. All patients were alive at last the follow-up.[136] De la Fuente et al. reported on 16 patients (13 with SCA) treated with haplo-SCT and PT-Cy. The median age was 10 years.[3-18] The conditioning regimen was modified adding thiotepa (10 mg/kg) and ATG (4.5 mg/kg), and all patients received primed BM as the stem cell source. Sirolimus was used instead of calcineurin inhibitors. All patients but one engrafted achieving a full-donor chimerism, without SCA-related clinical manifestations. Grade 2 or more aGVHD was observed in two patients (12%) and cGVHD in one; one patient died from macrophage activation syndrome.[137] Recently the NIH group published a phase 1/2 prospective study in patients with hemoglobinopathies (mostly SCA, 19/23) and several comorbidities. The conditioning regimen consisted of alemtuzumab and TBI 4 Gy, followed by PBSC from haploidentical donor. The GVHD prophylaxis consisted of sirolimus, in the cohort 1, and 3 out of 3 patients rejected their graft, and this arm was closed. In cohort 2 and 3, PT-Cy (50 mg/kg and 100 mg/kg, respectively) was added. In the first cohort, 25% of patients reversed SCA-phenotype. In the cohort 3, 83% engrafted and 50% obtained the SCA-free clinical state. While the OS was 87%, none of the patients had full-donor chimerism, with seven patients having primary graft failure and eight secondary graft failure. No severe aGVHD and GVHD were observed.[138] Finally, Anurathapan et al. treated 31 patients (median age 10 years) with severe β-thal with haploidentical donor. The conditioning regimen was modified to overcome the risk of graft failure using two courses of pharmacological pretransplant immunosuppressive therapy (PTIS) with fludarabine plus dexamethasone, followed by a busulfan-based MAC with ATG and PT-Cy. All patients were infused with PBSC. All patients but two achieved a full engraftment. They observed 2 DSA-related primary graft failure, and five patients did not have severe venoocclusive disease. The OS and EFS at 1 year were 95% and 94%, respectively. Only one patient died from aGVHD.[139]

All these studies are of outmost importance because they paved the way to an enhanced accessibility to allo-SCT for patients with hemoglobinopathies, without an evident loss of efficacy due to high toxicity–related mortality.

CONCLUSIONS

The development of T-cell replete platforms all around the world allowed to overcome the problems linked to the donor procurement because now virtually we can have one or more donors for each patients. Furthermore, the time to donor procurement probably does not matter in the clinical outcome because we can found a donor in a very short period. These two points have as consequence that when allogeneic transplantation is considered the best option for the patients; thus they will be transplanted in the right time without any delay. The adoption of one platform over others can be made arbitrarily by the transplantation program director, considering that huge differences are not detectable. Finally, in the near future, the results from randomized prospective studies can help physician and patient to do the best choice when transplantation is to program, even in a new-drug era in many hematological diseases.

REFERENCES

1. Thomas ED, Blume KG, Forman SJ. *Hematopoietic Cell Transplantation*. Malden, MA: Blackwell Sciences; 1999.
2. Henslee-Downey PJ, Abhyankar SH, Parrish RS, et al. Use of partially mismatched related donors extends access to allogeneic marrow transplant. *Blood*. 1997;89:3864–3872.
3. Anasetti C, Amos D, Beatty PG, et al. Effect of HLA compatibility on engraftment of bone marrow transplants in patients with leukemia or lymphoma. *N Engl J Med*. 1989;320(4):197–204.
4. Aversa F, Terenzi A, Carotti A, et al. Improved outcome with T-cell-depleted bone marrow transplantation for acute leukemia. *J Clin Oncol*. 1999;17:1545–1550.
5. Ji SQ, Chen HR, Wang HX, et al. G-CSF-primed haploidentical marrow transplantation without ex vivo T cell depletion: an excellent alternative for high-risk leukemia. *Bone Marrow Transpl*. 2002;30(12):861–866.
6. Huang XJ, Chang YJ, Zhao XY. Maintaining hyporesponsiveness and polarization potential of T cells after in vitro mixture of G-CSF mobilized peripheral blood grafts and G-CSF primed bone marrow grafts in different proportions. *Transpl Immunol*. 2007;17(3):193–197.
7. Lv M, Zhao XS, Hu Y, et al. Monocytic and promyelocytic myeloid-derived suppressor cells may contribute to G-CSF-induced immune tolerance in haplo-identical allogeneic hematopoietic stem cell transplantation. *Am J Hematol*. 2015;90(1):E9–E16.
8. Hu Y, He GL, Zhao XY, et al. Regulatory B cells promote graft-versus-host disease prevention and maintain graft-versus-leukemia activity following allogeneic bone marrow transplantation. *Onco Immunol*. 2017;6(3):e1284721.
9. Xu LP, Liu KY, Liu DH, et al. The inferiority of G-PB to rhG-CSF-mobilized blood and marrow grafts as a stem cell source in patients with high-risk acute leukemia who underwent unmanipulated HLA-mismatched/haploidentical transplantation: a comparative analysis. *Bone Marrow Transpl*. 2010;45(6):985–992.
10. Chang YJ, Xu LP, Wang Y, et al. Controlled, randomized, open-label trial of risk-stratified corticosteroid prevention of acute graft-versus-host disease after haploidentical transplantation. *J Clin Oncol*. 2016;34(16):1855–1863.
11. Luo XH, Chang YJ, Xu LP, Liu DH, Liu KY, Huang XJ. The impact of graft composition on clinical outcomes in unmanipulated HLA-mismatched/haploidentical hematopoietic SCT. *Bone Marrow Transpl*. 2009;43(1):29–36.
12. Zhao XY, Chang YJ, Xu LP, Liu DH, Liu KY, Huang XJ. Association of natural killer cells in allografts with transplant outcomes in patients receiving G-CSF-mobilized PBSC grafts and G-CSF-primed BM grafts from HLA-haploidentical donors. *Bone Marrow Transpl*. 2009;44(11):721–728.
13. Soiffer RJ, Lerademacher J, Ho V, et al. Impact of immune modulation with anti-T-cell antibodies on the outcome of reduced-intensity allogeneic hematopoietic stem cell transplantation for hematologic malignancies. *Blood*. 2011;117(25):6963–6970.
14. Wang Y, Fu HX, Liu DH, et al. Influence of two different doses of antithymocyte globulin in patients with standard-risk disease following haploidentical transplantation: a randomized trial. *Bone Marrow Transpl*. 2014;49(3):426–433.
15. Chang YJ, Wang Y, Mo XD, et al. Optimal dose of rabbit thymoglobulin in conditioning regimens for unmanipulated, haploidentical, hematopoietic stem cell transplantation: long-term outcomes of a prospective randomized trial. *Cancer*. 2017;123(15):2881–2892.
16. Wang Y, Wu DP, Liu QF, et al. Donor and recipient age, gender and ABO incompatibility regardless of donor source: validated criteria for donor selection for haematopoietic transplants. *Leukemia*. 2018;32(2):492–498.
17. Yan CH, Xu LP, Wang FR, et al. Causes of mortality after haploidentical hematopoietic stem cell transplantation and the comparison with HLA-identical sibling hematopoietic stem cell transplantation. *Bone Marrow Transpl*. 2016;51(3):391–397.
18. Girmenia C, Barosi G, Piciocchi A, et al. Primary prophylaxis of invasive fungal diseases in allogeneic stem cell transplantation: revised recommendations from a consensus process by Gruppo Italiano Trapianto Midollo Osseo (GITMO). *Biol Blood Marrow Transpl*. 2014;20(8):1080–1088.
19. Sun YQ, Xu LP, Liu DH, et al. The incidence and risk factors of invasive fungal infection after haploidentical haematopoietic stem cell transplantation without in vitro T-cell depletion. *Clin Microbiol Infect*. 2012;18(10):997–1003.
20. Huang X, Chen H, Han M, et al. Multicenter, randomized, open-label study comparing the efficacy and safety of micafungin versus itraconazole for prophylaxis of invasive fungal infections in patients undergoing hematopoietic stem cell transplant. *Biol Blood Marrow Transpl*. 2012;18(10):1509–1516.

21. Lu DP, Dong L, Wu T, et al. Conditioning including antithymocyte globulin followed by unmanipulated HLA-mismatched/haploidentical blood and marrow transplantation can achieve comparable outcomes with HLA-identical sibling transplantation. *Blood.* 2006;107(8):3065–3073.

22. Liu J, Kong J, Chang YJ, et al. Patients with refractory cytomegalovirus (CMV) infection following allogeneic haematopoietic stem cell transplantation are at high risk for CMV disease and non-relapse mortality. *Clin Microbiol Infect.* 2015;21(12): 1121.e9–e15.

23. Pei XY, Zhao XY, Chang YJ, et al. Cytomegalovirus-specific T-cell transfer for refractory cytomegalovirus infection after haploidentical stem cell transplantation: the quantitative and qualitative immune recovery for cytomegalovirus. *J Infect Dis.* 2017;216(8):945–956.

24. Chang YJ, Zhao XY, Xu LP, et al. Donor-specific anti-human leukocyte antigen antibodies were associated with primary graft failure after unmanipulated haploidentical blood and marrow transplantation: a prospective study with randomly assigned training and validation sets. *J Hematol Oncol.* 2015;8:84.

25. Shi MM, Kong Y, Song Y, et al. Atorvastatin enhances endothelial cell function in posttransplant poor graft function. *Blood.* 2016;128(25):2988–2999.

26. Kong Y, Wang YT, Cao XN, et al. Aberrant T cell responses in the bone marrow microenvironment of patients with poor graft function after allogeneic hematopoietic stem cell transplantation. *J Transl Med.* 2017;15(1):57.

27. Wang Y, Chang YJ, Xu LP, et al. Who is the best donor for a related HLA haplotype-mismatched transplant? *Blood.* 2014;124(6):843–850.

28. Xu L, Chen H, Chen J, et al. The consensus on indications, conditioning regimen, and donor selection of allogeneic hematopoietic cell transplantation for hematological diseases in China-recommendations from the Chinese Society of Hematology. *J Hematol Oncol.* 2018;11(1):33.

29. Xu LP, Wu DP, Han MZ, et al. A review of hematopoietic cell transplantation in China: data and trends during 2008–2016. *Bone Marrow Transpl.* 2017;52(11):1512–1518.

30. Wang Y, Liu QF, Xu LP, et al. Haploidentical vs identical-sibling transplant for AML in remission: a multicenter, prospective study. *Blood.* 2015;125(25):3956–3962.

31. Sun Y, Beohou E, Labopin M, et al. Acute Leukemia Working Party of the EBMT. Unmanipulated haploidentical versus matched unrelated donor allogeneic stem cell transplantation in adult patients with acute myelogenous leukemia in first remission: a retrospective pair-matched comparative study of the Beijing approach with the EBMT database. *Haematologica.* 2016;101(8):e352–e354.

32. Huang XJ, Zhu HH, Chang YJ, et al. The superiority of haploidentical related stem cell transplantation over chemotherapy alone as postremission treatment for patients with intermediate- or high-risk acute myeloid leukemia in first complete remission. *Blood.* 2012;119(23):5584–5590.

33. Chang YJ, Wang Y, Liu YR, et al. Haploidentical allograft is superior to matched sibling donor allograft in eradicating pre-transplantation minimal residual disease of AML patients as determined by multiparameter flow cytometry: a retrospective and prospective analysis. *J Hematol Oncol.* 2017;10(1):134.

34. Yan CH, Jiang Q, Wang J, et al. Superior survival of unmanipulated haploidentical hematopoietic stem cell transplantation compared with chemotherapy alone used as post-remission therapy in adults with standard-risk acute lymphoblastic leukemia in first complete remission. *Biol Blood Marrow Transpl.* 2014;20(9):1314–1321.

35. Chen H, Liu KY, Xu LP, et al. Haploidentical hematopoietic stem cell transplantation without in vitro T cell depletion for the treatment of philadelphia chromosome-positive acute lymphoblastic leukemia. *Biol Blood Marrow Transpl.* 2015;21(6):1110–1116.

36. Wang Y, Liu QF, Xu LP, et al. Haploidentical versus matched-sibling transplant in adults with philadelphia-negative high-risk acute lymphoblastic leukemia: a biologically phase III randomized study. *Clin Cancer Res.* 2016;22(14):3467–3476.

37. Han LJ, Wang Y, Fan ZP, et al. Haploidentical transplantation compared with matched sibling and unrelated donor transplantation for adults with standard-risk acute lymphoblastic leukaemia in first complete remission. *Br J Haematol.* 2017;179(1):120–130.

38. Xu LP, Wang SQ, Wu DP, et al. Haplo-identical transplantation for acquired severe aplastic anaemia in a multicentre prospective study. *Br J Haematol.* 2016;175(2):265–274.

39. Xu LP, Jin S, Wang SQ, et al. Upfront haploidentical transplant for acquired severe aplastic anemia: registry-based comparison with matched related transplant. *J Hematol Oncol.* 2017;10(1):25.

40. Xu LP, Xu ZL, Wang FR, et al. Unmanipulated haploidentical transplantation conditioning with busulfan, cyclophosphamide and anti-thymoglobulin for adult severe aplastic anaemia. *Bone Marrow Transpl.* 2018;53(2):188–192.

41. Huang XJ, Liu DH, Liu KY, Xu LP, Chen H, Han W. Donor lymphocyte infusion for the treatment of leukemia relapse after HLA-mismatched/haploidentical T-cell-replete hematopoietic stem cell transplantation. *Haematologica.* 2007;92(3):414–417.

42. Wang Y, Liu DH, Xu LP, et al. Prevention of relapse using granulocyte CSF-primed PBPCs following HLA-mismatched/haploidentical, T-cell-replete hematopoietic SCT in patients with advanced-stage acute leukemia: a retrospective risk-factor analysis. *Bone Marrow Transpl.* 2012;47(8):1099–1104.

43. Ogawa H, Ikegame K, Yoshihara S, et al. 2-3 antigen-mismatched (haploidentical) stem cell transplantation using nonmyeloablative conditioning. *Biol Blood Marrow Transpl.* 2006;12(10):1073–1084.

44. Ogawa H, Ikegame K, Kaida K, et al. Kawase. Unmanipulated HLA 2-3 antigen-mismatched (haploidentical) bone marrow transplantation using only pharmacological GVHD prophylaxis. *Exp Hematol.* 2008;36(1):1–8.

45. Ikegame K, Yoshida T, Yoshihara S, et al. Unmanipulated haploidentical reduced-intensity stem cell transplantation using fludarabine, busulfan, low-dose antithymocyte globulin, and steroids for patients in non-complete remission or at high risk of relapse: a prospective multicenter phase I/II study in Japan. *Biol Blood Marrow Transpl.* 2015;21(8):1495–1505.

46. Lee KH, Lee JH, Lee JH, et al. Hematopoietic cell transplantation from an HLA-mismatched familial donor is feasible without ex vivo-T cell depletion after reduced-intensity conditioning with busulfan, fludarabine, and antithymocyte globulin. *Biol Blood Marrow Transpl.* 2009;15(1):61–72.

47. Lee KH, Lee JH, Lee JH, et al. Reduced-intensity conditioning therapy with busulfan, fludarabine, and antithymocyte globulin for HLA-haploidentical hematopoietic cell transplantation in acute leukemia and myelodysplastic syndrome. *Blood.* 2011;118(9):2609–2617.

48. Lee KH, Lee JH, Lee JH, et al. Reduced-intensity conditioning with busulfan, fludarabine, and antithymocyte globulin for hematopoietic cell transplantation from unrelated or haploidentical family donors in patients with acute myeloid leukemia in remission. *Biol Blood Marrow Transpl.* 2017;23(9):1555–1566.

49. Cho BS, Yoon JH, Shin SH, et al. Comparison of allogeneic stem cell transplantation from familial-mismatched/haploidentical donors and from unrelated donors in adults with high-risk acute myelogenous leukemia. *Biol Blood Marrow Transpl.* 2012;18(10):1552–1563.

50. Di Bartolomeo P, Santarone S, De Angelis G, et al. Haploidentical, unmanipulated, G-CSF-primed bone marrow transplantation for patients with high-risk hematologic malignancies. *Blood.* 2013;121(5):849–857.

51. Arcese W, Picardi A, Santarone S, et al. Rome Transplant Network. Haploidentical, G-CSF-primed, unmanipulated bone marrow transplantation for patients with high-risk hematological malignancies: an update. *Bone Marrow Transpl.* 2015;50(suppl 2):S24–S30.

52. De Felice L, Agostini F, Suriano C, et al. Hematopoietic, mesenchymal, and immune cells are more enhanced in bone marrow than in peripheral blood from granulocyte colony-stimulating factor primed healthy donors. *Biol Blood Marrow Transpl.* 2016;22(10):1758–1764.

53. Luznik L, Jalla S, Engstrom LW, Iannone R, Fuchs EJ. Durable engraftment of major histocompatibility complex–incompatible cells after nonmyeloablative conditioning with fludarabine, low-dose total body irradiation, and posttransplantation cyclophosphamide. *Blood.* 2001;98(12):3456–3464.

54. Berenbaum MC, Brown IN. Prolongation of homograft survival in mice with single doses of cyclophosphamide. *Nature.* 1963;200:84.

55. Santos GW, Owens AH. Production of graft-versus-host disease in the rat and its treatment with cytotoxic agents. *Nature.* 1966;210(5032):139–140.

56. Mayumi H, Good RA. Long-lasting skin allograft tolerance in adult mice induced across fully allogeneic (multimajor H-2 plus multiminor histocompatibility) antigen barriers by a tolerance inducing method using cyclophosphamide. *J Exp Med.* 1989;169(1):213–238.

57. Colson YL, Wren SM, Schuchert MJ, et al. A nonlethal conditioning approach to achieve durable multilineage mixed chimerism and tolerance across major, minor, and hematopoietic histocompatibility barriers. *J Immunol.* 1995;155(9):4179–4188.

58. Kanakry CG, Ganguly S, Zahurak M, et al. Aldehyde dehydrogenase expression drives human regulatory T cell resistance to posttransplantation cyclophosphamide. *Sci Transl Med.* 2013;5(211): 211ra157.

59. Luznik L, Engstrom LW, Iannone R, Fuchs EJ. Posttransplantation cyclophosphamide facilitates engraftment of major histocompatibility complex-identical allogeneic marrow in mice conditioned with low-dose total body irradiation. *Biol Blood Marrow Transplant.* 2002;8(3).

60. O'Donnell PV, Luznik L, Jones RJ, et al. Nonmyeloablative bone marrow transplantation from partially HLA-mismatched related donors using posttransplantation cyclophosphamide. *Biol Blood Marrow Transpl.* 2002;8:377–386.

61. Luznik L, O'Donnell PV, Symons HJ, et al. HLA-haploidentical bone marrow transplantation for hematologic malignancies using nonmyeloablative conditioning and high-dose, posttransplantation cyclophosphamide. *Biol Blood Marrow Transpl.* 2008;14(6):641–650.

62. Kasamon YL, Luznik L, Leffell MS, et al. Nonmyeloablative HLA-haploidentical bone marrow transplantation with high-dose posttransplantation cyclophosphamide: effect of HLA disparity on outcome. *Biol Blood Marrow Transpl.* 2010;16(4):482–489.

63. Solomon SR, Aubrey MT, Zhang X, et al. Selecting the best donor for haploidentical transplant: impact of HLA, killer cell immunoglobulin-like receptor genotyping, and other clinical variables. *Biol Blood Marrow Transpl.* 2018;24(4):789–798.

64. McCurdy SR, Zhang MJ, St Martin A, et al. Effect of donor characteristics on haploidentical transplantation with posttransplantation cyclophosphamide. *Blood Adv.* 2018;2(3):299–307.

65. Raiola AM, Risitano A, Sacchi N, et al. Impact of HLA disparity in haploidentical bone marrow transplantation followed by high-dose cyclophosphamide. *Biol Blood Marrow Transpl.* 2018;24(1):119–126.

66. Cesaro S, Crocchiolo R, Tridello G, et al. Comparable survival using a CMV-matched or a mismatched donor for CMV+ patients undergoing T-replete haplo-HSCT with PT-Cy for acute leukemia: a study of behalf of the infectious diseases and acute leukemia working parties of the EBMT. *Bone Marrow Transpl.* 2018;53(4):422–430.

67. Elmariah H, Kasamon YL, Zahurak M, et al. Haploidentical bone marrow transplantation with post-transplant cyclophosphamide using non-first-degree related donors. *Biol Blood Marrow Transpl.* 2018;24(5):1099–1102.

68. McCurdy SR, Kanakry CG, Tsai HL, et al. Acute graft-versus-host disease and higher nucleated cell graft dose improve progression-free survival after HLA-haploidentical transplant with post-transplant cyclophosphamide. *Biol Blood Marrow Transpl.* 2018;24(2):343–352.

69. Al-Homsi AS, Roy TS, Cole K, Feng Y, Duffner U. Post-transplant high-dose cyclophosphamide for the prevention of graft-versus-host disease. *Biol Blood Marrow Transpl.* 2015;21(4):604–611.

70. Takanashi M, Atsuta Y, Fujiwara K, et al. The impact of anti-HLA antibodies on unrelated cord blood transplantations. *Blood.* 2010;116(15):2839–2846.

71. Spellman S, Bray R, Rosen-Bronson S, et al. The detection of donor-directed, HLA-specific alloantibodies in recipients of unrelated hematopoietic cell transplantation is predictive of graft failure. *Blood.* 2010;115(13):2704–2708.

72. Cutler C, Kim HT, Sun L, et al. Donor-specific anti-HLA antibodies predict outcome in double umbilical cord blood transplantation. *Blood.* 2011;118(25):6691–6697.

73. Ciurea SO, Thall PF, Wang X, et al. Donor-specific anti-HLA Abs and graft failure in matched unrelated donor hematopoietic stem cell transplantation. *Blood.* 2011;118(22):5957–5964.

74. Ciurea SO, de Lima M, Cano P, et al. High risk of graft failure in patients with anti-HLA antibodies undergoing haploidentical stem-cell transplantation. *Transplantation.* 2009;88(8):1019–1024.

75. Ciurea SO, Cao K, Fernadez-Vina M, et al. The European society for blood and marrow transplantation (EBMT) consensus Guidelines for the detection and treatment of donor-specific anti-HLA antibodies (DSA) in haploidentical hematopoietic cell transplantation. *Bone Marrow Transpl.* 2018;53(5):521–534.

76. Armand P, Kim HT, Logan BR, et al. Validation and refinement of the Disease Risk Index for allogeneic stem cell transplantation. *Blood.* 2014;123(23):3664–3671.

77. McCurdy SR, Kanakry JA, Showel MM, et al. Risk stratified outcomes of nonmyeloablative HLA-haploidentical BMT with high-dose posttransplantation cyclophosphamide. *Blood.* 2015;125(19):3024–3031.

78. Roberto A, Castagna L, Zanon V, et al. Role of naive-derived T memory stem cells in T-cell reconstitution following allogeneic transplantation. *Blood.* 2015;125(18):2855–2864.

79. Roberto A, Castagna L, Gandolfi S, et al. B-cell reconstitution recapitulates B-cell lymphopoiesis following haploidentical BM transplantation and post-transplant CY. *Bone Marrow Transpl.* 2015;50(2):317–319.

80. Roberto A, Di Vito C, Zaghi E, et al. The early expansion of anergic NKG2Apos/CD56dim/CD16neg natural killer represents a therapeutic target in haploidentical hematopoietic stem cell transplantation. *Haematologica.* 2018;103(8):1390–1402.

81. Russo A, Oliveira G, Berglund S, et al. NK cell recovery after haploidentical HSCT with posttransplant cyclophosphamide: dynamics and clinical implications. *Blood.* 2018;131(2):247–262.

82. Crocchiolo R, Bramanti S, Vai A, et al. Infections after T-replete haploidentical transplantation and high-dose cyclophosphamide as graft-versus-host disease prophylaxis. *Transpl Infect Dis.* 2015;17(2):242–249.

83. Dietrich S, Finel H, Martinez C, et al. Post-transplant cyclophosphamide-based haplo-identical transplantation as alternative to matched sibling or unrelated donor transplantation for non-Hodgkin lymphoma: a registry study by the European society for blood and marrow transplantation. *Leukemia.* 2016;30(10):2086–2089.

84. Mariotti J, Devillier R, Bramanti S, et al. T cell-replete haploidentical transplantation with post-transplantation cyclophosphamide for Hodgkin lymphoma relapsed after autologous transplantation: reduced incidence of relapse and of chronic graft-versus-host disease compared with HLA-identical related donors. *Biol Blood Marrow Transpl.* 2018;24(3):627–632.

85. Raiola A, Dominietto A, Varaldo R, et al. Unmanipulated haploidentical BMT following non-myeloablative conditioning and post-transplantation CY for advanced Hodgkin's lymphoma. *Bone Marrow Transpl.* 2014;49(2):190–194.

86. Kanate AS, Mussetti A, Kharfan-Dabaja MA, et al. Reduced-intensity transplantation for lymphomas using haploidentical related donors vs HLA-matched unrelated donors. *Blood.* 2016;127(7):938–947.

87. Ghosh N, Karmali R, Rocha V, et al. Reduced-intensity transplantation for lymphomas using haploidentical related donors versus HLA-matched sibling donors: a center for international blood and marrow transplant research analysis. *J Clin Oncol.* 2016;34(26):3141–3149.

88. Kanakry JA, Kasamon YL, Gocke CD, et al. Outcomes of related donor HLA-identical or HLA-haploidentical allogeneic blood or marrow transplantation for peripheral T cell lymphoma. *Biol Blood Marrow Transpl.* 2013;19(4):602–606.

89. Kanakry JA, Gocke CD, Bolaños-Meade J, et al. Phase II study of nonmyeloablative allogeneic bone marrow transplantation for B cell lymphoma with post-transplantation Rituximab and donor selection based first on non-HLA factors. *Biol Blood Marrow Transpl.* 2015;21(12):2115–2122.

90. Burroughs LM, O'Donnell PV, Sandmaier BM, et al. Comparison of outcomes of HLA-matched related, unrelated, or HLA-haploidentical related hematopoietic cell transplantation following nonmyeloablative conditioning for relapsed or refractory Hodgkin lymphoma. *Biol Blood Marrow Transpl.* 2008;14(11):1279–1287.

91. Martínez C, Gayoso J, Canals C, et al. Lymphoma working party of the European group for blood and marrow transplantation. Post-transplantation cyclophosphamide-based haploidentical transplantation as alternative to matched sibling or unrelated donor

transplantation for Hodgkin lymphoma: a registry study of the lymphoma working party of the European society for blood and marrow transplantation. *J Clin Oncol.* 2017;35(30):3425–3432.

92. Castagna L, Bramanti S, Devillier R, et al. Haploidentical transplantation with post-infusion cyclophosphamide in advanced Hodgkin lymphoma. *Bone Marrow Transpl.* 2017;52(5):797.

93. Gayoso J, Balsalobre P, Pascual MJ, et al. Busulfan-based reduced intensity conditioning regimens for haploidentical transplantation in relapsed/refractory Hodgkin lymphoma: Spanish multicenter experience. *Bone Marrow Transpl.* 2016;51(10):1307–1312.

94. Gauthier J, Poiré X, Gac AC, et al. Better outcome with haploidentical over HLA-matched related donors in patients with Hodgkin's lymphoma undergoing allogeneic haematopoietic cell transplantation-a study by the Francophone Society of Bone Marrow Transplantation and Cellular Therapy. *Bone Marrow Transpl.* 2018;53(4):400–409.

95. Castagna L, Mussetti A, Devillier R, et al. Haploidentical allogeneic hematopoietic cell transplantation for multiple myeloma using post-transplantation cyclophosphamide graft-versus-host disease prophylaxis. *Biol Blood Marrow Transpl.* 2017;23(9):1549–1554.

96. Ciurea SO, Mulanovich V, Saliba RM, et al. Improved early outcomes using a T cell replete graft compared with T cell depleted haploidentical hematopoietic stem cell transplantation. *Biol Blood Marrow Transpl.* 2012;18(12):1835–1844.

97. Ciurea SO, Zhang MJ, Bacigalupo AA, et al. Haploidentical transplant with posttransplant cyclophosphamide vs matched unrelated donor transplant for acute myeloid leukemia. *Blood.* 2015;126(8):1033–1040.

98. Salvatore D, Labopin M, Ruggeri A, et al. Outcomes of hematopoietic stem cell transplantation from unmanipulated haploidentical versus matched sibling donor in patients with acute myeloid leukemia in first complete remission with intermediate or high-risk cytogenetics: a study from the Acute Leukemia Working Party of the European Society for Blood and Marrow Transplantation. *Haematologica.* 2018;103(8):1317–1328.

99. Versluis J, Labopin M, Ruggeri A, et al. Alternative donors for allogeneic hematopoietic stem cell transplantation in poor-risk AML in CR1. *Blood Adv.* 2017;1:477–485.

100. Piemontese S, Ciceri F, Labopin M, et al. A comparison between allogeneic stem cell transplantation from unmanipulated haploidentical and unrelated donors in acute leukemia. *J Hematol Oncol.* 2017;10(1):24.

101. Canaani J, Labopin M, Huang XJ, et al. T-cell replete haploidentical stem cell transplantation attenuates the prognostic impact of FLT3-ITD in acute myeloid leukemia: a report from the Acute Leukemia Working Party of the European Society for Blood and Marrow Transplantation. *Am J Hematol.* 2018;93(6):736–744.

102. Li Z, Labopin M, Ciceri F, et al. Haploidentical transplantation outcomes for secondary acute myeloid leukemia: acute leukemia working party (ALWP) of the European society for blood and marrow transplantation (EBMT) study. *Am J Hematol.* 2018;93(6):769–777.

103. Ruggeri A, Sun Y, Labopin M, et al. Post-transplant cyclophosphamide versus anti-thymocyte globulin as graft- versus-host disease prophylaxis in haploidentical transplant. *Haematologica.* 2017;102(2):401–410.

104. Srour SA, Milton DR, Bashey A, et al. Haploidentical transplantation with post-transplantation cyclophosphamide for high-risk acute lymphoblastic leukemia. *Biol Blood Marrow Transpl.* 2017;23(2):318–324.

105. Santoro N, Labopin M, Giannotti F, et al. Unmanipulated haploidentical in comparison with matched unrelated donor stem cell transplantation in patients 60 years and older with acute myeloid leukemia: a comparative study on behalf of the ALWP of the EBMT. *J Hematol Oncol.* 2018;11(1):55.

106. Tischer J, Stemmler HJ, Engel N, et al. Feasibility of clofarabine cytoreduction followed by haploidentical hematopoietic stem cell transplantation in patients with relapsed or refractory advanced acute leukemia. *Ann Hematol.* 2013;92(10):1379–1388.

107. Jaiswal SR, Zaman S, Chakrabarti A, et al. Improved outcome of refractory/relapsed acute myeloid leukemia after post-transplantation cyclophosphamide-based haploidentical transplantation with myeloablative conditioning and early prophylactic granulocyte colony-stimulating factor-mobilized donor lymphocyte infusions. *Biol Blood Marrow Transpl.* 2016;22(10):1867–1873.

108. How J, Slade M, Vu K, et al. T Cell-Replete T cell-replete peripheral blood haploidentical hematopoietic cell transplantation with post-transplantation cyclophosphamide results in outcomes similar to transplantation from traditionally matched donors in active disease acute myeloid leukemia. *Biol Blood Marrow Transpl.* 2017;23(4):648653.

109. Piemontese S, Ciceri F, Labopin M, et al. Acute Leukemia Working Party (ALWP) of the European Group for Blood and Marrow Transplantation (EBMT). A survey on unmanipulated haploidentical hematopoietic stem cell transplantation in adults with acute leukemia. *Leukemia.* 2015;29(5):1069–1075.

110. Lee CJ, Savani BN, Mohty M, et al. Haploidentical hematopoietic cell transplantation for adult acute myeloid leukemia: a position statement from the acute leukemia working party of the European society for blood and marrow transplantation. *Haematologica.* 2017;102(11):1810–1822.

111. Raiola AM, Dominietto A, Ghiso A, et al. Unmanipulated haploidentical bone marrow transplantation and posttransplantation cyclophosphamide for hematologic malignancies after myeloablative conditioning. *Biol Blood Marrow Transpl.* 2013;19(1):117–122.

112. Solomon SR, Sizemore CA, Sanacore M, et al. Haploidentical transplantation using T cell replete peripheral blood stem cells and myeloablative conditioning in patients with high-risk hematologic malignancies who lack conventional donors is well tolerated and produces excellent relapse-free survival: results of a prospective phase II trial. *Biol Blood Marrow Transpl.* 2012;18(12):1859–1866.

113. Bacigalupo A, Dominietto A, Ghiso A, et al. Unmanipulated haploidentical bone marrow transplantation and post-transplant cyclophosphamide for hematologic malignancies following a myeloablative conditioning: an update. *Bone Marrow Transpl.* 2015;50(suppl 2):S37–S39.

114. Rubio MT, Savani BN, Labopin M, et al. The impact of HLA-matching on reduced intensity conditioning regimen unrelated donor allogeneic stem cell transplantation for acute myeloid leukemia in patients above 50 years-a report from the EBMT acute leukemia working party. *J Hematol Oncol.* 2016;9(1):65.

115. Castagna L, Crocchiolo R, Furst S, et al. Bone marrow compared with peripheral blood stem cells for haploidentical transplantation with a nonmyeloablative conditioning regimen and post-transplantation cyclophosphamide. *Biol Blood Marrow Transpl.* 2014;20(5):724–729.

116. Bhamidipati PK, DiPersio JF, Stokerl-Goldstein K, et al. Haploidentical transplantation using G-CSF-mobilized T-cell replete PBSCs and post-transplantation CY after non-myeloablative conditioning is safe and is associated with favorable outcomes. *Bone Marrow Transpl.* 2014;49(8):1124–1126.

117. Raj K, Pagliuca A, Bradstock K, et al. Peripheral blood hematopoietic stem cells for transplantation of hematological diseases from related, haploidentical donors after reduced-intensity conditioning. *Biol Blood Marrow Transpl.* 2014;20(6):890–895.

118. Bradstock K, Bilmon I, Kwan J, et al. Influence of stem cell source on outcomes of allogeneic reduced-intensity conditioning therapy transplants using haploidentical related donors. *Biol Blood Marrow Transpl.* 2015;21(9):1641–1645.

119. Bashey A, Zhang MJ, McCurdy SR, et al. Mobilized peripheral blood stem cells versus unstimulated bone marrow as a graft source for T-cell-replete haploidentical donor transplantation using post-transplant cyclophosphamide. *J Clin Oncol.* 2017;35(26):3002–3009.

120. Ruggeri A, Labopin M, Bacigalupo A, et al. Bone marrow versus mobilized peripheral blood stem cells in haploidentical transplants using posttransplantation cyclophosphamide. *Cancer.* 2018;124(7):1428–1437.

121. Savani BN, Labopin M, Blaise D, et al. Peripheral blood stem cell graft compared to bone marrow after reduced intensity conditioning regimens for acute leukemia: a report from the ALWP of the EBMT. *Haematologica.* 2016;101(2):256–262.

122. O'Donnell PV, Eapen M, Horowitz MM, et al. Comparable outcomes with marrow or peripheral blood as stem cell sources for hematopoietic cell transplantation from haploidentical donors after non-ablative conditioning: a matched-pair analysis. *Bone Marrow Transpl.* 2016;51(12):1599–1601.

123. Castagna L, Bramanti S, Furst S, et al. Tacrolimus compared with cyclosporine A after haploidentical T-cell replete transplantation with post-infusion cyclophosphamide. *Bone Marrow Transpl.* 2016;51(3):470.

124. Kasamon YL, Fuchs EJ, Zahurak M, et al. Shortened-duration tacrolimus after nonmyeloablative, HLA-haploidentical bone marrow transplantation. *Biol Blood Marrow Transpl.* 2018;24(5):1022–1028.

125. Walter RB, Estey EH. Management of older or unfit patients with acute myeloid leukemia. *Leukemia.* 2015;29(4):770–775.

126. Kasamon YL, Bolaños-Meade J, Prince GT, et al. Outcomes of Nonmyeloablative HLA-Haploidentical Blood or Marrow Transplantation With High-Dose Post-Transplantation Cyclophosphamide in Older Adults. *J Clin Oncol.* 2015;33(28):3152–3161.

127. Blaise D, Fürst S, Crocchiolo R, et al. Haploidentical T cell-replete transplantation with post-transplantation cyclophosphamide for patients in or above the sixth decade of age compared with allogeneic hematopoietic stem cell transplantation from an human leukocyte antigen-matched related or unrelated donor. *Biol Blood Marrow Transpl.* 2016;22(1):119–124.

128. Devillier R, Legrand F, Rey J, et al. HLA-matched sibling versus unrelated versus haploidentical related donor allogeneic hematopoietic stem cell transplantation for patients aged over 60 Years with acute myeloid leukemia: a single-center donor comparison. *Biol Blood Marrow Transpl.* 2018;24(7):1449–1454.

129. Bashey ZA, Zhang X, Brown S, et al. Comparison of outcomes following transplantation with T-replete HLA-haploidentical donors using post-transplant cyclophosphamide to matched related and unrelated donors for patients with AML and MDS aged 60 years or older. *Bone Marrow Transpl.* 2018;53(6):756–763.

130. Ciurea SO, Shah MV, Saliba RM, et al. Haploidentical transplantation for older patients with acute myeloid leukemia and myelodysplastic syndrome. *Biol Blood Marrow Transpl.* 2018;24(6):1232–1236.

131. Slade M, DiPersio JF, Westervelt P, Vij R, Schroeder MA, Romee R. Haploidentical hematopoietic cell transplant with post-transplant cyclophosphamide and peripheral blood stem cell grafts in older adults with acute myeloid leukemia or myelodysplastic syndrome. *Biol Blood Marrow Transpl.* 2017;23(10):1736–1743.

132. Santoro N, Labopin M, Giannotti F, et al. Unmanipulated haploidentical in comparison with matched unrelated donor stem cell transplantation in patients 60 years and older with acute myeloid leukemia: a comparative study on behalf of the ALWP of the EBMT. *J Hematol Oncol.* 2018;11(1):55.

133. Clay J, Kulasekararaj AG, Potter V, et al. Nonmyeloablative peripheral blood haploidentical stem cell transplantation for refractory severe aplastic anemia. *Biol Blood Marrow Transpl.* 2014;20(11):1711–1716.

134. Esteves I, Bonfim C, Pasquini R, et al. Haploidentical BMT and post-transplant Cy for severe aplastic anemia: a multicenter retrospective study. *Bone Marrow Transpl.* 2015;50(5):685–689.

135. DeZern AE, Zahurak M, Symons H, Cooke K, Jones RJ, Brodsky RA. Alternative donor transplantation with high-dose post-transplantation cyclophosphamide for refractory severe aplastic anemia. *Biol Blood Marrow Transpl.* 2017;23(3):498–504.

136. Bolaños-Meade J, Fuchs EJ, Luznik L, et al. HLA-haploidentical bone marrow transplantation with posttransplant cyclophosphamide expands the donor pool for patients with sickle cell disease. *Blood.* 2012;120(22):4285–4291.

137. De la Fuente J, O'Boyle F, Harrington Y, et al. Haploidentical BMT with a post-infusion of stem cell cyclophosphamide approach is feasible and leads to a high rate of donor engraftment in hemoglobinopathies allowing universal application of transplantation. *Blood Abs.* 2015;126:4317.

138. Fitzhugh CD, Hsieh MM, Taylor T, et al. Cyclophosphamide improves engraftment in patients with SCD and severe organ damage who undergo haploidentical PBSCT. *Blood Adv.* 2017;1(11):652–661.

139. Anurathapan U, Hongeng S, Pakakasama S, et al. Hematopoietic stem cell transplantation for homozygous β-thalassemia and β-thalassemia/hemoglobin E patients from haploidentical donors. *Bone Marrow Transpl.* 2016;51(6):813–818.

140. Huang XJ, Liu DH, Liu KY, et al. Haploidentical hematopoietic stem cell transplantation without in vitro T-cell depletion for the treatment of hematological malignancies. *Bone Marrow Transpl.* 2006;38(4):291–297.

141. Xiao-Jun H, Lan-Ping X, Kai-Yan L, et al. Partially matched related donor transplantation can achieve outcomes comparable with unrelated donor transplantation for patients with hematologic malignancies. *Clin Cancer Res.* 2009;15:4777–4783.

142. Castagna L, Bramanti S, Furst S, et al. Nonmyeloablative conditioning, unmanipulated haploidentical SCT and post-infusion CY for advanced lymphomas. *Bone Marrow Transpl.* 2014;49(12):1475–1480.

143. Garciaz S, Castagna L, Bouabdallah R, et al. Familial haploidentical challenging unrelated donor Allo-SCT in advanced non-Hodgkin lymphomas when matched related donor is not available. *Bone Marrow Transpl.* 2015;50(6):880.

144. Lacerda MP, Arrais Rodrigues C, Pereira AD, et al. Transplantation for relapsed/refractory Hodgkin lymphoma: a multicenter analysis. *Biol Blood Marrow Transpl.* 2017;23(4):705–707.

145. Bashey A, Zhang X, Sizemore CA, et al. T-cell-replete HLA-haploidentical hematopoietic transplantation for hematologic malignancies using post-transplantation cyclophosphamide results in outcomes equivalent to those of contemporaneous HLA-matched related and unrelated donor transplantation. *J Clin Oncol.* 2013;31(10):1310–1316.

146. Di Stasi A, Milton DR, Poon LM, et al. Similar transplantation outcomes for acute myeloid leukemia and myelodysplastic syndrome patients with haploidentical versus 10/10 human leukocyte antigen-matched unrelated and related donors. *Biol Blood Marrow Transpl.* 2014;20(12):1975–1981.

147. Rashidi A, DiPersio JF, Westervelt P, et al. Comparison of outcomes after peripheral blood haploidentical versus matched unrelated donor allogeneic hematopoietic cell transplantation in patients with acute myeloid leukemia: a retrospective single center review. *Biol Blood Marrow Transpl.* 2016;22(9):1696–1701.

148. Bashey A, Zhang X, Jackson K, et al. Comparison of Outcomes of Hematopoietic Cell Transplants from T-Replete Haploidentical Donors Using Post-Transplantation Cyclophosphamide with 10 of 10 HLA-A, -B, -C, -DRB1, and -DQB1 Allele-Matched Unrelated Donors and HLA-Identical Sibling Donors: A Multivariable Analysis Including Disease Risk Index. *Biol Blood Marrow Transplant.* 2016;22:125–133.

149. Raiola AM, Dominietto A, di Grazia C, et al. Unmanipulated haploidentical transplants compared with other alternative donors and matched sibling grafts. *Biol Blood Marrow Transpl.* 2014;20(10):1573–1579.

150. Rashidi A, Slade M, DiPersio JF, Westervelt P, Vij R, Romee R. Post-transplant high-dose cyclophosphamide after HLA-matched vs haploidentical hematopoietic cell transplantation for AML. *Bone Marrow Transplant.* 2016;51(12):1561–1564.

151. Brunstein CG, Fuchs EJ, Carter SL, et al. Alternative donor transplantation after reduced intensity conditioning: results of parallel phase 2 trials using partially HLA mismatched related bone marrow or unrelated double umbilical cord blood grafts. *Blood.* 2011;118(2):282–288.

152. El-Cheikh J, Crocchiolo R, Furst S, et al. Unrelated cord blood compared with haploidentical grafts in patients with hematological malignancies. *Cancer.* 2015;121(11):1809–1816.

153. Ruggeri A, Labopin M, Sanz G, et al. Eurocord, Cord Blood Committee of Cellular Therapy and Immunobiology working party-EBMT; ALWP-EBMT study. Comparison of outcomes after unrelated cord blood and unmanipulated haploidentical stem cell transplantation in adults with acute leukemia. *Leukemia.* 2015;29(9):1891–1900.

154. Ringden O, Labopin M, Ciceri F, et al. Is there a stronger graft-versus-leukemia effect using HLA-haploidentical donors compared with HLA-identical siblings? *Leukemia.* 2016;30(2):447–455.

155. Devillier R, Bramanti S, Furst S, et al. T replete haploidentical allogeneic transplantation using post-transplantation cyclophosphamide in advanced AML and myelodysplastic syndromes. *Bone Marrow Transpl.* 2016;51(2):194–198.

156. Gladstone DE, Zachary AA, Fuchs EJ, et al. Partially mismatched transplantation and human leukocyte antigen donor-specific antibodies. *Biol Blood Marrow Transpl.* 2013;19(4):647–652.

CHAPTER 8

Umbilical Cord Blood Transplantation

KELLY G. ROSS, MD • LAUREN VELTRI, MD • ABRAHAM S. KANATE, MD

INTRODUCTION

Allogeneic transplantation of hematopoietic stem cells (HSCs) and hematopoietic progenitor cells (HPCs) derived from a donor is potentially a curative therapy for various benign and malignant hematological disorders. Traditionally a human leukocyte antigen (HLA)–matched sibling/related donor (MRD) is considered the optimal first choice for allogeneic hematopoietic cell transplantation (allo-HCT). However, only about 30% of eligible patients will have a suitable MRD. When an MRD is unavailable, in the current era, various alternative donor options including HLA-matched unrelated donor (MUD), mismatched related or unrelated (including haploidentical related donors) donors, and umbilical cord blood (UCB) may be considered. The establishment of robust donor registries such as the National Marrow Donor Program (NMDP) with more than 20 million registered volunteer donors have significantly improved the probability of identifying a suitable unrelated donor, especially for Caucasian patients. Unfortunately, likely due to the volunteer disparities, a significant proportion of ethnic/racial minorities will not have a suitable MUD available. In this context other alternative donor sources may be considered attractive options.[1] Umbilical cord blood transplantation (UCBT) has recently evolved as a safe and effective therapeutic strategy, thus broadening the availability of allo-HCT to more patients.

History

In the year 1982 Dr. Hal Broxmeyer first hypothesized the possibility that UCB may be a feasible HSC and HPC source. This led to the founding of Biocyte Corporation that funded the initial studies exploring the biology and cryopreservation of cord blood.[2] The scientific endeavor that ensued resulted in identifying cord blood as a suitable source of HPC for transplantation. These studies noted that cord blood–derived HPCs were sufficient for successful engraftment and could be obtained without causing danger to the newborn or mother and showed the methods for successful and long-term cryopreservation without losing viable progenitor cells.[3] The very first UCBT was performed in France in 1988, the recipient being a 5-year-old boy with severe aplastic anemia due to Fanconi anemia. He received a sibling-derived UBCT after undergoing conditioning with attenuated-dose cyclophosphamide (20 mg/kg) and total-body irradiation (TBI) of 5 Gy, resulting in complete trilineage engraftment and full donor chimerism.[4] Reports of stable engraftment with low incidence of acute and chronic graft-versus-host disease (GVHD) after UCBT from siblings with HLA-matched and with HLA disparity at one antigen (n = 44) confirmed the feasibility and safety of this strategy as an alternative donor source.[5] The first study to show the prospect of successful allogeneic transplantation from unrelated UCB in children (n = 25) reported a 100-day overall survival (OS) of 64%.[6] Since then several reports have confirmed UCB as a safe and effective donor source. The initial application of UCBT was largely restricted to pediatric patient population owing to the concern that the relatively lower cell dose in a single UCB unit may not be sufficient to ensure durable engraftment in adults. Indeed the initial studies evaluating single-unit UCB transplantation in an adult cohort reported high early deaths (35 of 68 patients died by day 100) associated with transplantation but interestingly noticed that higher infused cell dose was associated with a superior event-free survival.[7] This observation led to studies evaluating the simultaneous use of two umbilical cord units (so-called "double" or "dual" UCBT) for an individual patient to optimize the cell dose in the graft. As a result of published data showing its benefit in children and adult patients, the number of UCBT performed yearly has continuously increased since 2003 and remained uninterrupted until 2011.[8] A recent decline in the number of yearly UCBT performed is likely attributed to the resurgence of haploidentical related donor transplantation using posttransplant cyclophosphamide.

Cord Blood Collection, Processing, and Storage

UCB may be collected after the vaginal or surgical delivery of a healthy term baby without interference or complications in the postdelivery obstetric or neonatal care.

Hematopoietic Cell Transplantation for Malignant Conditions. https://doi.org/10.1016/B978-0-323-56802-9.00008-0

Cord blood can be stored in a cryopreserved state for more than 20 years and still allow for efficient recovery of functional hematopoietic progenitor cells on thawing.[9] The ability to collect and cryopreserve these units is vital for UCB banking and transplantation. Since its inception, public and private UCB banks have been established across the world with the majority of UCB units utilized for hematopoietic transplantation coming from public banking.

Public banks are subject to national regulations, and the United States (US) requires that a UCB unit be licensed by the Food and Drug Administration or used under an Investigational New Drug protocol. These regulations significantly increase the operational cost of the product but ensures that minimum standards are met for UCB processing to improve the safety, potency, and therapeutic potential of the graft. Cord blood banking practices do have significant institutional variations and have evolved over the past several years. Dana Farber reviewed specific processing techniques of UCB units provided to 133 patients undergoing double UCBT (dUCBT).[10] UCB units were received from 48 different banks, and significant variation was noted in the processing procedures, with many centers using automated processing and red blood cell depletion. However, after controlling for patient-related variables in the multivariate analysis, no impact on survival was noted. The criteria for storage of UCB units have also been questioned because majority of the stored units will not be used for HCT but continue to drive up the costs of banking. A review of the NMDP inventory in the US showed that the median total nucleated cell (TNC) count of the inventory is 104×10^7 and that the median TNC of units shipped is 176×10^7.[11] Over a 5-year period the likelihood of a unit with at least 175×10^7 TNC being selected for use will be 29% compared with only 8% for the total NMDP inventory. Currently no specific criteria for discontinuation of banking and storage of UCB units exists.

Private UCB banks have been instituted mainly for families to store for future autologous or allogeneic use for an affected family member when such a clinical scenario arise. In this case the respective families are responsible for the cost of collection and annual cost of storage. In general, these units are collected and stored regardless of the size or cell content as the potential use of the product in the future is yet to be defined. Private UCB banks have been subject to controversy and raise the ethical dilemma of having families pay for these units and encouraging them to store an infant's UCB as a form of "biological insurance," without a well-defined role of its clinical utility.

CORD BLOOD UNIT SELECTION

The outcomes of UCBT rely on characteristics of the graft, including cell dose and HLA match. TNC dose is an established determinant of engraftment and impacts transplantation outcomes.[12-15] dUCBT utilizing two partially HLA-matched UCB units helps overcome the cell-dose barrier that otherwise would limit its use, especially in adult patients.[16] Despite its influence on transplantation, a standard TNC dose has not been defined, although a minimum TNC dose of $2.5-3 \times 10^7$/kg is recommended at freezing for a 5–6/6 HLA-matched UCBT, while higher numbers maybe preferred for greater HLA disparity.

CD34+ cell dose and colony-forming units (CFUs) are more likely to reflect the hematopoietic stem cell (HSC) and hematopoietic progenitor cell (HPC) content of a graft. The interlaboratory reliability of these variables make them difficult to use as an established standard.[17] Purtill et al. evaluated the precryopreservation and postthaw characteristics in 129 patients who underwent dUCBT.[18] The dominant unit CD34+ cell dose was the only characteristic identified that was associated with engraftment (HR, 1.43, $P = .002$). Importantly, postthaw CD34+ cell counts correlated more accurately with the precryopreservation CD34+ cell count than the prefreeze TNC count. Although postthaw CD34+ cell viability is associated with unit dominance and engraftment, the postthaw doses are not available until the time of unit infusion.[19] Wagner et al. reported an increased probability of survival in UCBT recipients when the graft contained at least 1.7×10^5 CD34+ cells/kg and had <2 HLA mismatches.[20] Although not established per standard guidelines, the majority of centers do use CD34+ cell dose as a factor in UCB unit selection.[21]

The degree of HLA match also impacts UCBT outcomes (Table 8.1).[13] The current standard for HLA matching for a UCBT includes antigen-level matching for HLA-A and HLA-B and allele-level matching for HLA-DRB-1 with consideration given for selection of a 4–6/6 match. The Cord Blood Transplantation Study retrospectively evaluated the significance of high-resolution (allele level) HLA matching between unrelated UCB units and recipients, although the UCB unit selection for the HCT was originally based on the current standards.[22] Of 179 patient–donor pairs, 32% were found to be disparate when typed for high resolution at all six alleles. Matching at the allele level by high-resolution typing was associated with decreased incidence of acute GVHD but did not influence engraftment. The NMDP has encouraged high-resolution typing of UCB units to facilitate future studies on its impact

TABLE 8.1
Select Studies Showing the Impact of Degree of HLA Matching on Posttransplant Outcomes After Umbilical Cord Blood Transplantation

Study	Typing	N	HLA Match	aGVHD n (%)	cGVHD n (%)	TRM (1-yr)	OS (1-yr)	Comment
Gluckman et al. NEJM. 1997	Antigen level for HLA-A HLA-B and allele level for HLA-DRB-1	70 related 65 (UR)	60 0MM 3 1MM 15≥2MM 9 0MM 43 1MM 13≥2MM	5/60 (9%) 0/3 (0%) 9/15 (60%) 3/9 (42%) 14/43 (38%) 4/13 (31%)	Related: 8/56 (14%) Unrelated: 0/23 (0%)	NA	73% in 0MM 33% in ≥1MM 29% (MM did not impact survival)	HLA MM in a related donor was the most important risk factor for developing aGVHD.
Rubinstein et al. NEJM. 1998	Antigen level for HLA-A and HLA-B and allele level for HLA-DRB-1[a]	562	40 0MM 218 1MM 301 ≥2MM	34/40 (85%) 156/218 (72%) 207/301 (69%)	39/158 (25%) for 180-day survivors	35/40 (88%) 153/218 (70%) 212/301 (70%) [TRE]	NA	Grafts with ≤2 HLA MM are effective. HLA disparity did not influence GVHD.
Wagner et al. Blood. 2002	Antigen level for HLA-A and, HLA-B and allele level for HLA-DRB-1	102	14 0MM 44 1MM 44 ≥2MM	39% (grade 2–4) 11% (grade 3–4)	9% (1-year)	30%	58%	CD34 cell dose impacted TRM and OS. Degree of HLA match only influenced OS but not GVHD or TRM.
Eapen et al. The Lancet. 2007	Antigen level for HLA-A and HLA-B and allele level for HLA-DRB-1	503	35 0MM 201 1MM 267 2MM	8/34 (24%) 78/165 (47%) 107/259 (41%) (grade 2–4)	10/33 (30%) 34/186 (18%) 38/247 (15%)	2/35 (6%) 64/201 (32%) 124/267 (46%)	NA	HLA disparity did not impact GVHD. Higher TRM noted with ≥2 HLA antigen mismatches.
Barker et al. Blood. 2010	Antigen level for HLA-A and HLA-B and allele level for HLA-DRB-1	1061	56 0MM 352 1MM 653 ≥2MM	43/56 (76%) 229/352 (65%) 423/653 (65%) (grade 3–4)	30/56 (54%) 150/352 (43%) 232/653 (36%)	0.4(0.2–0.9) 1.7 (1.1–2.6)[b]	NA	Both degree of HLA match and TNC dose shown to impact TRM.
Eapen et al. Lancet Oncol. 2011	Antigen level for HLA-A, HLA-B, and HLA-C and allele level for HLA-DRB-1	803	69 0MM 147 1MM 587 ≥2MM	Similar grade 2–4 aGVHD in all groups	Similar cGVHD except with >3 MM including HLA-A locus	MM at HLA-DRB1 and HLA-C increased TRM[c]	Similar 3-year OS expect with paired MM at -DRB1 & -C	Additional matching at HLA-C should be considered to minimize mortality risk

Continued

TABLE 8.1

Select Studies Showing the Impact of Degree of HLA Matching on Posttransplant Outcomes After Umbilical Cord Blood Transplantation—cont'd

Study	Typing	N	HLA Match	aGVHD n (%)	cGVHD n (%)	TRM (1-yr)	OS (1-yr)	Comment
Eapen et al. Blood. 2014	Allele level at HLA-A, HLA-B, HLA-C, and HLA-DRB-1	1568	117 0MM 230 1MM 1184 ≥2 MM	Grade 2–4 higher with MM but statistically NS	No difference by degree of HLA matching	9% (3-year)[d] 26% 26%–41%	54% (3-year) 42% 34%–47%	Allele-level HLA matching at HLA-A, HLA -B, HLA-C, and HLA-DRB-1 to be considered for better TRM
Brunstein CG et al. BBMT. 2016	Allele level at HLA-A, HLA-B, HLA-C, HLA-DRB-1, and HLA-DQB-1	342	2–5/10 (n = 108) 6–8/10 (n = 202) 9–10/10 (n = 32)	Grade 2–4 and 3–4 aGVHD not affected by degree of MM in	Degree of MM did not impact cGVHD	HLA mismatch did not impact TRM	NA	In dUCBT, the degree of allele-level HLA mismatch did not seem to adversely affect outcomes

aGVHD, acute graft-versus-host disease; *cGVHD,* chronic graft-versus-host disease; *dUCBT,* double umbilical cord blood transplantation; *HLA,* human leukocyte antigen; *MM,* mismatch; *N,* number; *NA,* not available; *NS,* not significant; *OR,* odds ratio; *OS,* overall survival; *TRE,* treatment-related event; *TRM,* treatment-related mortality; *UR,* unrelated.
[a]Exception in the first 14 cord units selected were not based on high resolution for DRB-1.
[b]Recipients of 0MM units had significantly lower TRM. Patients with 2MM units and a TNC dose in the same range as a 1MM unit had a significantly greater TRM. However, recipients of units with a high TNC dose with either 1 or 2MM did not differ in TRM risk (1 MM vs. 2 MM, RR = 0.8; 95% CI, 0.5–1.2; *P* = .223).
[c]When compared to transplantations matched at HLA-A, HLA-B, HLA-C, and HLA-DRB-1 (n = 69), TRM risk was higher after transplantations matched at HLA-A, HLA-B, and HLA-DRB-1 but mismatched at HLA-C (n = 23; HR 3.97, 95% CI 1.27–12.40; *P* = .018). TRM was also higher in those with a single mismatch and mismatched at HLA-C (n = 234, 1.70, 1.06–2.74; *P* = .029) compared to those matched at HLA-C with a single mismatch (n = 127).
[d]The degree of HLA MM was independently associated with increased risk of TRM. In evaluation of the risk estimates, mismatching at specific loci suggest that isolated allele-level mismatches at HLA-A, HLA-C, orHLA-DRB-1 but not HLA-B are associated with higher TRM risks.

on posttransplantation outcomes. Most centers do consider high-resolution typing of all three aforementioned loci in addition to HLA-C. In a large retrospective analysis from the Center for International Blood and Marrow Transplantation Research (CIBMTR) and Eurocord databases, 803 patients who underwent single-unit UCBT were retrospectively evaluated to assess the importance of additional HLA-C matching.[23] Treatment-related mortality (TRM) was higher in patients with HLA-A, HLA-B, and HLA-DRB-1–matched and HLA-C–mismatched single UCBT than in those matched at all four loci (HR 3.97, 95% CI 1.27–12.40, $P = .018$). TRM was also higher after transplantation with a single mismatch at HLA-A, HLA-B, or HLA-DRB-1 with a concomitant mismatched HLA-C versus those with a 5/6 match (single mismatch at HLA-A, HLA-B, or HLA-DRB-1) with a concomitant match at HLA-C (HR 1.70, 95% CI 1.06–2.74, $P = .029$). The degree of HLA disparity was not significantly associated with overall mortality risk; however, a single mismatch at HLA-DRB-1 and HLA-C (matched at HLA-A and HLA-B) was associated with a higher overall mortality than pairs mismatched at HLA-DRB-1 but matched at HLA-A, HLA-B, and HLA-C (HR 2.95, 95% CI 1.67–5.20, $P = .002$). A large registry study with data from CIBMTR, Netcord, Eurocord, and European Blood and Marrow Transplantation evaluated allele-level matching at HLA-A, HLA-B, HLA-C and HLA-DRB-1 for single-unit UCBT in patients (n = 1568) with acute leukemia and MDS.[24] Patients with an 8/8 allele-level match had the lowest TRM independent of the cell dose and patient age.

Barker et al. evaluated 1061 patients who received single-unit myeloablative UCB transplantation for leukemia or myelodysplasia and evaluated the outcomes based on prefreeze TNC dose and HLA match.[25] Regardless of the TNC dose, the best outcome for neutrophil and platelet engraftment, acute GVHD, TRM, treatment failure, and overall mortality was associated with a 6/6 HLA-matched cord. Recipients with a 5/6 HLA-matched cord with a TNC dose of 2.5×10^7/kg or greater or 4/6 HLA-matched units with a TNC dose of 5.0×10^7/kg or greater had the next best survival outcomes. Although the patients with a 4/6 HLA-matched cord with a TNC dose of 5.0×10^7/kg had earlier engraftment, this did not result in a lower TRM or better survival than in those with a single mismatch and TNC dose of 2.5×10^7/kg. It may be noted that not all studies have shown inferior outcomes with a higher degree of HLA mismatch. Brunstein et al., retrospectively evaluated the impact of allele-level HLA mismatch in 342 patients receiving dUCBT at the University of Minnesota.[26] In this study, 32 patients matched at 9–10/10,

202 at 6–8/10 and 108 at 2–5/10. Outcomes including engraftment, GVHD, TRM, and treatment failure were similar between the groups. A subgroup analysis performed in 174 patients with acute leukemia after adjusting for the length of first remission and cytogenetic risk group showed that the group associated with the lowest risk of relapse and treatment failure was in fact the 2–5/10 HLA-matched group.

Although the cell dose and degree of HLA match clearly impact transplantation outcomes, the exact or minimum cell dose required, acceptable degree of HLA disparity, and how to balance these two factors remains undefined. Patient and disease characteristics do play a role in this balancing act. For example, a higher cell dose ought to be considered for patients with significant risk of graft failure such as those with bone marrow failure syndromes or hemoglobinopathies who have not received as much pretransplant therapy.[27] The race and ethnicity of the patient likely play a role as well, when considering HLA disparity. A CIBMTR registry study evaluated the effects of race/ethnicity on UCBT in adults and children who received a single unrelated UCBT for leukemia or MDS.[28] A total of 885 patients including 612 whites, 145 blacks, and 128 Hispanics were considered in the study. While 40% of white and 42% of Hispanic patients received a 5–6/6 HLA-matched graft with a TNC of $\geq 2.5 \times 10^7$/kg, only 21% black patients received the same. In a multivariate analysis adjusting for disease and treatment factors, black patients had an inferior OS (RR of death = 1.31, $P = .02$) compared to white patients, likely due to the disparity in cell dose and degree of HLA matching. The survival rates were similar when the analysis was restricted to patients with well-matched cord units with an adequate cell dose.

Other factors may potentially impact UCBT outcomes but remain less defined are briefly described in the following. Takanashi et al. retrospectively evaluated 386 patients who received a single UCB unit after myeloablative conditioning (MAC) and evaluated the impact of anti-HLA antibodies on outcomes.[29] Eighty-nine patients tested positive for anti-HLA antibodies with 20 having donor-specific antibodies (DSAs) against the corresponding UCB HLA type. In a multivariate analysis the presence of DSAs was associated with significantly lower neutrophil recovery than those without antibodies (RR = 0.69, 95% CI, 0.49–0.96, $P = .027$). The presence of DSAs had no effect on acute GVHD, relapse, or TRM. The role of DSA in dUCBT is more controversial with studies reporting conflicting results. In one study among 73 patients who underwent dUCBT, 18 patients were noted to have detectable

DSAs which resulted in an increased incidence of graft failure, prolonged time to engraftment, and increased day 100 TRM which ultimately led to inferior long-term PFS and OS compared to those without DSA.[30] Contrary to the aforementioned fact, researchers from the University of Minnesota published outcomes in 126 dUCBT recipients including 18 patients with identified DSAs.[31] Engraftment did not seem affected by the presence of DSAs targeting one or both UCB units. Ruggeri et al. evaluated 294 UCB transplant recipients undergoing reduced-intensity conditioning (RIC) in which 23% (n = 62) had anti-HLA antibodies before transplantation with 14 having DSAs.[32] The cumulative incidence of day 60 neutrophil engraftment was 81% in those without DSAs and 44% for those with DSAs ($P = .006$), whereas the CI of 1-year TRM was 32% versus 46%, respectively ($P = .06$). The presence of DSAs was associated with a trend toward decreased survival (42% vs. 29%, $P = .07$). As the presence of DSAs in recipients of unrelated UCB transplant may be associated with graft failure and higher mortality, screening patients before transplantation is recommended.

The HLA of the UCB unit's mother is now being captured by many cord blood banks to provide information on noninherited maternal antigens (NIMAs). Retrospective analysis has demonstrated that matching with the donor's NIMA was associated with improved engraftment, lower TRM, and improved survival.[33,34] Blood group (ABO) matching has not been widely established as a significant factor that impacts transplantation outcomes, although some retrospective studies have found an association between ABO mismatch and survival outcomes.[35,36] The influence of donor killer-cell immunoglobulin-like receptor (KIR) ligand matching is also considered more controversial with some studies suggesting improved outcomes with KIR–ligand incompatibility,[37] whereas others suggest inferior outcomes[38] or no significant difference.[39,40]

Conditioning Regimens

Two main goals are considered in the selection of conditioning regimens for allo-HCT including UCBT treating any residual disease at the time of HCT and suppressing the recipient immune system to allow engraftment of HPC/HSCs. MAC regimens are usually associated with an increased regimen-/treatment-related morbidity and mortality compared with RIC and nonmyeloablative (NMA) regimens. This difference is offset by higher risk of relapse of the primary malignancy seen with RIC/NMA conditioning.

MAC regimens

MAC regimens, discussed in Chapters 3 and 4, are either high-dose TBI based or chemotherapy based. TBI-based regimens were among the first studied, using radiation doses of 12–13.4 Gy. One of the first and commonly reported TBI-based regimens is fludarabine (Flu) 75 mg/m², cyclophosphamide (Cy) 120 mg/kg, and TBI 13.2 Gy. Barker et al., in the Minnesota group's first evaluation of dUCBT in adults, found sustained neutrophil engraftment at a median of 23 days, a TRM of 22% at 6 months, and a 1-year disease-free survival (DFS) of 57%.[41] Most MAC regimens for UCBT use TBI, so there are limited data on chemotherapy-only regimens. As in other donor/graft source allo-HCT, most chemotherapy-based regimens use an alkylator backbone such as busulfan (Bu), melphalan (Mel), or cyclophosphamide (Cy). Busulfan is myeloablative but not particularly immunosuppressive. This has resulted in many chemotherapy-based conditioning regimens being studied with concurrent ATG for in vivo cell depletion, the use of which in UCBT is controversial, as discussed elsewhere in this chapter.

Reduced-intensity conditioning and non-myeloablative regimens

With the advent of less-intensive conditioning regimens, curative allogeneic HCT has become available to a wider population of patients with life-threatening hematological disorders and malignancies, including older and medically infirm patients. The tradeoff in this scenario is the increased rates of relapse noted with RIC/NMA conditioning.[42] As the potency or intensity of the conditioning regimen decreases, the transplant relies more heavily on the graft-versus-tumor effect for its curative potential. As such, the immunosuppressive characteristics of the conditioning regimen remain of utmost importance. The use of busulfan is associated with low rates of engraftment in UCBT and thus is generally not used in RIC/NMA regimens.[41,43] Popular regimens for UCBT generally include fludarabine (Flu), cyclophosphamide (Cy), and a low-dose TBI, either 2 or 4 Gy. Barker et al. evaluated Flu 200 mg/m², Cy 50 mg/m², and TBI 2 Gy in 22 patients and found 94% engraftment at a median of 10 days, 28% TRM at day +100, and 41% DFS at 1 year.[41] Brunstein et al. evaluated the same regimen in 110 patients and found 92% neutrophil engraftment at a median of 12 days, 26% TRM at 3 years, and OS of 45%.[44] The cumulative incidence of sustained engraftment, defined as neutrophil recovery with stable donor chimerism, was 85%. In this study, graft failure was noted in a total of 15 patients with no predictors found in regression analysis. The cumulative incidence of disease relapse was 31%. The 3-year event-free survival of 38% was positively impacted by the absence of preexisting high-risk clinical features, defined as poor organ function, Aspergillus in prior 4 months, Karnofsky ≤60, extensive prior therapy, ($P<0.01$) with a trend toward better EFS in recipients of 2 UCB units ($P=.07$).[44]

Evaluation of a higher TBI dose of 3 Gy in eight such patients had favorable results, with median time to engraftment of 17 days and 53% 1-year OS.[45] Somers et al. used the same chemotherapy backbone but with 4 Gy of TBI (n = 52) and noted rapid neutrophil engraftment in 92% of patients at a median of 36 days. The 2-year progression-free survival (PFS) and OS were 42% and 57%, respectively.[46] Building on the reduced-intensity Flu/Cy/TBI regimens, Ponce et al. evaluated a novel combination (n = 30) consisting of fludarabine 150 mg/m², cyclophosphamide 50 mg/kg, thiotepa 10 mg/kg, and TBI 4 Gy as an alternative to MAC regimens. Sustained engraftment was noted in 97% of patients at a median of 26 days. Other posttransplant outcomes included grade II–IV acute GVHD of 67% at day 180, chronic GVHD of 10% at 1-year, TRM of 20% at day 180, and relapse of 11% at 2-year. The 2-year OS was 60%.[47] While the combination of fludarbine/cyclophosphamide/TBI is probably the most commonly used RIC conditioning, single-institution studies using other alkylators have been reported.[48]

Antithymocyte globulin

Implementation of an appropriate GVHD prophylaxis strategy is of paramount importance in any allo-HCT and can have important ramifications in post-HCT outcomes including engraftment, immune reconstitution, and possibly mortality. As pioneered by the Minnesota group, the most widely used prophylactic combination include a calcineurin inhibitor such as cyclosporine in combination with mycophenolate mofetil.[49] Antithymocyte globulin (ATG), a polyclonal antibody used for in vivo T-cell depletion, was used in many initial studies (discussed under GVHD) to improve engraftment and prevent GVHD.[50] However, this has come under scrutiny of late. However, the delays in immune reconstitution, increase in viral infections,[51,52] and increase in posttransplant lymphoproliferative disorder[53,54] have caused the use of ATG in UCBT to be questioned. Pascal et al. reported two studies evaluating the impact of ATG in UCBT recipients after undergoing ablative conditioning (n = 91) and RIC conditioning with Flu/Cy/2 Gy TBI (n = 661).[55,56] In multivariate analysis, the use of ATG improved GVHD but was associated with higher TRM and decreased OS compared with those

who did not receive ATG. These results suggest caution in the routine use of ATG, especially close to graft infusion in UCBT recipients.

Posttransplantation Outcomes of UCBT
Engraftment
The use of UCB as a graft source has advantages and disadvantages. One of the initial problems with UCBT was the time to and rate of engraftment. Although UCB has a higher concentration of stem cells than peripheral blood from an adult donor source, there are 1–2 log fewer total cells in each unit. As discussed previously, the first studies in UCBT were performed with single-cord blood units in children. Wagner et al. demonstrated 100% engraftment in single-unit UCBT performed in children, with an average weight of the recipient of 15.4 kg and a minimum TNC dose of 1×10^7/kg body weight.[57] In another study that evaluated a larger population of 102 children, the rate of engraftment was 88% by day 42. Moreover, this study demonstrated a significant correlation between cell dose and engraftment.[58] Initial cord blood transplants in adults were also performed with single-cord blood units, but the larger size of the adults proved challenging, and engraftment rates were lower than those seen in children. Rubenstein et al. evaluated 562 patients including children and adults, who underwent single-unit UCBT and found that 81% of patients engrafted their neutrophils by day 42, with the median time to neutrophil engraftment being 28 days. Successful engraftment was associated with younger age, higher cell dose, and lesser degree of HLA disparity.[59] In one study evaluating adult patients (n = 68) undergoing single-unit UCBT, the median time to neutrophil recovery was 27 days, and of the 60 patients who survived beyond 28 days, five experienced primary graft failure.[60]

In an effort to overcome the disadvantage of low cell dose in cord blood units as compared to adult donor source, in 2001 Barker et al. performed the first dUCBT in a 53-year-old woman with CML, and hematopoietic engraftment occurred at day 25. The patient died at day 68 of disseminated aspergillosis, but this paved the way for the use of two units of cord blood in adults as a means to improve cell dose and thus engraftment rates.[61] Studies using two units to enhance engraftment soon followed, showing sustained neutrophil engraftment at a median of 23 days and high rates of engraftment by day 42 at 88%–100%.[16,41,49,62]

Interestingly, although two units are infused in dUCBT, in most patients, one unit will ultimately "win" and take over hematopoiesis, so-called "single-unit predominance." Barker et al. found hematopoiesis to be accounted for by a single unit in 76% of patients by day 21, 90% of patients by day 60, and >95% of patients by day 100.[63] True "mixed chimeras," or sustained presence of both cord blood units contributing to hematopoiesis, is rare and occurs in <5% of patients. No clear factors have emerged to allow for prediction of which unit will predominate, including cell dose size, order of infusion, CD3 cell dose, ABO type, HLA mismatch, and sex of the cords.[46,64,65] The mechanism of single-unit predominance is likely immune mediated. In addition to mediating graft-versus-tumor effect, the T-cells from the two units also battle for dominance in a graft-versus-graft effect. This can lead to "preengraftment syndrome," a poorly characterized syndrome consisting of fever and rash in the absence of infection starting around 7 days after transplantation. This may be associated with higher acute GVHD and improved engraftment but does not seem to impact chronic GVHD or OS.[66] Other attempts to improve engraftment including injection of cord blood grafts directly into bone marrow,[67,68] third-party haploidentical donor coinfusion to boost cell dose,[69,70] ex vivo graft expansion,[71] and mesenchymal cell coinfusion[72] have all been used, with varying degrees of success. Currently these techniques remain experimental.

Graft-versus-host disease

GVHD is one of the most feared complications of allo-HCT as it may be associated with significant recipient morbidity and mortality. As such, one of the focuses of graft selection for allogeneic HCT is circumventing the risk of both acute and chronic GVHD. The evaluation, pathophysiology, and management of GVHD are discussed elsewhere in this textbook (see Chapter 22). Here we will focus on the incidence of GVHD with UCBT compared with other donor/graft sources.

Acute GVHD. The majority of UCBTs done in adults use two cord blood units. Single-unit UCBT has the lowest risk of acute GVHD of all donor sources, whereas dUCBT has the highest risk, regardless of the degree of HLA match. Lazaryan et al. compared 469 MRD allogeneic transplants, 295 single UBCTs, and 416 dUCBTs and found rates of grade II–IV acute GVHD of 37%, 26%, and 56%, respectively, and rates of grade III-IV acute GVHD of 16%, 7%, and 21%, respectively. Acute GVHD did not impact relapse risk, TRM, or survival among UCBT recipients but did result in higher TRM among MRD allo-HCT recipients.[73] Patients undergoing dUCBT tend to experience acute GVHD earlier in the course of their transplant than those undergoing single UCBT. The lower incidence of acute GVHD in

single UCBT is likely related to the lower overall cell dose, and in addition, the higher incidence of acute GVHD in dUCBT is thought to be related to immune activation of the graft-versus-graft effect of the two cord blood units, with the tissues affected by acute GVHD as collateral damage in the immune activation.

Chronic GVHD. One of the greatest advantages of the use of UCBT is the low rates of chronic GVHD, which in its most severe forms can be a devastating, life-long illness. Lazaryan et al. also evaluated the same cohort of patients for rates of chronic GVHD and found that the incidence of chronic GVHD was 40% for MRD allo-HCT compared with 7% for single UCBT and 26% for dUCBT.[73] Gutman et al. compared 51 dUCBT recipients with 57 MUD transplant recipients and found that at 3 years after transplantation the incidence of moderate-to-severe chronic GVHD was 44% after MUD HCT and 8% after dual UCBT.[74] No difference in OS was noted between the groups. The reasons for the lower incidence of chronic GVHD in the UCBT population are thought to be related to the immature alloreactive immune cells of the umbilical cord blood. The T-cells in the graft, which mediate acute GVHD, can also play a role in the pathophysiology of chronic GVHD, and in UCBT these cells are less likely to have prior antigen exposure and activation and allow for coexistence of graft and host, even in the face of HLA mismatch.

Immune reconstitution

Patients undergoing allo-HCT are at increased risk for infection in the peritransplant period, due to conditioning regimens and neutropenia. However, the complexity of the immune system is not reflected solely in the white blood cell or neutrophil count, and patients undergoing UCBT have delayed immune reconstitution compared with those having other graft sources. The relatively naïve immune system of the UCB, which incidentally contribute to the lower rates of chronic GVHD, also result in a lack of robust innate immunity. This puts UCBT recipients at a higher risk for both opportunistic and viral infections.

The use of ATG in conditioning regimens for cord blood transplantation, discussed previously, is controversial and likely contributes to delayed immune reconstitution through in vivo T-cell depletion. Thomson et al. evaluated 30 children undergoing myeloablative UCBT and found that CD4, CD8, CD19, and NK cell recovery was achieved at 12, 9, 6, and 2 months, respectively.[75] This is significantly longer compared to allografts from other adult donor sources.[75-79] The risk of increased TRM as a result of slow immune reconstitution in UCBT and subsequent infection is an area of valid concern. Recipients of UCBT are at higher risk for viral infections with cytomegalovirus (CMV), Epstein–Barr virus, varicella zoster virus, adenovirus, human herpes virus-6 (HHV-6), and polyoma virus (BK virus). In patients undergoing UCBT (n = 52), prior reports have noted a peak incidence of bacterial and fungal infections occurred during the time of neutropenia in the first 30 days of transplantation as expected, but the peak incidence of viral infections was in days 31–60 after transplantation, affecting 30% of patients.[52] The most common viral infection was CMV. Additionally, within the first 120 days of transplantation, viral infections were unrelated to GVHD incidence, but after that period, viral infections occurred exclusively in the context of GVHD and immunosuppressive therapy. This leads to an interesting point concerning the close association between chronic GVHD and late risk of infections. In a small study comparing MUD (n = 57) versus UCBT (n = 51), Gutman et al. found less incidence of late infections and hospitalizations in the UCBT cohort, likely due to significant difference in the incidence of moderate-to-severe chronic GVHD in UCBT group (8%) compared with MUD group (44%, P = .0006). The higher incidence of chronic GVHD in the MUD group resulted in prolonged immunosuppressive therapy compared with UCBT, likely contributing to the increased late infection risk, although no differences in survival was noted.[74]

FUTURE OF CORD BLOOD TRANSPLANTATION

The inherent limitations of UCBT include delayed engraftment, increased risk of graft failure, and delayed immune reconstitution. As noted previously, these adverse effects are felt to reflect the lower cell dose within the UCB unit, especially when considering adult recipients. Several strategies have been explored to overcome these limitations by enhancing UCB expansion and improving the homing capacity of the UCB-derived progenitor cells.[2] Initial studies with ex vivo expansion in culture with cytokines[80,81] did not demonstrate significant improvement in engraftment felt to be at least partially reflective of cytokine-induced differentiation.[82] This has led to the exploration of different agents to block the differentiation of early progenitor cells (EPCs). Strategies that have been explored include the use of copper chelation,[83] constitutive notch signaling,[84,85] nicotinamide,[86,87] stem-regenin-1,[88] and culture with mesenchymal stem cells.[89] The use of notch ligand Delta-1–mediated expansion of short-term

repopulating cells resulted in early neutrophil engraftment at 16 days.[85] The use of ex vivo coculture with mesenchymal progenitor cells in UCBT (n = 31) reported by the MD Anderson group noted a 30-fold expansion in CD34+ count and a median time to engraftment of 15 days.[89]

While trials are ongoing to improve the cell dose with expansion of the graft, specific techniques to improve homing of the UCB progenitor cells to the bone marrow have shown additional benefit in enhancing engraftment. To ensure the successful migration and adhesion of HPCs to the bone marrow, interactions of E- and P-selectins on endothelial cells with relevant ligands on HPCs are of importance. These ligands must be α1,3-fucosylated to form terminal glycan determinants, and one study evaluated enforced fucosylation of UCB-derived HPCs (n = 22) which resulted in early engraftment compared to historical controls.[90] The use of prostaglandin E2 exposure has also noted some engraftment benefit in a phase I study.[91] Dipeptidyl peptidase-4 (DDP-4) inhibition is another area of focus as DDP4 cleaves several proteins including stromal-derived factor-1α which combines with CXCR4 (chemokine receptor) and plays a key role in chemotaxis with initial trials being promising for improved engraftment.[92,93] However, it may be emphasized that these methods remain investigational presently and are limited to specialized centers with the ability to manipulate the UCB product. However, these techniques are yet to be validated and standardized for route implementation among the transplant community but may hold promise in the future for UCBT.

In the absence of an MRD, the optimal alternative donor remains an important question. Based on observational reports showing similar survival outcomes, several centers now opt for UCBT or haploidentical related donor allografts when an MRD is unavailable, bypassing the often time-consuming unrelated donor search. Others still consider matched (and sometimes mismatched) unrelated donor as the next best option in this scenario. No uniform consensus exits in this regard, likely due to paucity of phase III comparisons, and practices for donor selection is very much center/physician dependent. Although no randomized controlled trials are currently comparing UCBT with MRD/MUD allografts, the ongoing phase III BMT CTN 1101 (NCT01597778) study comparing UCB versus haploidentical related donor transplantation will hopefully provide some insight into the ideal alternative donor. Nevertheless, the use of UCB for allogeneic transplantation has evolved since the late 1980s when the first UCBT was performed. To date, more than 35,000 such transplantations have been conducted establishing UBCT as a feasible, effective, and safe therapeutic option for patients with life-threatening hematological disorders who may have been previously denied an allo-HCT for want of a suitable sibling or unrelated donor.

REFERENCES

1. Appelbaum FR. Pursuing the goal of a donor for everyone in need. *N Engl J Med.* 2012;367:1555–1556.
2. Ballen KK, Gluckman E, Broxmeyer HE. Umbilical cord blood transplantation: the first 25 years and beyond. *Blood.* 2013;122:491–498.
3. Broxmeyer HE, et al. Human umbilical cord blood as a potential source of transplantable hematopoietic stem/progenitor cells. *Proc Natl Acad Sci USA.* 1989;86: 3828–3832.
4. Gluckman E, et al. Hematopoietic reconstitution in a patient with Fanconi's anemia by means of umbilical-cord blood from an HLA-identical sibling. *N Engl J Med.* 1989;321:1174–1178.
5. Wagner J, Steinbuch M, Kernan N, Broxmayer H, Gluckman E. Allogeneic sibling umbilical-cord-blood transplantation in children with malignant and non-malignant disease. *Lancet.* 1995;346:214–219.
6. Kurtzberg J, et al. Placental blood as a source of hematopoietic stem cells for transplantation into unrelated recipients. *N Engl J Med.* 1996;335:157–166.
7. Laughlin MJ, et al. Hematopoietic engraftment and survival in adult recipients of umbilical-cord blood from unrelated donors. *N Engl J Med.* 2001;344:1815–1822.
8. D'Souza A, Zhu X. *Current Uses and Outcomes of Hematopoietic Cell Transplantation (HCT): CIBMTR Summary Slides;* 2016. Available at: http://www.cibmtr.org.
9. Broxmeyer HE, et al. Hematopoietic stem/progenitor cells, generation of induced pluripotent stem cells, and isolation of endothelial progenitors from 21- to 23.5-year cryopreserved cord blood. *Blood.* 2011;117:4773–4777.
10. Nikiforow S, et al. Lack of impact of umbilical cord blood unit processing techniques on clinical outcomes in adult double cord blood transplant recipients. *Cytotherapy.* 2017;19:272–284.
11. Bart T, et al. Impact of selection of cord blood units from the United States and swiss registries on the cost of banking operations. *Transfus Med Hemother Off Organ Dtsch Ges Transfusionsmedizin Immunhamatol.* 2013;40:14–20.
12. Rocha V, et al. Transplants of umbilical-cord blood or bone marrow from unrelated donors in adults with acute leukemia. *N Engl J Med.* 2004;351:2276–2285.
13. Rubinstein P, et al. Outcomes among 562 recipients of placental-blood transplants from unrelated donors. *N Engl J Med.* 1998;339:1565–1577.
14. Gluckman E, et al. Factors associated with outcomes of unrelated cord blood transplant: guidelines for donor choice. *Exp Hematol.* 2004;32:397–407.
15. Laughlin MJ, et al. Hematopoietic engraftment and survival in adult recipients of umbilical-cord blood from unrelated donors. *N Engl J Med.* 2001;344:1815–1822.
16. Barker JN, et al. Transplantation of 2 partially HLA-matched umbilical cord blood units to enhance engraftment in adults with hematologic malignancy. *Blood.* 2005;105:1343–1347.
17. Spellman S, et al. Guidelines for the development and validation of new potency assays for the evaluation of umbilical cord blood. *Cytotherapy.* 2011;13:848–855.
18. Purtill D, et al. Dominant unit CD34+ cell dose predicts engraftment after double-unit cord blood transplantation and is influenced by bank practice. *Blood.* 2014;124: 2905–2912.
19. Scaradavou A, et al. Cord blood units with low CD34+ cell viability have a low probability of engraftment after double unit transplantation. *Biol Blood Marrow Transpl J Am Soc Blood Marrow Transpl.* 2010;16:500–508.
20. Wagner JE, et al. Transplantation of unrelated donor umbilical cord blood in 102 patients with malignant and nonmalignant diseases: influence of CD34 cell dose and HLA disparity on treatment-related mortality and survival. *Blood.* 2002;100:1611–1618.
21. Barker JN, et al. Optimal practices in unrelated donor cord blood transplantation for hematologic malignancies. *Biol Blood Marrow Transpl.* 2017;23:882–896.
22. Kurtzberg J, et al. Results of the Cord Blood Transplantation Study (COBLT): clinical outcomes of unrelated donor umbilical cord blood transplantation in pediatric patients with hematologic malignancies. *Blood.* 2008;112: 4318–4327.
23. Eapen M, et al. Effect of donor-recipient HLA matching at HLA A, B, C, and DRB1 on outcomes after umbilical-cord blood transplantation for leukaemia and myelodysplastic syndrome: a retrospective analysis. *Lancet Oncol.* 2011;12:1214–1221.
24. Eapen M, et al. Impact of allele-level HLA matching on outcomes after myeloablative single unit umbilical cord blood transplantation for hematologic malignancy. *Blood.* 2014;123:133–140.
25. Barker JN, Scaradavou A, Stevens CE. Combined effect of total nucleated cell dose and HLA match on transplantation outcome in 1061 cord blood recipients with hematologic malignancies. *Blood.* 2010;115:1843–1849.
26. Brunstein CG, et al. Impact of allele level HLA mismatch on outcomes in recipients of double umbilical cord blood transplantation. *Biol Blood Marrow Transpl J Am Soc Blood Marrow Transpl.* 2016;22:487–492.
27. Broxmeyer HE, Farag SS, Rocha V. Cord blood hematopoietic cell transplantation. In: *Thomas' Hematopoietic Cell Transplantation.* Vol. 1. Wiley & Sons Ltd.; 2016: 437–451.
28. Ballen KK, et al. Relationship of race/ethnicity and survival after single umbilical cord blood transplantation for adults and children with leukemia and myelodysplastic syndromes. *Biol Blood Marrow Transpl J Am Soc Blood Marrow Transpl.* 2012;18.

29. Takanashi M, et al. The impact of anti-HLA antibodies on unrelated cord blood transplantations. *Blood.* 2010;116:2839–2846.
30. Cutler C, et al. Donor-specific anti-HLA antibodies predict outcome in double umbilical cord blood transplantation. *Blood.* 2011;118:6691–6697.
31. Brunstein CG, et al. Anti-HLA antibodies in double umbilical cord blood transplantation. *Biol Blood Marrow Transpl J Am Soc Blood Marrow Transpl.* 2011;17:1704–1708.
32. Ruggeri A, et al. Impact of donor-specific anti-HLA antibodies on graft failure and survival after reduced intensity conditioning-unrelated cord blood transplantation: a Eurocord, Societe Francophone d'Histocompatibilite et d'Immunogenetique (SFHI) and Societe Francaise de Greffe de Moelle et de Therapie Cellulaire (SFGM-TC) analysis. *Haematologica.* 2013;98:1154–1160.
33. van Rood JJ, et al. Reexposure of cord blood to noninherited maternal HLA antigens improves transplant outcome in hematological malignancies. *Proc Natl Acad Sci.* 2009;106:19952–19957.
34. Rocha V, et al. Effect of HLA-matching recipients to donor noninherited maternal antigens on outcomes after mismatched umbilical cord blood transplantation for hematologic malignancy. *Biol Blood Marrow Transpl J Am Soc Blood Marrow Transpl.* 2012;18:1890–1896.
35. Arcese W, et al. Unrelated cord blood transplants in adults with hematologic malignancies. *Haematologica.* 2006;91:223–230.
36. Kurtzberg J, et al. Results of the Cord Blood Transplantation Study (COBLT): clinical outcomes of unrelated donor umbilical cord blood transplantation in pediatric patients with hematologic malignancies. *Blood.* 2008;112:4318–4327.
37. Willemze R, et al. KIR-ligand incompatibility in the graft-versus-host direction improves outcomes after umbilical cord blood transplantation for acute leukemia. *Leukemia.* 2009;23:492–500.
38. Brunstein CG, et al. Negative effect of KIR alloreactivity in recipients of umbilical cord blood transplant depends on transplantation conditioning intensity. *Blood.* 2009;113:5628–5634.
39. Tanaka J, et al. Effects of KIR ligand incompatibility on clinical outcomes of umbilical cord blood transplantation without ATG for acute leukemia in complete remission. *Blood Cancer J.* 2013;3:e164.
40. Rocha V, et al. Killer cell immunoglobulin-like receptor–ligand matching and outcomes after unrelated cord blood transplantation in acute myeloid leukemia. *Biol Blood Marrow Transpl.* 2016;22:1284–1289.
41. Barker JN, et al. Rapid and complete donor chimerism in adult recipients of unrelated donor umbilical cord blood transplantation after reduced-intensity conditioning. *Blood.* 2003;102:1915–1919.
42. Oran B, Wagner JE, DeFor TE, Weisdorf DJ, Brunstein CG. Effect of conditioning regimen intensity on acute myeloid leukemia outcomes after umbilical cord blood transplantation. *Biol Blood Marrow Transpl J Am Soc Blood Marrow Transpl.* 2011;17:1327–1334.
43. Komatsu T, et al. Successful engraftment of mismatched unrelated cord blood transplantation following reduced intensity preparative regimen using fludarabine and busulfan. *Ann Hematol.* 2007;86:49–54.
44. Brunstein CG, et al. Umbilical cord blood transplantation after nonmyeloablative conditioning: impact on transplantation outcomes in 110 adults with hematologic disease. *Blood.* 2007;110:3064–3070.
45. Ostronoff F, et al. Double umbilical cord blood transplantation in patients with hematologic malignancies using a reduced-intensity preparative regimen without antithymocyte globulin. *Bone Marrow Transpl.* 2013;48:782–786.
46. Somers JAE, et al. Rapid induction of single donor chimerism after double umbilical cord blood transplantation preceded by reduced intensity conditioning: results of the HOVON 106 phase II study. *Haematologica.* 2014;99:1753–1761.
47. Ponce DM, et al. A novel reduced-intensity conditioning regimen induces a high incidence of sustained donor-derived neutrophil and platelet engraftment after double-unit cord blood transplantation. *Biol Blood Marrow Transpl J Am Soc Blood Marrow Transpl.* 2013;19:799–803.
48. Oran B, Shpall E. Umbilical cord blood transplantation: a maturing technology. *ASH Educ Program Book.* 2012;2012:215–222.
49. Ballen KK, et al. Double unrelated reduced-intensity umbilical cord blood transplantation in adults. *Biol Blood Marrow Transpl J Am Soc Blood Marrow Transpl.* 2007;13:82–89.
50. MacMillan ML, et al. Acute graft-versus-host disease after unrelated donor umbilical cord blood transplantation: analysis of risk factors. *Blood.* 2009;113:2410.
51. Lindemans CA, et al. Impact of thymoglobulin prior to pediatric unrelated umbilical cord blood transplantation on immune reconstitution and clinical outcome. *Blood.* 2014;123:126–132.
52. Sauter C, et al. Serious infection risk and immune recovery after double-unit cord blood transplantation without antithymocyte globulin. *Biol Blood Marrow Transpl J Am Soc Blood Marrow Transpl.* 2011;17:1460–1471.
53. Ballen KK, et al. Donor-derived second hematologic malignancies after cord blood transplantation. *Biol Blood Marrow Transpl J Am Soc Blood Marrow Transpl.* 2010;16:1025–1031.
54. Brunstein CG, et al. Marked increased risk of Epstein-Barr virus-related complications with the addition of antithymocyte globulin to a nonmyeloablative conditioning prior to unrelated umbilical cord blood transplantation. *Blood.* 2006;108:2874–2880.
55. Pascal L, et al. Impact of rabbit ATG-containing myeloablative conditioning regimens on the outcome of patients undergoing unrelated single-unit cord blood transplantation for hematological malignancies. *Bone Marrow Transpl.* 2015;50:45–50.
56. Pascal L, et al. Impact of ATG-containing reduced-intensity conditioning after single- or double-unit allogeneic cord blood transplantation. *Blood.* 2015;126:1027.

57. Wagner J, et al. Successful transplantation of HLA-matched and HLA-mismatched umbilical cord blood from unrelated donors: analysis of engraftment and acute graft-versus-host disease. *Blood*. 1996;88:795.

58. Wagner JE, et al. Transplantation of unrelated donor umbilical cord blood in 102 patients with malignant and nonmalignant diseases: influence of CD34 cell dose and HLA disparity on treatment-related mortality and survival. *Blood*. 2002;100:1611–1618.

59. Gluckman E, et al. Outcome of cord-blood transplantation from related and unrelated donors. Eurocord Transplant Group and the European Blood and Marrow Transplantation Group. *N Engl J Med*. 1997 Aug 7;337(6):373–381.

60. Laughlin MJ, et al. Hematopoietic engraftment and survival in adult recipients of umbilical-cord blood from unrelated donors. *N Engl J Med*. 2001;344:1815–1822.

61. Barker JN, Weisdorf DJ, Wagner JE. Creation of a double chimera after the transplantation of umbilical-cord blood from two partially matched unrelated donors. *N Engl J Med*. 2001;344:1870–1871.

62. Cutler C, et al. Double umbilical cord blood transplantation with reduced intensity conditioning and sirolimus-based GVHD prophylaxis. *Bone Marrow Transpl*. 2011;46:659–667.

63. Barker JN, et al. Transplantation of 2 partially HLA-matched umbilical cord blood units to enhance engraftment in adults with hematologic malignancy. *Blood*. 2005;105:1343–1347.

64. Ramirez P, et al. Factors predicting single-unit predominance after double umbilical cord blood transplantation. *Bone Marrow Transpl*. 2012;47:799–803.

65. Majhail NS, Brunstein CG, Wagner JE. Double umbilical cord blood transplantation. *Curr Opin Immunol*. 2006;18:571–575.

66. Park M, et al. Pre-engraftment syndrome after unrelated cord blood transplantation: a predictor of engraftment and acute graft-versus-host disease. *Biol Blood Marrow Transpl J Am Soc Blood Marrow Transpl*. 2013;19:640–646.

67. Frassoni F, et al. Direct intrabone transplant of unrelated cord-blood cells in acute leukaemia: a phase I/II study. *Lancet Oncol*. 2008;9:831–839.

68. Murata M, et al. Phase II study of intrabone single unit cord blood transplantation for hematological malignancies. *Cancer Sci*. 2017;108:1634–1639.

69. Kwon M, et al. Early peripheral blood and T-cell chimerism dynamics after umbilical cord blood transplantation supported with haploidentical cells. *Bone Marrow Transpl*. 2014;49:212–218.

70. Kwon M, et al. Haplo-cord transplantation using CD34+ cells from a third-party donor to speed engraftment in high-risk patients with hematologic disorders. *Biol Blood Marrow Transpl*. 2014;20:2015–2022.

71. Wagner JE, et al. Phase I/II trial of StemRegenin-1 expanded umbilical cord blood hematopoietic stem cells supports testing as a stand alone graft. *Cell Stem Cell*. 2016;18:144–155.

72. de Lima M, et al. Cord-blood engraftment with ex vivo mesenchymal-cell coculture. *N Engl J Med*. 2012;367:2305–2315.

73. Lazaryan A, et al. Risk factors for acute and chronic graft-versus-host disease after allogeneic hematopoietic cell transplantation with umbilical cord blood and matched related donors. *Biol Blood Marrow Transpl J Am Soc Blood Marrow Transpl*. 2016;22:134–140.

74. Gutman JA, et al. Chronic graft versus host disease burden and late transplant complications are lower following adult double cord blood versus matched unrelated donor peripheral blood transplantation. *Bone Marrow Transpl*. 2016;51:1588–1593.

75. Thomson BG, et al. Analysis of engraftment, graft-versus-host disease, and immune recovery following unrelated donor cord blood transplantation. *Blood*. 2000;96:2703–2711.

76. Mohty M. Mechanisms of action of antithymocyte globulin: T-cell depletion and beyond. *Leukemia*. 2007;21:1387–1394.

77. Ruggeri A, et al. Outcomes, infections, and immune reconstitution after double cord blood transplantation in patients with high-risk hematological diseases. *Transpl Infect Dis Off J Transpl Soc*. 2011;13:456–465.

78. Danby R, Rocha V. Improving engraftment and immune reconstitution in umbilical cord blood transplantation. *Front Immunol*. 2014;5:68.

79. Talvensaari K, et al. A broad T-cell repertoire diversity and an efficient thymic function indicate a favorable long-term immune reconstitution after cord blood stem cell transplantation. *Blood*. 2002;99:1458–1464.

80. Shpall EJ, et al. Transplantation of ex vivo expanded cord blood. *Biol Blood Marrow Transpl J Am Soc Blood Marrow Transpl*. 2002;8:368–376.

81. Hofmeister CC, Zhang J, Knight KL, Le P, Stiff PJ. Ex vivo expansion of umbilical cord blood stem cells for transplantation: growing knowledge from the hematopoietic niche. *Bone Marrow Transpl*. 2007;39:11–23.

82. Hofmeister CC, Zhang J, Knight KL, Le P, Stiff PJ. Ex vivo expansion of umbilical cord blood stem cells for transplantation: growing knowledge from the hematopoietic niche. *Bone Marrow Transpl*. 2007;39:11–23.

83. Montesinos P, et al. StemEx® (copper chelation based) ex vivo expanded umbilical cord blood stem cell transplantation (UCBT) accelerates engraftment and improves 100 Day survival in myeloablated patients compared to a registry cohort undergoing double unit UCBT: results of a multicenter study of 101 patients with hematologic malignancies. *Blood*. 2013;122:295.

84. Varnum-Finney B, et al. Pluripotent, cytokine-dependent, hematopoietic stem cells are immortalized by constitutive Notch1 signaling. *Nat Med*. 2000;6:1278–1281.

85. Delaney C, et al. Notch-mediated expansion of human cord blood progenitor cells capable of rapid myeloid reconstitution. *Nat Med*. 2010;16:232–236.

86. Peled T, et al. Nicotinamide, a SIRT1 inhibitor, inhibits differentiation and facilitates expansion of hematopoietic progenitor cells with enhanced bone marrow homing and engraftment. *Exp Hematol.* 2012;40:342–355.e1.

87. Horwitz ME, et al. Umbilical cord blood expansion with nicotinamide provides long-term multilineage engraftment. *J Clin Investig.* 2014;124:3121–3128.

88. Boitano AE, et al. Aryl hydrocarbon receptor antagonists promote the expansion of human hematopoietic stem cells. *Science.* 2010;329:1345–1348.

89. de Lima M, et al. Cord-blood engraftment with ex vivo mesenchymal-cell coculture. *N Engl J Med.* 2012;367: 2305–2315.

90. Popat U, et al. Enforced fucosylation of cord blood hematopoietic cells accelerates neutrophil and platelet engraftment after transplantation. *Blood.* 2015;125:2885–2892.

91. Cutler C, et al. Prostaglandin-modulated umbilical cord blood hematopoietic stem cell transplantation. *Blood.* 2013;122:3074.

92. Farag SS, et al. In vivo DPP-4 inhibition to enhance engraftment of single-unit cord blood transplants in adults with hematological malignancies. *Stem Cells Dev.* 2013;22:1007–1015.

93. Vélez de Mendizábal N, et al. Modelling the sitagliptin effect on dipeptidyl peptidase-4 activity in adults with haematological malignancies after umbilical cord blood haematopoietic cell transplantation. *Clin Pharmacokinet.* 2014;53:247–259.

94. Eapen M, et al. Outcomes of transplantation of unrelated donor umbilical cord blood and bone marrow in children with acute leukaemia: a comparison study. *Lancet.* 2007 Jun 9;369(9577):1947–1954.

CHAPTER 9

Allogeneic Hematopoietic Stem Cell Transplantation for Acute Myeloid Leukemia

BENJAMIN TOMLINSON, MD • MARCOS DE LIMA, MD

INTRODUCTION

Allogeneic hematopoietic stem cell transplant (allo-HSCT) plays a critical role in the management of acute myeloid leukemia (AML), offering curative potential for patients who have incurable disease with standard forms of chemotherapy. Allo-HSCT incorporates a conditioning regimen of chemotherapy with or without radiation to eradicate residual leukemia and provide recipient immunosuppression. Potent alkylating agents such as busulfan, melphalan, as well as high doses of total-body irradiation (TBI) are highly effective agents against AML, but without marrow rescue with hematopoietic progenitor cells, it can result in prolonged or fatal myelosuppression. Historically, autologous HSCT was studied as a form of consolidation, but improvements over standard consolidation have not been demonstrated.[1] Allogenic transplant requires recipients to be immunosuppressed to limit graft rejection and have additional risks for treatment-related mortality from graft-versus-host disease (GVHD), infection, and primary and secondary graft failure. Nevertheless, allo-HSCT capitalizes on an allogeneic immune effect of graft-versus-leukemia (GVL) that adds synergistically to the cytotoxic effects of the conditioning regimen. Here, we review AML risk stratification, selection of appropriate candidates for allo-HSCT, conditioning regimens, and outcomes of transplantation using matched related or unrelated donors, and alternative donor allo-HSCTs.

MECHANISMS OF ALLO-HSCT IN AML

The curative potential of allo-HSCT was recognized by early studies showing cures even in a small proportion of refractory patients.[2] A significant portion of the responses can be attributed to the GVL effect. The earliest implications of this were seen in murine models in which transplanted marrow eliminated leukemia even before cytotoxic irradiation was applied.[3] Early studies of sibling donor transplants noted that non–T cell–depleted grafts had improved rates of leukemia relapse.[4] By the early 1990s retrospective analyses of international transplant registries clearly demonstrated that the presence of acute or chronic GVHD was linked to a reduced risk of relapse.[5,6] Furthermore, the activity of donor lymphocyte infusion (DLI) in treating posttransplant recurrence has further cemented this observation. The concept of "adoptive immunotherapy" was developed by Mathé as he treated a leukemia patient with increasing doses of donor leukocytes.[7] A syndrome, later recognized to be GVHD, developed, but the patient never relapsed. Susceptibility to the GVL effect may be higher in CML, but still significant in AML.[8]

Allogeneic T cells are critical to GVL. Their importance was clearly demonstrated when T cell depletion was introduced as a possible means to manage and prevent GVHD.[9] Relapse rates for multiple hematologic malignancies, including AML, were notably higher in T cell–depleted grafts.[5] The primary mechanism for GVL is felt to be initiated by antigen presentation by host dendritic cells. These antigen-presenting cells are responsible for the activation and maintenance of donor CD4+ T cells and cytotoxic CD8+ T cells that result in long-term disease control.[10–12] As a result, some degree of donor engraftment is expected, and DLI can result in increased activation and antileukemic efficacy.

Hematopoietic Cell Transplantation for Malignant Conditions. https://doi.org/10.1016/B978-0-323-56802-9.00004-3

ACUTE MYELOID LEUKEMIA—DISEASE AND CLASSIFICATION

AML results from clonal proliferation and differentiation blockade of hematopoietic progenitor cells. The resulting cells infiltrate the bone marrow and other tissues and lead to the clinical manifestations of leukocytosis, frequently with anemia and thrombocytopenia, coagulation disorders, and high infection risk.[13] The diagnosis of AML is based off morphologic and immunophenotypic assessment of bone marrow and peripheral blood, with karyotype analysis, fluorescent in situ hybridization (FISH) of common cytogenetic changes, and polymerase chain reaction (PCR) or next-generation sequencing to identify common molecular abnormalities. AML is still often given a morphologic description based off the French-American-British classification system, but final diagnosis today should include genetic markers and assignment to the WHO classification system, last revised in 2016.[14–16] Incorporation of genetically defined AML started with the recognition of t(15; 17) as disease defining in the case of acute promyelocytic leukemia, followed quickly by the core-binding factor leukemias t(8; 21), t(16; 16), and inv(16), and finally translocations of *KMT2A* (previously known as *MLL*).[17,18] The most recent iteration takes genomic classification further than before, specifically recognizing AML with mutations in *NPM1* and biallelic *CEBPα* as separate entities, and provisionally recognizing AML with RUNX1 mutations.[15] Therapy-related neoplasms remain separately recognized given the known risks of ionizing radiation along with cytotoxic chemotherapy. The 2016 WHO revisions for AML are summarized in Table 9.1.

An increasing number of germline mutations are now recognized as predisposing to AML, including *RUNX1*, *CEBPα*, and *GATA2*, with more potential genes emerging, and need to be considered during transplant evaluation. Families with *RUNX1* present with family platelet disorders in additional to high incidences of leukemia.[19] Germline *CEBPα* mutations inherit a "first hit" for the risk of AML in an autosomal dominant pattern.[20] Despite the inherited gene, *CEBPα* mutations still appear to be correlated with a favorable outcome to standard therapy even in families with a known genetic predisposition. Inherited bone marrow failure syndromes including telomere biology disorders and Fanconi's anemia required special attention and need to be considered in any younger individual with a family history of AML or aplastic anemia.[21,22] AML is a common secondary malignancy in this setting, and transplant is required for long-term disease control.

TABLE 9.1

WHO 2016 Revision–Current Classification of Acute Myeloid Leukemia[15]

Classification	Subcategories
AML with Recurrent Genetic Abnormalities	AML with t(8; 21); *RUNX1-RUNX1T1* AML with inv16 or t(16; 16); *CBFB-MYH11* APL with *PML-RARα* AML with t(9; 11);*MLLT3-KMT2A* AML with t(6; 9);*DEK-NUP214* AML with inv(3) or t(3; 3); *GATA2, MECOM* AML (megakaryoblastic) with t(1; 22);*RBM15-MKL1* AML with mutated *NPM1* AML with biallelic mutations of *CEBPα* Provisional: AML with mutated *RUNX1* Provisional: AML with BCR-ABL1
AML with MDS-related changes	*none*
Therapy-related myeloid neoplasms	*none*
AML NOS	AML with minimal differentiation AML without maturation AML with maturation Acute myelomonocytic leukemia Acute monoblastic/monocytic leukemia Pure erythroid leukemia Acute megakaryoblastic leukemia Acute basophilic leukemia Acute panmyelosis with myelofibrosis
Myeloid sarcoma	*none*

AML, acute myeloid leukemia; *MDS*, myelodysplastic syndrome; *NOS*, not otherwise specified.

These patients can have severe side effects to alkylating agents and high doses of radiation. Special attention is required including consideration of nonmyeloablative conditioning as a standard.[23]

Even in the absence of germline mutations, the development of somatic mutations that can lead to AML is now better understood. A variety of founder mutations have been implicated and impact the cytogenetic and molecular heterogeneity of AML.[24] Work has suggested that founder mutations are present in up to 10% of the population, and the presence of these mutations impacts risks for disease other than malignancy, such as atherosclerotic disease.[25,26]

RISK STRATIFICATION OF ACUTE MYELOID LEUKEMIA

Accurate prediction of outcomes for specific AML patients is critically linked to developing postremission strategies for consolidation, including allo-HSCT. Both disease- and patient-related factors impact these decisions. Within patients, advancing age, presence of comorbidities, and poor performance status are linked to worse outcomes with intensive therapy including treatment-related mortality.[27] Specific cutoffs for defining "elderly" in the AML population are a moving target, as age is a continuum that does not perfectly describe all attributes of a specific patient. In general, patients aged 60 years and older are reasonably defined as elderly.[28] Selection of appropriate candidates for induction continues to be a clinical challenge despite available tools to predict treatment-related outcomes.[29] The hematopoietic cell therapy-comorbidity index (HCT-CI) is frequently used to estimate peritransplant mortality risk.[30,31]

Disease-specific factors include genetic changes within the group. Consensus guidelines from several groups including European Leukemia Net (ELN), National Comprehensive Cancer Center Network (NCCN), and the United Kingdom's Medical Research Council (MRC) have significant overlap and are summarized in Table 9.2.[32,33] One of the most notable changes is the modification of the ELN risk stratification to exclude separate categories for intermediate-1 and intermediate-2 AML.[34]

Specific cytogenetic abnormalities within AML have long been recognized as strong prognostic factors. Examples include core-binding factor AMLs t(8; 21), t(16; 16), and inv(16) with the known fusion genes, as well as the poor prognosis of a number of additional fusion genes such as t(6; 9), DEK-NUP214. Patients with cytogenetically normal AML with mutations in NPM1 have improved prognosis. Pertinently, there is no significant improvement in outcome with allo-HSCT in young patients with NPM1 mutation.[35] More recent updates to the NCCN and ELN risk stratification have included recognition of the favorable risk of CEBPα double mutations, whereas p53 and ASXL1 mutations are now recognized as poor prognostic variables. A more nuanced understanding of FLT3-ITD mutations is now incorporated, indicating that a high ratio of mutant to wild-type FLT3 carries a strong negative impact in survival.[36]

Therapy-related AML (tAML) and AML arising from antecedent hematologic malignancies are generally considered of poor prognosis, and allo-HSCT is usually used, although post-HSCT outcome is worse than de novo AML.[37] Secondary AML arising from MDS

TABLE 9.2
AML Risk Stratification[33]

Risk Category	Cytogenetic and molecular abnormalities
Favorable	t(8; 21) RUNX1-RUNX1T1 inv(16) or t(16; 16) CBFB-MYH11 mutated NPM1 without FLT3-ITD or with FLT3-ITD^{low} Biallelic mutated CEBPα
Intermediate	Mutated NPM1 and FLT3-ITD^{high} Wild-type NPM1 without FLT3-ITD or with FLT3-ITD^{low} t(9; 11); MLLT3-KMT2A Undefined cytogenetic abnormalities
Adverse	t(6; 9); DEK-NUP214 t(v; 11q23.3); KMT2A rearranged t(9; 22); BCR-ABL1 inv(3) or t(3; 3); GATA2, MECOM(EVI1) −5 or del(5q); −7; −17/abn(17p) Complex karyotype Monosomal karyotype Wild-type NPM1 and FLT3-ITD^{high} Mutated RUNX1 Mutated ASXL1 Mutated TP53

AML, acute myeloid leukemia.

(myelodysplastic syndrome) may fare better than AML arising from other antecedent malignancies but is still considered a high-risk disease.[38]

DYNAMIC RISK PROGNOSTICATION

Disease status is a well-known determinant of survival in AML. Primary refractory disease, also known as primary induction failure (PIF) is associated with a worse prognosis.[39] Moreover, patients with longer first remissions have improved prognosis at the time of relapse.[40] These observations suggest that sensitive testing of disease responsiveness to initial therapy may further improve risk stratification and the potential benefit of allo-HSCT. The concept of minimal or measurable residual disease (MRD) is now being adapted into current measures of response, beyond the traditional morphologic assessment.[33,41] MRD can be detected through evaluation of leukemia-specific immunophenotypes by flow cytometry, quantitative reverse transcriptase (RQ-PCR) for specific leukemia-associated mutations, or next-generation sequencing to detect persistent changes associated with disease.[42–44] Moreover, the association of MRD with increased relapsed risk has been

TABLE 9.3
Strategies to Monitor Minimal Residual Disease in AML

Method	Description/Examples	Limit of Detection	Examples of Transplant Risk Stratification
Multi-color Flow Cytometry	• Detects small numbers of cells with aberrant surface marker expression • Identifies a "leukemia-associated immunopheno-type (LAIP)"	Variable depends on degree of difference in the LAIP	1. Relapse risk similar to active disease, if positive before trans-plantation. • Buckley et al. 2017[54] • Zhou et al. 2016[50] 2. Reappearance highly predictive of relapse. • Miyazaki et al. 2012[148]
Quantitative reverse transcriptase PCR—fusion genes and mutated genes	• Requires knowledge of mu-tation, appropriate primers • Well validated for acute promyelocytic leukemia • Fusion genes: • t(8; 21) • t(16; 16), inv16 • t(9; XX) • t(9; 22), *BCR-ABL* • Mutated genes • NPM1 • FLT3	<0.01% or better	1. Reappearance of detectable t(8; 21) and t(16; 16) highly predic-tive of relapse • Wang et al. 2014[149] • Elmaagacli et al. 1998[150] 2. Monitoring of NPM1 transcripts can predict relapse • Bacher et al. 2008[151]
Next-generation sequencing	• Detection of large number of potentially mutant genes	Variable—depends on number of genes	1. Detectable MRD by NGS addi-tive to predictive value of flow cytometry • Jongen et al. 2018[43]

AML, acute myeloid leukemia; *PCR*, polymerase chain reaction; *NGS*, next-generation sequencing.

repeatedly demonstrated.[45–48] The significance of spe-cific mutations is a work in progress. *DNMT3A, TET2, and ASXL1* mutations may persist even in the absence of relapse risk after achievement of CR, whereas *NPM1, IDH2, and FLT3-ITD* mutations may prove much more reliable markers of MRD.[43] Different techniques to monitor MRD are enumerated in Table 9.3.

In some settings MRD may have a higher predictive power for AML outcome than the traditional pretreat-ment parameters, although as expected, a variety of well-known poor prognosticators are associated with persistent MRD.[46,48,49] A retrospective analysis of 279 patients with AML who underwent allo-HSCT showed that the presence of MRD at the time of transplant was associated with an increased overall mortality, even when adjusted for classic risk factors. Though prospec-tive trials will be required, these single-institution data suggest that MRD presence at HSCT may be overcome with myeloablative conditioning.[50] Ustun et al. found that flow cytometry positive status was associated with increased rates of relapse and worse overall survival

(OS) in patients receiving reduced intensity condition-ing (RIC).[51] Therefore a more stringent definition of CR may be important if RIC is to be used.[52] Other data suggest that a high level of MRD before allo-HSCT may be associated with outcomes similar to active disease, even with ablative conditioning.[53] Meta-analysis of published trials has found that both MRD detected by molecular and flow cytometry techniques are associ-ated with increased risk of relapse.[54]

INDICATIONS FOR ALLO-HSCT

The earliest reports of allo-HSCT were for patients with active, advanced-phase AML.[2] For patients relapsing after first complete remission, the long-term prognosis is known to be poor without allo-HSCT, taking into con-sideration remission duration and other covariables. As a result, allo-HSCT is nearly universally recommended for eligible patients in second CR. As expected, how-ever, results are better earlier in the disease course. Rea-sons for this include better physical dispositions with less chemotherapy exposure as well as lower likelihood of AML resistance to chemotherapy.

As a result, allo-HSCT in first CR may be ideal for selected patients in which the risk of relapse and general physical condition are adequate. Appropriate selection of these patients is critical, as there are subsets that are potentially cured with chemotherapy alone sparing them potential risks of treatment related mortality (TRM) and quality-of-life issues with chronic GVHD. It is generally accepted that patients with favorable risk AML should avoid allo-HSCT in first remission given the high potential for cure with standard chemotherapy. On the other end of the spectrum, AML with unfavorable risk in first CR is also considered a clear indication to move to transplant.

Patients in the intermediate risk category present the biggest challenge in determining transplant eligibility. Historically, the role of transplantation has been studied in a 'donor versus no donor' fashion, proposing a genetic randomization that used only fully matched sibling or unrelated donors. Limitations of the trials performed in the 90s and early 2000s include the absence of alternative donors (haploidentical and cord blood) and the high TRM rates associated with alloHSCT, which frequently denied the possible survival advantage conferred by the GVL effect. In a prospective trial, the European Organization of Research and Treatment of Cancer— Leukemia Group/Gruppo Italiano Malattie Ematologiche dell'Adulto (EORTC-LG/GIMEMA) assigned patients with HLA-matched siblings to allo-HSCT and others to autologous HSCT. Not all patients were able to proceed to their assigned treatment, with 69% of patients in the allo-HSCT group proceeding to receive it and 56% proceeding to autologous HSCT. OS was similar between the two groups.[55] The UK MRC AML10 trial for patients under the age of 55 years compared 419 patients with a matched sibling and 644 without. On a strict donor/no donor basis, relapse risk and DFS were improved, but OS was statistically similar (55% vs. 50%, $P=.1$). However, there was a survival benefit within the group of intermediate risk patients (55% vs. 44%; $P=.02$).[56] Overall, particularly for younger patients with intermediate risk disease, the trend has been toward a survival benefit for those with an HLA-matched donor.

Results of four studies that evaluated postremission strategies in a donor/no donor fashion from the Bordeaux Grenoble Marseille Toulouse (BGMT) cooperative group have been reported. With good adherence to assigned treatment arms, 182 patients assigned to receive matched sibling donor (MSD) allo-HSCT were compared with 290 patients in the no donor group. Ten-year OS favored allo-HSCT (51% vs. 43% survival).

Patients with intermediate risk disease were statistically likely to benefit even when examined in isolation.[57] HOVAN-SAKK evaluated 1032 first CR AML patients treated from 1987 through 2004; 326 patients had an MSD, of which 82% adhered to the assigned treatment plan and underwent allo-HSCT. DFS was significantly better in the donor group (48% vs. 37%, $P<.001$), with subgroup analysis indicating benefits for both intermediate- and poor-risk patients.[58]

A meta-analysis by Koreth et al. of over 6000 patients enrolled in 24 separate clinical trials showed a hazard ration (HR) of relapse or death for patients who received allo-HSCT in first CR of 0.80. Subset analysis indicated a significant protective effect in intermediate- and poor-risk AML patients with HR of 0.69 (0.57–0.84) and 0.76 (0.68–0.85), respectively. Patients with favorable risk disease in first CR did not appear to benefit.[59] Notably, this meta-analysis specifically analyzed studies based on donor versus no donor status and largely included younger patients. It is largely accepted that the outcome of matched unrelated donor HSCT is similar to that of MSD transplants, although this assumption is based on single-institution studies.[60] Many providers will consider patients with a well-matched unrelated donor as similarly likely to benefit, and so transplant should be considered for intermediate- and poor-risk patients in first CR with a well-matched sibling or with an unrelated donor (matched at HLA-A, -B, –C, and DRB1 by high-resolution methods).

The propensity of data favoring transplant in first CR for intermediate- and poor-risk AML patients favors the ongoing use of upfront risk stratification (as outlined in Table 9.1), whereas consolidation with chemotherapy alone should be considered for favorable risk disease. Indeed, allo-HSCT should be avoided in the favorable risk setting. In the current era this means both corebinding factor AMLs but also cytogenetically normal AML with *NPM1* and double *CEBPα* mutations. There is poor consensus for cytogenetically normal AML with *FLT3-ITD* mutations, where some authors suggest that presence of a low mutant to wild-type allele burden ratio may not have a poor prognosis and may not benefit from allo-HSCT, whereas others strongly suggest allo-HSCT regardless of allele burden.[61] Accepted indications for allo-HSCT are listed in Table 9.2.

Higher levels of MRD before transplant are linked to increased relapse and lower survival rates.[62] In one retrospective study the presence of any level of MRD by multiparametric flow cytometry had a 2-year OS rate of 30% compared with 76% without MRD.[48] Although it is commonly accepted that presence of MRD determines a worse prognosis and is an indication for HSCT, it is less clear if allo-HSCT rescues these patients in a systematic way. Furthermore, it is largely unknown if patients in morphologic CR with MRD benefit from further pre-HSCT therapy because often effective therapy is not available. Prospective studies are lacking.

In another example of widening indications, older patients are now common recipients of allo-HSCT. Aging is associated with lower CR rates and shorter CR duration. In the past, advanced age was considered a contraindication to HSCT, but with the wider utilization of reduced intensity and nonmyeloablative (NMA) conditioning, patients up to the age of 75 years are often considered for the intervention. Moreover, while donor/no donor strategies may have dictated who was able to receive a transplant, in the modern era, the availability of related haploidentical donors along with umbilical cord blood means that nearly everyone has a potential donor, and the consideration for candidacy for allo-HSCT depends more than ever on patient-specific factors, disease-related factors, and to some degree, donor-related risks over the simple availability of donors. As discussed in the following sections, it is unclear, however, if alternative donor transplants lead to similar survival and DFS as those performed using well-matched donors, especially among patients older than 60 years.

CONDITIONING REGIMENS

Original conditioning or preparative regimens were universally myeloablative, in that autologous hematopoietic recovery was unlikely or would take weeks to occur. RIC was developed to allow older patients or those with comorbidities to tolerate therapy and is more dependent on a successful GVL effect for leukemia control. It is assumed that autologous recovery could occur after such regimens, in a relatively short period of time. RIC regimens have permitted patients in their 50, 60, and 70s to receive allo-HSCT. Nonmyeloablative regimens, as exemplified by the combination of fludarabine and 200 cGy of TBI, provide enough immunosuppression for engraftment of well-matched donor cells, at the expense of minimal myelosuppression and disease control. As discussed below, AML relapse rates are higher with less regimen dose intensity.

MYELOABLATIVE CONDITIONING

Three regimens are commonly employed: (1) cyclophosphamide with TBI (Cy-TBI), (2) busulfan with cyclophosphamide (BuCy), and (3) busulfan with fludarabine (BuFlu).[2,63,64] Early ablative conditioning regimens focused on the use of high doses of TBI as a critical part of the conditioning regimen. Busulfan was proposed by Santos et al. as a replacement for TBI.[63] Several authors in the 90s compared large numbers of patients receiving TBI versus busulfan found evidence suggesting that TBI may be the superior choice. Ringden et al. compared Cy-TBI to BuCy in patients with a variety of different primary malignancies including AML, ALL, and CML, and Blaise et al. evaluated a younger population of AML patients.[65,66] Notable findings included that the use of TBI in conditioning appeared to better control advanced disease and appeared to lessen long-term complications, including rates of debilitating conditions such as bronchiolitis obliterans. Nevertheless, these early studies primarily reported patients using oral busulfan.[67-70] Some of these worse outcomes may be attributed to the route of busulfan administration. Busulfan was generally given as fixed doses orally, which resulted in substantial variability in plasma levels, as shown by the Seattle group. Dosing based on pharmacokinetic analysis results in more predictable drug levels and lower rates of toxicity. This strategy minimizes the risk of under-dosing and over-dosing which is associated with higher relapse risk and sinusoidal obstructive syndrome (SOS), respectively.[71] Toxicity rates have been further reduced with IV busulfan. Since the drug was solubilized by Andersson et al., multiple retrospective studies have found lower SOS rates as plasma concentrations are more predictable.[67,69,70]

As a result of the wider use of IV busulfan, it is not possible to conclude that TBI is a superior conditioning regimen, and several more recent studies suggest the opposite conclusion. A prospective registration cohort study by Bredeson et al. evaluated IV busulfan ablative regimens compared with TBI-based ablative regimens specifically for AML patients (N = 1473 patients). OS was improved with the use of IV busulfan.[72] A CIBMTR retrospective study of 1230 AML patients evaluated BuCy versus Cy-TBI conditioning for first allo-HSCT and found that TRM and relapse were improved with IV busulfan compared to TBI.[73] A similar study from the EBMT in 1659 AML patients in first or second remission transplanted from 2004 to 2010 found no statistical difference between IV busulfan versus TBI in combination with cyclophosphamide.[74] A prospective cohort from 2009 to 2011 of 1483 patients, a majority of whom had AML, found that IV busulfan in combination with cyclophosphamide was associated with improved OS.[72] In contrast the EBMT also performed a retrospective analysis on 842 patients with advanced and refractory AML, 514 of which received IV busulfan, and the remaining patients received TBI. No differences in 2-year outcomes including OS and LFS were found (33.4% vs. 37.8%, P = .65).[74]

Whether fludarabine and busulfan can be used as an alternative for BuCy has also been studied. The logic for this approach is that use of fludarabine appears to increase the safety of the regimen without sacrificing efficacy. Fludarabine is a purine analog that is highly lymphotoxic and may decrease graft rejection, as well as increasing the sensitivity of leukemia cells to alkylating agents.[75]

Investigators at the MD Anderson Cancer Center developed the concept of reduced toxicity conditioning, based on once-daily ablative doses of busulfan in combination to fludarabine. Subsequently, the initial observations were confirmed in an Italian prospective, randomized trial, comparing BuFlu versus BuCy. Eligible were patients (n = 252) with AML in CR. TRM was significantly higher (17.2% vs. 7.9%) in patient receiving BuCy.[76] In addition, retrospective studies improved results when IV busulfan is dosed based on pharmacokinetic studies.[72] Andersson et al. retrospectively evaluated outcomes of AML and MDS patients receiving allo-HSCT and found an improved TRM in patients receiving fludarabine over alternative combinations with busulfan, resulting in improvement in median EFS of 19.1 months versus 8.4 months.[64] As a matter of practice, use of TBI-based ablative regimens in AML is decreasing.

REDUCED INTENSITY CONDITIONING
A strategy to reduce TRM is to simply reduce the dose while ideally maintaining immunosuppression to allow engraftment. Purine analogs fludarabine and cladribine were combined with melphalan or low-dose TBI in early RIC regimens and elicited durable remissions, based on the initial experiences at the MD Anderson Cancer Center, Hadassah Hospital, and in Seattle.[77]

The tradeoff when reducing the regimen intensity is a higher relapse rate than ablative conditioning, although this concept has been challenged as well. Despite this caveat, donor versus no-donor analyses have clearly demonstrated superiority of RIC allo-HSCT over chemotherapy only for elderly patients with AML.[78]

A genetically randomized donor versus no-donor prospective trial in France compared 95 patients with AML in CR receiving RIC allo-HSCT versus conventional chemotherapy. Both relapse and OS rates were substantially improved.[79] An additional time-dependent analysis from four prospective phase III

trials from the Dutch-Belgian Hemato-Oncology Cooperative Group and the Swiss Group for Clinical Cancer Research (HOVON-SAKK) collaborative study group compared postremission strategies for AML patients ≥60 years of age. RIC HSCT was found to have improved 5-year OS compared with other strategies, which included chemotherapy, auto-HSCT, and no further therapy.[80,81]

Retrospective studies have suggested that RIC is a reasonable approach for all AML patients in remission, as there was a suggestion that despite the increased risk of relapse, the OS of patients after RIC was the same as that observed after ablative conditioning.[82,83] These observations led to prospective clinical studies. The LAM2001 phase 3 trial compared AML patients older than 50 years receiving matched sibling donor RIC allo-HSCT versus patients younger than 50 years receiving MAC. OS at 108 months was 65.8% for RIC and 63.4% for MAC.[84] In contrast, the BMT Clinical Trial Network performed a prospective randomized trial of myeloablative versus RIC conditioning in which accrual was ended early as myeloablative conditioning was associated with improved RFS for MDS and AML patients. Within the AML subgroup, there was a statistically significant trend toward OS benefit at 18 months (76.5% vs. 63.4% favoring myeloablative conditioning, P = .035.)[85] The combination of available data would suggest that for eligible patients with AML in CR1 up to the age of 65 years, myeloablative conditioning should be considered the standard of care.

Nevertheless, RIC has permitted many patients who would not be candidates for ablative conditioning to benefit from allo-HSCT. This is especially important for older patients, where the cure rates with standard therapy are very low. The primary strategy to reduce the intensity of therapy is to reduce alkylating agent dose and combine this with fludarabine or low-dose TBI to facilitate engraftment.[86] Several dosing regimens of TBI, cyclophosphamide, busulfan, and melphalan have been used.[77,87–89] In vivo T cell depletion, usually with rabbit antithymocyte globulin, is often used to improve engraftment. In myeloablative conditioning, in vivo T cell depletion may be associated with increased relapse risk, but it is not clear if this is the case with RIC.[90,91]

Large retrospective studies have confirmed encouraging outcomes with the approach. The CIBMTR analyzed 545 AML and 535 MDS patients aged 40–79 years who received RIC allo-HSCT. Two-year OS was not impacted by age and included 2-year OS of 34% and 36% in patients aged 60–64 and ≥65 years.[92] EBMT compared RIC allo-HSCT with a matched sibling donor to autologous transplant for patients in CR2 and found a reduced relapse risk (RR of 0.77; 95% CI, 0.63–0.95; $P = .013$). In multivariate analysis, RIC was associated with improved OS as well.[93]

NONMYELOABLATIVE CONDITIONING

NMA conditioning regimens should result in minimal cytopenias. Even if administered without stem cell support, autologous recovery of hematopoiesis is expected. Nevertheless, the therapy intensity results in a recovery pattern that is both uncertain and unpredictable, and thus, stem cell administration is still required.[94] Longer times are required to generate full donor chimerism. Hematologic recovery after conditioning is often a mix of donor-recipient cells, and a well-defined pattern of T cell engraftment followed by myeloid cell engraftment is followed. This also means that often GVHD onset is delayed.[87,88]

The benefits of NMA conditioning for elderly patients with AML is well reported. One large review of patients enrolled on 18 multicenter studies of hematologic malignancies undergoing NMA conditioning allo-HSCT included 109 patients with AML a 5-year demonstrated OS of 40% (95% CI of 30%–49%). No detrimental effect of age was identified.[30]

Comparisons of RIC and NMA regimens are limited. Part of this stems from the multiple different regimens in use, as the intensity of the preparative chemotherapy falls on a spectrum.[95] For MDS and AML patients, the MD Anderson group retrospectively compared NMA conditioning of fludarabine, cytarabine, and idarubicin with fludarabine and melphalan (RIC) in a population with median ages of 52 and 61 years, respectively. Relapse rates were higher with NMA, but OS was similar due to higher TRM in the RIC subgroup. In patients transplanted in remission, there was a nonsignificant trend toward improved OS with RIC.[96] Generally speaking, it is recommended that the higher tolerable intensity should be used to treat AML. Determining dose intensity is as much an art as it is a science incorporating frailty and comorbidities assessment, as well as disease characteristics and center experience and preference.

ALTERNATIVE DONOR TRANSPLANTATION

The efficacy and superiority of allo-HSCT for AML was largely proven in patients with HLA-matched sibling and matched anonymous donors. However, not all patients will have a matched donor, and timing of unrelated donor search may not fit the patient's need given relapse risk. Only 30%–35% of patients will have a matched sibling who can potentially donate, and the odds of having a matched unrelated donor (MUD) is dependent on a patient's ethnicity. Close to all patients will have a donor if sources of hematopoietic stem cells are extended to include umbilical cord blood (UCB) and haploidentical related donors. It has been postulated, but yet to be proven in prospective studies, that the outcome for AML patients is similar when using different stem cell donors.

UCB transplants are associated with less severe GVHD and therefore do not require the same degree of HLA-match as adult-derived bone marrow or peripheral blood. Mismatches at up to two-three HLA-A, B, C and DRB1 loci are permitted, though outcomes are improved with better donor-recipient matching. The earliest report of UCB graft for adult AML came from Kurtzberg et al. who reported on a series of 25 patients that received a single UCB unit.[97] Early UCB transplant universally used myeloablative conditioning, with encouraging 5-year survival rates of 46%–65%.[98,99] Double UCB have been proposed especially in the USA to increase cell dose and decrease TRM.[100] Here, one of the transplanted units will predominate and provide the majority of hematopoiesis by 100 days after transplant.[101] Double cord blood transplants with ablative conditioning appear to have 3-year LFS rates exceeding 50% in single center studies.[102] NMA conditioning has also been used, with encouraging engraftment outcomes, with LFS of 38% at 3-year in the largest series.[103] In registry studies, overall outcomes for AML actually appear similar between UCB and matched adult donors.[104,105] A single center retrospective analysis suggested UCB may have an advantage in patients with MRD over other stem cell sources, with less relapses.[106]

Haploidentical donors provide the promise of a donor to most patients in need, with a shorter procurement time. Historically, T-cell depleted, CD34 selected haploidentical transplants were associated with high risk of engraftment failure and limited immune reconstitution. Ex vivo depletion of T cells is effective, but not reproducible outside centers with high experience in this approach, and has been limited due to increased risks of relapse and infections. There is now widely acceptance to the use of T cell replete bone marrow or peripheral blood with posttransplant cyclophosphamide-based GVHD prophylaxis. Immune reconstitution seems faster than after UCB transplants, and this practice has now gained worldwide acceptance. In AML, both prospective studies and retrospective studies are encouraging as OS appears to be similar to that observed after unrelated donor transplantation Table 9.4.[107]

Given possible similarity of outcomes between haploidentical and unrelated donor transplants along with the broad availability of the former, the traditional

TABLE 9.4

Comparative Studies Evaluating Outcomes of AML Patients Undergoing Hematopoietic Stem Cell Transplant With Haploidentical Donors Versus Matched Related and Matched Unrelated Donors

Author/ Year	Data Source	Description	Patient Number	CI of cGVHD	NRM	Relapse	OS
Ciurea 2015[107]	CIBMTR	MA and RIC comparison of Haplo using Post-Tx Cy versus MUD for AML in CR1	Haplo: 192 MUD: 1982	MA: 3-year Haplo versus MUD 30% versus 53% (P<.0001) RIC: 3-year Haplo versus MUD 34% versus 52% (P=.002)	MA: 3-year NRM Haplo versus MUD 14% versus 20% (P=.14) RIC: 3-year NRM 9% versus 23% (P=.0001)	MA: 3-year relapse risk Haplo versus MUD 44% versus 39% (P=.37) RIC: 3-year relapse risk 58% versus 42% (P=.006)	MA: 3-year 45% versus 50% (P=.38) Haplo versus MUD RIC: 3-year 46% versus 44% (P=.71)
Versluis 2017[152]	EBMT	MRD versus (10/10) MUD versus (9/10) MUD versus UCB versus Haplo for AML in CR1	Haplo: 193 MUD: 549 UCB: 333	At any time Haplo versus MUD versus UCB: 29% versus 30% versus 19% (p not reported)	2-year NRM (HR vs. MRD) Haplo: 26% (1.98, P<.001) versus MUD 20% (1.39, P<.001) versus UCB 29% (2.41, P<.001)	2-year CIR (HR vs. MRD): Haplo 22% (0.6, P=.001) versus MUD 27% (0.74, P<.001) versus UCB 30% (0.96, P=.69)	2-year OS (HR vs. MRD): Haplo 57% (1.12, P=.34) versus MUD 57% (0.99, P=.89) versus UCB 44% (1.54, P<.001)
Piemontese 2017[153]	EBMT	Unmanipulated haplo versus (10/10) MUD and (9/10) MUD for acute leukemia in 1st or 2nd CR	Haplo – 265 (10/10) MUD – 2490 (9/10) MUD - 813	3-year Haplo versus (10/10)MUD versus (9/10) MUD 34% versus 40% versus 33%	3-year NRM (HR vs. Haplo) Haplo versus (10/10)MUD versus (9/10) MUD 29% versus 21% (0.636, P=.001) versus. 29% 0.991, P=.957)	3-year CIR (HR vs. Haplo) Haplo versus (10/10)MUD versus (9/10) MUD 30% versus 29% (0.862, P=.259) versus. 25% 0.843, P=.245)	3-year OS (HR vs. Haplo) Haplo versus (10/10)MUD versus (9/10) MUD 46% versus 56% (0.707, P=.001) versus. 48% 0.930, P=.560)
Sun 2016[154]	Single institution paired with EBMT data.	AML Patients in CR1 Ablative conditioning; GCSF primed haplo marrow, T cell replete with intensive immunosuppression versus 10/10 MUD	Haplo: 87 10/10 MUD: 87	Not reported	5-year (haplo vs. MUD) 13.8% versus 15.7%, P=.962	5-year: (haplo vs. MUD) 12.7% versus 24% P=.083	5-year OS (haplo vs. MUD): 78.2% versus 63.3%, P=.148

Continued

TABLE 9.4

Comparative Studies Evaluating Outcomes of AML Patients Undergoing Hematopoietic Stem Cell Transplant With Haploidentical Donors Versus Matched Related and Matched Unrelated Donors—cont'd

Author/ Year	Data Source	Description	Patient Number	CI of cGVHD	NRM	Relapse	OS
Wang 2015[155]	Multi-center	AML patients in CR1 MRD versus T-cell replete Haplo with aggressive immunosuppression. Methods: prospective trial with genetic randomization	Haplo: 231 MRD: 219	1-year: Haplo versus MRD 42% versus 15%, $P<.001$	3-year NRM: Haplo versus MRD 13% versus 8%, $P=.13$	3-year CIR: Haplo versus MRD 15% versus 15%, $P=.98$	3-year Haplo versus MRD 79% versus 82%, $P=.36$
Rashidi 2016[156]	Single Institution	AML patients undergoing first HCT (41% with active AML) MUD versus T-cell replete Haplo with post-Tx Cy	Haplo: 52 MUD: 88	1.5 years Haplo versus MUD 10% versus 9% $P=.91$	1.5 years Haplo versus MUD 27% versus 27%, $P=.54$	1.5 years Haplo versus MUD 29% versus 43%, $P=.08$	1.5 years Haplo versus MUD 42% versus 37%, $P=.17$
How 2017[157]	Single Institution	AML patients with active leukemia MUD and MRD versus Haplo with post-Tx Cy	Haplo: 24 MRD: 32 MUD: 43	1 year Haplo versus MRD versus MUD 13% versus 17% versus 20%, $P=.73$	2-year TRM: Haplo versus MRD versus MUD 26% versus 42% versus 29%, $P=.49$	1 year CIR: Haplo versus MRD versus MUD 33% versus 28% versus 48%, $P=.40$	2 year Haplo versus MRD versus MUD 36% versus 28% versus 29%, $P=.21$
Salvatore 2018[158]	EBMT	AML patients in CR1 of unmanipulated Haplo versus MRD	Haplo: 185 MRD: 2469	2 year Haplo versus MRD 33% versus 35% $P=.05$	2 year NRM: Haplo versus MRD 23% versus 10%, $P<.01$	2 year CIR: Haplo versus MRD 19% versus 24%, $P=.10$	2 year Haplo versus MRD 68% versus 76%, $P<.01$

AML, acute myeloid leukemia; *PCR*, polymerase chain reaction; *NGS*, next-generation sequencing; *UCB*, umbilical cord blood.

'donor versus no donor' design has been challenged. Classically, an available donor was defined as having a matched sibling or unrelated donor. If outcomes of alternative donor transplants are similar, most patients will indeed have a donor.[107] However, despite multiple single center and registry studies, the hypothesis of similar outcomes with different donor types remains to be proven in prospective studies. A prospective BMT CTN is in preparation to address the question of haploidentical versus MUD transplantation. In addition, the BMT CTN is currently conducting a prospective study comparing UCB to haploidentical donors for hematologic malignancies (NCT01597778).

TRANSPLANTATION IN INDUCTION FAILURE OR IN RELAPSE

Patients that fail to achieve CR and are in primary induction failure (PIF) have no expectation of long-term disease control without allo-HSCT. Nevertheless, if further rounds of induction chemotherapy are administered, only a minority of patients will enter a CR and a substantial percentage develop infections or have a decline in performance status that will make allo-HSCT unfeasible. MD Anderson performed a retrospective study comparing outcomes of first salvage after failed high-dose cytarabine induction chemotherapy. OS at 2 years was substantially higher (39% vs. 2%) for patients that received an allogeneic transplant.[108] Many transplant physicians consider PIF to be an urgent situation where allo-HSCT should be performed, especially for those with AML that is not rapidly proliferating and have a preserved general condition. A retrospective analysis of 1673 AML patients who received myeloablative conditioning and stem cell transplant when not in CR found a 3-year OS rate of 19%. Notably, patients in PIF who immediately had allo-HSCT actually fared better than patients who were transplanted with relapsed disease after CR that lasted less than 6 months. Other significant risk factors included AML risk category, presence of circulating blasts, and degree of HLA match.[109] This retrospective analysis did not include alternative donor transplants (UCB or haploidentical) We consider any patient with PIF a potential candidate for emergent allo-HSCT, preferably in the setting of a clinical trial. Absence of circulating blasts, and a relatively indolent course of disease seem to identify the small but significant minority of candidates here.

Novel strategies to improve outcomes are being investigated. Both chemoimmunoradioconjugates and immunoradioconjugates are being employed in investigative settings to increase antitumor effect of conditioning prior to transplant. Antibodies conjugated with potent alkylating agents can selective result in leukemia cytotoxicity. Earlier attempts of targeted cytoxin delivery with antibodies targeting CD33 to cytoreduce active AML prior to transplant with gemtuzumab ozogamicin and vadastuximab talirine resulted in increased risks for hepatotoxicity and sinusoidal obstructive syndrome (NCT02614560).[110] Antibodies targeting CD45 conjugated to iodine 131 have shown promise as a minimally toxic regimen tolerable by older patients with acute myeloid leukemia.[111] Anti-CD45 antibody conjugated with cytotoxins has shown promise in murine models while avoiding cytopenias.[112] Supplementation of the graft with ex vivo expanded NK cells to improve GVL has been explored in very high-risk settings.[113] Finally, numerous post-transplant therapies have been suggested to improved outcomes and will be discussed below.

MANAGEMENT OF POSTTRANSPLANT RELAPSE

AML relapse is the major cause of allo-HSCT treatment failure, and to date, there is no standard management given the overall limited success of available therapies. Approaches almost invariable include additional cellular therapy with DLI or a second transplant.[114] Long-term survival rates vary from 5% to 30%, depending primarily on post-HSCT remission duration, PS, comorbidities and donor availability. DLI alone is usually inadequate and unanswered questions about this strategy remain, including role of therapy before and after DLI, timing, and ideal disease status to optimize outcome. Induction chemotherapy is often given as DLI performed in CR is more efficacious, but there are no standard salvage therapies in this setting.[115,116] Novel therapeutic agents may have additional roles in the post-allo-HSCT setting providing both direct cytotoxicity and increased tumor immunogenicity, either through activation of T cells and NK cells or increased expression of tumor antigens.[117] Azacitidine and decitabine have both have demonstrated limited efficacy in relapse after allo-HSCT and are usually combined with DLI.[118,119]

Cytokines and immunotherapy to enhance GVL are also being explored. Interferon-α can augment cytotoxic T-lymphocytes.[120] In small studies of relapsed acute leukemia, CR rates of up to 75% have been reported, including in the absence of additional cytotoxic therapy.[121] Immune checkpoint inhibition with the CTLA-4 antibody ipilimumab has been used with some efficacy in a small series of four patients with extramedullary AML relapsed after allo-HSCT.[122] Interleukin (IL)-15 activates NK cells and T cells and has the potential to enhance GVL. ALT-803 is a recombinant IL-15 complexed with a circulating receptor to extend the otherwise short half-life of the free cytokine. In a phase 1 trial of hematologic malignancies relapsing after allo-HSCT, ALT-803 induced a CR in myeloid malignancy and clinical benefit in patients with AML.[123]

Second allogeneic stem cell transplants have been performed. Registry outcome data suggest that 2-year OS is as high as 30%.[124] As with AML prior to transplant, the length of time in remission appears to be a major determinant in outcome for any treatment for AML relapsing after allo-HSCT.[125]

PREVENTING AML RELAPSE WITH POST-HSCT MAINTENANCE THERAPY

As discussed previously, AML relapsing after HSCT is associated with very poor outcomes. As a result, a number of maintenance strategies have been proposed to reduce the risk of relapse. A summary of maintenance therapies are presented in Table 9.5.

TABLE 9.5
Strategies to Prevent Relapse After Allo-HSCT

Strategy	Proposed Mechanism	Examples
Targeted maintenance therapies	• Small molecular inhibitors against driver mutations	• Sorafenib,[127,159] midostaurin,[160] gilteritinib,[61] quizartinib[129] for *FLT3* mutant disease • Imatinib, dasatinib, nilotinib for *BCR-ABL* positive AML[139,161]
Epigenetic maintenance therapy	• Reexpression of leukemia antigens, enhanced GVL • Suppression of leukemia driver mutations	• Azacitidine[132] • Decitabine[133] • Vorinostat[162] • Panobinostat[136]
Prophylactic donor lymphocyte infusion	• Enhanced GVL	• Wang et al.[142] • Yan et al.[143]
Preemptive treatment based on MRD monitoring	• Identification of high-risk patients for relapse	• Immune withdrawal[163] • Initiation of maintenance therapy on detection of MRD • MRD based prophylactic DLI[164]

Allo-HSCT, allogeneic hematopoietic stem cell transplant; *AML*, acute myeloid leukemia; *DLI*, donor lymphocyte infusion; *GVL*, graft-versus-leukemia.

For patients with FLT3-ITD, maintenance administration of FLT3 inhibitors is under active investigation. The earliest published examples were single-institution reports of sorafenib, a multi-targeted TKI including inhibition of FLT3. A phase 1 trial of 22 patients treated with up to 400 mg twice daily found a 1 year LFS of 85% with a median follow-up of 16.7 months.[126] Another study has preliminarily reported on 28 patients with FLT3-ITD AML given sorafenib before and after transplant. After a median of 14.8 months follow-up, only 5 relapses have been observed, and three of these patients were off therapy at the time of recurrence.[127] Challenges of this approach include drug toxicities and interactions. Other FLT3 inhibitors such as midostaurin, quizartinib, gilteritinib, and crenolanib are under active investigation. A phase II study of midostaurin maintenance therapy reported a low 12-month relapse rate of 9.2%.[128] A phase 1 study of post-HSCT quizartinib (n = 13 patients) observed only one relapse with over 12 months of median follow-up.[129,130] The BMT CTN is conducting a multicenter randomized, placebo controlled maintenance trial of gilteritinib after allo-HSCT for FLT3+ AML patients (clinicaltrials.gov identifier NCT02997202).

We and others have proposed that GVL and GVHD may be modulated by epigenetic modulation.[131] Hypomethylating agents (HMAs) that have been used after allo-HSCT include both azacitidine and decitabine. Concerns with HMAs are the additive toxicity, as myelosuppression and gastrointestinal side effects are common. Maximum tolerated doses for maintenance post-allo-HSCT are typically lower than standard doses given for active disease. A phase 1 study of Azacitidine found dosing at 32 mg/m^2 for 5 days to be safe.[132] Decitabine at doses up to 15 mg/m^2 for 5 days also seems tolerable after allo-HSCT.[119,133] A multicenter phase I/II trial of the oral azacitidine formulation (CC486) defined the dose of 200 mg PO daily for 14 days (in 28 da cycles) as well tolerated and devoid of major drug interactions. One-year OS was in excess of 80% (n = 30).[132,134,135]

Epigenetic modulation is also thought to be the primary mechanism of histone deacetylase (HDAC) inhibitors, and both vorinostat and panobinostat have been used after allo-HSCT. The former has been studied as GVHD prophylaxis in a phase 1–2 study in combination with tacrolimus and mycophenolate. The authors enrolled 50 patients (AML, n = 19). The cumulative incidence of grade II-IV acute GVHD and relapse was 22%, and 16%, respectively. Panobinostat was investigated in a phase 1/2 study as maintenance for AML and MDS patients, including 37 patients with high-risk AML. The 2 year cumulative incidence of relapse was 20%, whereas 2-year OS rate was 81%. An alternate week dosing scheduled was found to be the most tolerable.[136] Combination of HDAC inhibition and HMAs may further improve epigenetic modulation, though to date, concerns remain about toxicity and immunosuppression. A phase 1 study demonstrated the feasibility of the combination of panobinostat with decitabine, as well as low-dose DLI in very poor risk AML patients (n = 54). OS survival at 12 months was 81%, with 41 of 54 patients receiving epigenetic therapy. Despite DLI, a low rate of chronic GVHD was observed.[137]

AML with BCR-ABL is a rare entity generally considered to be of poor prognosis. Imatinib, dasatinib, nilotinib, and bosutinib are frequently used and case reports suggest efficacy.[138] Single-institution series suggest that imatinib maintenance results in durable remissions and potential cures.[139] Moreover, the EBMT published the outcomes of 57 patients undergoing allo-HSCT for BCR-ABL positive AML and found a 54% overall survival at 5 years, speculating that TKIs have been instrumental in improving survival.

Currently post-HSCT maintenance is considered experimental, and the decision to offer this treatment modality should take into consideration the risk of relapse, availability of clinical trials, and patient preference. Frequent monitoring is needed, and as in other transplant scenarios reviewed previously, prospective clinical trials are lacking or the results not available yet.

In addition to maintenance strategies, prophylactic DLI has been proposed to reduce relapse risk.[140,141] A risk-stratified approach has been suggested, with selective administration of additional donor cells for patients at very high risk of relapse. Retrospective series suggest that prophylactic DLI lead to significantly higher LFS in selected patients.[142] In a prospective fashion, Yan et al. evaluated prophylactic DLI in 100 high-risk AML patients after allo-HSCT. In the absence of GVHD, multiple DLIs were pursed. At 3 years, LFS was an encouraging 50.3%, though rates of GVHD were high as expected.[143]

FUTURE DIRECTION

GVL is frequently associated with GVHD, and separating these entities has been a major goal of investigating in our field for more than 30 years. As discussed, TRM has been significantly reduced, and relapse is the main cause of treatment failure. The education of recipient or donor lymphocytes by means of genetic engineering holds the promise of abolishing GVHD while increasing GVL efficacy. The success of chimeric antigen receptor cells (CAR T) targeting CD19 in acute lymphocytic leukemia is yet to be reproduced in AML.[144] Most of the initially investigated target antigens are broadly expressed in the hematopoietic system (CD33, CD123, for example), and therefore CAR T cells against these epitopes may lead to severe myelosuppression and graft failure.[145,146] Other targets are under investigation.

As with the field of AML treatment without treatment, it is hoped that identification of new molecularly driven targets will occur and lead to new agents, such as it has happened with FLT3 and IDH1/2.[147] Therefore, it is expected that these new agents will be also investigated as posttransplant maintenance or in the treatment of relapse.

Combination of cell therapy and pharmacologic agents is likely to play a role in the transplant setting, as exemplified by the newly renewed interest in NK cells and IL-15, for example, or with the use of HMA to increase tumor antigen expression, priming AML for immune checkpoint blockade. Therefore, it is expected that allogeneic transplantation for AML will benefit from findings in the immunology and pharmacologic arenas. The next 5 years will bring a variety of new approaches to the time honored allogeneic immune therapy camp, capitalizing on major achievements observed in the last 3 decades.

REFERENCES

1. Nathan PC, Sung L, Crump M, Beyene J. Consolidation therapy with autologous bone marrow transplantation in adults with acute myeloid leukemia: a meta-analysis. *JNCI J Natl Cancer Inst.* 2004;96(1):38–45.
2. Thomas ED, Buckner CD, Banaji M, et al. One hundred patients with acute leukemia treated by chemotherapy, total body irradiation, and allogeneic marrow transplantation. *Blood.* 1977;49(4):511–533.
3. Barnes DW, Corp MJ, Loutit JF, Neal FE. Treatment of murine leukaemia with X rays and homologous bone marrow; preliminary communication. *Br Med J.* 1956;2(4993):626–627.
4. Maraninchi D, Gluckman E, Blaise D, et al. Impact of T-cell depletion on outcome of allogeneic bone-marrow transplantation for standard-risk leukaemias. *Lancet.* 1987;2(8552):175–178.
5. Horowitz MM, Gale RP, Sondel PM, et al. Graft-versus-leukemia reactions after bone marrow transplantation. *Blood.* 1990;75(3):555–562.
6. Weiden PL, Sullivan KM, Flournoy N, Storb R, Thomas ED. Antileukemic effect of chronic graft-versus-host disease: contribution to improved survival after allogeneic marrow transplantation. *N Engl J Med.* 1981;304(25):1529–1533.
7. Mathe G, Amiel JL, Schwarzenberg L, et al. Successful allogenic bone marrow transplantation in man: chimerism, induced specific tolerance and possible anti-leukemic effects. *Blood.* 1965;25:179–196.
8. Radujkovic A, Guglielmi C, Bergantini S, et al. Donor lymphocyte infusions for chronic myeloid leukemia relapsing after allogeneic stem cell transplantation: may we predict graft-versus-leukemia without graft-versus-host disease? *Biol Blood Marrow Transplan.* 2015;21(7):1230–1236.
9. Kolb HJ, Rieder I, Rodt H, et al. Antilymphocytic antibodies and marrow transplantation. VI. Graft-versus-host tolerance in DLA-incompatible dogs after in vitro treatment of bone marrow with absorbed antithymocyte globulin. *Transplantation.* 1979;27(4):242–245.
10. Ridge JP, Di Rosa F, Matzinger P. A conditioned dendritic cell can be a temporal bridge between a CD4+ T-helper and a T-killer cell. *Nature.* 1998;393(6684):474–478.

11. Kolb HJ, Schattenberg A, Goldman JM, et al. Graft-versus-leukemia effect of donor lymphocyte transfusions in marrow grafted patients. *Blood.* 1995;86(5):2041–2050.

12. Chakraverty R, Eom HS, Sachs J, et al. Host MHC class II+ antigen-presenting cells and CD4 cells are required for CD8-mediated graft-versus-leukemia responses following delayed donor leukocyte infusions. *Blood.* 2006;108(6):2106–2113.

13. Dohner H, Weisdorf DJ, Bloomfield CD. Acute myeloid leukemia. *N Engl J Med.* 2015:373.

14. Bennett JM, Catovsky D, Daniel MT, et al. Proposed revised criteria for the classification of acute myeloid leukemia. A report of the French-American-British Cooperative Group. *Ann Intern Med.* 1985;103(4):620–625.

15. Arber DA, Orazi A, Hasserjian R, et al. The 2016 revision to the World Health Organization classification of myeloid neoplasms and acute leukemia. *Blood.* 2016;127(20):2391–2405.

16. Vardiman JW, Thiele J, Arber DA, et al. The 2008 revision of the World Health Organization (WHO) classification of myeloid neoplasms and acute leukemia: rationale and important changes. *Blood.* 2009;114(5):937–951.

17. Harris NL, Jaffe ES, Diebold J, et al. World Health Organization classification of neoplastic diseases of the hematopoietic and lymphoid tissues: report of the Clinical Advisory Committee meeting-Airlie House, Virginia, November 1997. *J Clin Oncol.* 1999;17(12):3835–3849.

18. Winters AC, Bernt KM. MLL-rearranged leukemias—an update on science and clinical approaches. *Front Pediatr.* 2017;5:4.

19. Churpek JE, Garcia JS, Madzo J, Jackson SA, Onel K, Godley LA. Identification and molecular characterization of a novel 3' mutation in RUNX1 in a family with familial platelet disorder. *Leukemia Lymphoma.* 2010;51(10):1931–1935.

20. Pabst T, Eyholzer M, Haefliger S, Schardt J, Mueller BU. Somatic CEBPA mutations are a frequent second event in families with germline CEBPA mutations and familial acute myeloid leukemia. *J Clin Oncol.* 2008;26(31):5088–5093.

21. Kee Y, D'Andrea AD. Molecular pathogenesis and clinical management of Fanconi anemia. *J Clin Investig.* 2012;122(11):3799–3806.

22. Nickels EM, Soodalter J, Churpek JE, Godley LA. Recognizing familial myeloid leukemia in adults. *Ther Adv Hematol.* 2013;4(4):254–269.

23. Peffault de Latour R, Peters C, Gibson B, et al. Recommendations on hematopoietic stem cell transplantation for inherited bone marrow failure syndromes. *Bone Marrow Transplant.* 2015;50(9):1168–1172.

24. Welch JS, Ley TJ, Link DC, et al. The origin and evolution of mutations in Acute Myeloid Leukemia. *Cell.* 2012;150(2):264–278.

25. Steensma DP, Baer MR, Slack JL, et al. Multicenter study of decitabine administered daily for 5 days every 4 Weeks to adults with myelodysplastic syndromes: the alternative dosing for outpatient treatment (ADOPT) trial. *J Clin Oncol.* 2009;27(23):3842–3848.

26. Jaiswal S, Natarajan P, Silver AJ, et al. Clonal hematopoiesis and risk of atherosclerotic cardiovascular disease. *N Engl J Med.* 2017;377(2):111–121.

27. Buchner T, Berdel WE, Haferlach C, et al. Age-related risk profile and chemotherapy dose response in acute myeloid leukemia: a study by the German Acute Myeloid Leukemia Cooperative Group. *J Clin Oncol.* 2009;27(1):61–69.

28. Appelbaum FR, Gundacker H, Head DR, et al. Age and acute myeloid leukemia. *Blood.* 2006;107(9):3481–3485.

29. Krug U, Rollig C, Koschmieder A, et al. Complete remission and early death after intensive chemotherapy in patients aged 60 years or older with acute myeloid leukaemia: a web-based application for prediction of outcomes. *Lancet.* 2010;376(9757):2000–2008.

30. Sorror ML, Sandmaier BM, Storer BE, et al. Long-term outcomes among older patients following nonmyeloablative conditioning and allogeneic hematopoietic cell transplantation for advanced hematologic malignancies. *JAMA.* 2011;306(17):1874–1883.

31. Sorror ML, Storb RF, Sandmaier BM, et al. Comorbidity-age index: a clinical measure of biologic age before allogeneic hematopoietic cell transplantation. *J Clin Oncol.* 2014;32(29):3249–3256.

32. Grimwade D, Hills RK, Moorman AV. Refinement of cytogenetic classification in acute myeloid leukaemia: determination of prognostic significance of rarer recurring chromosomal abnormalities amongst 5,876 younger adult patients treated in the UK Medical Research Council trials. *Blood.* 2010:116.

33. Döhner H, Estey E, Grimwade D, et al. Diagnosis and management of AML in adults: 2017 ELN recommendations from an international expert panel. *Blood.* 2017;129(4):424–447.

34. Dohner H, Estey EH, Amadori S. Diagnosis and management of acute myeloid leukemia in adults: recommendations from an international expert panel, on behalf of the European LeukemiaNet. *Blood.* 2010:115.

35. Schlenk RF, Döhner K, Krauter J, et al. Mutations and treatment outcome in cytogenetically normal acute myeloid leukemia. *N Engl J Med.* 2008;358(18):1909–1918.

36. Schlenk RF, Kayser S, Bullinger L, et al. Differential impact of allelic ratio and insertion site in FLT3-ITD-positive AML with respect to allogeneic transplantation. *Blood.* 2014;124(23):3441.

37. Kayser S, Dohner K, Krauter J, et al. The impact of therapy-related acute myeloid leukemia (AML) on outcome in 2853 adult patients with newly diagnosed AML. *Blood.* 2011;117(7):2137–2145.

38. Granfeldt Ostgard LS, Medeiros BC, Sengelov H, et al. Epidemiology and clinical significance of secondary and therapy-related acute myeloid leukemia: a national population-based cohort study. *J Clin Oncol.* 2015;33(31):3641–3649.

39. Ravandi F. Primary refractory acute myeloid leukaemia – in search of better definitions and therapies. *Br J Haematol.* 2011;155(4):413–419.

40. Breems DA, Van Putten WLJ, Huijgens PC, et al. Prognostic index for adult patients with acute myeloid leukemia in first relapse. *J Clin Oncol*. 2005;23(9):1969–1978.

41. Cheson BD, Bennett JM, Kopecky KJ, et al. Revised recommendations of the international working group for diagnosis, standardization of response criteria, treatment outcomes, and reporting standards for therapeutic trials in acute myeloid leukemia. *J Clin Oncol*. 2003;21(24):4642–4649.

42. Al-Mawali A, Gillis D, Lewis I. The role of multiparameter flow cytometry for detection of minimal residual disease in acute myeloid leukemia. *Am J Clin Pathol*. 2009;131(1):16–26.

43. Jongen-Lavrencic M, Grob T, Hanekamp D, et al. Molecular minimal residual disease in acute myeloid leukemia. *N Engl J Med*. 2018;378(13):1189–1199.

44. Gabert J, Beillard E, van der Velden VH, et al. Standardization and quality control studies of 'real-time' quantitative reverse transcriptase polymerase chain reaction of fusion gene transcripts for residual disease detection in leukemia - a Europe against Cancer program. *Leukemia*. 2003;17(12):2318–2357.

45. Terwijn M, van Putten WL, Kelder A, et al. High prognostic impact of flow cytometric minimal residual disease detection in acute myeloid leukemia: data from the HOVON/SAKK AML 42A study. *J Clin Oncol*. 2013;31(31):3889–3897.

46. Ivey A, Hills RK, Simpson MA, et al. Assessment of minimal residual disease in standard-risk AML. *N Engl J Med*. 2016;374(5):422–433.

47. Freeman SD, Virgo P, Couzens S, et al. Prognostic relevance of treatment response measured by flow cytometric residual disease detection in older patients with acute myeloid leukemia. *J Clin Oncol*. 2013;31(32):4123–4131.

48. Walter RB, Gooley TA, Wood BL, et al. Impact of pretransplantation minimal residual disease, as detected by multiparametric flow cytometry, on outcome of myeloablative hematopoietic cell transplantation for acute myeloid leukemia. *J Clin Oncol*. 2011;29(9):1190–1197.

49. Chen Y, Kantarjian H, Pierce S, et al. Prognostic significance of 11q23 aberrations in adult acute myeloid leukemia and the role of allogeneic stem cell transplantation. *Leukemia*. 2013;27(4):836–842.

50. Zhou Y, Othus M, Araki D, et al. Pre- and post-transplant quantification of measurable ('minimal') residual disease via multiparameter flow cytometry in adult acute myeloid leukemia. *Leukemia*. 2016;30(7):1456–1464.

51. Ustun C, Courville E, DeFor T, et al. Myeloablative, but not reduced-intensity, conditioning overcomes the negative effect of flow-cytometric evidence of leukemia in Aml. *Biol Blood Marrow Transplant*. 2016;22(4):669–675.

52. Ustun C, Wiseman AC, Defor TE, et al. Achieving stringent CR is essential before reduced-intensity conditioning allogeneic hematopoietic cell transplantation in AML. *Bone Marrow Transplant*. 2013;48(11):1415–1420.

53. Araki D, Wood BL, Othus M, et al. Allogeneic hematopoietic cell transplantation for acute myeloid leukemia: time to move toward a minimal residual disease-based definition of complete remission? *J Clin Oncol*. 2016; 34(4):329–336.

54. Buckley SA, Wood BL, Othus M, et al. Minimal residual disease prior to allogeneic hematopoietic cell transplantation in acute myeloid leukemia: a meta-analysis. *Haematologica*. 2017;102(5):865–873.

55. Suciu S, Mandelli F, de Witte T, et al. Allogeneic compared with autologous stem cell transplantation in the treatment of patients younger than 46 years with acute myeloid leukemia (AML) in first complete remission (CR1): an intention-to-treat analysis of the EORTC/GIMEMAAML-10 trial. *Blood*. 2003;102(4):1232–1240.

56. Burnett AK, Wheatley K, Goldstone AH, et al. The value of allogeneic bone marrow transplant in patients with acute myeloid leukaemia at differing risk of relapse: results of the UK MRC AML 10 trial. *Br J Haematol*. 2002;118(2):385–400.

57. Jourdan E, Boiron J-M, Dastugue N, et al. Early allogeneic stem-cell transplantation for young adults with acute myeloblastic leukemia in first complete remission: an intent-to-treat long-term analysis of the BGMT experience. *J Clin Oncol*. 2005;23(30):7676–7684.

58. Cornelissen JJ, Putten WL, Verdonck LF. Results of a HOVON/SAKK donor versus no-donor analysis of myeloablative HLA-identical sibling stem cell transplantation in first remission acute myeloid leukemia in young and middle-aged adults: benefits for whom? *Blood*. 2007:109.

59. Koreth J, Schlenk R, Kopecky KJ. Allogeneic stem cell transplantation for acute myeloid leukemia in first complete remission: systematic review and meta-analysis of prospective clinical trials. *JAMA*. 2009:301.

60. Flomenberg N, Baxter-Lowe LA, Confer D, et al. Impact of HLA class I and class II high-resolution matching on outcomes of unrelated donor bone marrow transplantation: HLA-C mismatching is associated with a strong adverse effect on transplantation outcome. *Blood*. 2004;104(7):1923–1930.

61. Pratz KW, Levis M. How I treat FLT3-mutated AML. *Blood*. 2017;129(5):565.

62. Leung W, Pui C-H, Coustan-Smith E, et al. Detectable minimal residual disease before hematopoietic cell transplantation is prognostic but does not preclude cure for children with very-high-risk leukemia. *Blood*. 2012;120(2):468–472.

63. Santos GW, Tutschka PJ, Brookmeyer R, et al. Marrow transplantation for acute nonlymphocytic leukemia after treatment with busulfan and cyclophosphamide. *N Engl J Med*. 1983;309(22):1347–1353.

64. Andersson BS, de Lima M, Thall PF, et al. Once daily i.v. busulfan and fludarabine (i.v. Bu-Flu) compares favorably with i.v. busulfan and cyclophosphamide (i.v. BuCy2) as pretransplant conditioning therapy in AML/MDS. *Biol Blood Marrow Transplant*. 2008;14(6):672–684.

65. Ringden O, Remberger M, Ruutu T, et al. Increased risk of chronic graft-versus-host disease, obstructive bronchiolitis, and alopecia with busulfan versus total body irradiation: long-term results of a randomized trial in allogeneic marrow recipients with leukemia. Nordic Bone Marrow Transplantation Group. *Blood.* 1999;93(7):2196–2201.

66. Blaise D, Maraninchi D, Michallet M, et al. Long-term follow-up of a randomized trial comparing the combination of cyclophosphamide with total body irradiation or busulfan as conditioning regimen for patients receiving HLA-identical marrow grafts for acute myeloblastic leukemia in first complete remission. *Blood.* 2001;97(11):3669–3671.

67. Kashyap A, Wingard J, Cagnoni P, et al. Intravenous versus oral busulfan as part of a busulfan/cyclophosphamide preparative regimen for allogeneic hematopoietic stem cell transplantation: decreased incidence of hepatic venoocclusive disease (HVOD), HVOD-related mortality, and overall 100-day mortality. *Biol Blood Marrow Transplant.* 2002;8(9):493–500.

68. Lee JH, Choi SJ, Lee JH, et al. Decreased incidence of hepatic veno-occlusive disease and fewer hemostatic derangements associated with intravenous busulfan vs oral busulfan in adults conditioned with busulfan + cyclophosphamide for allogeneic bone marrow transplantation. *Ann Hematol.* 2005;84(5):321–330.

69. Nath CE, Shaw PJ. Busulphan in blood and marrow transplantation: dose, route, frequency and role of therapeutic drug monitoring. *Curr Clin Pharmacol.* 2007;2(1):75–91.

70. Sobecks RM, Rybicki L, Yurch M, et al. Intravenous compared with oral busulfan as preparation for allogeneic hematopoietic progenitor cell transplantation for AML and MDS. *Bone Marrow Transplant.* 2012;47(5):633–638.

71. McCune JS, Gibbs JP, Slattery JT. Plasma concentration monitoring of busulfan: does it improve clinical outcome? *Clin Pharmacokinetics.* 2000;39(2):155–165.

72. Bredeson C, LeRademacher J, Kato K, et al. Prospective cohort study comparing intravenous busulfan to total body irradiation in hematopoietic cell transplantation. *Blood.* 2013;122(24):3871–3878.

73. Copelan EA, Hamilton BK, Avalos B, et al. Better leukemia-free and overall survival in AML in first remission following cyclophosphamide in combination with busulfan compared with TBI. *Blood.* 2013;122(24):3863–3870.

74. Nagler A, Rocha V, Labopin M, et al. Allogeneic hematopoietic stem-cell transplantation for acute myeloid leukemia in remission: comparison of intravenous busulfan plus cyclophosphamide (Cy) versus total-body irradiation plus Cy as conditioning regimen–a report from the acute leukemia working party of the European Society for blood and marrow transplantation. *J Clin Oncol.* 2013;31(28):3549–3556.

75. de Lima M, Couriel D, Thall PF, et al. Once-daily intravenous busulfan and fludarabine: clinical and pharmacokinetic results of a myeloablative, reduced-toxicity conditioning regimen for allogeneic stem cell transplantation in AML and MDS. *Blood.* 2004;104(3):857–864.

76. Rambaldi A, Grassi A, Masciulli A, et al. Busulfan plus cyclophosphamide versus busulfan plus fludarabine as a preparative regimen for allogeneic haemopoietic stem-cell transplantation in patients with acute myeloid leukaemia: an open-label, multicentre, randomised, phase 3 trial. *Lancet Oncol.* 2015;16(15):1525–1536.

77. Giralt S, Thall PF, Khouri I, et al. Melphalan and purine analog-containing preparative regimens: reduced-intensity conditioning for patients with hematologic malignancies undergoing allogeneic progenitor cell transplantation. *Blood.* 2001;97(3):631–637.

78. Estey E, de Lima M, Tibes R, et al. Prospective feasibility analysis of reduced-intensity conditioning (RIC) regimens for hematopoietic stem cell transplantation (HSCT) in elderly patients with acute myeloid leukemia (AML) and high-risk myelodysplastic syndrome (MDS). *Blood.* 2007;109(4):1395–1400.

79. Mohty M, de Lavallade H, El-Cheikh J, et al. Reduced intensity conditioning allogeneic stem cell transplantation for patients with acute myeloid leukemia: long term results of a 'donor' versus 'no donor' comparison. *Leukemia.* 2009;23(1):194–196.

80. Versluis J, Hazenberg CL, Passweg JR. Post-remission treatment with allogeneic stem cell transplantation in patients aged 60 years and older with acute myeloid leukaemia: a time-dependent analysis. *Lancet Haematol.* 2015;2.

81. de Lima M. Aging and transplanting graciously. *Lancet Haematol.* 2015;2(10):e398–e399.

82. Scott BL, Sandmaier BM, Storer B, et al. Myeloablative vs nonmyeloablative allogeneic transplantation for patients with myelodysplastic syndrome or acute myelogenous leukemia with multilineage dysplasia: a retrospective analysis. *Leukemia.* 2006;20(1):128–135.

83. Alyea EP, Kim HT, Ho V. Comparative outcome of nonmyeloablative and myeloablative allogeneic hematopoietic cell transplantation for patients older than 50 years of age. *Blood.* 2005:105.

84. Lioure B, Bene MC, Pigneux A, et al. Early matched sibling hematopoietic cell transplantation for adult AML in first remission using an age-adapted strategy: long-term results of a prospective GOELAMS study. *Blood.* 2012;119(12):2943–2948.

85. Scott BL, Pasquini MC, Logan BR, et al. Myeloablative versus reduced-intensity hematopoietic cell transplantation for acute myeloid leukemia and myelodysplastic syndromes. *J Clin Oncol.* 2017;35(11):1154–1161.

86. Sengsayadeth S, Savani BN, Blaise D, Malard F, Nagler A, Mohty M. Reduced intensity conditioning allogeneic hematopoietic cell transplantation for adult acute myeloid leukemia in complete remission - a review from the Acute Leukemia Working Party of the EBMT. *Haematologica.* 2015;100(7):859–869.

87. Childs R, Clave E, Contentin N, et al. Engraftment kinetics after nonmyeloablative allogeneic peripheral blood stem cell transplantation: full donor T-cell chimerism precedes alloimmune responses. *Blood*. 1999;94(9):3234–3241.

88. Slavin S, Nagler A, Naparstek E, et al. Nonmyeloablative stem cell transplantation and cell therapy as an alternative to conventional bone marrow transplantation with lethal cytoreduction for the treatment of malignant and nonmalignant hematologic diseases. *Blood*. 1998;91(3):756–763.

89. Baron F, Maris MB, Sandmaier BM, et al. Graft-versus-tumor effects after allogeneic hematopoietic cell transplantation with nonmyeloablative conditioning. *J Clin Oncol*. 2005;23(9):1993–2003.

90. Kottaridis PD, Milligan DW, Chopra R, et al. In vivo CAMPATH-1H prevents graft-versus-host disease following nonmyeloablative stem cell transplantation. *Blood*. 2000;96(7):2419–2425.

91. Bayraktar UD, de Lima M, Saliba RM, et al. Ex vivo T cell-depleted versus unmodified allografts in patients with acute myeloid leukemia in first complete remission. *Biol Blood Marrow Transplant*. 2013;19(6):898–903.

92. McClune BL, Weisdorf DJ, Pedersen TL, et al. Effect of age on outcome of reduced-intensity hematopoietic cell transplantation for older patients with acute myeloid leukemia in first complete remission or with myelodysplastic syndrome. *J Clin Oncol*. 2010;28(11):1878–1887.

93. Herr AL, Labopin M, Blaise D, et al. HLA-identical sibling allogeneic peripheral blood stem cell transplantation with reduced intensity conditioning compared to autologous peripheral blood stem cell transplantation for elderly patients with de novo acute myeloid leukemia. *Leukemia*. 2007;21(1):129–135.

94. Bacigalupo A, Ballen K, Rizzo D, et al. Defining the intensity of conditioning regimens: working definitions. *Biol Blood Marrow Transplant*. 2009;15(12):1628–1633.

95. Deeg HJ, Sandmaier BM. Who is fit for allogeneic transplantation? *Blood*. 2010;116(23):4762–4770.

96. de Lima M, Anagnostopoulos A, Munsell M, et al. Nonablative versus reduced-intensity conditioning regimens in the treatment of acute myeloid leukemia and high-risk myelodysplastic syndrome: dose is relevant for long-term disease control after allogeneic hematopoietic stem cell transplantation. *Blood*. 2004;104(3):865.

97. Kurtzberg J, Laughlin M, Graham ML, et al. Placental blood as a source of hematopoietic stem cells for transplantation into unrelated recipients. *N Engl J Med*. 1996;335(3):157–166.

98. Ooi J, Iseki T, Takahashi S, et al. Unrelated cord blood transplantation for adult patients with de novo acute myeloid leukemia. *Blood*. 2004;103(2):489.

99. Sanz J, Boluda JC, Martin C, et al. Single-unit umbilical cord blood transplantation from unrelated donors in patients with hematological malignancy using busulfan, thiotepa, fludarabine and ATG as myeloablative conditioning regimen. *Bone Marrow Transplant*. 2012;47(10):1287–1293.

100. Laughlin MJ, Barker J, Bambach B, et al. Hematopoietic engraftment and survival in adult recipients of umbilical-cord blood from unrelated donors. *N Engl J Med*. 2001;344(24):1815–1822.

101. Ballen KK, Spitzer TR, Yeap BY, et al. Double unrelated reduced-intensity umbilical cord blood transplantation in adults. *Biol Blood Marrow Transplant*. 2007;13(1):82–89.

102. Barker JN, Fei M, Karanes C, et al. Results of a prospective multicentre myeloablative double-unit cord blood transplantation trial in adult patients with acute leukaemia and myelodysplasia. *Br J Haematol*. 2015;168(3):405–412.

103. Brunstein CG, Gutman JA, Weisdorf DJ, et al. Allogeneic hematopoietic cell transplantation for hematologic malignancy: relative risks and benefits of double umbilical cord blood. *Blood*. 2010;116(22):4693–4699.

104. Peffault de Latour R, Brunstein CG, Porcher R, et al. Similar overall survival using sibling, unrelated donor, and cord blood grafts after reduced-intensity conditioning for older patients with acute myelogenous leukemia. *Biol Blood Marrow Transplant*. 2013;19(9):1355–1360.

105. Rocha V, Labopin M, Sanz G, et al. Transplants of umbilical-cord blood or bone marrow from unrelated donors in adults with acute leukemia. *N Engl J Med*. 2004;351(22):2276–2285.

106. Milano F, Gooley T, Wood B, et al. Cord-blood transplantation in patients with minimal residual disease. *N Engl J Med*. 2016;375(10):944–953.

107. Ciurea SO, Zhang MJ, Bacigalupo AA, et al. Haploidentical transplant with posttransplant cyclophosphamide vs matched unrelated donor transplant for acute myeloid leukemia. *Blood*. 2015;126(8):1033–1040.

108. Jabbour E, Daver N, Champlin R, et al. Allogeneic stem cell transplantation as initial salvage for patients with acute myeloid leukemia refractory to high-dose cytarabine-based induction chemotherapy. *Am J Hematol*. 2014;89(4):395–398.

109. Duval M, Klein JP, He W, et al. Hematopoietic stem-cell transplantation for acute leukemia in relapse or primary induction failure. *J Clin Oncol*. 2010;28(23):3730–3738.

110. Wang ES, Zeidan A, Tan W, et al. Cytoreduction with gemtuzumab ozogamicin and cytarabine prior to allogeneic stem cell transplant for relapsed/refractory acute myeloid leukemia. *Leukemia Lymphoma*. 2012;53(10):2085–2088.

111. Pagel JM, Gooley TA, Rajendran J, et al. Allogeneic hematopoietic cell transplantation after conditioning with 131I-anti-CD45 antibody plus fludarabine and low-dose total body irradiation for elderly patients with advanced acute myeloid leukemia or high-risk myelodysplastic syndrome. *Blood*. 2009;114(27):5444.

112. Palchaudhuri R, Saez B, Hoggatt J, et al. Non-genotoxic conditioning for hematopoietic stem cell transplantation using a hematopoietic-cell-specific internalizing immunotoxin. *Nat Biotechnol*. 2016;34(7):738–745.

113. Ciurea SO, Schafer JR, Bassett R, et al. Phase 1 clinical trial using mbIL21 ex vivo-expanded donor-derived NK cells after haploidentical transplantation. *Blood*. 2017;130(16):1857–1868.

114. van den Brink MR, Porter DL, Giralt S, et al. Relapse after allogeneic hematopoietic cell therapy. *Biol Blood Marrow Transplant.* 2010;16(suppl 1):S138–S145.

115. Levine JE, Braun T, Penza SL, et al. Prospective trial of chemotherapy and donor leukocyte infusions for relapse of advanced myeloid malignancies after allogeneic stem-cell transplantation. *J Clin Oncol.* 2002;20(2):405–412.

116. Schmid C, Labopin M, Nagler A, et al. Treatment, risk factors, and outcome of adults with relapsed AML after reduced intensity conditioning for allogeneic stem cell transplantation. *Blood.* 2012;119(6):1599–1606.

117. Goodyear O, Agathanggelou A, Novitzky-Basso I, et al. Induction of a CD8+ T-cell response to the MAGE cancer testis antigen by combined treatment with azacitidine and sodium valproate in patients with acute myeloid leukemia and myelodysplasia. *Blood.* 2010;116(11):1908–1918.

118. Schroeder T, Czibere A, Platzbecker U, et al. Azacitidine and donor lymphocyte infusions as first salvage therapy for relapse of AML or MDS after allogeneic stem cell transplantation. *Leukemia.* 2013;27(6):1229–1235.

119. Schroeder T, Rautenberg C, Haas R, Kobbe G. Hypomethylating agents after allogeneic blood stem cell transplantation. *Stem Cell Invest.* 2016;3:84.

120. Robb RJ, Kreijveld E, Kuns RD, et al. Type I-IFNs control GVHD and GVL responses after transplantation. *Blood.* 2011;118(12):3399–3409.

121. Tang X, Zhou Q, Jin Z, et al. Novel therapy with interferon-α in combination with donor lymphocyte infusion for high risk acute leukemia patients who relapsed after allogeneic hematopoietic stem cell transplantation. *Blood.* 2011;118(21):658.

122. Davids MS, Kim HT, Bachireddy P, et al. Ipilimumab for patients with relapse after allogeneic transplantation. *N Engl J Med.* 2016;375(2):143–153.

123. Romee R, Cooley S, Berrien-Elliott MM, et al. First-in-human phase 1 clinical study of the IL-15 superagonist complex ALT-803 to treat relapse after transplantation. *Blood.* 2018.

124. Shaw BE, Mufti GJ, Mackinnon S, et al. Outcome of second allogeneic transplants using reduced-intensity conditioning following relapse of haematological malignancy after an initial allogeneic transplant. *Bone Marrow Transplant.* 2008;42(12):783–789.

125. Bejanyan N, Weisdorf DJ, Logan BR, et al. Survival of AML patients relapsing after allogeneic hematopoietic cell transplantation: a CIBMTR study. *Biol Blood Marrow Transplant.* 2015;21(3):454–459.

126. Chen YB, Li S, Lane AA, et al. Phase I trial of maintenance sorafenib after allogeneic hematopoietic stem cell transplantation for fms-like tyrosine kinase 3 internal tandem duplication acute myeloid leukemia. *Biol Blood Marrow Transplant.* 2014;20(12):2042–2048.

127. Pratz KW, Gojo I, Karp JE, et al. Prospective study of peri-transplant use of sorafenib as remission maintenance for FLT3-ITD patients undergoing allogeneic transplantation. *Blood.* 2015;126(23):3164.

128. Schlenk R, Döhner K, Salih H, et al. Midostaurin in combination with intensive induction and as single agent maintenance therapy after consolidation therapy with allogeneic hematopoietic stem cell transplantation or high-dose cytarabine (NCT01477606). *Blood.* 2015;126(23):322.

129. Sandmaier BM, Khaled S, Oran B, Gammon G, Trone D, Frankfurt O. Results of a phase 1 study of quizartinib as maintenance therapy in subjects with acute myeloid leukemia in remission following allogeneic hematopoietic stem cell transplant. *Am J Hematol.* 2018;93(2):222–231.

130. Collins R, Kantarjian HM, Ravandi F, et al. Full doses of crenolanib, a type I FLT3 inhibitor, can be safely administered in AML patients post allogeneic stem cell transplant. *Blood.* 2015;126(23):4359.

131. Bashir Q, William BM, Garcia-Manero G, de Lima M. Epigenetic therapy in allogeneic hematopoietic stem cell transplantation. *Rev Bras Hematol Hemoter.* 2013;35(2):126–133.

132. de Lima M, Giralt S, Thall PF, et al. Maintenance therapy with low-dose azacitidine after allogeneic hematopoietic stem cell transplantation for recurrent acute myelogenous leukemia or myelodysplastic syndrome: a dose and schedule finding study. *Cancer.* 2010;116(23):5420–5431.

133. Pusic I, Choi J, Fiala MA, et al. Maintenance therapy with decitabine after allogeneic stem cell transplantation for acute myelogenous leukemia and myelodysplastic syndrome. *Biol Blood Marrow Transplant.* 2015;21(10):1761–1769.

134. de Lima M, Porter DL, Battiwalla M, et al. Proceedings from the National Cancer Institute's Second International Workshop on the biology, prevention, and treatment of relapse after hematopoietic stem cell transplantation: part III. Prevention and treatment of relapse after allogeneic transplantation. *Biol Blood Marrow Transplant.* 2014;20(1):4–13.

135. de Lima M, Oran B, Papadopoulos EB, et al. CC-486 (oral azacitidine) maintenance therapy is well tolerated after allogeneic hematopoietic stem cell transplantation (AlloHSCT) in patients with myelodysplastic syndromes (MDS) or acute myeloid leukemia (AML). *Biol Blood Marrow Transplant.* 2016;22(3):S312–S313.

136. Bug G, Burchert A, Wagner EM, et al. Phase I/II study of the deacetylase inhibitor panobinostat after allogeneic stem cell transplantation in patients with high-risk MDS or AML (PANOBEST trial). *Leukemia.* 2017;31(11):2523–2525.

137. Cornelissen JJ, van Norden Y, van Gelder M, et al. Early post-transplant epigenetic therapy by panobinostat and decitabine followed by donor lymphocyte infusion (DLI): interim results of the HOVON-116 phase I/II feasibility study in poor-risk AML recipients of allogeneic stem cell transplantation (alloHSCT). *Blood.* 2016;128(22):832.

138. Neuendorff NR, Burmeister T, Dorken B, Westermann J. BCR-ABL-positive acute myeloid leukemia: a new entity? Analysis of clinical and molecular features. *Ann Hematol.* 2016;95(8):1211–1221.

139. Bhatt VR, Akhtari M, Bociek RG, et al. Allogeneic stem cell transplantation for Philadelphia chromosome-positive acute myeloid leukemia. *J Natl Compr Cancer Netw.* 2014;12(7):963–968.

140. Eefting M, Halkes CJ, de Wreede LC, et al. Myeloablative T cell-depleted alloSCT with early sequential prophylactic donor lymphocyte infusion is an efficient and safe post-remission treatment for adult ALL. *Bone Marrow Transplant.* 2014;49(2):287–291.

141. Krishnamurthy P, Potter VT, Barber LD, et al. Outcome of donor lymphocyte infusion after T cell-depleted allogeneic hematopoietic stem cell transplantation for acute myelogenous leukemia and myelodysplastic syndromes. *Biol Blood Marrow Transplant.* 2013;19(4):562–568.

142. Wang Y, Liu DH, Fan ZP, et al. Prevention of relapse using DLI can increase survival following HLA-identical transplantation in patients with advanced-stage acute leukemia: a multi-center study. *Clin Transplant.* 2012;26(4):635–643.

143. Yan CH, Liu QF, Wu DP, et al. Prophylactic donor lymphocyte infusion (DLI) followed by minimal residual disease and graft-versus-host disease-guided multiple DLIs could improve outcomes after allogeneic hematopoietic stem cell transplantation in patients with refractory/relapsed acute leukemia. *Biol Blood Marrow Transplant.* 2017;23(8):1311–1319.

144. Park JH, Rivière I, Gonen M, et al. Long-term follow-up of CD19 CAR therapy in acute lymphoblastic leukemia. *N Engl J Med.* 2018;378(5):449–459.

145. Rafiq S, Purdon TJ, Schultz LM, Brentjens RJ. CD33-Directed chimeric antigen receptor (CAR) T cells for the treatment of acute myeloid leukemia (AML). *Blood.* 2016;128(22):2825.

146. Luo Y, Chang L-J, Hu Y, Dong L, Wei G, Huang H. First-in-Man CD123-specific chimeric antigen receptor-modified T cells for the treatment of refractory acute myeloid leukemia. *Blood.* 2015;126(23):3778.

147. Stein EM, DiNardo CD, Pollyea DA, et al. Enasidenib in mutant-IDH2 relapsed or refractory acute myeloid leukemia. *Blood.* 2017.

148. Miyazaki T, Fujita H, Fujimaki K, et al. Clinical significance of minimal residual disease detected by multidimensional flow cytometry: serial monitoring after allogeneic stem cell transplantation for acute leukemia. *Leukemia Res.* 2012;36(8):998–1003.

149. Wang Y, Wu DP, Liu QF, et al. In adults with t(8;21)AML, posttransplant RUNX1/RUNX1T1-based MRD monitoring, rather than c-KIT mutations, allows further risk stratification. *Blood.* 2014;124(12):1880–1886.

150. Elmaagacli AH, Beelen DW, Kroll M, Trzensky S, Stein C, Schaefer UW. Detection of CBFbeta/MYH11 fusion transcripts in patients with inv(16) acute myeloid leukemia after allogeneic bone marrow or peripheral blood progenitor cell transplantation. *Bone Marrow Transplant.* 1998;21(2):159–166.

151. Bacher U, Badbaran A, Fehse B, Zabelina T, Zander AR, Kroger N. Quantitative monitoring of NPM1 mutations provides a valid minimal residual disease parameter following allogeneic stem cell transplantation. *Exp Hematol.* 2009;37(1):135–142.

152. Versluis J, Labopin M, Ruggeri A, et al. Alternative donors for allogeneic hematopoietic stem cell transplantation in poor-risk AML in CR1. *Blood Adv.* 2017;1(7):477–485.

153. Piemontese S, Ciceri F, Labopin M, et al. A comparison between allogeneic stem cell transplantation from unmanipulated haploidentical and unrelated donors in acute leukemia. *J Hematol Oncol.* 2017;10:24.

154. Sun Y, Beohou E, Labopin M, et al. Unmanipulated haploidentical versus matched unrelated donor allogeneic stem cell transplantation in adult patients with acute myelogenous leukemia in first remission: a retrospective pair-matched comparative study of the Beijing approach with the EBMT database. *Haematologica.* 2016;101(8):e352–e354.

155. Wang Y, Liu Q-F, Xu L-P, et al. Haploidentical vs identical-sibling transplant for AML in remission: a multicenter, prospective study. *Blood.* 2015;125(25):3956–3962.

156. Rashidi A, DiPersio JF, Westervelt P, et al. Comparison of outcomes after peripheral blood haploidentical versus matched unrelated donor allogeneic hematopoietic cell transplantation in patients with acute myeloid leukemia: a retrospective single-center review. *Biol Blood Marrow Transplant.* 2016;22(9):1696–1701.

157. How J, Slade M, Vu K, et al. T cell-replete peripheral blood haploidentical hematopoietic cell transplantation with post-transplantation cyclophosphamide results in outcomes similar to transplantation from traditionally matched donors in active disease acute myeloid leukemia. *Biol Blood Marrow Transplant.* 2017;23(4):648–653.

158. Salvatore D, Labopin M, Ruggeri A, et al. Outcomes of hematopoietic stem cell transplantation from unmanipulated haploidentical versus matched sibling donor in patients with acute myeloid leukemia in first complete remission with intermediate or high-risk cytogenetics: a study from the Acute Leukemia Working Party of the European Society for Blood and Marrow Transplantation. *Haematologica.* 2018.

159. Battipaglia G, Ruggeri A, Massoud R, et al. Efficacy and feasibility of sorafenib as a maintenance agent after allogeneic hematopoietic stem cell transplantation for Fms-like tyrosine kinase 3-mutated acute myeloid leukemia. *Cancer.* 2017;123(15):2867–2874.

160. Maziarz RT, Patnaik MM, Scott BL, et al. Radius: a phase 2, randomized trial of standard of care (SOC) with or without midostaurin to prevent relapse following allogeneic hematopoietic stem cell transplant (alloHSCT) in patients (pts) with FLT3-Itd-Mutated acute myeloid leukemia (AML). *Blood.* 2016;128(22):2248.

161. Lazarevic VL, Labopin M, Depei W, et al. Relatively favorable outcome after allogeneic stem cell transplantation for BCR-ABL1-positive AML: a survey from the acute leukemia working party of the European Society for blood and marrow transplantation (EBMT). *Am J Hematol.* 2018;93(1):31–39.

162. Choi SW, Braun T, Chang L, et al. Vorinostat plus tacrolimus and mycophenolate to prevent graft-versus-host disease after related-donor reduced-intensity conditioning allogeneic haemopoietic stem-cell transplantation: a phase 1/2 trial. *Lancet Oncol.* 2014;15(1):87–95.

163. Rein LAM, Sung AD, Rizzieri DA. New approaches to manipulate minimal residual disease after allogeneic

stem cell transplantation. *Int J Hematol Oncol.* 2013;2(1). https://doi.org/10.2217/ijh.2213.2214.

164. Dominietto A, Pozzi S, Miglino M, et al. Donor lymphocyte infusions for the treatment of minimal residual disease in acute leukemia. *Blood.* 2007;109(11):5063–5064.

Hematopoietic Cell Transplantation for Acute Lymphoblastic Leukemia

L.M. POON • PARTOW KEBRIAEI MD

INTRODUCTION

Acute lymphoblastic leukemia (ALL) is a neoplasm originating from B or T lymphocyte precursors which undergo malignant transformation. ALL accounts 10% of all leukemia cases in adults and an annual incidence of 1.7 per 100,000 men and women per year.[1] Unlike the dramatic advances made in the treatment of childhood ALL with 5-year survival at more than 90%,[2] therapeutic progress for adult ALL remains considerably inferior, with only 30%–40% patients achieving long-term leukemia-free survival.[3-6] Although complete remission rates are high (80%–90%) with modern induction regimens,[4,6] the major barrier to improved results in adult ALL treatment remains the high relapse rates after first complete remission (CR1). Allogeneic transplantation remains the most effective modality for consolidation and prevention of relapse. Unfortunately, the efficacy of allo-HCT is balanced by significantly higher acute and long-term toxicity, with allo-HSCT.[7] Thus, identifying prognostic markers which could help determine the appropriate timing of allo-HCT in the treatment algorithm of ALL is paramount to ensure optimal utilization of this treatment modality. This decision-making algorithm is made more complicated in the current treatment landscape of ALL. Advances include the increasing use of alternative donor transplants and reduced intensity-conditioning regimens which have increased the accessibility of allogeneic transplantation versus the advent of pediatric chemotherapy protocols and incorporation of novel agents into ALL treatment protocols which have improved cure rates in adult ALL and brought into question the adverse prognosis of some traditional high-risk factors for ALL.

In this chapter, we aim to focus on the role of allo-HCT for adult ALL in CR1 and beyond based on a risk-oriented paradigm, which takes into account the increasing utilization of minimal residual disease (MRD) monitoring. We also explore advances in the field of allo-HCT including the use of alternative donors and the development of reduced intensity conditioning regimens and their impact on the ALL treatment algorithm.

Allo-HCT in CR1 for Ph-Negative ALL

After achieving complete remission with induction therapy, consolidation options include continued chemotherapy or allogeneic transplantation. Historically, the role of allo-HCT for ALL in CR1 has been controversial.

Conventional adverse prognostic factors identified have included white blood cell (WBC) counts, age >40 years, immunophenotype, cytogenetics, and postinduction treatment response. What constitutes a high WBC count appears dependent on the ALL subtype, with a WBC count greater than 30,000/μL for B-lineage ALL and greater than 100,000/μL for T-lineage ALL predicting for poorer prognosis. Increasing age has also been shown to portend a worse prognosis with OS ranging from 34% to 57% for patients aged less than 30 years compared with only 15%–17% for patients older than 50 years.[8] With regards to immunophenotype, T lineage ALL also appears to have better outcomes than B lineage ALL, whereas among T lineage ALL, patients with cortical T ALL appeared to have the best outcomes.[9] In contrast, a recently recognized subtype of T-ALL/LBL derived from thymic cells at the early T-cell precursor (ETP) differentiation stage has been found to be associated with poor outcomes especially when treated with conventional adult regimens.[10,11] Specific cytogenetic abnormalities have also been found to have a major impact on prognosis. Some well-accepted adverse prognostic cytogenetics include the Ph chromosome, t(4; 11) (q21; q23), as well as t(8; 14) (q24.1; q32), complex karyotype defined as >5 chromosomal abnormalities, or low hypodiploidy/near triploidy.[12-14]

Finally, the achievement of CR and time to CR after induction therapy also carries significant implications, with patients who require more than 4 weeks to achieve a CR having a lower likelihood of being cured.

Hematopoietic Cell Transplantation for Malignant Conditions. https://doi.org/10.1016/B978-0-323-56802-9.00010-9

Although stratification for high-risk disease has varied between the different studies, historically, most of the early studies carried out based on biologic randomization, including the French LALA-87[15] and LALA94,[3] as well as the GOELAL02 trial,[16] have shown a survival advantage for patients with adverse prognostic factors who were treated with allo-HCT compared with adult ALL chemotherapy regimens. The French LALA-87[15] which looked at 257 ALL patients in CR1 in a biologic randomization fashion and with an intention to treat analysis showed that patients with adverse prognostic markers who had an HLA-compatible donor had a significant survival advantage compared with patients without a donor (5-year OS 44% vs. 20%). In a follow-up study, the LALA94 trial,[3] which stratified only high-risk patients with donors to allo-HSCT, a similar survival advantage was again seen in the patients with donors. (5-year leukemia-free survival [LFS] 45% in those with donors compared with 23% for those without). Similar findings were also demonstrated by the GOELAL02 trial[16] in which almost twofold improvement in OS was seen in the group with available donors (6-year OS 75% vs. 39%).

Even among the trials that were not able to demonstrate overall survival benefit for the high-risk group assigned to allo-HCT, it was clear that the relapse rates in the allo-HCT arms were superior compared with the chemotherapy or ASCT arm suggesting that the conflicting results were due to the high nonrelapse mortality in the high-risk groups, abrogating the overall survival benefits from allo-HCT rather than the lack of efficacy of the graft-versus-leukemia effect.[17,18]

Table 10.1 summarizes some of the largest prospective trials looking at upfront transplantation for standard and high-risk ALL based on a donor versus no-donor analysis.

As pediatric regimens for treating ALL gains wider acceptance in recent years, however, the continued relevance of these traditional risk factors as decision-making tools for allo-HCT have been challenged. Instead, markers like disease response and minimal residual monitoring (MRD) has shown promise and may trump these conventional markers, changing the decision-making paradigm for allo-HCT for ALL. As MRD is inherently a response-based assessment, it may serve as an in vivo test for chemosensitivity and disease biology that pretreatment markers along may not be able to help. More recent reports have also suggested that MRD stratification may be combined with molecular subtyping to provide better risk stratification. In a recent study by the Group for Research on Adult Acute Lymphoblastic Leukemia (GRAALL),[19]

522 transplant-eligible Ph-negative ALL patients (aged between 15–55 years) who were stratified as high risk based on at least one traditional adverse risk factor and who were treated with a pediatric-intensive chemotherapy regimen, were evaluated. No relapse-free or overall survival benefit was demonstrated in the allo-HCT (N = 282, either with a 10/10 matched related [matched RD] or unrelated donor [MUD], n = 231, or a 9/10 MUD or umbilical cord blood [UCB] transplant, n = 51), compared to the chemotherapy arm (N = 240). Of note however, postinduction MRD of >10(-3) and presence of the IKZF1 deletion were able to identify a subgroup of particularly high risk of relapse who would benefit from allogeneic stem cell transplantation (allo-SCT) in CR1. Importantly, these markers were found to be better for risk stratification than analysis of pretreatment characteristics alone. This finding that has also been supported by similar results from other large cooperative group studies. Though using different technical aspects for MRD quantification, different protocol designs and selection criteria for MRD-directed therapy, the Spanish PETHEMA group[20] and North Italian Leukemia group (NILG)[21] have also shown that MRD negativity identifies a low-risk group of patients for whom chemotherapy-alone approaches alone may be associated with prolonged disease-free survival. Within the NILG, Bassan et al. performed an MRD-oriented therapy for Ph-negative patients (excluding those with the t(4; 11) translocation) and were able to identify a low-risk MRD-negative population, with bone marrow relapse rates of less than 20%, and DFS nearly 80%, in whom SCT in CR1 was unnecessary. Similarly, the PETHEMA group demonstrated that in high-risk patients (based on pretreatment characteristics) with rapid MRD clearance, avoiding HCT was safe, with 5-year DFS and OS of 55% and 59%, respectively, from chemotherapy alone. Of note, in both the studies, multivariate analysis showed that the pattern of MRD clearance was the most significant prognostic factor for CR duration and OS, as compared to classic risk factors.

Moving forward, MRD is likely to play a more pertinent role in the allo-HCT decision-making algorithm, superseding conventional pretreatment risk factors. More work is however necessary in determining the optimal MRD method and appropriate time points for testing before MRD can be incorporated into risk-adapted therapies.

Allo-HCT in CR1 for Ph-Positive ALL

Historically, the prognosis of patients with Ph+ ALL has been poor with long-term DFS rates of 10%–20%.[22] In the preimatinib era, allo-HCT has been standard of care

TABLE 10.1

Prospective Trials of Upfront Allo-HSCT Versus No Allo-HSCT for Standard-Risk and High-Risk ALL in the Pre-MRD and MRD Era

				PROSPECTIVE DONOR VERSUS NO-DONOR STUDIES IN STANDARD-RISK AND HIGH-RISK ALL				
				5-YEAR OVERALL SURVIVAL %				
					NO DONOR			
Study	Accrual Period	Patients, n	Donor, Allo-HSCT	Overall	Chemo	Auto-HSCT	P Value	Other Findings
Pre-MRD Era								
LALA-87[15]	1986–1991	SR: N = 161	51	45	DNS	DNS	NS	
		HR: N = 96	44	20	DNS	DNS	0.03	
MRC/ ECOG[17]	1993–2006	SR: N = 562	62	52	56	46	0.02	
		HR[b]: N = 465	41	35	31	37	NS	
HOVON trials[48]	1992–2005	SR: N = 138	69	49	NA	49	0.05	
		HR: N = 119	53	41	NA	41	NS	
LALA-94[3,a]	1994–2002	HR[b] N = 259	45	23	DNS	DNS	0.007	
MRD Era								
GRAALL, 2003/2005[19]	2003–2011	HR[b]: N = 522	3-year OS: (donor allo-HCT group): 70% 3-yr OS: HR, 0.76 (95% CI, 0.57 to 1.02) was not significantly improved in the SCT group				$P = .07$	47% of cases MRDneg at 6 weeks after induction. Allo-HSCT was associated with longer RFS in patients MRD-pos >10^{-3} after induction (hazard ratio, 0.40) but not in good MRD responders
GMALL 06/09 and 07/03[92]	1999–2009	HR[b]/SR with MRD-positive wk 16, N = 580	5-year leukemia-free survival for SR/ HR patients with MRDpos at week 16 (N = 120): 44% (allo-HSCT) versus 11% (no allo-[HCT]				$P < .001$	Allo-HSCT benefit in both high and standard risk with MRDpos. No allo-HSCT benefit in MRDneg group.

Auto-HSCT, autologous stem cell transplant; *DNS*, data not stated; *HR*, high risk; *LFS*, leukemia-free survival; *MRD*, minimal residual disease; *MRDneg*, negative minimal residual disease; *MRDpos*, positive minimal residual disease; *NA*, not applicable; *NS*, not significant; *OS*, overall survival; *SR*, standard risk.
[a]5-year leukemia-free survival.
[b]High risk excluding Ph-positive ALL cases.

for consolidation, with 30%–65% long-term survival for patients transplanted in CR1.[23–25]

In the post-TKI era, the incorporation of imatinib into standard ALL therapy has resulted in significantly improved remission induction rates, as well as improved depth of remissions,[26–29] enabling more HSCT in CR. Three-year OS rates of between 50% and

65% have been reported in patients transplanted with myeloablative conditioning[26,30–32] in this setting.

With the improved outcomes in the post-TKI era, a number of questions have arose about the use of allo-HCT and role of maintenance TKI after allo-HCT, as well as the role of auto-HCT in patients with good MRD response and who are without a donor.

Question 1: Is Transplant Mandatory for all Ph-Positive ALL Patients?

Before the development of tyrosine kinase inhibitors (TKIs), Philadelphia-positive ALL carried a poor prognosis even with allo-HCT.[25,33] The incorporation of TKIs into chemotherapy regimens has led to improved response rates and depth of responses and allowed more patients to be able to undergo allo-HCT with better remission states.

With TKIs/chemotherapy allowing complete molecular remission in a significant subset of patients, there has been debate in recent years whether allo-HCT is still mandatory. Table 10.2 summarizes some of the largest prospective studies looking at allo-HCT for Ph-positive ALL in first remission. Although allo-SCT is still regarded as the best treatment option for patients with Ph-positive ALL in CR1, the long-term results of regimens combining chemotherapy with TKIs suggest the possibility of long-term survival in a proportion of patients who do not undergo a transplant This concept was first inspired by a study from the Children's Oncology Group which reviewed pediatric patients with ALL treated with imatinib and chemotherapy.[34,35] Patients with matched related donors were offered allo-HCT. In the long-term

---

TABLE 10.2

Prospective Studies of Upfront Allo-HSCT in Ph-Positive Patients in the TKI Era

Study	Accrual Period	Regimen	Patients, n	CR Rates	Percentage Undergoing Allo-HSCT in CR1	Outcomes	Allo-HSCT Effect in CR Patients
MRC/ECOG[38]	2003–2014	UKALL chemoregimen + imatinib; allo-HSCT if donor	N = 175	92%	46%	4-yr OS, 38% overall; 4-yr EFS, 33% overall.	4-yr OS 50% for the per-protocol allo-HSCT versus 19% in those who achieved CR but did not undergo allo-HSCT
GRAALL, 2005[39]	2006–2011	Randomization to induction regimen: VCR/Dex + imatinib ×28 days (arm A) versus Hyper-CVAD + imatinib ×14 days (arm B); allo-HCT or auto-HCT based on donor availability if patients achieved MMR after cycle 2	N = 268	98% arm A versus 91% arm B; (MMR 66% v. 65%)	77% (63% allo-HSCT, 14% auto-HSCT)	5-yr OS 46%; 5-yr EFS 37%; no differences between induction arms	Significant benefit to allo-HSCT in RFS and OS; no benefit in MRDneg patients
SWOG, 0805[40]	2009–2013	HyperCVAD + dasatinib; allo-HSCT if donor	N = 94	88%	49%	3-yr EFS, 54% overall; 3-yr EFS, 76% for allo-HSCT	Landmark analysis 175 days after CR: significantly better RFS ($P = 0.037$) and OS ($P = 0.036$)
MDACC group[93]	2011–13	Hyper-CVAD + ponatinib; No planned allo-HSCT	N = 37	97%	24%	2-yr EFS 80%; 2-yr OS 81%	No benefit to allo-HSCT at median 26 months follow-up; all allo-HSCT in MRDneg state

CR, complete remission; Dex, dexamethasone; EFS, event-free survival; MMR, major molecular remission; MRD, minimal residual disease; Neg, negative; OS, overall survival; RFS, relapse-free survival; VCR, vincristine.

follow-up, there was no superiority in the DSF between the matched related donor allo-HCT arm and the chemotherapy plus imatinib-alone arm (5-year DFS 65% vs. 70%). However, this study cannot be considered definitive, given the small number of patients in both the arms (28 treated with imatinib and 21 patients received sibling-donor BMT), as well as a high nonprotocol MUD allo-HCT rates. In the adult population, there has been conflicting results. The ALL202 trial from the Japanese Adult Leukemia Study Group reported on 80 patients who received a combination of imatinib and chemotherapy.[31] Of these patients, 31 did not undergo allo-HCT. Outcomes among the chemotherapy-only versus the allo-HCT group were similar, albeit with short follow-up data. In contrast data from the MD Anderson cancer centre (MDACC) demonstrated that patients <40 years old who underwent allo-HCT showed a trend toward improved survival compared with patients treated with second-generation TKIs/chemotherapy, though statistical significance was not reached, likely due to the limited patient numbers.[36,37] The UKALLXII/ECOG2993 trial reported on patients treated with imatinib added to standard BFM-type induction chemotherapy.[38] Transplant patients had significantly better overall survival (50% vs. 19%), event-free survival (46% vs. 14%), and relapse-free survival compared to the nontransplant patients (69% vs. 18%), though there were differences between the transplant versus nontransplant group suggesting potential selection biases affecting study results. The GRAALL group showed that allo-HCT was associated with a significant benefit in relapse-free survival (RFS) (hazard ratio [HR], 0.69 [95% confidence interval (CI), 0.49–0.98]; $P = .036$) and OS (HR, 0.64 [95% CI, 0.44–0.93]; $P = .02$) in their population of patients who were younger than 60 years and received imatinib-based therapy.[39] Interestingly, however, patients who achieved a molecular CR did not benefit from allo-HCT in terms of RFS, whereas those who had MRD did. Most recently, a multicenter US intergroup trial[40] showed superior RFS and OS for the transplanted patients, after induction with hyper-CVAD (fractionated cyclophosphamide, vincristine, doxorubicin, dexamethasone) and dasatinib.

These findings suggest second-generation TKIs may not be potent enough to eliminate the need for allo-HCT; however, MRD monitoring may select a small subgroup of patients who have excellent long-term outcomes even without allo-HCT in first remission. These results are further supported by the studies from the MDACC in their cohort of patients[41,42] treated with TKIs and hyper-CVAD regimen, where achievement of at least a major molecular response (MMR) was found to be independently prognostic for improved survival.

In addition, patients who achieved a complete molecular remission (CMR) (defined as absence of BCR-ABL1 transcripts with a sensitivity of 0.01%) by 3 months had an excellent long-term survival even without allo-HCT, with a 4-year OS rate for patients achieving CMR by 3 months of 66%, and a median OS of 10 years.

Moving forward, prospective trials using MRD-based risk stratification for patients with Ph-positive ALL are important to elucidate the optimal postremission management of these patients and to assess the appropriate time points for MRD assessments.

Question 2: Is Posttransplant TKI Maintenance Necessary?

Given the efficacy of TKIs and the continuing risks of relapse after allo-HCT, an important issue is the role of TKIs maintenance after transplantation. In patients who turn MRD-positive after allo-HCT, TKI may help convert some to molecular remission, allowing prolonged disease-free survival.[43] In patients who are MRD negative, however, the use of TKI remains unclear given the limitations in the literature with a paucity of prospective studies and conflicting results from retrospective studies, most of which have small patient numbers. In one of the largest retrospective studies of 113 patients with Ph-positive ALL undergoing allo-HSCT, neither TKI use before HSCT nor after HSCT was found to significantly impact transplant outcomes in univariate or multivariate analyses.[44] The GMALL performed a prospective multicenter randomized trial of prophylactic versus MRD-triggered imatinib after allo-HCT.[45] Incidence of molecular recurrence after allo-HCT was significantly reduced compared with imatinib given at detection of MRD (40% vs. 69%, respectively, $P = .046$). The probabilities of ongoing remission, DFS, OS, and EFS were 82.6%, 69.4%, 77.3%, and 62.5%, respectively, with no statistically significant difference between study arms. There was however premature discontinuation of imatinib in the majority of patients due to poor tolerability, and the numbers in both the arms were small (N = 26 and 29). Liew et al. performed a meta-analysis of the published studies comparing the outcomes of patients after allo-HSCT who did or did not receive TKIs.[46] This looked at 346 patients who received a TKI after alloSCT and 1095 patients who did not. There were no differences in relapse-free survival or overall survival in both the arms. Although the result from this meta-analysis needs to be interpreted with caution given the heterogeneity between the studies, these overall findings do suggest that TKIs might not be necessary and highlights the need for larger prospective controlled studies to address this issue.

In patients who become MRD positive after allo-HSCT, posttransplant TKI appears beneficial, being able to convert some of them to molecular remission and allow prolonged disease-free survival.

Until then, a panel of experts from the Acute Leukemia Working Party of the European Society for Blood and Marrow transplantation has prepared a consensus statement to guide the use of TKIs after allo-HCT.[47] Some key points of this recommendation include:

1 All Ph-positive ALL patients are candidates for TKI use after allo-HCT.
2 Patients with detectable MRD after allo-HCT should be started on TKI treatment as soon as possible.
3 For patients who are MRD negative after allo-HCT, both a prophylactic and preemptive strategy are valid options.
4 For patients transplanted in CR1, TKIs should be given for 12 months of continued MRD negativity, whereas if transplanted in CR2, TKIs should be continued indefinitely.

Question 3: Is There a Role for Autologous HCT for Ph-Positive Patients?

In patients with Ph-negative ALL, most of the studies using biologic randomization to compare autologous HCT (autoHCT) or chemotherapy versus allogeneic transplantation have found that for high-risk patients, allo-HCT led to superior DFS and OS compared with autologous HSCT or chemotherapy,[3,15–17,48] with no significant difference between chemotherapy and autologous HSCT.[3,15] In the MRC/ECOG trial[25] with the largest number of patients randomized to autologous versus chemotherapy (456 patients), the event-free survival of the autologous arm was significantly lower, and the relapse risk was significantly higher than that of chemotherapy. Thus, currently, there does not appear to be any benefit for autologous HSCT in the treatment of Ph-negative ALL.

In contrast, for Ph-positive ALL patients, there have been data suggesting a potential role for auto-HCT in these patients, especially those with MRD negativity at the time of transplant. The EBMT compared the outcomes of auto-HCT for Ph ALL, before and after the use of TKIs in 177 patients, and showed an improvement in overall survival and leukemia-free survival (LFS) in those transplanted in the TKI era.[49] Among the subgroup of 22 patients actually treated with TKIs and being in complete molecular remission at the time of auto-HCT, the LFS at 3 years was 65%. Similar results have been shown in other retrospective studies looking at auto-HCT in Ph-positive patients, especially in the setting of MRD negativity.

ALLOGENEIC HSCT BEYOND CR1

The outcome of patients with relapsed refractory ALL is dismal, with complete response rates to salvage therapy ranging from 40% to 45% and overall survival being usually less than 10%.[50–53] A number of multicenter trials have characterized prognosis and outcome of patients with ALL after relapse and shown that in patients with CR2, allo-HCT offers the best chance for potential cure. Data from the MRC UKALL12/ECOG2993 trial[52] showed that in patients with relapsed disease, 5-year survival after HSCT ranged from 15% to 23% depending on donor type (15% for autograft, 16% for MUD, 23% for MRD) and was significantly better than chemotherapy (4%) ($P < .05$). Similar findings were reported by the GMALL as well as the LALA and PET-HEMA group.[53–55] Gokbuget et al. reported outcomes of 547 ALL patients in first relapse.[53] Three-year OS was 38% for the patients who underwent transplantation, whereas none of the nontransplantation patients had long-term survival. In an analysis of 421 patients previously treated on LALA-94, who had disease relapse, CR2 was attained in 44% of patients, but the 5-year OS was again significantly better in the subset that was able to receive allo-HSCT (25% vs. 7% for the whole group).[54] Oriol et al. reported on the outcome of 263 adults with relapsed ALL, all of whom were previously treated on four consecutive PETHEMA trials with similar induction therapies.[55] Forty-five percent of patients achieved a second remission, and best outcome was noted for patients younger than 30 years with a long first remission duration transplanted in CR2, with an OS of 38% at 5 years. Significantly, outcomes of allo-HCT in CR2 are much poorer than those of allo-HCT performed in CR1 in all the studies, hence underscoring the importance of identifying high-risk patients who should be transplanted in first remission.

Many patients with relapsed and refractory disease do not reach allo-HCT stage, either due to treatment-related toxicities of salvage treatment which precludes subsequent transplantation or persistently refractory disease.[56] The treatment-related mortality associated with salvage chemotherapy in this setting may be as high as 20%.[57] Given these risks, some have argued that for patients with low-to-moderate disease burden and an available donor, reinduction chemotherapy may be omitted in preference for immediate allo-HCT. Terwey et al. performed one of the largest retrospective review addressing this and was able to show a 5-year OS rate of 47% in 19 patients with relapsed or refractory disease who received an allo-HSCT without prior reinduction chemotherapy, a result that was superior to the group that had received prior reinduction chemotherapy (5-year OS: 18%).[58] It should be noted that the patients who went transplantation immediately had very low tumor burden and that such results are not universally shared with other similar results suggesting that allo-HCT in CR2 is superior to allo-HCT in active disease.[59,60] The EBMT recently reviewed the results of patients with ALL transplanted in refractory disease and developed a prognostic score for LFS in this patient group.[61] Use of TBI and infusion of a female hematopoietic cells into male recipients were associated with improved outcomes. Patients with both the factors have a 5-year OS of 57% compared with patients with no prognostic factors present. Although this scoring system requires validation, it does provide a basis for future studies. Until more prospective data are available, recommendations regarding reinduction chemotherapy versus upfront transplant in patients with refractory disease or early relapse will have to be individualized depending on the patient, their disease behavior, and the availability of donors.

OPTIMAL CONDITIONING AND DONOR SELECTION FOR ALLO-HCT FOR ALL

From the data discussed, it is evident that there are patients for whom an allo-HSCT would allow best chances for long-term disease control. However, only about 30% of patients, however, will have a matched sibling donor. In addition, the toxicities associated with a myeloablative regimen limit its use to younger patients without comorbidities. The development of reduced-intensity conditioning (RIC) regimens and use of alternative donor allo-HSCTs increase the accessibility of this modality to patients who might need it most.

Choice of Myeloablative Conditioning

Myeloablative conditioning for ALL has generally included total-body irradiation (TBI) or busulfan. Given the ability of TBI-based myeloablative regimens to eradicate the leukemia cells in sanctuary sites, cyclophosphamide and TBI remain the preferred MA regimen for ALL. The frequent immediate and late complications such as azoospermia, diabetes, hypertension, as well as late secondary malignancies of TBI, however, has led to continued development of novel radiation-free myeloablative regimens, using busulfan as a backbone, to improve outcomes. These are associated with encouraging rates of PFS and OS as well as acceptable toxicity profiles and are reasonable alternatives to TBI-based regimens. In addition, in recent years, thiotepa has been added to these conditioning

regimens given its ability to cross the blood-brain barrier. A recent matched pair analysis from the EBMT[62] found that thiotepa conditioning was associated with higher relapse rates compared with Cy/TBI arm (HR = 1.78; 95% CI, 1.07–2.95; P = .03) but equivalent 2-year PFS and OS and supports the use of thiotepa-based conditioning as a valuable alternative to TBI-based conditioning.

Choice of RIC

The data for RIC for ALL are less mature than those for AML. Two large observational database retrospective registry studies from the EBMT and CIBMTR[63,64] have demonstrated the feasibility and efficacy of RIC for ALL. The optimal RIC conditioning also remains unclear with various regimens reported from various centers.[65–68] Importantly, most studies for RIC have shown that outcomes of patients transplanted in CR1 appear to be superior than those transplanted beyond CR1 (45% vs. 28% in CIBMTR study and 51% vs. 33% in the EBMT group). In contrast, patients transplanted with active disease did poor suggesting a limited role for RIC allo-HSCT for ALL not in CR.[69] Although awaiting more data from randomized studies, RIC HCT should be considered for ALL patients in CR1 with higher NRM risks, in the absence of clinical trials. In contrast, for younger patients without comorbidities with higher risks of relapse (e.g., disease in CR2 and beyond), MA conditioning should still be considered.

Alternative Donors

Only about one-third of patients who need a transplant will have a sibling donor. For others, alternative donors including matched unrelated, cord blood, and haploidentical donors have been investigated.

MUD Transplants

Prospective studies comparing allo-HSCT to chemotherapy have been based on the availability of a matched sibling donor. However, with the availability of allele-level HLA typing and improved supportive care over time, the safety of MUD transplants has improved, and there are increasing data suggesting comparable outcomes for MUD compared with sibling transplants. Some important studies include the following: (1) a multicenter retrospective review from Germany and Sweden that reported no significant difference in 5-year DFS in 221 patients with high-risk ALL that underwent an HLA-matched versus an HLA unrelated allo-HSCT (42% vs. 45% at 5 years for patients in CR1);[70] (2) Data from the Japanese registry that showed lower NRM (14% vs. 24% at 4 years, P = .0002), higher relapse rates (32% vs. 22% at 4 years, P = .03), and no difference in OS (65% vs. 62% at 4 years, P = .19) between the sibling and MUD transplants; and (3) Data from the CIBMTR on 672 ALL patients, which found no difference in leukemia-free survival between MUD and sibling allo-HSCT.[1] There have also been several other single-center studies which have reported their experience with MUD transplants for ALL and demonstrated comparable disease-free and overall survivals as compared with sibling transplants.[71,72]

For patients without MUD donors, cord blood and haploidentical transplants are alternatives.

UCB Transplants

Unlike sibling and MUD transplants, cord blood transplants allow for greater HLA disparity and hence matches are easier to find. The largest data sets supporting the use of UCB transplantation for ALL comes from registry data. In one of the largest studies, Eapen et al. reported data from 1500 patients from the CIBMTR and EBMT[73] and showed that LFS for UCB transplants was comparable with that after a 8/8 or 7/8 allele-matched peripheral blood stem cells (PBSC) or bone marrow transplantation, though NRM was higher after UCB transplantation than 8/8 allele-matched PBPC recipients (HR, 1.62; 95% CI, 1.18–2.23; P = .003) or bone-marrow transplantation (HR, 1.69; 95% CI, 1.19–2.39; P = .003).[73] Recent publications from the University of Minnesota[74,75] and Fred Hutchinson Cancer Research Center (FHCRC)[76] have also compared UCB transplants with alternative donor sources specifically for patients with ALL and found similar PFS and OS among the groups. Interestingly, results from the FHCRC have also suggested that for patients with MRD positivity, UCB transplants were associated with lower relapse rates than MUD transplants. Overall these findings suggest that for adult patients with high-risk ALL, UCB transplants are an acceptable alternative and have comparable outcomes to a well-matched unrelated donor.

Haploidentical Transplants

Another alternative door option is that of haploidentical transplantation. This has been increasingly used since haplo-donors are virtually available for all patients, and it allows almost all patients to undergo an allo-HCT if needed. Early use of haploidentical transplantation involved mainly T-cell depletion of the graft associated with higher incidences of graft failure and slow immune recovery and infective complications. In the last decade, there has been an increasing use of unmanipulated grafts with in vivo T-cell depletion using either the John Hopkins method using posttransplant cyclophosphamide[77,78] or the Beijing hospital strategy of intensive antithymocyte globulin (ATG)-based immunosuppression.[79,80]

Using a T-cell depletion strategy, Ciceri and colleagues reported a leukemia-free 2-year survival rate of 13% for patients with high-risk ALL undergoing haploidentical transplantation in first complete remission, 30% for those undergoing HSCT in second or further complete remission, and 7% in those undergoing HSCT in nonremission.[81] The Beijing group recently compared outcomes of haploidentical (N = 103) with matched sibling donor allografts (N = 83) in a cohort of high-risk Ph-negative ALL patients in CR1 (N = 210).[79] At 3 years, cumulative incidence of relapse (18 vs. 24%; P = .30), NRM (13 vs. 11%; P = .84), DFS (68 vs. 64%; P = .56), and OS (75 vs. 69%; P = .51) were similar between both the groups. In recent years, there have also been a number of multicenter or registry data specifically reviewing outcomes of posttransplant cyclophosphamide for ALL. In recent multicenter retrospective study by Srour et al.,[82] outcomes of 109 adults with ALL receiving haploidentical transplant with posttransplant cyclophosphamide were reported. Effective disease control and safety profile in concordance with outcomes of matched related and MUD transplants were demonstrated, including an encouraging DFS of 52% at 3 years. Similarly the EBMT published their data specifically looking at the use of unmanipulated haploidentical stem cell transplantation in 208 patients with ALL transplanted in EBMT centers from 2007–2014 (57% using posttransplantation cyclophosphamide and 43% using ATG plus standard prophylaxis).[83] No difference was found in the outcomes between the two types of graft versus host prophylaxis though there was a trend toward increased NRM in the ATG group. Patients transplanted in CR1 had a 3-year OS of 52% which appears comparable with results reported for matched related and MUD transplants, whereas patients transplanted with active disease did poorly with only a 5% OS at 3 years. Overall these findings suggest that for adult patients with high-risk ALL, haploidentical transplants are a valid alternative donor option; though for patients with active disease, given the poor outcomes, efforts should be made to achieve disease remission before transplantation.

ADVANCES IN THE FIELD OF ALL
Novel ALL Entities and Role of Allo-HCT for These Entities

In recent years, there have been 2 new distinct subsets of ALL identified with distinctive clinical behavior and prognosis, immunophenotype, as well as gene expression signatures.

These include the early T precursor acute lymphoblastic leukemia (ETP-ALL) and the Philadelphia-like ALL (Ph-like ALL). For transplant physicians, it is important to know about these new entities and how to incorporate transplantation into the treatment algorithm for these entities.

Early T precursor ALL

ETP ALL is a leukemia derived from thymic cells at the early T precursor differentiation stage.[10] These leukemic cells are believed to have a unique genetic makeup with multilineage pluripotency and characteristics of myeloid progenitors as well as hematopoietic stem cells at both the immunophenotypic and genetic level.[84] In the WHO 2016 classification, ETP ALL is recognized as a new provisional entity, defined based on immunophenotype with expression of CD7 but lacking CD1a and CD8 and with positivity for 1 or more of the myeloid/stem cell markers CD34, CD117, HLADR, CD13, CD33, CD11b, or CD65.[85] The prognostic significance of ETP ALL remains conflicting and appears to depend on the treatment provided. The use of a paediatrics-based approach with treatment intensification based on MRD appears to be able to abrogate the prognostic significance of ETP ALL. Favorable long-term outcomes have been seen in ETP ALL patients in the Children's Oncology Group and Medical Research Council Working Party on Leukaemia in Children UK National Acute Lymphoblastic Leukaemia 2003 study despite higher MRD rates after induction. In contrast, in ETP patients treated in the MD Anderson Cancer Centre with a mainly adult-type chemotherapy, outcomes appeared to be poorer than those of the patients with other T ALL subtypes.[11] More studies in this field will allow us to better determine the optimal management of this ALL subtype and whether there is a role for upfront allogeneic transplantation versus using a pediatric protocol in this disease entity.

Philadelphia-like ALL (BCR-ABL–like ALL)

Ph-like ALL is a novel entity first described by Mulligan et al. from the Children's Oncology group and St Jude's children's hospital[86] and by den Boer et al. from the Netherlands,[87] which had a gene expression profile that was very similar to Ph-positive ALL. Of note, this entity is found to be associated with a variety of genomic alternations that activate kinase and cytokine receptor signaling, including JAK/STAT signaling, as well as FGFR1, IL2RB, PDGFRA, and the RAS signaling pathway among others. In addition, this entity was also found to be associated with high frequency of deletions of the *IKZF1* gene which encodes IKAROS, the lymphoid transcription factors.[86–88] More studies are currently underway to identify options to improve outcomes in these patients including ways to more rapidly identify this entity, as well as studies of clinical or prognostic markers that can identify subsets who would benefit from the addition of tyrosine kinases to treatment regimens. The role of allo-HCT in improving outcomes of this high-risk ALL subset remains unclear and will also be an area of further research.

Incorporation of Novel Agents into the Treatment Algorithm of ALL

After many decades of little progress of new drugs, in recent years, there has been a rapid development of several immune-based therapies which has shown significant promise both as single agents as well as in combination with chemotherapy, for the treatment of ALL. Of these, the 2 leading compounds, inotuzumab and blinatumomab, have been recently approved by the FDA in the setting of relapsed refractory ALL.

Blinatumomab is a bi-specific T cell–engaging construct with dual specificity against CD19 and CD3, hence bringing cytotoxic T cells to close proximity with CD19 ALL cells and optimizing cell killing. It was first investigated with patients in CR1 with MRD positivity with encouraging results but has since been extensively investigated in the relapsed refractory setting where it has been shown to have superior outcomes than current standard of care chemotherapy (SOC). An open label multicenter clinical trial (TOWER NCT02013167) compared blinatumomab to SOC in 405 patients with relapsed refractory ALL[89] and showed a statistically significant improvement in overall survival for patients treated with blinatumomab compared with SOC (HR, 0.71; 95% CI: 0.55–0.93; $P = .012$). Median survival was also improved in the blinatumomab arm (7.7 months, 95% CI: 5.6–9.6) compared with that in the SOC arm (4.0 months, 95% CI: 2.9–5.3). The results of this trial led to approval for blinatumomab in the United States in 2014. Blinatumomab is currently also being investigated as maintenance therapy after allogenic transplantation. In addition, a US Intergroup (E910) is currently also assessing chemotherapy with and without blinatumomab in adult patients with newly diagnosed ALL.

Inotuzumab, a monoclonal antibody against CD22 and linked to calicheamicin, has also recently received approval for the treatment of ALL in the relapsed refractory setting, based on results from the randomized INO-VATE ALL (NCT01564784) trial[90] Of the initial 218 randomized patients, the rates of complete remission were significantly higher in the inotuzumab group (80.7% vs. 29.4%, $P < .001$).

Progression-free survival was also improved in the inotuzumab group (median 0.0 months vs. 1.8 months; HR, 0.4; $P < .001$), but responses appear shortlived and allo-HCT appears still necessary to consolidate clinical responses. Importantly, however, the use of inotuzumab has been associated with higher risks of venoocclusive disease (VOD) subsequently in patients undergoing allo-HCT, and in a series of 23 patients receiving an allo-HCT after salvage therapy with inotuzumab, Kebriaei et al.[91] reported a fatal VOD rate of 19% (n = 5). Of note, 4 of the 5 patients had received two alkylating agents in their conditioning regimen. These findings are a stark reminder to transplanters that novel agents may have an impact on allo-HCT outcomes and that understanding of drug toxicities and careful selection of preparative regimens and avoidance of other concomitant hepatotoxic drugs may be considered to reduce posttransplantation toxicities. There are also currently several other monoclonal antibodies in currently earlier phases of clinical development with promising initial results.

In recent years, one of the most exciting developments in the field of ALL treatment has been the development of chimeric antigenic T cells (CAR-T) for the treatment of relapsed refractory B cell malignancies. Currently there are more 240 trials of CAR-T cells worldwide and two CAR-T cells from Novartis and Gilead and KiTE Pharma, targeting the CD19 antigen found on B cells, have been approved for the treatment of B acute lymphoblastic leukemia and diffuse large B cell lymphoma, respectively. With a response rate of more than 80% among patients with relapsed refractory AL treated with the CD19 CART, tisagenlecleucel (Kymriah) from Novartis, the potential of this treatment is immense. However, the high rates of potentially fatal complications such as cytokine release syndrome and neurotoxicity associated with this treatment entity, as well the prohibitive costs of these CAR-T cell therapies have been barriers to the widespread use of this technology. Further work to improve upon the safety and affordability of CAR-T cells is currently ongoing and will hopefully allow this therapy to become a more broadly applicable treatment option.

More data and results are needed from ongoing clinical trials to determine the optimal patient population, sequence in treatment, and optimal role of these agents in ALL treatment. In addition, current results suggest that despite the efficacy of novel agents, allo-HCT remains relevant, and more studies will be needed to determine the optimal incorporation of these agents and allo-HCT into the treatment algorithm for ALL.

Conclusion

Allogeneic transplantation is associated with a strong GVL effect and remains an essential tool in the treatment of adult ALL. Despite the development of novel agents as well as pediatric styled protocols for adult patients, it remains a relevant modality of treatment and development of RIC protocols, and increasing use of alternative donors allows allo-HCT to be considered for more patients. A risk-adapted approach is needed for better selection of patients who would benefit from transplantation in CR1, and MRD is likely going to have a key role in this treatment algorithm.

REFERENCES

1. Ringden O, et al. The graft-versus-leukemia effect using matched unrelated donors is not superior to HLA-identical siblings for hematopoietic stem cell transplantation. *Blood.* 2009;113(13):3110–3118.
2. Hunger SP, Mullighan CG. Acute lymphoblastic leukemia in children. *N Engl J Med.* 2015;373(16):1541–1552.
3. Thomas X, et al. Outcome of treatment in adults with acute lymphoblastic leukemia: analysis of the LALA-94 trial. *J Clin Oncol.* 2004;22(20):4075–4086.
4. Kantarjian H, et al. Long-term follow-up results of hyperfractionated cyclophosphamide, vincristine, doxorubicin, and dexamethasone (Hyper-CVAD), a dose-intensive regimen, in adult acute lymphocytic leukemia. *Cancer.* 2004;101(12):2788–2801.
5. Gokbuget N, et al. Treatment of adult ALL according to protocols of the German multicenter study group for adult ALL (GMALL). *Hematol Oncol Clin North Am.* 2000;14(6):1307–1325.
6. Rowe JM, et al. Induction therapy for adults with acute lymphoblastic leukemia: results of more than 1500 patients from the international ALL trial: MRC UKALL XII/ECOG E2993. *Blood.* 2005;106(12):3760–3767.
7. Baker KS, et al. Late effects in survivors of acute leukemia treated with hematopoietic cell transplantation: a report from the Bone Marrow Transplant Survivor Study. *Leukemia.* 2010;24(12):2039–2047.
8. Pui CH, Evans WE. Acute lymphoblastic leukemia. *N Engl J Med.* 1998;339(9):605–615.
9. Marks DI, et al. T-cell acute lymphoblastic leukemia in adults: clinical features, immunophenotype, cytogenetics, and outcome from the large randomized prospective trial (UKALL XII/ECOG 2993). *Blood.* 2009;114(25):5136–5145.
10. Coustan-Smith E, et al. Early T-cell precursor leukaemia: a subtype of very high-risk acute lymphoblastic leukaemia. *Lancet Oncol.* 2009;10(2):147–156.
11. Jain N, et al. Early T-cell precursor acute lymphoblastic leukemia/lymphoma (ETP-ALL/LBL) in adolescents and adults: a high-risk subtype. *Blood.* 2016;127(15):1863–1869.

12. Czuczman MS, et al. Value of immunophenotype in intensively treated adult acute lymphoblastic leukemia: cancer and leukemia Group B study 8364. *Blood*. 1999;93(11):3931–3939.

13. Gokbuget N, Hoelzer D. Treatment of adult acute lymphoblastic leukemia. *Hematol Am Soc Hematol Educ Program*. 2006:133–141.

14. Moorman AV, et al. Karyotype is an independent prognostic factor in adult acute lymphoblastic leukemia (ALL): analysis of cytogenetic data from patients treated on the Medical Research Council (MRC) UKALLXII/Eastern Cooperative Oncology Group (ECOG) 2993 trial. *Blood*. 2007;109(8):3189–3197.

15. Sebban C, et al. Allogeneic bone marrow transplantation in adult acute lymphoblastic leukemia in first complete remission: a comparative study. French Group of Therapy of Adult Acute Lymphoblastic Leukemia. *J Clin Oncol*. 1994;12(12):2580–2587.

16. Hunault M, et al. Better outcome of adult acute lymphoblastic leukemia after early genoidentical allogeneic bone marrow transplantation (BMT) than after late high-dose therapy and autologous BMT: a GOELAMS trial. *Blood*. 2004;104(10):3028–3037.

17. Goldstone AH, et al. In adults with standard-risk acute lymphoblastic leukemia, the greatest benefit is achieved from a matched sibling allogeneic transplantation in first complete remission, and an autologous transplantation is less effective than conventional consolidation/maintenance chemotherapy in all patients: final results of the International ALL Trial (MRC UKALL XII/ECOG E2993). *Blood*. 2008;111(4):1827–1833.

18. Labar B, et al. Allogeneic stem cell transplantation in acute lymphoblastic leukemia and non-Hodgkin's lymphoma for patients <or=50 years old in first complete remission: results of the EORTC ALL-3 trial. *Haematologica*. 2004;89(7):809–817.

19. Dhedin N, et al. Role of allogeneic stem cell transplantation in adult patients with Ph-negative acute lymphoblastic leukemia. *Blood*. 2015;125(16):2486–2496; quiz 2586.

20. Ribera JM, et al. Treatment of high-risk Philadelphia chromosome-negative acute lymphoblastic leukemia in adolescents and adults according to early cytologic response and minimal residual disease after consolidation assessed by flow cytometry: final results of the PETHEMA ALL-AR-03 trial. *J Clin Oncol*. 2014;32(15):1595–1604.

21. Bassan R, et al. Different molecular levels of post-induction minimal residual disease may predict hematopoietic stem cell transplantation outcome in adult Philadelphia-negative acute lymphoblastic leukemia. *Blood Cancer J*. 2014;4:e225.

22. Wetzler M, et al. Prospective karyotype analysis in adult acute lymphoblastic leukemia: the cancer and leukemia Group B experience. *Blood*. 1999;93(11):3983–3993.

23. Laport GG, et al. Long-term remission of Philadelphia chromosome-positive acute lymphoblastic leukemia after allogeneic hematopoietic cell transplantation from matched sibling donors: a 20-year experience with the fractionated total body irradiation-etoposide regimen. *Blood*. 2008;112(3):903–909.

24. Snyder DS, et al. Long-term follow-up of 23 patients with Philadelphia chromosome-positive acute lymphoblastic leukemia treated with allogeneic bone marrow transplant in first complete remission. *Leukemia*. 1999;13(12):2053–2058.

25. Fielding AK, et al. Prospective outcome data on 267 unselected adult patients with Philadelphia chromosome-positive acute lymphoblastic leukemia confirms superiority of allogeneic transplantation over chemotherapy in the pre-imatinib era: results from the International ALL Trial MRC UKALLXII/ECOG2993. *Blood*. 2009;113(19):4489–4496.

26. Thomas DA, et al. Treatment of Philadelphia chromosome-positive acute lymphocytic leukemia with hyper-CVAD and imatinib mesylate. *Blood*. 2004;103(12):4396–4407.

27. Tanguy-Schmidt A, et al. Long-term results of the imatinib GRAAPH-2003 study in newly-diagnosed patients with de novo Philadelphia chromosome-positive acute lymphoblastic leukemia. *ASH Annu Meet Abstr*. 2009;114(22):3080.

28. Fielding AK, et al. Imatinib significantly enhances long-term outcomes in Philadelphia positive acute lymphoblastic leukaemia; final results of the UKALLXII/ECOG2993 trial. *ASH Annu Meet Abstr*. 2010;116(21): 169.

29. Brissot E, et al. Tyrosine kinase inhibitors improve long-term outcome of allogeneic hematopoietic stem cell transplantation for adult patients with Philadelphia chromosome positive acute lymphoblastic leukemia. *Haematologica*. 2015;100(3):392–399.

30. de Labarthe A, et al. Imatinib combined with induction or consolidation chemotherapy in patients with de novo Philadelphia chromosome-positive acute lymphoblastic leukemia: results of the GRAAPH-2003 study. *Blood*. 2007;109(4):1408–1413.

31. Yanada M, et al. High complete remission rate and promising outcome by combination of imatinib and chemotherapy for newly diagnosed BCR-ABL–Positive acute lymphoblastic leukemia: a phase II study by the Japan adult leukemia study group. *J Clin Oncol*. 2006;24(3):460–466.

32. Pfeifer H, et al. Long-term outcome of 335 adult patients receiving different schedules of imatinib and chemotherapy as front-line treatment for Philadelphia-positive acute lymphoblastic leukemia (Ph+ ALL). *ASH Annu Meet Abstr*. 2010;116(21): 173.

33. Dombret H, et al. Outcome of treatment in adults with Philadelphia chromosome-positive acute lymphoblastic leukemia–results of the prospective multicenter LALA-94 trial. *Blood*. 2002;100(7):2357–2366.

34. Schultz KR, et al. Improved early event-free survival with imatinib in Philadelphia chromosome-positive acute lymphoblastic leukemia: a children's oncology group study. *J Clin Oncol*. 2009;27(31):5175–5181.

35. Schultz KR, et al. Long-term follow-up of imatinib in pediatric Philadelphia chromosome-positive acute lymphoblastic leukemia: children's Oncology Group study AALL0031. *Leukemia*. 2014;28(7):1467–1471.

36. Daver N, et al. Final report of a phase II study of imatinib mesylate with hyper-CVAD for the front-line treatment of adult patients with Philadelphia chromosome-positive acute lymphoblastic leukemia. *Haematologica.* 2015;100(5):653–661.

37. Ravandi F, et al. Long-term follow-up of a phase 2 study of chemotherapy plus dasatinib for the initial treatment of patients with Philadelphia chromosome-positive acute lymphoblastic leukemia. *Cancer.* 2015;121(23):4158–4164.

38. Fielding AK, et al. UKALLXII/ECOG2993: addition of imatinib to a standard treatment regimen enhances long-term outcomes in Philadelphia positive acute lymphoblastic leukemia. *Blood.* 2014;123(6):843–850.

39. Chalandon Y, et al. Randomized study of reduced-intensity chemotherapy combined with imatinib in adults with Ph-positive acute lymphoblastic leukemia. *Blood.* 2015;125(24):3711–3719.

40. Ravandi F, et al. US intergroup study of chemotherapy plus dasatinib and allogeneic stem cell transplant in Philadelphia chromosome positive ALL. *Blood Adv.* 2016;1(3):250–259.

41. Ravandi F, et al. Detection of MRD may predict the outcome of patients with Philadelphia chromosome-positive ALL treated with tyrosine kinase inhibitors plus chemotherapy. *Blood.* 2013;122(7):1214–1221.

42. Short NJ, et al. Impact of complete molecular response on survival in patients with Philadelphia chromosome-positive acute lymphoblastic leukemia. *Blood.* 2016;128(4):504–507.

43. Wassmann B, et al. Early molecular response to post-transplantation imatinib determines outcome in MRD+ Philadelphia-positive acute lymphoblastic leukemia (Ph+ ALL). *Blood.* 2005;106(2):458–463.

44. Kebriaei P, et al. Long-term follow-up of allogeneic hematopoietic stem cell transplantation for patients with Philadelphia chromosome-positive acute lymphoblastic leukemia: impact of tyrosine kinase inhibitors on treatment outcomes. *Biol Blood and Marrow Transplant.* 2012;18.

45. Pfeifer H, et al. Randomized comparison of prophylactic and minimal residual disease-triggered imatinib after allogeneic stem cell transplantation for BCR-ABL1-positive acute lymphoblastic leukemia. *Leukemia.* 2013;27(6):1254–1262.

46. Liew E, Ghosh S, Saini L. Use of tyrosine kinase inhibitors post-allogeneic stem cell transplant in patients with Philadelphia or BCR-ABL positive acute lymphoblastic leukemia: a systematic review and meta-analysis. *Blood.* 2016;128(22):2778.

47. Giebel S, et al. Use of tyrosine kinase inhibitors to prevent relapse after allogeneic hematopoietic stem cell transplantation for patients with Philadelphia chromosome-positive acute lymphoblastic leukemia: a position statement of the Acute Leukemia Working Party of the European Society for Blood and Marrow Transplantation. *Cancer.* 2016;122(19):2941–2951.

48. Cornelissen JJ, et al. Myeloablative allogeneic versus autologous stem cell transplantation in adult patients with acute lymphoblastic leukemia in first remission: a prospective sibling donor versus no-donor comparison. *Blood.* 2009;113(6):1375–1382.

49. Giebel S, et al. Improving results of autologous stem cell transplantation for Philadelphia-positive acute lymphoblastic leukaemia in the era of tyrosine kinase inhibitors: a report from the Acute Leukaemia Working Party of the European Group for Blood and Marrow Transplantation. *Eur J Cancer.* 2014;50(2):411–417.

50. Bassan R, Lerede T, Barbui T. Strategies for the treatment of recurrent acute lymphoblastic leukemia in adults. *Haematologica.* 1996;81(1):20–36.

51. Garcia-Manero G, Thomas DA. Salvage therapy for refractory or relapsed acute lymphocytic leukemia. *Hematol Oncol Clin North Am.* 2001;15(1):163–205.

52. Fielding AK, et al. Outcome of 609 adults after relapse of acute lymphoblastic leukemia (ALL); an MRC UKALL12/ECOG 2993 study. *Blood.* 2007;109(3):944–950.

53. Gokbuget N, et al. Outcome of relapsed adult lymphoblastic leukemia depends on response to salvage chemotherapy, prognostic factors, and performance of stem cell transplantation. *Blood.* 2012;120(10):2032–2041.

54. Tavernier E, et al. Outcome of treatment after first relapse in adults with acute lymphoblastic leukemia initially treated by the LALA-94 trial. *Leukemia.* 2007;21(9):1907–1914.

55. Oriol A, et al. Outcome after relapse of acute lymphoblastic leukemia in adult patients included in four consecutive risk-adapted trials by the PETHEMA Study Group. *Haematologica.* 2010;95(4):589–596.

56. Martino R, et al. Allogeneic or autologous stem cell transplantation following salvage chemotherapy for adults with refractory or relapsed acute lymphoblastic leukemia. *Bone Marrow Transplant.* 1998;21(10):1023–1027.

57. Thomas DA, et al. Primary refractory and relapsed adult acute lymphoblastic leukemia: characteristics, treatment results, and prognosis with salvage therapy. *Cancer.* 1999;86(7):1216–1230.

58. Terwey TH, et al. Allogeneic SCT in refractory or relapsed adult ALL is effective without prior reinduction chemotherapy. *Bone Marrow Transplant.* 2008;42(12):791–798.

59. Cornelissen JJ, et al. Unrelated marrow transplantation for adult patients with poor-risk acute lymphoblastic leukemia: strong graft-versus-leukemia effect and risk factors determining outcome. *Blood.* 2001;97(6):1572–1577.

60. Doney K, et al. Predictive factors for outcome of allogeneic hematopoietic cell transplantation for adult acute lymphoblastic leukemia. *Biol Blood Marrow Transplant.* 2003;9(7):472–481.

61. Pavlu J, et al. Allogeneic hematopoietic cell transplantation for primary refractory acute lymphoblastic leukemia: a report from the Acute Leukemia Working Party of the EBMT. *Cancer.* 2017;123(11):1965–1970.

62. Eder S, et al. Thiotepa-based conditioning versus total body irradiation as myeloablative conditioning prior to allogeneic stem cell transplantation for acute lymphoblastic leukemia: a matched-pair analysis from the Acute Leukemia Working Party of the European Society for Blood and Marrow Transplantation. *Am J Hematol.* 2017;92(10):997–1003.

63. Marks DI, et al. The outcome of full-intensity and reduced-intensity conditioning matched sibling or unrelated donor transplantation in adults with Philadelphia chromosome-negative acute lymphoblastic leukemia in first and second complete remission. *Blood.* 2010;116(3):366–374.

64. Mohty M, et al. Reduced-intensity versus conventional myeloablative conditioning allogeneic stem cell transplantation for patients with acute lymphoblastic leukemia: a retrospective study from the European Group for Blood and Marrow Transplantation. *Blood.* 2010;116(22):4439–4443.

65. Stein AS, et al. Reduced-intensity conditioning followed by peripheral blood stem cell transplantation for adult patients with high-risk acute lymphoblastic leukemia. *Biol Blood Marrow Transpl.* 2009;15(11):1407–1414.

66. Cho BS, et al. Reduced-intensity conditioning allogeneic stem cell transplantation is a potential therapeutic approach for adults with high-risk acute lymphoblastic leukemia in remission: results of a prospective phase 2 study. *Leukemia.* 2009;23(10):1763–1770.

67. Santarone S, et al. Fludarabine and pharmacokinetic-targeted busulfan before allografting for adults with acute lymphoid leukemia. *Biol Blood Marrow Transplant.* 2011;17(10):1505–1511.

68. Russell JA, et al. Allogeneic transplantation for adult acute leukemia in first and second remission with a novel regimen incorporating daily intravenous busulfan, fludarabine, 400 CGY total-body irradiation, and thymoglobulin. *Biol Blood Marrow Transplant.* 2007;13(7):814–821.

69. Arnold R, et al. Nonmyeloablative stem cell transplantation in adults with high-risk ALL may be effective in early but not in advanced disease. *Leukemia.* 2002;16(12):2423–2428.

70. Kiehl MG, et al. Outcome of allogeneic hematopoietic stem-cell transplantation in adult patients with acute lymphoblastic leukemia: no difference in related compared with unrelated transplant in first complete remission. *J Clin Oncol.* 2004;22(14):2816–2825.

71. Lee S, et al. Allogeneic stem cell transplantation in first complete remission enhances graft-versus-leukemia effect in adults with acute lymphoblastic leukemia: antileukemic activity of chronic graft-versus-host disease. *Biol Blood Marrow Transplant.* 2007;13(9):1083–1094.

72. Dahlke J, et al. Comparable results in patients with acute lymphoblastic leukemia after related and unrelated stem cell transplantation. *Bone Marrow Transplant.* 2006;37(2):155–163.

73. Eapen M, et al. Effect of graft source on unrelated donor haemopoietic stem-cell transplantation in adults with acute leukaemia: a retrospective analysis. *Lancet Oncol.* 2010;11(7):653–660.

74. Bachanova V, et al. Prolonged survival in adults with acute lymphoblastic leukemia after reduced-intensity conditioning with cord blood or sibling donor transplantation. *Blood.* 2009;113(13):2902–2905.

75. Tomblyn MB, et al. Myeloablative hematopoietic cell transplantation for acute lymphoblastic leukemia: analysis of graft sources and long-term outcome. *J Clin Oncol.* 2009;27(22):3634–3641.

76. Milano F, Appelbaum FR, Delaney C. Cord-blood transplantation in patients with minimal residual disease. *N Engl J Med.* 2016;375(22):2204–2205.

77. Luznik L, et al. HLA-haploidentical bone marrow transplantation for hematologic malignancies using nonmyeloablative conditioning and high-dose, posttransplantation cyclophosphamide. Biology of blood and marrow transplantation. *Journal Am Soc Blood Marrow Transplant.* 2008;14(6):641–650.

78. Luznik L, et al. High-dose cyclophosphamide as single-agent, short-course prophylaxis of graft-versus-host disease. *Blood.* 2010;115(16):3224–3230.

79. Wang Y, et al. Haploidentical versus matched-sibling transplant in adults with Philadelphia-negative high-risk acute lymphoblastic leukemia: a biologically phase III randomized study. *Clin Cancer Res.* 2016;22(14):3467–3476.

80. Huang XJ, Chang YJ. Unmanipulated HLA-mismatched/haploidentical blood and marrow hematopoietic stem cell transplantation. *Biol Blood Marrow Transplant.* 2011;17(2):197–204.

81. Ciceri F, et al. A survey of fully haploidentical hematopoietic stem cell transplantation in adults with high-risk acute leukemia: a risk factor analysis of outcomes for patients in remission at transplantation. *Blood.* 2008;112(9):3574–3581.

82. Srour SA, et al. Haploidentical transplantation with posttransplantation cyclophosphamide for high-risk acute lymphoblastic leukemia. *Biol Blood Marrow Transplant.* 2017;23(2):318–324.

83. Santoro N, et al. Unmanipulated haploidentical stem cell transplantation in adults with acute lymphoblastic leukemia: a study on behalf of the Acute Leukemia Working Party of the EBMT. *J Hematol Oncol.* 2017;10(1):113.

84. Zhang J, et al. The genetic basis of early T-cell precursor acute lymphoblastic leukaemia. *Nature.* 2012;481(7380):157–163.

85. Arber DA, et al. The 2016 revision to the World Health Organization classification of myeloid neoplasms and acute leukemia. *Blood.* 2016;127(20):2391–2405.

86. Mullighan CG, et al. Deletion of IKZF1 and prognosis in acute lymphoblastic leukemia. *N Engl J Med.* 2009;360(5):470–480.

87. Den Boer ML, et al. A subtype of childhood acute lymphoblastic leukaemia with poor treatment outcome: a genome-wide classification study. *Lancet Oncol.* 2009;10(2):125–134.

88. Boer JM, et al. Expression profiling of adult acute lymphoblastic leukemia identifies a BCR-ABL1-like subgroup characterized by high non-response and relapse rates. *Haematologica.* 2015;(7):100: e261–e264.

89. Kantarjian H, et al. Blinatumomab versus chemotherapy for advanced acute lymphoblastic leukemia. *N Engl J Med.* 2017;376(9):836–847.

90. Kantarjian HM, et al. Inotuzumab ozogamicin versus standard therapy for acute lymphoblastic leukemia. *N Engl J Med.* 2016;375(8):740–753.

91. Kebriaei P, et al. Feasibility of allografting in patients with advanced acute lymphoblastic leukemia after salvage therapy with inotuzumab ozogamicin. *Clin Lymphoma Myeloma Leuk.* 2013;13(3):296–301.

92. Gokbuget N, et al. Adult patients with acute lymphoblastic leukemia and molecular failure display a poor prognosis and are candidates for stem cell transplantation and targeted therapies. *Blood.* 2012;120(9):1868–1876.

93. Jabbour E, et al. Combination of hyper-CVAD with ponatinib as first-line therapy for patients with Philadelphia chromosome-positive acute lymphoblastic leukaemia: a single-centre, phase 2 study. *Lancet Oncol.* 2015;16(15):1547–1555.

Hematopoietic Cell Transplantation for Myeloproliferative Neoplasms

REBECCA DEVLIN, PHD • VIKAS GUPTA, MD, FRCP, FRCPATH

INTRODUCTION

Myeloproliferative neoplasms (MPNs) are a group of Philadelphia-negative clonal hematological disorders, characterized by hematopoietic proliferation. The three major classical MPN subgroups are essential thrombocythemia (ET), polycythemia vera (PV), and myelofibrosis (MF), the latter of which can be primary (PMF) or evolved from PV (post-PV MF, PPV-MF) or ET (post-ET MF, PET-MF). In this chapter, patients with PMF, PPV-MF, and PET-MF will be referred as MF.

All three disorders are chronic in nature, with an initial chronic phase (CP), defined as a blast count <10%, increased risk of complications such as thrombosis and bleeding, a variable degree of symptom burden of the disease related to organomegaly, and cytokine-driven constitutional symptoms. The chronic phase is typically longer in PV and ET than in MF, with some patients whose ET/PV is well controlled that they are able to live a near-normal life. Transformation to acute myeloid leukemia (AML) is seen in a small proportion ET and PV patients. Estimates range from 0.7% to 4% at 10 years for ET and 2.3%–14.4% at 10 years for PV[1] and higher for patients with MF in the range of 20%–30%.[2] Survival of AML evolved from MPN is dismal, with median overall survival ranging from 3 to 6 months,[3–5] having improved little in the past 20 years.[6]

Recent years have seen a rapid expansion in mutations identified in MPN patients and, to some extent, in our understanding of their prognostic value. The first identified and most common driver mutation present in MPN patients is in the JAK2 gene (*JAK2 V617F*).[7,8] The vast majority of remaining MPN patients harbor a mutation in the calreticulin (CALR)[7,9] or MPL genes.[10]

In PMF, *CALR* has been found to be associated with a milder disease phenotype and superior overall survival (OS) relative to *JAK2/MPL*-positive patients.[11] However, when *CALR* patients are categorized into type I or type I like and type II or type II like, only *CALR* type I or type I like is associated with superior survival compared with

JAK2 V617F.[12] Patients who do not harbor a detectable *JAK2*, *MPL*, or *CALR* driver mutation (so called "triple-negative" patients) are an additional group identified as high-risk associated with decreased survival and increased risk of transformation to AML.[11,13]

Several other subclonal mutations such as *ASLX1*, *SRSF2*, *IDH1/2*, and *EZH2* are of prognostic value in MF.[14–16] The number of detrimental mutations also has a prognostic role in PMF. Guglielmelli et al.[17] analyzed survival and leukemia-free survival based on the presence and number of "prognostically detrimental" (nondriver) mutations (*ASXL1*, *EZH2*, *SRSF2*, and *IDH1/2*). Presence of any of these mutations shortened survival (7 years for one mutation vs. 12.3 years for no mutations), and the presence of two or more of these mutations predicted the worst survival (median, 2.6 years) and shortened leukemia-free survival. A study of 359 patients with PET-MF and PPV-MF suggests that secondary MF differs from that of PMF in terms of mutational prognostication.[18] In contrast to PMF, the type of driver mutation did not influence survival in PET-MF or PPV-MF, though triple-negative PET patients had a lower OS. The high molecular risk (HMR) genes *ASXL1*, *EZH2*, *SRSF2*, and *IDH1/2* were analyzed, but only *SRSF2* associated with reduced survival in PET-MF.

NONTRANSPLANT THERAPIES IN MF

The key discovery of the *JAK2 V617F* mutation in patients with myeloproliferative neoplasms (MPNs) paved the way for development of JAK 1/2 inhibitors (JAKi) designed to suppress the cytokine-signaling cascade caused by constitutively activated JAK2.

Ruxolitinib is the only approved JAKi therapy for MF and can result in significant improvement of splenomegaly, constitutional symptoms, performance status, and quality of life (QoL).[19–21] Anemia and thrombocytopenia are two major toxicities. Long-term follow-up data are available on COMFORT-I and COMFORT-II trials, and no additional safety concerns have arisen on the use of ruxolitinib in MF patients.[22,23] Although there is no debate on the salutary effects of ruxolitinib in decreasing the disease symptom burden, the issue of improvement on survival is contentious. Moreover, ruxolitinib has limited activity against JAK2-mutant clones, and there are no convincing data on the resolution of fibrosis. Long-term data show that ~50% of patients discontinue ruxolitinib by 3 years due to either side effects or loss of response.[22]

However, some patient subgroups are difficult to treat with ruxolitinib, such as those with severe thrombocytopenia and heavily transfusion-dependent patients, whereas others such as those with *ASXL1/EZH2* or ≥3 mutations may have shorter time to treatment failure.[24,25] Other investigational JAKi or combination therapies may be an appropriate alternative in some of these patients.

HCT IN MF

HCT is the only curative modality for MPNs. However, owing to the significant morbidity and mortality associated with transplant, HCT is not usually indicated in patients with PV or ET, unless the disease transforms to MF or AP/BP. In a multicenter retrospective study of HCT for ET and PV,[26] 39% patients had transformed to MF by the time of HCT, illustrating the advanced nature of disease in these patients. Owing to the comparative rarity of use of HCT in other MPNs, the remainder of this chapter will focus on HCT for patients with MF.

HCT in Chronic Phase of MPN

Significant nonrelapse mortality related to graft failure (GF), regimen-related toxicities, and graft-versus-host disease (GVHD) remain substantial issues in HCT for MF.[27,28] Table 11.1 summarizes the outcomes of large studies (>100 patients) of HCT in MF published in the past 10 years.

TABLE 11.1
Outcomes of HCT in MF in Recent Studies Reporting ≥100 Patients

Study	Timeline of HCT	Number of Patients	Overall Survival	Overall Survival by Donor Type
Rampal et al. 2017[75]	2007–2015	101	52% at 5 years	Details not provided by donor type
Ali et al. 2017[28]	2004–2017	110	74% at 2 years; 65% at 5 years	Details not provided not provided by donor type
Robin et al. 2016[76]	2005–2014	160	Flu-Mel: 52% at 7 years; Flu-Bu: 59% at 7 years	Details not provided
Shanavas et al. 2016[56]	2009–2014	100	61% at 2 years	Details not provided
Gupta et al. 2014[33]	1997–2010	233	47% at 5 years	MSD: 56% at 5 years; well-matched URD: 48% at 5 years; Partially matched/mismatched URD: 34% at 5 years
Scott et al. 2012[77]	1990–2009	170	57% at 5 years	Details not provided
Robin et al. 2011[78]	1997–2008	147	39% at 4 years	Details not provided
Alchalby et al. 2010[79]	1999–2009	162	62% at 5 years	Matched: 67%; mismatched: 36%
Ballen et al. 2010[29]	1989–2002	289	Details not provided	MRD: 37% at 5 years; URD 30% at 5 years; HLA-identical: 40% at 5 years
Kroger et al. 2009[42]	2002–2007	103	67% at 5 years	Details not provided

Flu-Bu, fludarabine-busulphan; *Flu-Mel*, fludarabine-melphalan; *HLA*, human leukocyte antigen-identical; *MRD*, matched related donor; *URD*, unrelated donor.

As mentioned, significant rates of GF, nonrelapse mortality (NRM), graft-versus-host disease (GVHD), and regimen-related toxicities all contribute to the significant morbidity and mortality of HCT for MF. Poor performance status[29] and severe comorbidities[30,31] are both associated with increased NRM. Though the median age of transplantation for MF increased by a decade between 2000 and 2014 (49 vs. 59 years),[27] there are conflicting data regarding the effect of age on transplant outcomes.[32–34] Advanced age adversely impacts HCT outcomes[32,35] but is important to note the correlation that exists between increasing age and comorbidities[36] likely contributing to this observation. Patients with MF are at significantly higher risk of developing regimen-related hepatotoxicity, which may be related to underlying portal hypertension.[37] Some studies have reported higher-than-expected rates of GVHD in MF patients,[30,38–41] though some studies report rates similar to other hematologic malignancies.[29,42] The factors influencing GVHD in MF patients are not clear. Inflammatory cytokines, which are elevated in MF, may contribute to the higher mortality, as well as the constitutional symptoms of MF.[43] Reported incidence of GF in MF is 5%–25%,[29,40,41] with at least one prospective study reporting a significantly higher rate of primary GF in unrelated donor (URD) versus matched sibling donor (MSD).[40] The risk factors related to GF in MF are poorly understood. However, one possibility is that the higher rates of tumor necrosis factor alpha (TNF-α) in patients with more advanced disease[43] may play a role, rather than donor factors alone. TNF-α negatively regulates normal hematopoietic stem cell expansion[44,45] and might have a differential effect on MPN versus normal hematopoietic stem cells. There is a wide variation in treatment options for MF, from conservative options such as hydroxyurea to more intense therapies such as HCT. Risk-stratification tools can aid in navigating the MF therapeutic landscape.

Risk Stratification of MF

It is important to understand that MF is a highly heterogenous disease with survival ranging from in excess of a decade to a few months. An accurate assessment of disease risk status is essential in choosing the appropriate therapy for an individual patient that allows the careful evaluation of the risk-benefit ratio. A variety of prognostic scoring systems based on clinical and laboratory characteristics have been created with the aim of teasing out higher risk individuals, who may benefit from more aggressive treatment options such as HCT, and shielding those with lower risk disease from transplant-related risk.

In the last decade, several modern prognostic scores have been described. In a 2009 multicenter study, the international prognostic scoring system (IPSS) was published.[46] In this scoring system the independent risk factors for survival include age > 65 years, hemoglobin ≤ 100 g/L, white blood cells ≥ 25×10^9/L, circulating blasts ≥1%, and presence of constitutional symptoms at the time of diagnosis. The scores of 0, 1, 2, and ≥3 correlated with low, intermediate-1, intermediate-2, and high-risk groups, with survival of 135, 95, 48, and 27 months, respectively. The same risk factors were evaluated in a time-dependent manner, resulting in formulation of the dynamic IPSS (DIPSS).[47] The main difference in this scoring system is that anemia is assigned a score of 2 as opposed to 1, as the hazard ratio of mortality with anemia was double compared with other risk factors. Other prognostic risk factors such as adverse karyotype, platelet count of $<100 \times 10^9$/L, and transfusion dependence were further incorporated in the DIPSS to create the DIPSS-Plus.[2]

Based on these scores, patients with intermediate-2/high-risk disease with survival less than 5 years are usually considered appropriate candidates for HCT. More recently, the role of phenotypic driver mutations as well as other mutations has been described in predicting the survival and risk of leukemic transformation (LT).[13] Of particular note, type I *CALR* mutations are associated with superior prognosis.[48] In addition, *ASLX1*, *EZH2*, *IDH1*, *IDH2*, and *SRSF2* mutations are associated with decreased survival and increased risk of LT and considered HMR mutations.[49] In addition, the prognostic value of degree of fibrosis has recently been described.[50]

A molecular enhanced prognostic scoring system in patients under the age of 70 years (MIPSS70) has been recently published by collaboration of investigators from Mayo clinic and multiple Italian centers.[51] The median survival of MIPSS70 low-, intermediate-, and high-risk category patients is 27.7, 7.1, and 2.3 years, respectively. Incorporation of cytogenetics data along with mutation data led to development of MIPSS70 plus score. Other scoring systems incorporating genetic information include the genetically inspired prognostic scoring system,[52] the scoring of which differs from MIPSS70, most notably by inclusion of *U2AF1Q157* as an adverse mutation.

All of the scoring systems discussed thus far are described in PMF. The only tool the authors are aware of specifically for risk stratification in secondary MF was published by Passamonti et al.[53] Myelofibrosis secondary to PV and ET-prognostic model is for risk stratification in PPV-MF and PET-MF. The model assigns 2 points to each of hemoglobin <110 g/L, peripheral blasts ≥3%,

TABLE 11.2
European Leukemia Net (ELN)
Recommendations on HCT for MF

ELN Guideline Expert Recommendation[80]

High-risk patients (IPSS/DIPSS/DIPSS-plus)
Consider HCT in all transplant-eligible patients

Int-2 risk patients (IPSS/DIPSS/DIPSS-plus)
Consider HCT in all transplant-eligible patients

Int-1 risk patients (IPSS/DIPSS/DIPSS-plus)
(i) Consider HCT in transplant-eligible patients who have:
- Refractory, transfusion-dependent anemia;
- OR > 2% peripheral blasts in at least two repeated manual measurements;
- OR adverse cytogenetics;
- OR high-risk mutations

Low risk
Transplant not recommended

CALR-unmutated genotype, and 1 point to each of platelet count $<150 \times 10^9/L$ and constitutional symptoms. Unique among the risk-stratification systems for MF, it also assigns 0.15 points for each year of age.

The growing number of risk-stratification systems has caused confusion among practitioners about which to adopt in patient care. DIPSS is currently the most commonly used risk-stratification system used in clinical practice as well as clinical trials. We suggest the use of MIPSS70 for risk stratification when advanced mutation data are available. However, when advanced mutation data are not available, as is often the case at present, we suggest using DIPSS. We anticipate there will be shift toward MIPSS70 as accessibility of next-generation sequencing in routine clinical work flow increases.

MIPSS70 provides further sophistication to risk stratification in MF patients eligible for transplant. While DIPSS is based solely on clinical features and basic laboratory investigations, MIPSS70 also integrates bone marrow histology and molecular profiling results. Using the rationale of expert guidelines (Table 11.2), data from the MIPSS70 study indicate that the only clear indication for transplant according to this score is high-risk patients as they have survival ≤3 years when treated with supportive therapy or JAKi therapy. In contrast, risks associated with HCT do not justify the use of HCT in low-risk patients. In intermediate-risk patients, the use of HCT must be individualized according to additional risk factors. European Leukemia Net

guidelines also recommend that transplants be carried out as part of patient registries or clinical trials.

JAKi Therapy versus HCT

Therapeutic decision-making regarding the use of JAKi therapy versus HCT is complex. As mentioned, the only approved JAKi is ruxolitinib, and its use can result in significant decrease in disease symptom burden and improvement in QoL for patients.[54] However, ruxolitinib is not curative and has limited effect on prolongation of survival, and there is no convincing evidence of an effect on bone marrow fibrosis. Of particular relevance to transplant-eligible patients, ruxolitinib also does not decrease the risk of LT. On the other hand, HCT is a curative therapy but is associated with significant risk of morbidity and mortality. Therefore one has to carefully weigh the risk-benefit ratio of offering a curative treatment with increased risk of complications versus a relatively simpler treatment associated with decreased symptom burden and improvement in QoL.

Patients at high risk of LT are preferred candidates for HCT, such as those with adverse cytogenetics, a high-risk mutation profile, high peripheral blood blasts, or severe thrombocytopenia (platelet count $<50 \times 10^9/L$). Patients with severe thrombocytopenia are not suitable candidates for ruxolitinib therapy.

In current clinical practice, the majority of patients considered for HCT are already on JAKi therapy. This can present a dilemma of how to proceed when a patient is responding well to JAKi therapy. At present, there are no data comparing outcomes of HCT versus nontransplant therapies to assist in decision-making in such scenarios. Careful consideration is needed to balance the risks associated with proceeding with transplant against the risks of delaying transplant, including treatment failure, worsening splenomegaly, transfusion-associated iron overload, and LT. It is also necessary to consider patient age in a delayed transplant strategy, as many centers have age restrictions for HCT.

Mutational data may help optimize HCT decisions in such cases. Fig. 11.1 illustrates a potential framework for selection of JAKi versus HCT therapy. It is noteworthy that this framework is the authors' personal opinion and has not been validated prospectively at present. We recommend that all treatment decisions should be individualized and made after careful consideration of patient-, disease-, and transplant-related factors. The framework illustrates that HCT decisions are generally more straightforward for low- and high-risk patients. Transplant in low-risk patients may lead to significant treatment-related mortality and decrease in QoL in

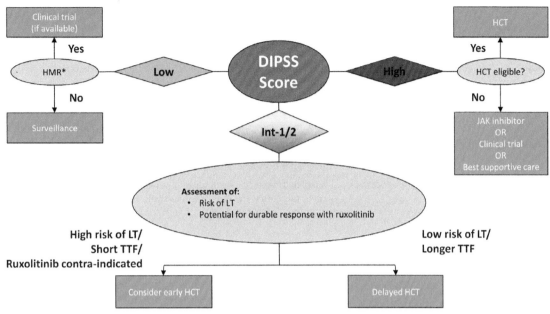

FIG. 11.1 A suggested framework* integrating the role of high molecular risk (HMR) profile in HCT decision-making. *DIPSS*, dynamic international prognostic scoring system; *HCT*, hematopoietic cell transplant; *HMR*, high molecular risk; *LT*, leukemic transformation; *TTF*, time to treatment failure.*the suggested framework is the personal opinion of the authors and has not been validated in prospective studies. (From Aldauij W, McNamara C, Schuh A, et al. Clinical utility of next generation sequencing in the management of myeloproliferative neoplasms: a single-centre experience. *Hemasphere.* 2018;2(3):e44.)

patients who have an otherwise longer predicted life expectancy and could maintain a reasonable QoL with non-HCT therapies. Therefore, transplant is not recommended for low-risk patients. High-risk patients have shorter duration of response to JAKi therapy and may benefit from early consideration of transplant. It is in treatment decisions for int-1/2 patients where mutational data may be of use. Two key considerations are the risk of LT and the potential for a durable response with ruxolitinib. Severe thrombocytopenia, increased peripheral blood blasts, and high-risk cytogenetics are associated with a higher risk of LT,[55] whereas pre-JAKi transfusion dependence, high DIPSS score, and *ASXL1* or *EZH2* mutations are all predictors of shorter time to JAKi treatment failure and shorter OS.[25]

Role of JAK Inhibitors in HCT

When considering HCT in patients currently on JAKi therapy, retrospective data suggest that transplant outcomes are superior in patients who were responding to JAK inhibitors, with regard to spleen size, than in those who have failed or lost response.[56] However, at present, there are not enough conclusive data.

Use of JAKi therapy in HCT is a topic of active interest as the effect of JAKi therapy in decreasing disease symptom burden is especially attractive in a pre-HCT setting. However, controversial data exist on integration of JAKi therapy in HCT for MF. Preliminary results from a prospective study (JAK-ALLO) to examine JAK inhibitors in the HCT setting showed serious adverse events (SAEs), including cardiogenic shock and tumor lysis syndrome, resulting in a temporary hold on participant recruitment.[57] It is speculated that sudden discontinuation of JAK inhibitor before HCT and splenectomy procedure may have contributed to some of these SAEs. In contrast, several retrospective studies did not observe such SAEs, and no harmful effect on early posttransplant outcomes was observed in these studies (Table 11.3).[56,58–62] Furthermore, in the largest retrospective study to date,[56] SAEs occurred in 2 patients out of a total of 66 patients who continued JAKi therapy close to HCT (Table 11.3). Both patients experiencing SAEs discontinued JAKi therapy 6 days before conditioning therapy, whereas very few patients experienced adverse symptoms when JAKi therapy was continued close to conditioning therapy.

TABLE 11.3
Summary of Retrospective Studies Describing Combining JAK Inhibitors in HCT Protocols

Study	Number of Patients	Study Design	Results	Conclusions
Kröger et al. (2018)[61]	12	Prospective	No graft failure. Median leukocyte engraftment 12 days. 8% incidence of aGVHD (grade II–IV) at day +100 (n = 2). CMV reactivation in 41% of patients (n = 5) and ruxolitinib discontinued in 2 patients due to cytopenias. One patient developed fever after ruxolitinib withdrawal.	Peritransplant ruxolitinib until stable engraftment is well tolerated and may reduce aGVHD but results in higher CMV reactivation.
Gupta et al. (2018)[62]	19	Prospective	Ruxolitinib tapered off successfully in all 19/19 patients without any "withdrawal symptoms" or delay in HCT	Continuing ruxolitinib therapy until close to start conditioning therapy resulted in no adverse impact on HCT outcomes
Shanavas et al. (2016)[56]	100	Retrospective	No adverse impact on early outcomes of HCT	Continuing JAKi therapy near to start of conditioning therapy is associated with very low risk of withdrawal symptoms
Stübig et al. (2014)[59]	22	Retrospective	1-year OS of 100% in patients with a good response to ruxolitinib versus 60% in others	Continuing ruxolitinib until conditioning without taper resulted in no unexpected SAEs
Jaekel et al. (2014)[58]	14	Retrospective	Engraftment in 13 patients (93%); graft fibrosis (n = 1) and treatment-related sepsis (n = 1)	Tapering ruxolitinib until conditioning did not result in unexpected SAEs
Lebon et al. (2013)[60]	11	Retrospective	Good engraftment rates	Differing schedules of ruxolitinib tapering associated with high engraftment rates

aGVHD, acute graft-versus-host disease; *CMV*, cytomegalovirus; *HCT*, hematopoietic cell transplantation; *JAK*, Janus kinase; *OS*, overall survival; *SAE*, severe adverse event.

There is likely no role for JAK inhibitors in post-HCT maintenance in MF. The primary reason for this is the minimal effect of JAK inhibitors on the malignant clone, as evidenced by their lack of effect on allele burden and bone marrow histopathology.[22,54,63,64] In addition, the on-target effect of these agents results in suppression of hematopoiesis, which can be very severe in the post-transplant setting. Owing to CYP3A4 inhibition, there is also the potential for various drug interactions, especially with azole antifungals and calcineurin inhibitors. However, a small pilot study (n = 12) reported reduced acute GVHD (aGVHD) in patients receiving peritransplant ruxolitinib.[61] Only 1 patient experienced aGVHD grade I or II, and there was an 8% incidence of aGVHD grade II–IV at day +100. However, major side effects

were increased cytomegalovirus reactivation (n = 5) and cytopenias, with the latter resulting in discontinuation of ruxolitinib treatment in 2 patients.

Optimal Conditioning Therapy for HCT for MF

There has been increasing interest in the use of reduced intensity conditioning (RIC) regimens in patients with MF in recent years.[27,33] Age is likely one of the most important factors in the decision-making regarding conditioning therapy intensity. The majority of patients with MF are not candidates for full-intensity conditioning (FIC) due to advanced age. However, in younger patients, an important question is what is the optimal conditioning intensity, especially in those aged

<50 years without any comorbidities. Several retrospective studies have compared RIC with FIC in MF.[41,65,66] Even though the patients in the RIC cohort were significantly older in comparison to FIC cohorts in these studies, none of these studies showed superiority of FIC over RIC. In fact, one study reported favorable outcomes with RIC even after adjusting for age.[65] There are several limitations to these studies such as their retrospective nature and lack of statistical power. Other potential biases limiting the interpretation of these studies include possible selection bias for candidacy for transplantation for very fit older patients and period effect as the RIC cohort was transplanted more recently. Although a comparative prospective study in younger patients is desirable to answer this question, rarity of disease poses logistical challenges. Ongoing observational studies in the transplant registries may however provide an answer in the near future. In the meantime, it is reasonable to restrict RIC to patients aged ≥50 years unless in a clinical trial setting.

Among the various RIC regimens, registry trends show that fludarabine (flu) in combination with busulfan or melphalan (mel) are the two most commonly used regimens for HCT in MF.[33] An RIC regimen consisting of flu/bu was investigated prospectively in 103 patients in a study from the European Group of Blood and Marrow Transplantation (EBMT).[42] The probability of overall and progression-free survival at 5 years was 67% and 51%, respectively. There was no significant difference in outcomes of matched sibling versus well-matched URDs, whereas the results of mismatched URDs were significantly inferior. Myeloproliferative Neoplasm–Research Consortium (MPN-RC) prospectively investigated RIC consisting of flu/mel.[40] Although very encouraging results similar to flu/bu combination were reported in the MSD cohort, the results of the URD cohort were of concern. A high risk of GF was observed in the URD arm in this study. Another retrospective study from the Center for Blood and Marrow Transplantation (CIBMTR) evaluated the outcomes of RIC transplantation for MF, and a trend toward better outcomes was observed in flu/mel cohort.[33] Though it is difficult to make comparisons between these studies, patient selection, rather than conditioning therapy, may be the cause of differences in outcomes. In our opinion, none of the commonly used RIC regimens has yet been proven superior, and a prospective study is required to define the optimal RIC regimen for MF.

What is the preferred graft source in MF?
As with other diseases, recent transplants are predominantly performed using peripheral blood stem cells (PBSCT) rather than bone marrow (BM) grafts. A published retrospective series with a significant proportion of both PBSCT and BM failed to show superiority of one source of graft over the other. The incidence of GF is significant in MF, but no clear association with the source of stem cells has been reported. However, PBSCT is generally associated with a lower incidence of GF, and the majority of transplant physicians prefer to use PBSCT in MF due to this theoretical advantage.

Splenectomy in the era of JAK inhibitors
Splenomegaly is a frequent finding in patients with MF and often is associated with debilitating symptoms and complications including abdominal pain, difficulty in bending and walking, early satiety leading to weight loss, cytopenias, and in some cases, portal hypertension and splenic infarction. Splenectomy is an effective therapeutic option that may relieve symptoms, but it is not without complications. Splenectomy carries the risk of postoperative thrombocytosis, thrombohemorrhagic complications, and infectious complications resulting in significant postoperative morbidity and mortality.

The role of splenectomy before transplant has been extensively debated and has remained a controversial issue. Earlier studies failed to demonstrate a survival advantage for splenectomy before HCT. Several recent studies have suggested that splenectomy may enhance survival in selected HCT patients. In a French study, men who had not undergone splenectomy had a higher mortality rate (hazard ratio, 3.45) even when adjusted for the Lille score that was still highly statistically significant.[67] In the CIBMTR study published by Ballen et al.,[29] there was a trend toward increased disease-free survival in splenectomized patients (relative risk, 0.77). A recent large series of patients who underwent splenectomy before HCT was reported,[68] reporting that patients who underwent splenectomy before HCT had a lower mortality rate than patients with an intact spleen. However, a major issue in these studies is lack of information on the patients who underwent splenectomy before HCT and never proceeded to HCT due to an adverse event related to splenectomy.

The availability of JAKi therapy has largely replaced the need for surgery and with it also the consequences of surgical procedure. However, after JAKi therapy, some patients may still have large spleens or develop splenomegaly after failure of JAKi therapy. The role of splenectomy in such patients is controversial. In the JAKi era, splenectomy may be considered on case-by-case basis in those for whom JAKi therapy is no longer of benefit or who never showed a response. In our opinion, splenectomy before HCT is not required for those patients responding to JAK inhibitor therapy. Decisions regarding splenectomy in patients loosing clinical benefit or refractory to JAKi therapy should be considered on individual basis by careful assessment of the risk-benefit ratio.

Alternative Donor Transplantation in Myelofibrosis

Owing to improvements in human leukocyte antigen matching and supportive care, the difference in outcomes between fully matched related donors and matched URDs are generally getting smaller. However, substantial differences exist between matched donor and mismatched donor transplant outcomes. A prospective study of RIC in MF from the EBMT group reported a higher NRM with mismatched donors than that with well-matched donors (38% vs. 12% at 1 year). Higher mortality in mismatched transplant was also reported in a CIBMTR study, with a hazard ratio of mortality almost more than double compared with that reported in mismatched donor transplant, compared to MSD or well-matched URD donor transplants.[33]

There are minimal data on use of umbilical cord blood (UCB) or haploidentical transplants in patients with MF. A retrospective review of the Japanese registry that included 11 cases of unrelated UCB[69] revealed that these patients had a lower probability of hematopoietic recovery than those having related donor bone marrow transplantation. The difference in OS was not statistically significant, and definite conclusions cannot be made due to the small sample size. A larger study from Eurocord analyzed the role of UCB transplants (UCBTs) in HCT in 35 patients with MF.[70] There were seven patients with secondary AML from previous MF in this study. Two-year OS and progression-free survival were 44% and 30%, respectively. Although these studies have demonstrated the feasibility of UCBTs in patients with MF, results appear significantly inferior in comparison to sibling donor or well-matched URD transplantation.

Poor outcomes of mismatched URD and UCBT may influence decision of timing of transplantation in patients responding well to JAKi therapy. In our opinion, mismatched URD or UCBT should be considered in patients when JAKi therapy fails in those patients at high risk of leukemic transformation, those unable to tolerate JAKi therapy due to severe cytopenias, and the patient who does not have an MSD or well-matched URD.

Transplantation for MPN in AP/BP

HCT is currently the only curative therapy for AML evolving from MF, but few studies have been carried

out on this treatment due to the rarity of its occurrence. A retrospective study identifying 46 AML-transformed PMF patients by the EBMT registry demonstrated that HCT can be curative in such patients.[71] Treatment-related mortality at 1 year was 28%, with 47% of patients relapsing by 3 years, and the overall survival rate was 33%. Response to chemotherapy before transplantation was important for survival (69% vs. 22%). Other studies have echoed these results, demonstrating long-term survival is possible, but that complete remission before HCT is a major factor. A study by the M.D. Anderson Cancer Center (n = 14) reported 49% of patients undergoing HCT after MF leukemic transformation survived long term.[72] Similarly, the Mayo Clinic reported 75% 2-year progression-free survival, and all six patients (n = 13) who achieved complete remission before transplantation were alive at follow-up (median, 20.3 months).[73] A recent retrospective study of HCT for MF in BP analyzed outcomes of 410 patients from the Mayo Clinic (n = 249) and Italy (n = 162).[74] Reflecting previous studies, the median survival of patients after BP (all therapies) was poor at 3.6 months. In analysis of the Mayo cohort, the 3-year survival rate for patients receiving HCT was 32% (n = 24) versus 19% for patients achieving complete remission/complete remission 1 but not transplanted (n = 24). High-risk karyotype, platelet count $<100 \times 10^9/L$, age >65 years, and transfusion need were identified as independent risk factors for survival. Similar findings were observed in the Italian cohort.

CONCLUSIONS

HCT for MF is an arduous therapeutic modality that warrants careful selection of patients. The timing of HCT, optimal conditioning, pre-HCT management of splenomegaly, and careful evaluation of risk-benefit ratio are important factors warranting consideration. Poor outcomes of mismatched donors or alternative donors make nontransplant treatment options seem more appealing, especially in patients lacking a well-matched donor. Continued enrollment in clinical trials and studies comparing HCT to nontransplant options will help in optimizing the outcomes and define the position of HCT in the evolving MF therapeutic landscape.

DISCLOSURE STATEMENT

VG received grants for research studies from Incyte and Novartis through his institution, and has served as a consultant on advisory board for Incyte and Novartis. RD has nothing to declare.

REFERENCES

1. Cerquozzi S, Tefferi A. Blast transformation and fibrotic progression in polycythemia vera and essential thrombocythemia: a literature review of incidence and risk factors. *Blood Cancer J.* 2015;5:e366.
2. Gangat N, Caramazza D, Vaidya R, et al. DIPSS plus: a refined Dynamic International Prognostic Scoring System for primary myelofibrosis that incorporates prognostic information from karyotype, platelet count, and transfusion status. *J Clin Oncol.* 2011;29(4):392–397.
3. Thepot S, Itzykson R, Seegers V, et al. Treatment of progression of Philadelphia-negative myeloproliferative neoplasms to myelodysplastic syndrome or acute myeloid leukemia by azacitidine: a report on 54 cases on the behalf of the Groupe Francophone des Myelodysplasies (GFM). *Blood.* 2010;116(19):3735–3742.
4. Mesa RA, Li CY, Ketterling RP, Schroeder GS, Knudson RA, Tefferi A. Leukemic transformation in myelofibrosis with myeloid metaplasia: a single-institution experience with 91 cases. *Blood.* 2005;105(3):973–977.
5. Kennedy JA, Atenafu EG, Messner HA, et al. Treatment outcomes following leukemic transformation in Philadelphia-negative myeloproliferative neoplasms. *Blood.* 2013;121(14):2725–2733.
6. McNamara C, Panzarella T, Kennedy J, et al. *Mutational Landscape and its Impact on Outcomes in Accelerated and Blast Phase of Myeloproliferative Neoplasms (Abstract #PF619).* 23rd Congress of the European Hematology Association; 2018.
7. Klampfl T, Gisslinger H, Harutyunyan AS, et al. Somatic mutations of calreticulin in myeloproliferative neoplasms. *N Engl J Med.* 2013;369(25):2379–2390.
8. Levine RL, Wadleigh M, Cools J, et al. Activating mutation in the tyrosine kinase JAK2 in polycythemia vera, essential thrombocythemia, and myeloid metaplasia with myelofibrosis. *Cancer Cell.* 2005;7(4):387–397.
9. Nangalia J, Massie CE, Baxter EJ, et al. Somatic CALR mutations in myeloproliferative neoplasms with nonmutated JAK2. *N Engl J Med.* 2013;369(25):2391–2405.
10. Pardanani AD, Levine RL, Lasho T, et al. MPL515 mutations in myeloproliferative and other myeloid disorders: a study of 1182 patients. *Blood.* 2006;108(10):3472–3476.
11. Tefferi A, Lasho TL, Finke CM, et al. CALR vs JAK2 vs MPL-mutated or triple-negative myelofibrosis: clinical, cytogenetic and molecular comparisons. *Leukemia.* 2014;28(7):1472–1477.
12. Tefferi A, Lasho TL, Finke C, et al. Type 1 vs type 2 calreticulin mutations in primary myelofibrosis: differences in phenotype and prognostic impact. *Leukemia.* 2014;28(7):1568–1570.
13. Rumi E, Pietra D, Pascutto C, et al. Clinical effect of driver mutations of JAK2, CALR, or MPL in primary myelofibrosis. *Blood.* 2014;124(7):1062–1069.
14. Tefferi A, Guglielmelli P, Lasho TL, et al. CALR and ASXL1 mutations-based molecular prognostication in primary myelofibrosis: an international study of 570 patients. *Leukemia.* 2014;28(7):1494–1500.
15. Guglielmelli P, Biamonte F, Score J, et al. EZH2 mutational status predicts poor survival in myelofibrosis. *Blood.* 2011;118(19):5227–5234.
16. Lasho TL, Jimma T, Finke CM, et al. SRSF2 mutations in primary myelofibrosis: significant clustering with IDH mutations and independent association with inferior overall and leukemia-free survival. *Blood.* 2012;120(20):4168–4171.
17. Guglielmelli P, Lasho TL, Rotunno G, et al. The number of prognostically detrimental mutations and prognosis in primary myelofibrosis: an international study of 797 patients. *Leukemia.* 2014;28(9):1804–1810.
18. Rotunno G, Pacilli A, Artusi V, et al. Epidemiology and clinical relevance of mutations in postpolycythemia vera and postessential thrombocythemia myelofibrosis: a study on 359 patients of the AGIMM group. *Am J Hematol.* 2016;91(7):681–686.
19. Verstovsek S, Mesa RA, Gotlib J, et al. A double-blind, placebo-controlled trial of ruxolitinib for myelofibrosis. *N Engl J Med.* 2012;366(9):799–807.
20. Harrison C, Kiladjian JJ, Al-Ali HK, et al. JAK inhibition with ruxolitinib versus best available therapy for myelofibrosis. *N Engl J Med.* 2012;366(9):787–798.
21. Mesa R, Jamieson C, Bhatia R, et al. Myeloproliferative neoplasms, version 2.2017, NCCN clinical practice guidelines in Oncology. *J Natl Compr Canc Netw.* 2016;14(12):1572–1611.
22. Cervantes F, Vannucchi AM, Kiladjian JJ, et al. Three-year efficacy, safety, and survival findings from COMFORT-II, a phase 3 study comparing ruxolitinib with best available therapy for myelofibrosis. *Blood.* 2013;122(25):4047–4053.
23. Vannucchi AM, Kantarjian HM, Kiladjian JJ, et al. A pooled analysis of overall survival in COMFORT-I and COMFORT-II, 2 randomized phase III trials of ruxolitinib for the treatment of myelofibrosis. *Haematologica.* 2015;100(9):1139–1145.
24. Patel KP, Newberry KJ, Luthra R, et al. Correlation of mutation profile and response in patients with myelofibrosis treated with ruxolitinib. *Blood.* 2015;126(6):790–797.
25. Spiegel JY, McNamara C, Kennedy JA, et al. Impact of genomic alterations on outcomes in myelofibrosis patients undergoing JAK1/2 inhibitor therapy. *Blood Adv.* 2017;1(20):1729–1738.
26. Ballen KK, Woolfrey AE, Zhu X, et al. Allogeneic hematopoietic cell transplantation for advanced polycythemia vera and essential thrombocythemia. *Biol Blood Marrow Transplant.* 2012;18(9):1446–1454.
27. Devlin R, Gupta V. Myelofibrosis: to transplant or not to transplant? *Hematol Am Soc Hematol Ed Program.* 2016;2016(1):543–551.
28. Ali H, Aldoss I, Yang D, et al. *Long-term Survival in Myelofibrosis after Allogeneic Hematopoietic Cell Transplantation Using Fludarabine/Melphalan Conditioning Regimen (Abstract #199).* Atlanta, GA: American Society of Hematology 59th Annual Meeting & Exposition; 2017.
29. Ballen KK, Shrestha S, Sobocinski KA, et al. Outcome of transplantation for myelofibrosis. *Biol Blood Marrow Transplant.* 2010;16(3):358–367.

30. Kerbauy DMB, Gooley TA, Sale GE, et al. Hematopoietic cell transplantation as curative therapy for idiopathic myelofibrosis, advanced polycythemia vera, and essential thrombocythemia. *Biol Blood Marrow Transpl.* 2007;13(3):355–365.
31. Barosi G, Bacigalupo A. Allogeneic hematopoietic stem cell transplantation for myelofibrosis. *Curr Opin Hematol.* 2006;13(2):74–78.
32. Lussana F, Rambaldi A, Finazzi MC, et al. Allogeneic hematopoietic stem cell transplantation in patients with polycythemia vera or essential thrombocythemia transformed to myelofibrosis or acute myeloid leukemia: a report from the MPN Subcommittee of the Chronic Malignancies Working Party of the European Group for Blood and Marrow Transplantation. *Haematologica.* 2014;99(5):916–921.
33. Gupta V, Malone AK, Hari PN, et al. Reduced-intensity hematopoietic cell transplantation for patients with primary myelofibrosis: a cohort analysis from the center for international blood and marrow transplant research. *Biol Blood Marrow Transplant.* 2014;20(1):89–97.
34. Deeg HJ, Bredeson C, Farnia S, et al. Hematopoietic cell transplantation as curative therapy for patients with myelofibrosis: long-term success in all age groups. *Biol Blood Marrow Transplant.* 2015;21(11):1883–1887.
35. Alchalby H, Yunus DR, Zabelina T, Ayuk F, Kroger N. Incidence and risk factors of poor graft function after allogeneic stem cell transplantation for myelofibrosis. *Bone Marrow Transplant.* 2016;51(9):1223–1227.
36. Extermann M. Measurement and impact of comorbidity in older cancer patients. *Crit Rev Oncol Hematol.* 2000;35(3):181–200.
37. Wong KM, Atenafu EG, Kim D, et al. Incidence and risk factors for early hepatotoxicity and its impact on survival in patients with myelofibrosis undergoing allogeneic hematopoietic cell transplantation. *Biol Blood Marrow Transplant.* 2012;18(10):1589–1599.
38. Deeg HJ, Gooley TA, Flowers ME, et al. Allogeneic hematopoietic stem cell transplantation for myelofibrosis. *Blood.* 2003;102(12):3912–3918.
39. Guardiola P, Anderson JE, Bandini G, et al. Allogeneic stem cell transplantation for agnogenic myeloid metaplasia: a European Group for Blood and Marrow Transplantation, Societe Francaise de Greffe de Moelle, Gruppo Italiano per il Trapianto del Midollo Osseo, and Fred Hutchinson Cancer Research Center Collaborative Study. *Blood.* 1999;93(9):2831–2838.
40. Rondelli D, Goldberg JD, Isola L, et al. MPD-RC 101 prospective study of reduced-intensity allogeneic hematopoietic stem cell transplantation in patients with myelofibrosis. *Blood.* 2014;124(7):1183–1191.
41. Gupta V, Kroger N, Aschan J, et al. A retrospective comparison of conventional intensity conditioning and reduced-intensity conditioning for allogeneic hematopoietic cell transplantation in myelofibrosis. *Bone Marrow Transplant.* 2009;44(5):317–320.
42. Kroger N, Holler E, Kobbe G, et al. Allogeneic stem cell transplantation after reduced-intensity conditioning in patients with myelofibrosis: a prospective, multicenter study of the Chronic Leukemia Working Party of the European Group for Blood and Marrow Transplantation. *Blood.* 2009;114(26):5264–5270.
43. Tefferi A, Vaidya R, Caramazza D, Finke C, Lasho T, Pardanani A. Circulating interleukin (IL)-8, IL-2R, IL-12, and IL-15 levels are independently prognostic in primary myelofibrosis: a comprehensive cytokine profiling study. *J Clin Oncol.* 2011;29(10):1356–1363.
44. Bryder D, Ramsfjell V, Dybedal I, et al. Self-renewal of multipotent long-term repopulating hematopoietic stem cells is negatively regulated by FAS and tumor necrosis factor receptor activation. *J Exp Med.* 2001;194(7):941–952.
45. Dybedal I, Bryder D, Fossum A, Rusten LS, Jacobsen SEW. Tumor necrosis factor (TNF)–mediated activation of the p55 TNF receptor negatively regulates maintenance of cycling reconstituting human hematopoietic stem cells. *Blood.* 2001;98(6):1782–1791.
46. Cervantes F, Dupriez B, Pereira A, et al. New prognostic scoring system for primary myelofibrosis based on a study of the International Working Group for Myelofibrosis Research and Treatment. *Blood.* 2009;113(13):2895–2901.
47. Passamonti F, Cervantes F, Vannucchi AM, et al. A dynamic prognostic model to predict survival in primary myelofibrosis: a study by the IWG-MRT (International Working Group for Myeloproliferative Neoplasms Research and Treatment). *Blood.* 2010;115(9):1703–1708.
48. Guglielmelli P, Rotunno G, Fanelli T, et al. Validation of the differential prognostic impact of type 1/type 1-like versus type 2/type 2-like CALR mutations in myelofibrosis. *Blood Cancer J.* 2015;5:e360.
49. Vannucchi AM, Lasho TL, Guglielmelli P, et al. Mutations and prognosis in primary myelofibrosis. *Leukemia.* 2013;27(9):1861–1869.
50. Guglielmelli P, Vannucchi AM. The prognostic impact of bone marrow fibrosis in primary myelofibrosis. *Am J Hematol.* 2016;91(10):E454–E455.
51. Guglielmelli P, Lasho TL, Rotunno G, et al. MIPSS70: mutation-enhanced international prognostic score system for transplantation-age patients with primary myelofibrosis. *J Clin Oncol.* 2018;36(4):310–318.
52. Tefferi A, Guglielmelli P, Nicolosi M, et al. GIPSS: genetically inspired prognostic scoring system for primary myelofibrosis. *Leukemia.* 2018 (ePub ahead of print).
53. Passamonti F, Giorgino T, Mora B, et al. A clinical-molecular prognostic model to predict survival in patients with post polycythemia vera and post essential thrombocythemia myelofibrosis. *Leukemia.* 2017;31(12):2726–2731.
54. Harrison CN, Vannucchi AM, Kiladjian JJ, et al. Long-term findings from COMFORT-II, a phase 3 study of ruxolitinib vs best available therapy for myelofibrosis. *Leukemia.* 2016;30(8):1701–1707.
55. Tefferi A, Pardanani A, Gangat N, et al. Leukemia risk models in primary myelofibrosis: an International Working Group study. *Leukemia.* 2012;26(6):1439–1441.

56. Shanavas M, Popat U, Michaelis LC, et al. Outcomes of allogeneic hematopoietic cell transplantation in patients with myelofibrosis with prior exposure to Janus kinase 1/2 inhibitors. *Biol Blood Marrow Transplant.* 2016;22(3):432–440.

57. Robin M, Francois S, Huynh A, et al. Ruxolitinib before allogeneic hematopoietic stem cell transplantation (HSCT) in patients with myelofibrosis: a preliminary descriptive report of the JAK ALLO study, a phase II trial sponsored by goelams-FIM in collaboration with the Sfgmtc. *Blood.* 2013;122(21):306.

58. Jaekel N, Behre G, Behning A, et al. Allogeneic hematopoietic cell transplantation for myelofibrosis in patients pretreated with the JAK1 and JAK2 inhibitor ruxolitinib. *Bone Marrow Transplant.* 2014;49(2):179–184.

59. Stubig T, Alchalby H, Ditschkowski M, et al. JAK inhibition with ruxolitinib as pretreatment for allogeneic stem cell transplantation in primary or post-ET/PV myelofibrosis. *Leukemia.* 2014;28(8):1736–1738.

60. Lebon D, Rubio MT, Legrand F, et al. Ruxolitinib for patients with primary or secondary myelofibrosis before allogeneic hematopoietic stem cell transplantation (allo-HSCT): a retrospective study of the Société Française de Greffe de Moelle et de Thérapie Cellulaire (SFGM-TC). *Blood.* 2013;122(21):2111.

61. Kroger N, Shahnaz Syed Abd Kadir S, Zabelina T, et al. Peritransplant ruxolitinib prevents acute GVHD in myelofibrosis patients undergoing allogenic stem cell transplantation. *Biol Blood Marrow Transplant.* 2018. online ahead of print.

62. Gupta V, Kosiorek HE, Mead A, et al. Ruxolitinib therapy followed by reduced intensity conditioning for hematopoietic cell transplantation for myelofibrosis - myeloproliferative disorders research consortium 114 study. *Biol Blood Marrow Transplant.* 2018. (In Press).

63. Pardanani A, Harrison C, Cortes JE, et al. Safety and efficacy of fedratinib in patients with primary or secondary myelofibrosis: a randomized clinical trial. *JAMA Oncol.* 2015;1(5):643–651.

64. Gupta V, Mesa RA, Deininger MW, et al. Circulating cytokines and markers of iron metabolism in myelofibrosis patients treated with momelotininb: correlatives from the Ym-387-II study. *Blood.* 2015;126(23):1600.

65. Abelsson J, Merup M, Birgegard G, et al. The outcome of allo-HSCT for 92 patients with myelofibrosis in the Nordic countries. *Bone Marrow Transplant.* 2011;47(3):380–386.

66. Patriarca F, Bacigalupo A, Sperotto A, et al. Allogeneic hematopoietic stem cell transplantation in myelofibrosis: the 20-year experience of the Gruppo Italiano Trapianto di Midollo Osseo (GITMO). *Haematologica.* 2008;93(10):1514–1522.

67. Robin M, Espérou H, De Latour RP, et al. Correspondence: splenectomy after allogeneic haematopoietic stem cell transplantation in patients with primary myelofibrosis. *Br J Haematol.* 2010;150(6):721–724.

68. Scott BL, Gooley TA, Linenberger ML, et al. International working group scores predict post-transplant outcomes in patients with myelofibrosis. *Blood.* 2010;116(21):3085.

69. Murata M, Nishida T, Taniguchi S, et al. Allogeneic transplantation for primary myelofibrosis with BM, peripheral blood or umbilical cord blood: an analysis of the JSHCT. *Bone Marrow Transplant.* 2014;49(3):355–360.

70. Giannotti F, Deconinck E, Mohty M, et al. Outcomes after unrelated cord blood transplantation for adults with primary or secondary myelofibrosis: a retrospective study on behalf of Eurocord and chronic malignancy working party-EBMT. *Blood.* 2013;122(21):2156.

71. Alchalby H, Zabelina T, Stubig T, et al. Allogeneic stem cell transplantation for myelofibrosis with leukemic transformation: a study from the myeloproliferative neoplasm subcommittee of the CMWP of the European group for blood and marrow transplantation. *Biol Blood Marrow Transplant.* 2014;20(2):279–281.

72. Ciurea SO, de Lima M, Giralt S, et al. Allogeneic stem cell transplantation for myelofibrosis with leukemic transformation. *Biol Blood Marrow Transplant.* 2010;16(4):555–559.

73. Cherington C, Slack JL, Leis J, et al. Allogeneic stem cell transplantation for myeloproliferative neoplasm in blast phase. *Leuk Res.* 2012;36(9):1147–1151.

74. Tefferi A, Mudireddy M, Mannelli F, et al. Blast phase myeloproliferative neoplasm: Mayo-AGIMM study of 410 patients from two separate cohorts. *Leukemia.* 2018;32(5):1200–1210.

75. Rampal RK, Tamari R, Zhang N, et al. Impact of genomic alterations on outcomes in myelofibrosis patients undergoing allogeneic hematopoietic cell transplantation. *Blood.* 2016;128(22):2301.

76. Robin M, Porcher R, Wolschke C, et al. Outcome after transplantation according to reduced intensity conditioning regimen in patients transplanted for myelofibrosis. *Biol Blood Marrow Transplant.* 2016;22(7):1206–1211.

77. Scott BL, Gooley TA, Sorror ML, et al. The Dynamic International Prognostic Scoring System for myelofibrosis predicts outcomes after hematopoietic cell transplantation. *Blood.* 2012;119(11):2657–2664.

78. Robin M, Tabrizi R, Mohty M, et al. Allogeneic haematopoietic stem cell transplantation for myelofibrosis: a report of the Société Française de Greffe de Moelle et de Thérapie Cellulaire (SFGM-TC). *Br J Haematol.* 2011;152(3):331–339.

79. Alchalby H, Badbaran A, Zabelina T, et al. Impact of JAK2V617F mutation status, allele burden, and clearance after allogeneic stem cell transplantation for myelofibrosis. *Blood.* 2010;116(18):3572–3581.

80. Barbui T, Tefferi A, Vannucchi AM, et al. Philadelphia chromosome-negative classical myeloproliferative neoplasms: revised management recommendations from European LeukemiaNet. *Leukemia.* 2018;32(5):1057–1069.

81. Aldauij W, McNamara C, Schuh A, et al. Clinical utility of next generation sequencing in the management of myeloproliferative neoplasms: a single-centre experience. *Hemasphere.* 2018;2(3):e44.

CHAPTER 12

Hematopoietic Cell Transplantation for Chronic Lymphocytic Leukemia

FARRUKH T. AWAN, MD • MOHAMED A. KHARFAN-DABAJA MD, MBA

INTRODUCTION

Chronic lymphocytic leukemia (CLL) represents the most prevalent leukemia in the western hemisphere. It is anticipated that 20,110 cases of CLL will be diagnosed in the United States in 2017.[1] Recent advances in our understanding of the biologic, genetic, and molecular aspects of the disease have resulted in the emergence of more effective therapies, even for high-risk CLL cases harboring Del17p and/or mutations in the *TP53* gene or others.[2–7] For instance, the Bruton's tyrosine kinase inhibitor ibrutinib is approved as front-line therapy in patients with Del17p CLL and for those who have failed prior therapies.[5,6,8] Moreover, venetoclax, which inhibits *BCL-2*, a gene known to play an important role in regulating cell death, is also approved in CLL with Del17p who have received at least one prior therapy.[7] Although these therapies represent a welcomed addition to the therapeutic armamentarium of CLL, cure remains unattainable unless eligible patients are offered an allogeneic hematopoietic cell transplant (allo-HCT).

Recently, the American Society for Blood and Marrow Transplantation (ASBMT) published clinical practice recommendations on the use of allo-HCT in patients with CLL.[9] These recommendations acknowledge the growing role of new therapies within the newly proposed allo-HCT algorithms.[9] Below, we provide a comprehensive appraisal of the published literature on the current role of HCT for patients with CLL, with especial emphasis on allo-HCT. We also describe new and upcoming therapies at various phases of development.

AUTOLOGOUS HEMATOPOIETIC CELL TRANSPLANT

Several published randomized controlled trials (RCTs) and a meta-analysis failed to show a survival benefit of high-dose therapy, followed by autologous HCT (auto-HCT) in patients with CLL.[10–13] In our opinion, auto-HCT, in its current form, has been abandoned as a treatment option for patients with CLL whether as a front-line consolidation strategy or in the relapsed disease setting.

ALLOGENEIC HEMATOPOIETIC CELL TRANSPLANT

Allogeneic Hematopoietic Cell Transplant (Allo-HCT) can offer durable remissions in approximately 50% of patients with relapsed CLL who undergo this procedure.[14,15] Use of allo-HCT provides the advantage of infusing leukemia-free hematopoietic cells. Several studies have demonstrated that T cell–replete allografts can eradicate CLL even when high-risk disease features are present.[16–19] However, to our knowledge, no RCT comparing allo-HCT to conventional chemotherapy or chemoimmunotherapy(ies) or new therapies have been ever conducted. Three published studies demonstrated an advantage favoring allo-HCT over nontransplant therapies. Kharfan-Dabaja et al. published a Markov decision analysis showing a 10-month improved life expectancy (35 vs. 25 months) after allo-HCT.[20] Similarly, Herth et al. reported results of a donor versus no-donor analysis showing an advantage for allo-HCT in transplant-eligible CLL when offered the procedure earlier in the course of the disease.[21] Also, investigators from the MD Anderson Cancer Center showed that referral of patients with Del17p CLL for allo-HCT (vs. no referral) yields over twofold (64% vs. 25%) improvement in 2-year OS (64% vs. 25%).[22] These findings, however, are limited by the fact that these studies preceded availability of new therapies such as ibrutinib, idelalisib, and venetoclax.

There are several new disease-risk stratification models that have been developed for the purpose of helping prognosticate outcomes in patients with CLL.[23,24] Specifically for allo-HCT, Brown et al. reported a prognostic model using four pretransplant variables (disease status, serum lactate dehydrogenase enzyme level, a comorbidity score, and the absolute lymphocyte count).[25] Although this model was successful in discriminating four different prognostic subgroups with significantly varying OS rates (5-year OS for score 0 = 91% vs. score 1 = 78% vs. score 2 = 63% vs. score ≥3 = 22%, P < .0001), it is important to note that these findings are limited to using reduced intensity conditioning (RIC) allo-HCT regimens[25]; and this model remains to be validated in larger multicenter studies. Also, this model predates newly approved therapies, hence limiting its applicability at this time.

A single-institution study has shown that presence of bulky adenopathy (defined as ≥5 cm) is an adverse predictor of disease relapse after allo-HCT[26]; another study showed that patients receiving an RIC allo-HCT were at higher risk of CLL relapse if patients had less than a partial response (PR) at the time of allografting.[27] These and other predictors of outcome in the setting of RIC allo-HCT are summarized in a recently published extensive review.[28]

Who Is Considered a Candidate for Allo-HCT in the Era of Novel Therapies?

ASBMT clinical practice recommendations define standard-risk CLL as absence of Del17p and/or *TP53* mutations, complex karyotype, and Del11q at time of allo-HCT and recommended allo-HCT if there is lack of response or evidence of disease progression after B-cell receptor (BCR) inhibitors.[9] In the case of high-risk CLL, it is defined as presence of Del17p and/or *TP53* mutations and presence of complex karyotype. In this high-risk group, an allo-HCT is recommended in patients who demonstrate evidence of objective response to BCR inhibitors or to *BCL2* inhibitors or to a clinical trial.[9] As noted by the authors, these disease-risk definitions caused an unclear gap pertaining to patients harboring Del11q, but in the end, the authors suggested that patients harboring this mutation may be more appropriately allocated within the standard risk algorithm.[9] This is because new therapies such as ibrutinib or conventional chemoimmunotherapy combinations have demonstrated comparable efficacy in Del11q CLL versus established standard risk cases.[8,29]

Richter Syndrome

Approximately 10% of CLL cases transform into a more aggressive disease, known as Richter syndrome (RS), normally a diffuse large B-cell (DLBCL) or less often Hodgkin lymphoma (HL).[30–34] Several risk factors have been associated with development of RS including cytogenetic (presence of Del17p and Del11q), molecular (*IGHV*-unmutated, NOTCH 1), and clinical (bulky extensive adenopathy), among others.[30,31,33,35] Patients with RS have dismal outcomes with ibrutinib therapy, with median overall survival of less than 6 months.[36,37]

To our knowledge, there are a handful of studies which have evaluated the role of HCT in patients with RS.[38–40] A retrospective registry study from the European Society for Blood and Marrow Transplantation (EBMT) described 3-year OS of 59% after auto-HCT in a relative small sample of 34 RS patients. Relapses occurred in 11 (65%) patients manifesting as RS and in 6 (35%) others with CLL recurrence.[38] The relatively high relapse rates with auto-HCT for RS and CLL limits wider applicability of this treatment. On the other hand, allo-HCT is a well-established treatment option in CLL yielding 3-year OS exceeding 50%.[14,15]

EBMT described outcomes of 25 patients who received an allo-HCT for RS showing 3-year OS of 36% and an NRM of 26%.[38] Offering allo-HCT in the setting of progressive disease (PD) was associated with a lower 3-year OS compared to those in CR/PR (17% vs. 41%).[38] We caution the readers to note that a higher proportion of patients receiving an allo-HCT (vs. an auto-HCT) in the EBMT study had PD at time of transplantation (36% vs. 9%), suggesting a physician bias in allocating patients with more adverse clinical features to allo-HCT.[38] ASBMT recommends allo-HCT in patients with RS who demonstrate an objective response to anthracycline-based chemotherapy.[9] It is unclear whether patients who are deemed ineligible for allo-HCT may be considered for auto-HCT with the understanding that one-third of cases are at risk of CLL relapse. This scenario may represent an area of unmet need to study research strategies aiming at mitigating CLL relapse risk by incorporating new therapies.

Does the Intensity of the Condition Regimen Matter?

To our knowledge, no RCT has been ever performed comparing RIC versus myeloablative (MAC) preparative regimens in patients with CLL undergoing an allo-HCT. The Center for International Blood and Marrow Transplant Research (CIBMTR) compared outcomes of 912 patients who received an RIC against 426 conditioned with a MAC allo-HCT regimen, showing a significantly higher 3-year probability of survival in the RIC group (58% ± 2% vs. 50% ± 3%, P < .001).[15] It is highly probable that the higher nonrelapse mortality

(NRM) associated with MAC allo-HCT, which at times exceeds 35%, is the main reason for the inferior OS in this group.[14,41] A systematic review comparing outcomes of RIC versus MAC allo-HCT also showed higher OS pooled rated favoring RIC regimens (62% [95% CI = 49%–75%] versus 51% [95% CI = 42%–61%]).[42] In our opinion, it remains unclear if MAC allo-HCT ought to be preferred in younger and fit patients with bulky disease. Also, pertaining to RIC allo-HCT, there is no particular regimen that is considered standard and choice of a particular regimen over another is mostly due to physician and center experience.

Novel Therapies in the Current Era

Because the advent of novel therapies for CLL has had a significant impact on the utilization of HCT for CLL, it is important to briefly discuss the clinical outcomes associated with the use of these agents. Most important among these are therapies targeting the various components of the B-cell receptor pathway which plays an integral part in the development and maturation of B-cells. Constitutive activation of the BCR is one of the most important survival signals for the propagation of CLL B-cells.[43] Targeting the various kinases involved in the BCR pathway has resulted in significant improvements in the therapeutic options for this disease. Early results from studies carried out with BTK, PI3K, and SYK inhibitors have all shown excellent efficacy and tolerability, and these agents are currently being used in various combinations to further improve disease outcomes.

Ibrutinib

Ibrutinib is an irreversible inhibitor of BTK and covalently binds to Cys-481 near the ATP-binding domain of the BTK molecule and abrogates enzyme activity and BCR-mediated survival signals. In the initial phase I/II trial a 420-mg daily oral dose of ibrutinib demonstrated an ORR of 86% with 10% CR in patients with relapsed disease and an ORR of 84% with 29% CR in patients with previously untreated disease.[44] Most importantly, however, these responses are sustained and resulted in 60-month PFS of 92% in the untreated group and 43% in the relapsed group.[8] Patients with Del17p had an ORR of 55.9% with a median duration of response of 25 months.[44,45] Historical comparisons have also revealed a significantly improved response rate and PFS when ibrutinib was compared to either cyclin-dependent kinase inhibitors or other conventional therapies used in the past for patients with del17p.[46] Ibrutinib is generally well tolerated with the most common side effects being mild diarrhea, nausea, fatigue, bleeding, and atrial fibrillation. Ibrutinib is also being combined

with multiple other agents to further improve patient outcomes especially in patients with high-risk Del17p disease because it appears that Del17p still retains its role as a poor prognostic factor even in the ibrutinib era.

Idelalisib

Idelalisib is an oral delta isoform selective phosphatidylinositol-4,5-bisphosphate 3-kinase (PI3K)-δ inhibitor[47] that has shown promising activity against CLL patients. After promising early results from a phase I trial of 54 patients, with relapsed/refractory high-risk CLL patients, where it resulted in an ORR of 72% (including PR + L) and a median PFS of 15.8 months[48]; idelalisib was combined with rituximab and compared to rituximab and placebo in a phase 3 trial. The combination resulted in an ORR of 81% versus 13% and PFS at 1 year in excess of 90% versus 5.5% in the rituximab and placebo arm, respectively.[49] Similar to ibrutinib, idelalisib appears to be effective in patients with Del17p disease. Idelalisib, however, does cause transaminitis, diarrhea with colitis, pneumonitis, and infections that have resulted in a limited use. Idelalisib treatment in previously untreated patients also results in increased mortality secondary to infectious issues and serious transaminitis and should not be used in this setting.

Venetoclax

Venetoclax is an oral Bcl-2–targeting agent that has shown impressive activity with deep remissions in patients with relapsed and refractory CLL including those who have Del17p.[50,51] In a recent pooled analysis of patients with Del17p disease the estimated median PFS after venetoclax was in excess of 24 months.[7,52] Venetoclax use does result in cytopenias and tumor lysis which complicates its use to a certain extent. However, given its promising activity, it was approved for use in patients with Del17p disease after failing initial therapy.

Treatment with these agents, although more effective, is not curative, and patients who discontinue treatment with kinase inhibitors often experience rapid disease progression. Moreover, chronic exposure to kinase inhibitors also occasionally results in the emergence of resistant malignant cell clones.[53,54] Therefore, consideration for an allo-HCT can be made for the appropriate candidate with relapsed CLL who experiences a deep response to salvage therapy with novel agents.

Chimeric Antigen Receptor–T Cells

Chimeric antigen receptor–T (CAR-T) cells are engineered, autologous, lentiviral modified T-cells that contain an altered T-cell receptor targeting a specific surface antigen (e.g., CD19) on the surface of CLL B-cells. The modified T-cell receptor has a higher affinity and specificity toward the target antigen and is not MHC restricted. Multiple CAR-T cells are being evaluated in clinical trials with exciting early results.[55,56] Their use in CLL have shown that they can persist in vivo for an extended period and are able to induce prolonged clinical responses in the majority of patients.[57] However, their treatment is associated with severe cytokine release syndrome and macrophage activation syndrome that require aggressive and intensive supportive care and anti–IL-6 directed therapy. These modified CAR-T cells also result in the sustained elimination of normal B-cells and subsequent sustained hypogammaglobulinemia that require ongoing supportive care and infection prophylaxis to limit the incidence of infectious complications in these patients.[56] Development of these agents on a larger scale is ongoing to allow for larger studies to confirm their promising effect and could be a therapeutic entity that could result in sustained disease-free states or even cures.

Other Experimental Agents

Multiple other agents are being developed for use in CLL. Prominent among them is the second-generation BTK inhibitor acalabrutinib which has minimal off-target effects as compared with ibrutinib, hence limiting its adverse events.[58] It has already shown efficacy in patients with relapsed disease but lacks the depth of response seen with venetoclax. Other agents include umbralisib, a novel PI3K inhibitor which appears to be well tolerated in comparison to previous PI3K inhibitors from early results.[59] Nivolumab with or without ibrutinib has also preliminarily demonstrated promising activity in patients with RS and can be a useful option in patients who otherwise have a dismal prognosis.[60]

DISCUSSION

Treatment of CLL has undergone dramatic progress in recent times, and novel therapeutics options have started to replace conventional chemoimmunotherapeutic strategies. This has resulted in a paradigm shift in the field as more and more patients are now being treated with these agents rather than conventional chemotherapy-based treatments. However, long-term disease control data from these agents (including CAR-T cells) are limited, and cure of CLL still remains elusive. Moreover, patients with CLL are diagnosed at a median age of 72 years, and thus the vast majority of patients

are ineligible for allo-HCT due to presence of associated comorbidities in this age group. Furthermore, significant disease burden characterized as bulky lymphadenopathy, significant residual bone marrow disease, and older age predict worse outcomes in patients with CLL undergoing allo-HCT. Although these prognostic factors remain to be validated in larger multi-institutional studies, they pose an important issue in the era of novel therapies because the majority of these agents, apart from venetoclax, are unable to effect a deep remission and may not be suitable as a debulking strategy for patients planning to proceed with allo-HCT. In addition, these therapeutic modalities need to be continued indefinitely and are associated with significant adverse impact on quality-of-life issues and societal costs. Recent data also demonstrate that patients progressing on ibrutinib or harboring BTK resistance mutations comprise a group of patients with a particularly poor prognosis. Specifically for these patients, the goal of subsequent therapy should be to proceed with allo-HCT, in eligible patients, when they attain a remission to subsequent treatment such as venetoclax. These recommendations, however, need to be evaluated in light of the transplant-related morbidity and mortality associated with allo-HCT and the increasing availability of CAR-T cell treatment which can also potentially result in sustained remissions.

REFERENCES

1. Siegel RL, Miller KD, Jemal A. Cancer statistics, 2017. *CA Cancer J Clin.* 2017;67:7–30.
2. Dohner H, Stilgenbauer S, Benner A, et al. Genomic aberrations and survival in chronic lymphocytic leukemia. *N Engl J Med.* 2000;343:1910–1916.
3. Puente XS, Pinyol M, Quesada V, et al. Whole-genome sequencing identifies recurrent mutations in chronic lymphocytic leukaemia. *Nature.* 2011;475:101–105.
4. Kharfan-Dabaja MA, Chavez JC, Khorfan KA, et al. Clinical and therapeutic implications of the mutational status of IgVH in patients with chronic lymphocytic leukemia. *Cancer.* 2008;113:897–906.
5. Burger JA, Keating MJ, Wierda WG, et al. Safety and activity of ibrutinib plus rituximab for patients with high-risk chronic lymphocytic leukaemia: a single-arm, phase 2 study. *Lancet Oncol.* 2014;15:1090–1099.
6. Farooqui MZ, Valdez J, Martyr S, et al. Ibrutinib for previously untreated and relapsed or refractory chronic lymphocytic leukaemia with TP53 aberrations: a phase 2, single-arm trial. *Lancet Oncol.* 2015;16:169–176.
7. Stilgenbauer S, Eichhorst B, Schetelig J, et al. Venetoclax in relapsed or refractory chronic lymphocytic leukaemia with 17p deletion: a multicentre, open-label, phase 2 study. *Lancet Oncol.* 2016;17:768–778.

8. Byrd JC, Furman RR, Coutre SE, et al. Targeting BTK with ibrutinib in relapsed chronic lymphocytic leukemia. *N Engl J Med.* 2013;369:32–42.

9. Kharfan-Dabaja MA, Kumar A, Hamadani M, et al. Clinical practice recommendations for use of allogeneic hematopoietic cell transplantation in chronic lymphocytic leukemia on behalf of the guidelines committee of the American Society for Blood and Marrow Transplantation. *Biol Blood Marrow Transpl.* 2016;22:2117–2125.

10. Magni M, Di Nicola M, Patti C, et al. Results of a randomized trial comparing high-dose chemotherapy plus Auto-SCT and R-FC in CLL at diagnosis. *Bone Marrow Transpl.* 2014;49:485–491.

11. Brion A, Mahe B, Kolb B, et al. Autologous transplantation in CLL patients with B and C Binet stages: final results of the prospective randomized GOELAMS LLC 98 trial. *Bone Marrow Transpl.* 2012;47:542–548.

12. Michallet M, Dreger P, Sutton L, et al. Autologous hematopoietic stem cell transplantation in chronic lymphocytic leukemia: results of European intergroup randomized trial comparing autografting versus observation. *Blood.* 2011;117:1516–1521.

13. Reljic T, Kumar A, Djulbegovic B, et al. High-dose therapy and autologous hematopoietic cell transplantation as front-line consolidation in chronic lymphocytic leukemia: a systematic review. *Bone Marrow Transpl.* 2015;50:1069–1074.

14. Kharfan-Dabaja MA, Bazarbachi A. Hematopoietic stem cell allografting for chronic lymphocytic leukemia: a focus on reduced-intensity conditioning regimens. *Cancer Control.* 2012;19:68–75.

15. Pasquini MC, Zhu X. *Current Uses and Outcomes of Hematopoietic Stem Cell Transplantation: 2014 CIBMTR Summary Slides*; 2014. Available at: http://www.cibmtr.org.

16. Dreger P, Schnaiter A, Zenz T, et al. TP53, SF3B1, and NOTCH1 mutations and outcome of allotransplantation for chronic lymphocytic leukemia: six-year follow-up of the GCLLSG CLL3X trial. *Blood.* 2013;121:3284–3288.

17. Schetelig J, van Biezen A, Brand R, et al. Allogeneic hematopoietic stem-cell transplantation for chronic lymphocytic leukemia with 17p deletion: a retrospective European Group for Blood and Marrow Transplantation analysis. *J Clin Oncol.* 2008;26:5094–5100.

18. Caballero D, Garcia-Marco JA, Martino R, et al. Allogeneic transplant with reduced intensity conditioning regimens may overcome the poor prognosis of B-cell chronic lymphocytic leukemia with unmutated immunoglobulin variable heavy-chain gene and chromosomal abnormalities (11q- and 17p-). *Clin Cancer Res.* 2005;11:7757–7763.

19. Ritgen M, Stilgenbauer S, von Neuhoff N, et al. Graft-versus-leukemia activity may overcome therapeutic resistance of chronic lymphocytic leukemia with unmutated immunoglobulin variable heavy-chain gene status: implications of minimal residual disease measurement with quantitative PCR. *Blood.* 2004;104:2600–2602.

20. Kharfan-Dabaja MA, Pidala J, Kumar A, et al. Comparing efficacy of reduced-toxicity allogeneic hematopoietic cell transplantation with conventional chemo-(immuno) therapy in patients with relapsed or refractory CLL: a Markov decision analysis. *Bone Marrow Transpl.* 2012;47:1164–1170.

21. Herth I, Dietrich S, Benner A, et al. The impact of allogeneic stem cell transplantation on the natural course of poor-risk chronic lymphocytic leukemia as defined by the EBMT consensus criteria: a retrospective donor versus no donor comparison. *Ann Oncol.* 2014;25:200–206.

22. Poon ML, Fox PS, Samuels BI, et al. Allogeneic stem cell transplant in patients with chronic lymphocytic leukemia with 17p deletion: consult-transplant versus consult- no-transplant analysis. *Leuk Lymphoma.* 2015;56:711–715.

23. Pflug N, Bahlo J, Shanafelt TD, et al. Development of a comprehensive prognostic index for patients with chronic lymphocytic leukemia. *Blood.* 2014;124:49–62.

24. International CLLIPIwg. An international prognostic index for patients with chronic lymphocytic leukaemia (CLL-IPI): a meta-analysis of individual patient data. *Lancet Oncol.* 2016;17:779–790.

25. Brown JR, Kim HT, Armand P, et al. Long-term follow-up of reduced-intensity allogeneic stem cell transplantation for chronic lymphocytic leukemia: prognostic model to predict outcome. *Leukemia.* 2013;27:362–369.

26. Sorror ML, Storer BE, Sandmaier BM, et al. Five-year follow-up of patients with advanced chronic lymphocytic leukemia treated with allogeneic hematopoietic cell transplantation after nonmyeloablative conditioning. *J Clin Oncol.* 2008;26:4912–4920.

27. Dreger P, Brand R, Hansz J, et al. Treatment-related mortality and graft-versus-leukemia activity after allogeneic stem cell transplantation for chronic lymphocytic leukemia using intensity-reduced conditioning. *Leukemia.* 2003;17:841–848.

28. Kharfan-Dabaja MA. Predictors of outcome in reduced intensity allogeneic hematopoietic cell transplantation for chronic lymphocytic leukemia: summarizing the evidence and highlighting the limitations. *Immunotherapy.* 2015;7:47–56.

29. Hallek M, Fischer K, Fingerle-Rowson G, et al. Addition of rituximab to fludarabine and cyclophosphamide in patients with chronic lymphocytic leukaemia: a randomised, open-label, phase 3 trial. *Lancet.* 2010;376:1164–1174.

30. Rossi D, Spina V, Deambrogi C, et al. The genetics of Richter syndrome reveals disease heterogeneity and predicts survival after transformation. *Blood.* 2011;117:3391–3401.

31. Parikh SA, Rabe KG, Call TG, et al. Diffuse large B-cell lymphoma (Richter syndrome) in patients with chronic lymphocytic leukaemia (CLL): a cohort study of newly diagnosed patients. *Br J Haematol.* 2013;162:774–782.

32. Rossi D, Spina V, Forconi F, et al. Molecular history of Richter syndrome: origin from a cell already present at the time of chronic lymphocytic leukemia diagnosis. *Int J Cancer.* 2012;130:3006–3010.

33. Fabbri G, Khiabanian H, Holmes AB, et al. Genetic lesions associated with chronic lymphocytic leukemia transformation to Richter syndrome. *J Exp Med.* 2013;210:2273–2288.

34. Richter MN. Generalized reticular cell sarcoma of lymph nodes associated with lymphatic leukemia. *Am J Pathol.* 1928;4:285–292 7.

35. Rossi D, Cerri M, Capello D, et al. Biological and clinical risk factors of chronic lymphocytic leukaemia transformation to Richter syndrome. *Br J Haematol.* 2008;142:202–215.

36. Maddocks KJ, Ruppert AS, Lozanski G, et al. Etiology of ibrutinib therapy discontinuation and outcomes in patients with chronic lymphocytic leukemia. *JAMA Oncol.* 2015;1:80–87.

37. Jain P, Keating M, Wierda W, et al. Outcomes of patients with chronic lymphocytic leukemia after discontinuing ibrutinib. *Blood.* 2015;125:2062–2067.

38. Cwynarski K, van Biezen A, de Wreede L, et al. Autologous and allogeneic stem-cell transplantation for transformed chronic lymphocytic leukemia (Richter's syndrome): a retrospective analysis from the chronic lymphocytic leukemia subcommittee of the chronic leukemia working party and lymphoma working party of the European Group for Blood and Marrow Transplantation. *J Clin Oncol.* 2012;30:2211–2217.

39. Tsimberidou AM, O'Brien S, Khouri I, et al. Clinical outcomes and prognostic factors in patients with Richter's syndrome treated with chemotherapy or chemoimmunotherapy with or without stem-cell transplantation. *J Clin Oncol.* 2006;24:2343–2351.

40. El-Asmar J, Kharfan-Dabaja MA. Hematopoietic cell transplantation for Richter syndrome. *Biol Blood Marrow Transpl.* 2016;22:1938–1944.

41. Kharfan-Dabaja MA, El-Asmar J, Awan FT, et al. Current state of hematopoietic cell transplantation in CLL as smart therapies emerge. *Best Pract Res Clin Haematol.* 2016;29:54–66.

42. El-Asmar J, Reljic T, Kumar A, et al. Reduced intensity conditioning yields superior overall survival rates compared to myeloablative regimens for allogeneic HCT in chronic lymphocytic leukemia: a side-by-side systematic review/meta-analysis. *Biol Blood Marrow Transpl.* 2017;23:S269.

43. Duhren-von Minden M, Ubelhart R, Schneider D, et al. Chronic lymphocytic leukaemia is driven by antigen-independent cell-autonomous signalling. *Nature.* 2012;489:309–312.

44. O'Brien SM, Furman RR, Coutre SE, et al. Five-year experience with single-agent ibrutinib in patients with previously untreated and relapsed/refractory chronic lymphocytic leukemia/small lymphocytic leukemia. *Blood.* 2016;128. 233–233.

45. O'Brien S, Furman R, Coutre S, et al. Independent evaluation of ibrutinib efficacy 3 years post-initiation of monotherapy in patients with chronic lymphocytic leukemia/small lymphocytic leukemia including deletion 17p disease. *J Clin Oncol.* 2014;32:5s.

46. Stephens DM, Ruppert AS, Jones JA, et al. Impact of targeted therapy on outcome of chronic lymphocytic leukemia patients with relapsed del(17p13.1) karyotype at a single center. *Leukemia.* 2014;28:1365–1368.

47. Herman SE, Gordon AL, Wagner AJ, et al. Phosphatidylinositol 3-kinase-delta inhibitor CAL-101 shows promising preclinical activity in chronic lymphocytic leukemia by antagonizing intrinsic and extrinsic cellular survival signals. *Blood.* 2010;116:2078–2088.

48. Brown JR, Byrd JC, Coutre SE, et al. Idelalisib, an inhibitor of phosphatidylinositol 3-kinase p110delta, for relapsed/refractory chronic lymphocytic leukemia. *Blood.* 2014;123:3390–3397.

49. Furman RR, Sharman JP, Coutre SE, et al. Idelalisib and rituximab in relapsed chronic lymphocytic leukemia. *N Engl J Med.* 2014;370:997–1007.

50. ABT-199 shows effectiveness in CLL. *Cancer Discov.* 2014;4:OF7.

51. Roberts AW, Davids MS, Pagel JM, et al. Targeting BCL2 with venetoclax in relapsed chronic lymphocytic leukemia. *N Engl J Med.* 2016;374:311–322.

52. Roberts AW, Seymour JF, Eichhorst B, et al. Pooled multitrial analysis of venetoclax efficacy in patients with relapsed or refractory chronic lymphocytic leukemia. *Blood.* 2016;128:3230–3230.

53. Awan FT, Byrd JC. New strategies in chronic lymphocytic leukemia: shifting treatment paradigms. *Clin Cancer Res.* 2014 Dec 1;20(23):5869–74.

54. Woyach JA, Furman RR, Liu TM, et al. Resistance mechanisms for the Bruton's tyrosine kinase inhibitor ibrutinib. *N Engl J Med.* 2014;370:2286–2294.

55. Porter DL, Levine BL, Kalos M, et al. Chimeric antigen receptor-modified T cells in chronic lymphoid leukemia. *N Engl J Med.* 2011;365:725–733.

56. Gill S, June CH. Going viral: chimeric antigen receptor T-cell therapy for hematological malignancies. *Immunol Rev.* 2015;263:68–89.

57. Kalos M, Levine BL, Porter DL, et al. T cells with chimeric antigen receptors have potent antitumor effects and can establish memory in patients with advanced leukemia. *Sci Transl Med.* 2011;3:95ra73.

58. Byrd JC, Harrington B, O'Brien S, et al. Acalabrutinib (ACP-196) in relapsed chronic lymphocytic leukemia. *N Engl J Med.* 2016;374:323–332.

59. Zinzani PL, Broccoli A. Possible novel agents in marginal zone lymphoma. *Best Pract Res Clin Haematol.* 2017;30:149–157.

60. Jain N, Basu S, Thompson PA, et al. Nivolumab combined with ibrutinib for CLL and Richter transformation: a phase II trial. *Blood.* 2016;128:59–59.

Allogeneic Hematopoietic Cell Transplantation in Patients With Myelodysplastic Syndrome

IBRAHIM YAKOUB-AGHA, MD, PHD

INTRODUCTION

With the advent of molecular biology, the understanding of the pathogenesis of myelodysplastic syndrome (MDS) has dramatically increased in past 2 decades. Although the new therapeutic agents have improved disease control and, to a lesser extent, prolonged life of MDS patients,[1] the only curative option is still allogeneic hematopoietic cell transplantation (allo-HCT).[2–6] Since the late 90s, the introduction of reduced-intensity conditionaing (RIC)/toxicity conditioning regimens has extended the indication for allo-HCT to older patients as well as those with comorbidities. In addition, the availability of more and more unrelated donors and the advent of haploidentical transplantations has also contributed to the continuing increase in the number of allo-HCT options for MDS patients.[7–11]

Despite its curative potential and offering a better management of transplanted patients, allo-HCT cannot be a standard of treatment for all MDS patients because of posttransplant complications responsible for significant morbidity and mortality risks.[5,12]

When considering allo-HCT as an option for patients with MDS, several factors must be taken into consideration in the decision-making process. On the one hand, the disease characteristics that impact the risk of transformation into acute myeloid leukemia (AML) and survival must be considered. On the other hand, patient-related factors, such as age and comorbidities, must be taken into account.

This chapter discusses the role of allo-HCT in patients with MDS and the management of select patients who are potential allo-HCT candidates.

WHO IS A CANDIDATE FOR ALLO-HCT?

To refer a patient diagnosed with MDS for transplantation, several factors have to be taken into account.

Fig. 13.1 describes the decision-making flowchart according to patient-related factors and disease characteristics. Because MDS is a chronic progressive disease, the decision in favor of transplantation can be made at diagnosis or at any stage of the evolution of the disease. (Table 13.1).

Patient-Related Factors

Although there is no international consensus regarding the upper age limit to offer allogeneic transplantation to patients with MDS, a panel of international experts has recommended 70-years old as a reasonable limit to receive allo-HCT.[13] However, the first step in transplantation decision-making has to be the evaluation of transplant feasibility regardless of conditioning intensity. In fact, age, health status, and functional ability (performance status) and comorbidities are important factors that impact allo-HCT outcomes.[3,14]

To identify patients who are suitable to receive allo-HCT, several risk indexes have been established; however, none of them were sufficiently specific for MDS as they do not include specific disease characteristics such as number of cytopenias, percentage of marrow blasts, and cytogenetic risk groups.[15,16]

For decades, having been identified as a risk factor in univariate analyses, the cutoff age of 60 years was thought to be a poor prognostic factor for the feasibility of allo-HCT.[17–19] However, age alone is not a poor prognostic marker. Koreth et al. observed that, according to the International Prognostic Scoring System (IPSS), higher risk patients aged from 60 to 70 years benefited from transplantation following RIC than those who received nontransplant treatments.[20]

The comorbidity index (HCT-CI) developed by Sorror et al.[21] has been recognized as the most relevant clinical index to be considered to judge the feasibility of allo-HCT in a given patient.[22,23] In addition,

Hematopoietic Cell Transplantation for Malignant Conditions. https://doi.org/10.1016/B978-0-323-56802-9.00013-4

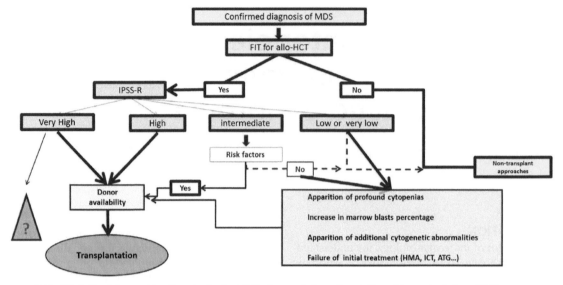

FIG. 13.1 Decision-making flowchart. *allo-HCT*, allogeneic hematopoietic cell transplantation; *HMA*, hypomethylating agent; *IPSS-R*, revised International Prognostic Scoring System; *ITC*, induction-type chemotherapy; *MDS*, myelodysplastic syndrome. (Adapted from Dewitte, et al. *Blood.* 2017;(13).)

TABLE 13.1
Decision-Making Algorithm Based on Disease Characteristics and Patient Age and Comorbidities

	DISEASE CHARACTERISTICS				
Patient Condition	**Cytogenetics**	**Marrow Blasts %**	**ICT**	**HMA**	**Upfront Allo-HCT**
Fit patients (without comorbidities)	< High risk	<5	No	BO	possible
		5–10	possible	BO	possible
		>10	BO	possible	possible
	High risk	<5	No	possible	BO[a]
		5–10	No	possible	BO[a]
		>10	possible	possible	BO[a]

[a]if allo-HCT can be performed rapidly within 4 months.
Adapted from Yakoub-Agha I, Deeg J. Are hypomethylating agents replacing induction-type chemotherapy before allogeneic stem cell transplantation in patients with myelodysplastic syndrome? *Biol Blood Marrow Transplant.* 2014;20(12):1885–1890. https://doi.org/10.1016/j.bbmt.2014.06.023.

age (≥40 years) assigned a weight of 1 and added to the HCT-CI constituted a composite comorbidity/age index.[21] Thus patients with comorbidity/age scores of 0–2 had comparable mortality risks regardless of conditioning regimens, whereas those patients with scores of 3–4 and ≥5 had statistically significant higher mortality risks after myeloablative (MA) and RIC versus nonmyeloablative (NMA) regimens. Therefore the decision of allo-HCT can be easily made for patients with low scores (<5) who are considered as "fit", whereas it is more difficult for those with higher scores because the estimated nonrelapse mortality (NRM) incidence can be as high as 50%.[21]

Disease Characteristics

The second step in the decision-making is to evaluate the risk of transformation toward AML and the survival of MDS patients. Since the late 90s, several scoring systems have been established to assess the prognosis of these patients, namely the IPSS,[24] the World Health Organization (WHO)[25] Classification-Based Prognostic Scoring System (WPSS), and more recently the revised IPSS (IPSS-R).[22]

The European Leukemia Network (ELN) and the National Comprehensive Cancer Network formulated the general recommendation for allo-HCT at diagnosis based on the IPSS, which is based on the number of cytopenias, percentage of marrow blasts, and cytogenetics.[22,23] Using a Markov statistical model, two studies have shown that postponing allo-HCT was beneficial for patients with low/intermediate-1 IPSS risk score, whereas immediate transplantation was associated with maximal life expectancy in patients with intermediate-2/high-risk disease.[20,26]

Given a certain heterogeneity that was observed in IPSS subgroups, in particular in patients with low/intermediate-1 risk scores, an international expert panel from the EBMT, ELN, and the International MDS Foundation adjusted this general recommendation to the IPSS-R risk score.[13] This revised scoring system is based on marrow blast percentage, modified cytogenetic risk groups,[27] and the severity of cytopenias. In addition, it is an age-adjusted risk score.[28]

IPSS-R identifies the following 5 risk categories: very low (score≤1.5), low (>1.5≤3.0), intermediate (>3≤4.5), high (>4≤6), and very high (>6). The 25% AML progression/median survival in the absence of therapy was (not reached/8.8), (10.8/5.3), (3.2/3), (1.4/1.6), and (0.7/0.8) years for patients with very low, low, intermediate, high, and very high risk, respectively.[28] The IPSS-R risk categories can function as the platform for disease-related factors. To simplify its clinical use, patients can be categorized into three risk groups when considering allo-HCT: lower risk—including low and very low risk groups, intermediate risk, and higher risk—including high and very high-risk groups.

As shown in Fig. 13.1, those patients who are not candidates for allo-HCT—patients considered "unfit" (regardless of the IPSS-R score) for allo-HCT and those with lower IPSS-R risk—should be offered nontransplant treatment.

The decision-making becomes more difficult for patients belonging to the intermediate IPSS-R group. In fact, these patients have a median survival of 3 years without treatment and 25% AML progression at 3.2 years.[28] Patients in the intermediate IPSS-R risk group who present at diagnosis more than 5% marrow blasts, poor karyotype, profound cytopenias (i.e., Hb < 8 g/dL, absolute neutrophil count <0.8 G/L,

platelets <50 G/L), or severe BM fibrosis can be referred for allo-HCT right away. Otherwise, patients in this risk group should be offered nontransplant options in the first place.[13,29]

Patients with higher risk scores have to be referred for allo-HCT as soon as possible. However, given their poor outcome even after allo-HCT, patients with very poor cytogenetics (i.e., complex karyotype and/or monosomal karyotype) should be considered for clinical trials.[30,31] This is especially the case for those with complex karyotypes and TP53 mutations.[13,32] In addition, patients with higher IPSS-R risk and aged more than 60 years may be considered for clinical trials.[13]

In patients with lower risk and intermediate risk who are not candidates for transplant at diagnosis, allo-HCT should be considered if they develop profound cytopenias, increasing marrow blasts, or additional cytogenetic abnormalities. Allo-HCT should also be considered in the case of initial treatment failure. Especially in the case where the following initial treatments have failed: hypomethylating agents (HMA), induction-type chemotherapy (ITC), and immunotherapy with antithymocyte globulin (ATG).[13]

Molecular abnormalities play a significant role in the prognosis of MDS[33-35] and in patient response to allo-HCT.[32] Some genetic abnormalities such as SF3B1 mutation generally have a favorable prognosis in contrast to SRSF2-mutated cases. In addition, multilineage dysplasias are generally associated with DNMT3A, TET2, IDH1, and IDH2 mutations. Furthermore, RUNX1-, U2AF1-, ASXL-, and TP53-mutated cases appear to be associated with poor prognosis.[36] With the exception of the combination of complex karyotype and TP53 mutations being associated with very poor outcome after allo-HCT, to date, there is no international consensus that incorporates molecular abnormalities as factors into the treatment decision-making process.

Other Subtypes of MDS
Chronic myelomonocytic leukemia
Two different types of chronic myelomonocytic leukemia (CMML) are distinguished in the WHO classification: CMML-1 with less than 5% of blasts in the peripheral blood (PB) and less than 10% in the bone marrow (BM); CMML-2 with 5%–19% of blasts in the PB and 10%–19% in the BM.[37] The use of the CMML-specific scoring system (CPSS) is recommended for allo-HCT,[38] whereas IPSS-R can be used for patients with the dysplastic type of CMML. It is recommended upfront allo-HCT in patients with CPSS intermediate-2 or high-risk

scores. Pretransplant treatment with HMAs in patients with proliferative CMML-MP could be an option despite the absence of prospective clinical trial evidence.[13]

Treatment-related MDS

In general the prognosis of Treatment-related MDS (t-MDS) is poorer than the prognosis of de novo MDS.[39] However, t-MDS was found more often to be associated with poor-risk cytogenetics than de novo MDS in a study by Cheng et al. of 257 patients with t-MDS/transformed AML. The 5-year relapse-free survival in this group was 29%. Multivariate analyses failed to show significant differences in the outcome when the t-MDS cohort was compared with a cohort of 339 patients who underwent allo-HCT for de novo MDS.[40] Overall, patients with t-MDS should follow the recommendations developed for de novo MDS according to the IPSS-R.[13]

Hypoplastic MDS

Here also, the IPSS-R risk score should be used to identify hypoplastic MDS patients who may benefit from allo-HCT. Indeed, the IPSS-R risk score does predict survival well in patients with hypoplastic MDS.[41]

MDS originating from congenital mutations

Patients with dyskeratosis congenita, Fanconi anemia, and disorders with mutations in the genes of telomerase complex who develop MDS are candidates for allo-HCT at an early stage of the disease should be referred to specific centers. Germline mutations of RUNX1 or GATA-2 may occur in family with this form of diseases.

DONOR SELECTION

Approximately 30% of patients have a human leukocyte antigen (HLA)–identical sibling donor that has been established as the "gold standard" for malignant and nonmalignant diseases.[42,43] In addition, outcomes after transplantation from high-resolution HLA-A–, HLA-B–, HLA-C–, HLA-DR–, and HLA-DQ–matched unrelated donors (so called 10/10) were similar to outcomes observed with HLA-identical sibling donors.[44–46] Therefore both HLA-identical sibling and 10/10 HLA-matched unrelated donor are equal and should be considered as a first choice.

Although allo-HCT from syngeneic donors are reputed to lack graft-versus-leukemia effect, results of such transplantations have similarly shown that they are responsible for lower posttransplant toxicity leading to similar or even better outcomes than HLA-matched related or unrelated donors.[47,48] Indeed, in an EBMT

study, a trend for better overall survival was observed in the twin group probably because of lower NRM with comparable relapse incidence.[49]

In the absence of an HLA-matched donor, allo-HCT from an alternative donor including haploidentical donor, HLA-mismatched related or unrelated donor, and unrelated cord blood can be considered.[10,11,50–52] Of note, in a study that included 3857 patients, Lee et al. reported that mismatching at a single HLA-A, HLA-B, HLA-C, or HLA-DRB-1 locus (7/8) was associated with lower survival and disease-free survival and higher treatment-related mortality than 8/8 HLA-matched pairs.[53] Therefore alternative donor transplants may be considered for young and fit patients with higher risk MDS for whom no HLA-matched donor can be identified within a reasonable search period.[13]

Overall, in the absence of an HLA-matched donor for a given patient, a prolonged search to identify a fully HLA-matched donor must be balanced against the risk of disease progression and the occurrence of cytopenia-related complications while the search is underway. Depending on the stage of the disease, rapid transplantation with the best available donor, even if allele- or antigen-level mismatched, may offer the best chance for survival.

SELECTING HEMATOPOIETIC CELL SOURCE

Numerous studies have compared mobilized peripheral blood stem cells (PBSCs) with BM for allo-HCT.[54–58] Although PBSC could be a preferred graft source for many types of allogeneic transplants from sibling HLA-matched donors, the potential benefits with this source are still unclear for unrelated donor transplantation. As a matter of fact, PBSC has been associated with a high rate of extensive chronic GVHD.[54–56,58–60]

In a prospective multicenter randomized trial that enrolled 551 unrelated transplantations, Anasetti et al. showed a 2-year incidence of chronic GVHD of 53% in PBSC group as compared with 41% in the BM group ($P = .01$).[54] The absence of the use of ATG as a GVHD prophylaxis in PBSC patients could be an explanation for these results because 72% of the patients had not received ATG within the conditioning. Indeed, the quantity of donor-derived lymphocytes in PBSC grafts could be up to 30-fold greater than in BM grafts.[61,62] In addition, the absence of ATG was observed to be an independent risk factor for both acute and chronic GVHD in a prospective randomized study that included 201 patients, of whom 164 had received PBSC.[63] In other studies, incorporating ATG into conditioning regimens for unrelated transplantations has decreased the incidence of GVHD without compromising survival or increasing posttransplant relapse rates.[59,60]

In a retrospective study that included 234 MDS patients and compared PBSC with BM using HLA-identical sibling donors, survival was significantly better among recipients of PBSC, except for patients with either refractory anemia or high-risk cytogenetics.[64] Although there is no international consensus regarding the preferred source of hematopoietic cells between PBSC and BM, ATG should be incorporated within the conditioning regimen whenever PBSC graft is used.

Unrelated cord blood can be chosen in the absence of an HLA-matched donor in certain centers in countries with easy access to this source.[52,65] However, ATG within conditioning should be avoided because it seems to have a detrimental impact on the outcome in transplants with either an MA or RIC pretransplant regimen.[66,67]

THE ROLE OF PRETRANSPLANT DEBULKING TREATMENT

Large studies have shown that the percentage of BM blasts at transplant significantly impact the posttransplant outcome for MDS patients, thus justifying the use of pretransplant cytoreduction treatment.[5,18,64] In addition, as a bridging strategy, before transplant therapy, MDS patients can take time to transplantation. However, debulking treatment before allo-HCT which aims to reduce the incidence of posttransplant relapse in patients with MDS is still debated. The achievement of complete remission (CR) before transplant has been shown to improve outcome, although one might question whether this better outcome reflects the selection of "responsive" patients or is related to a reduction in disease burden.

Patients with MDS who are candidates for allo-HCT can be offered three pretransplant strategies including ICT, HMA, or upfront transplant.

While ICT is the preferred pretransplant treatment in patients with more than 10% marrow blasts and an absence of poor cytogenetic abnormalities,[23,68,69] HMA is usually offered to older patients who have less than 10% marrow blasts.[70] In a retrospective comparison of ICT and HMA, Damage et al. observed similar posttransplant outcome with both strategies when patients received either ICT or HMA alone.[71] Patients who received ICT and HMA before transplant had higher NRM rate but similar incidence of posttransplant relapse compared to patients who received only ICT or HMA, reflecting an additional toxicity rather than a selection of

poor prognostic patients.[71] Furthermore, pretransplant debulking treatment can be responsible for morbidity and mortality that can prevent some patients to undergo allo-HCT. Indeed, in a prospective study comparing donor versus no donor in patients with higher risk MDS, Robin et al. observed that up to 25% of patients died before transplantation mainly because of pretransplant treatment toxicity.[6] In a large retrospective comparison, Damage et al. observed no difference in terms of overall survival, relapse-free survival, relapse mortality, and NRM between patients who received HMA before allo-HCT for MDS and those who did not.[72]

Given the absence of prospective data demonstrating a definite benefit of pretransplant treatment for posttransplant outcome, another approach would be to simply proceed to transplantation right away after the diagnosis of MDS with higher IPSS-R risk score. Indeed, with improvements in HLA typing techniques and the increased number of unrelated donors, the time to transplant is becoming shorter in most transplant centers worldwide.

According to all arguments aforementioned, Yakoub-Agha and Deeg propose a decision-making algorithm based on the percentage of marrow blasts and the presence of poor-risk cytogenetic in patients who are "fit" for allo-HCT.[73]

SELECTION OF THE INTENSITY OF CONDITIONING REGIMENS

The intensity of conditioning regimen can be defined by Martino et al.[74] with some modifications that have been suggested by an international panel of experts:[13]

1. conventional MA conditioning regimens containing total-body irradiation (TBI ≥ 8 Gy) or busulphan (Bu: ≥ 8 mg/kg orally or ≥) and new regimens, such as treosulfan ($42 g/m^2$) and fludarabine (Flu: $150 mg/m^2$)[75]
2. intermediate RIC, usually based on Bu (<8 mg/kg oral dose or < 6.4 mg/kg intravenously)
3. NMA RIC, e.g., 2 Gy TBI and fludarabine
4. preparative regimens in special situations, such as high-dose cyclophosphamide after allo-HCT with halo-identical family donors[76]
5. Sometimes, sequential conditioning regimens such as the Fludarabine, amsacrine, Aracytine and Melphalan (FLAMSA-MEL) protocol are used in patients with progressive disease.[77] However, this approach is based on few data from phase 2 studies.

The impact of conditioning intensity on patient outcome after allo-HCT for MDS is still controversial. However, some retrospective studies comparing MA with RIC regimens did not show a difference in survival when patients were transplanted in CR1, while none of the patients transplanted with active disease survived after RIC regimens.[78] Similarly, the results of a prospective randomized study that compared MA versus RIC in patients with AML or MDS were clearly in favor of an MA regimen.[79] Therefore MA conditioning should be the preferred regimen whenever possible. However, age-adjusted HCT/CI as well as disease characteristics should be taken into account before making the decision regarding conditioning intensity for a given patient.[13,21]

POSTTRANSPLANTATION STRATEGIES

Monitoring Residual Disease and Mixed Chimerism

New techniques based on polymerase chain reaction using whole BM or sorted subpopulations have been used to monitor posttransplant chimerism.[80-82] Declining donor chimerism after allo-HCT are usually considered as a marker of imminent relapse.[83] In some patients with MDS, the expression of Wilms' tumor 1 (WT1) can be a good quantitative marker for monitoring minimal residual disease after allo-HCT.[84]

Prevention of Relapse after Allo-HCT

Relapse remains the main cause of transplant failure,[19,30] especially following RIC regimens.[74] Although there is no solid prospective data to support posttransplant prophylaxis, many phase 2 studies have reported promising results with the use of HMA alone or associated with donor lymphocyte infusion (DLI) after allo-HCT.[85-88] Therefore the Francophone Society of Bone Marrow Transplantation and Cellular Therapy (SFGM-TC) recommends the use of azacitidine as a relapse prophylaxis at a low dose (32 mg/m[2]/day, 5 days a month) in patients transplanted for high-risk MDS (in press).

Management of Posttransplant Relapse

Option for MDS patients relapsing after allo-HCT includes best supportive care, cytoreduction treatment with either ICT or HMA, and immunotherapy (i.e., DLI and/or second transplant). Guieze et al. reported a retrospective study on 147 MDS patients who relapsed after allo-HCT.[89] They observed that early posttransplant relapse <6 months, history of GVHD, platelet count <50 G/L, and progression to AML at the time of relapse were the most important factors determining poor outcome. In addition, better 2-year postrelapse survival was observed in patients who received immunotherapy with or without cytoreduction treatment than in patients who received best supportive care or cytoreduction treatment alone.[89]

The international panel recommended a type of immune modulation (DLI or second autologous hematopoietic cell transplant) in case relapse occurred 6 months after allo-HCT.[13]

Management of Posttransplant Iron Overload

Iron overload (IOL) is an important issue after allo-HCT especially for MDS patients who accumulate iron mainly as a result of ineffective hematopoiesis and frequent red blood cell transfusion.[90] IOL can be responsible for posttransplant complications.[90-92]

Assessment of serum ferritin level is the easiest test to perform in this setting. However, new magnetic resonance imaging seems to be the most appropriate test to confirm IOL in the liver and heart.[93,94] Myocardial T2* values < 20 ms indicate increased myocardial iron, and values < 10 ms are associated with high risk of heart failure within the next 12 months.[95]

Although difficult, pretransplant iron chelation should be offered to patients with transfusion history of more than 20 units who are candidate for allo-HCT.[13,23,93,96]

IOL after allo-HCT may be treated by phlebotomies or by iron chelation.[13,93,97,98]

REFERENCES

1. Fenaux P, Mufti GJ, Hellstrom-Lindberg E, et al. Efficacy of azacitidine compared with that of conventional care regimens in the treatment of higher-risk myelodysplastic syndromes: a randomised, open-label, phase III study. *Lancet Oncol.* 2009;10(3):223–232. https://doi.org/10.1016/S1470-2045(09)70003-8. Published Online First: Epub Date.
2. Jurado M, Deeg HJ, Storer B, et al. Hematopoietic stem cell transplantation for advanced myelodysplastic syndrome after conditioning with busulfan and fractionated total body irradiation is associated with low relapse rate but considerable nonrelapse mortality. *Biol Blood Marrow Transplant.* 2002;8(3):161–169. Published Online First: Epub Date.
3. Lim Z, Brand R, Martino R, et al. Allogeneic hematopoietic stem-cell transplantation for patients 50 years or older with myelodysplastic syndromes or secondary acute myeloid leukemia. *J Clin Oncol.* 2010;28(3):405–411.
4. Warlick ED, Cioc A, Defor T, Dolan M, Weisdorf D. Allogeneic stem cell transplantation for adults with myelodysplastic syndromes: importance of pretransplant disease burden. *Biol Blood Marrow Transplant.* 2009;15(1):30–38. https://doi.org/10.1016/j.bbmt.2008.10.012. Published Online First: Epub Date.

5. Yakoub-Agha I, de La Salmoniere P, Ribaud P, et al. Allogeneic bone marrow transplantation for therapy-related myelodysplastic syndrome and acute myeloid leukemia: a long-term study of 70 patients-report of the French society of bone marrow transplantation. *J Clin Oncol*. 2000;18(5):963–971.

6. Robin M, Porcher R, Ades L, et al. Outcome of patients with IPSS intermediate (int) or high risk myelodysplastic syndrome (MDS) according to donor availability: a multicenter prospective non interventional study for the SFGM-TC and GFM. *Blood*. 2013;122:301.

7. Passweg JR, Baldomero H, Bader P, et al. Hematopoietic stem cell transplantation in Europe 2014: more than 40 000 transplants annually. *Bone Marrow Transplant*. 2016;51(6):786–792. https://doi.org/10.1038/bmt.2016.20. Published Online First: Epub Date.

8. Kroger N. From nuclear to a global family: more donors for MDS. *Blood*. 2013;122(11):1848–1850. https://doi.org/10.1182/blood-2013-07-515494. Published Online First: Epub Date.

9. Blaise D, Furst S, Crocchiolo R, et al. Haploidentical T cell-replete transplantation with post-transplantation cyclophosphamide for patients in or above the sixth decade of age compared with allogeneic hematopoietic stem cell transplantation from an human leukocyte antigen-matched related or unrelated donor. *Biol Blood Marrow Transplant*. 2016;22(1):119–124. https://doi.org/10.1016/j.bbmt.2015.08.029. Published Online First: Epub Date.

10. Blaise D, Nguyen S, Bay JO, et al. Allogeneic stem cell transplantation from an HLA-haploidentical related donor: SFGM-TC recommendations (Part 1). *Pathol Biol Paris*. 2014;62(4):180–184. https://doi.org/10.1016/j.patbio.2014.05.004. Published Online First: Epub Date.

11. Nguyen S, Blaise D, Bay JO, et al. Allogeneic stem cell transplantation from an HLA-haploidentical related donor: SFGM-TC recommendations (part 2). *Pathol Biol Paris*. 2014;62(4):185–189. https://doi.org/10.1016/j.patbio.2014.05.002. Published Online First: Epub Date.

12. Garcia-Manero G. Myelodysplastic syndromes: 2011 update on diagnosis, risk-stratification, and management. *Am J Hematol*. 2011;86(6):490–498. https://doi.org/10.1002/ajh.22047. Published Online First: Epub Date.

13. de Witte T, Bowen D, Robin M, et al. Allogeneic hematopoietic stem cell transplantation for MDS and CMML: recommendations from an international expert panel. *Blood*. 2017;129(13):1753–1762. https://doi.org/10.1182/blood-2016-06-724500. Published Online First: Epub Date.

14. Sorror ML, Sandmaier BM, Storer BE, et al. Comorbidity and disease status based risk stratification of outcomes among patients with acute myeloid leukemia or myelodysplasia receiving allogeneic hematopoietic cell transplantation. *J Clin Oncol*. 2007;25(27):4246–4254. https://doi.org/10.1200/JCO.2006.09.7865. Published Online First: Epub Date.

15. Armand P, Gibson CJ, Cutler C, et al. A disease risk index for patients undergoing allogeneic stem cell transplantation. *Blood*. 2012;120(4):905–913. https://doi.org/10.1182/blood-2012-03-418202. Published Online First: Epub Date.

16. Gratwohl A, Stern M, Brand R, et al. Risk score for outcome after allogeneic hematopoietic stem cell transplantation: a retrospective analysis. *Cancer*. 2009;115(20):4715–4726. https://doi.org/10.1002/cncr.24531. Published Online First: Epub Date.

17. McClune BL, Weisdorf DJ, Pedersen TL, et al. Effect of age on outcome of reduced-intensity hematopoietic cell transplantation for older patients with acute myeloid leukemia in first complete remission or with myelodysplastic syndrome. *J Clin Oncol*. 2010;28(11):1878–1887. https://doi.org/10.1200/JCO.2009.25.4821. Published Online First: Epub Date.

18. Sierra J, Perez WS, Rozman C, et al. Bone marrow transplantation from HLA-identical siblings as treatment for myelodysplasia. *Blood*. 2002/9/15;100(6):1997–2004.

19. de WT, Hermans J, Vossen J, et al. Haematopoietic stem cell transplantation for patients with myelo-dysplastic syndromes and secondary acute myeloid leukaemias: a report on behalf of the Chronic Leukaemia Working Party of the European Group for Blood and Marrow Transplantation (EBMT). *Br J Haematol*. 2000/9;110(3):620–630.

20. Koreth J, Pidala J, Perez WS, et al. Role of reduced-intensity conditioning allogeneic hematopoietic stem-cell transplantation in older patients with de novo myelodysplastic syndromes: an international collaborative decision analysis. *J Clin Oncol*. 2013;31(21):2662–2670. https://doi.org/10.1200/JCO.2012.46.8652. Published Online First: Epub Date.

21. Sorror ML, Storb RF, Sandmaier BM, et al. Comorbidity-age index: a clinical measure of biologic age before allogeneic hematopoietic cell transplantation. *J Clin Oncol*. 2014;32(29):3249–3256. https://doi.org/10.1200/JCO.2013.53.8157. Published Online First: Epub Date.

22. Greenberg PL, Attar E, Bennett JM, et al. Myelodysplastic syndromes: clinical practice guidelines in oncology. *J Natl Compr Cancer Netw*. 2013;11(7):838–874. Published Online First: Epub Date.

23. Malcovati L, Hellstrom-Lindberg E, Bowen D, et al. Diagnosis and treatment of primary myelodysplastic syndromes in adults: recommendations from the European LeukemiaNet. *Blood*. 2013;122(17):2943–2964. https://doi.org/10.1182/blood-2013-03-492884. Published Online First: Epub Date.

24. Greenberg P, Cox C, LeBeau MM, et al. International scoring system for evaluating prognosis in myelodysplastic syndromes. *Blood*. 1997;89(6):2079–2088.

25. Malcovati L, Porta MG, Pascutto C, et al. Prognostic factors and life expectancy in myelodysplastic syndromes classified according to WHO criteria: a basis for clinical decision making. *J Clin Oncol*. 2005;23(30):7594–7603. https://doi.org/10.1200/JCO.2005.01.7038. Published Online First: Epub Date.

26. Cutler CS, Lee SJ, Greenberg P, et al. A decision analysis of allogeneic bone marrow transplantation for the myelodysplastic syndromes: delayed transplantation for low-risk myelodysplasia is associated with improved outcome. *Blood.* 2004;104(2):579–585. https://doi.org/10.1182/blood-2004-01-0338 2004-01-0338. Published Online First: Epub Date.

27. Schanz J, Tuchler H, Sole F, et al. New comprehensive cytogenetic scoring system for primary myelodysplastic syndromes (MDS) and oligoblastic acute myeloid leukemia after MDS derived from an international database merge. *J Clin Onco.* 2012;30(8):820–829. https://doi.org/10.1200/JCO.2011.35.6394. Published Online First: Epub Date.

28. Greenberg PL, Tuechler H, Schanz J, et al. Revised international prognostic scoring system for myelodysplastic syndromes. *Blood.* 2012;120(12):2454–2465. https://doi.org/10.1182/blood-2012-03-420489. Published Online First: Epub Date.

29. Della Porta MG, Malcovati L, Boveri E, et al. Clinical relevance of bone marrow fibrosis and CD34-positive cell clusters in primary myelodysplastic syndromes. *J Clin Oncol.* 2009;27(5):754–762. https://doi.org/10.1200/JCO.2008.18.2246. Published Online First: Epub Date.

30. Deeg HJ, Scott BL, Fang M, et al. Five-group cytogenetic risk classification, monosomal karyotype, and outcome after hematopoietic cell transplantation for MDS or acute leukemia evolving from MDS. *Blood.* 2012;120(7):1398–1408. https://doi.org/10.1182/blood-2012-04-423046. Published Online First: Epub Date.

31. Gauthier J, Damaj G, Langlois C, et al. Contribution of revised international prognostic scoring system cytogenetics to predict outcome after allogeneic stem cell transplantation for myelodysplastic syndromes: a study from the French society of bone marrow transplantation and cellular therapy. *Transplantation.* 2015;99(8):1672–1680. https://doi.org/10.1097/TP.0000000000000649. Published Online First: Epub Date.

32. Bejar R, Stevenson KE, Caughey B, et al. Somatic mutations predict poor outcome in patients with myelodysplastic syndrome after hematopoietic stem-cell transplantation. *J Clin Oncol.* 2014;32(25):2691–2698. https://doi.org/10.1200/JCO.2013.52.3381. Published Online First: Epub Date.

33. Bejar R, Stevenson K, Abdel-Wahab O, et al. Clinical effect of point mutations in myelodysplastic syndromes. *N Engl J Med.* 2011;364(26):2496–2506. https://doi.org/10.1056/NEJMoa1013343. Published Online First: Epub Date.

34. Bejar R, Levine R, Ebert BL. Unraveling the molecular pathophysiology of myelodysplastic syndromes. *J Clin Oncol.* 2011;29(5):504–515. https://doi.org/10.1200/JCO.2010.31.1175. Published Online First: Epub Date.

35. Nikoloski G, Langemeijer SM, Kuiper RP, et al. Somatic mutations of the histone methyltransferase gene EZH2 in myelodysplastic syndromes. *Nat Genet.* 2010/8;42(8):665–667.

36. Malcovati L, Papaemmanuil E, Ambaglio I, et al. Driver somatic mutations identify distinct disease entities within myeloid neoplasms with myelodysplasia. *Blood.* 2014;124(9):1513–1521. https://doi.org/10.1182/blood-2014-03-560227. Published Online First: Epub Date.

37. Orazi A, Germing U. The myelodysplastic/myeloproliferative neoplasms: myeloproliferative diseases with dysplastic features. *Leukemia.* 2008;22(7):1308–1319. https://doi.org/10.1038/leu.2008.119. Published Online First: Epub Date.

38. Such E, Germing U, Malcovati L, et al. Development and validation of a prognostic scoring system for patients with chronic myelomonocytic leukemia. *Blood.* 2013;121(15):3005–3015. https://doi.org/10.1182/blood-2012-08-452938. Published Online First: Epub Date.

39. Borthakur G, Estey AE. Therapy-related acute myelogenous leukemia and myelodysplastic syndrome. *Curr Oncol Rep.* 2007;9(5):373–377.

40. Chang C, Storer BE, Scott BL, et al. Hematopoietic cell transplantation in patients with myelodysplastic syndrome or acute myeloid leukemia arising from myelodysplastic syndrome: similar outcomes in patients with de novo disease and disease following prior therapy or antecedent hematologic disorders. *Blood.* 2007;110(4):1379–1387. https://doi.org/10.1182/blood-2007-02-076307. Published Online First: Epub Date.

41. Huang TC, Ko BS, Tang JL, et al. Comparison of hypoplastic myelodysplastic syndrome (MDS) with normo-/hypercellular MDS by International Prognostic Scoring System, cytogenetic and genetic studies. *Leukemia.* 2008;22(3):544–550. https://doi.org/10.1038/sj.leu.2405076. Published Online First: Epub Date.

42. Armitage JO. Bone marrow transplantation. *N Engl J Med.* 1994;330(12):827–838. https://doi.org/10.1056/NEJM199403243301206. Published Online First: Epub Date.

43. Dalle JH, Donadieu J, Paillard C, et al. SFGM-TC recommendation on indications for allogeneic stem cell transplantation in children with congenital neutropenia. *Pathol Biol Paris.* 2014;62(4):209–211. https://doi.org/10.1016/j.patbio.2014.05.008. Published Online First: Epub Date.

44. Hows JM, Passweg JR, Tichelli A, et al. Comparison of long-term outcomes after allogeneic hematopoietic stem cell transplantation from matched sibling and unrelated donors. *Bone Marrow Transplant.* 2006;38(12):799–805. https://doi.org/10.1038/sj.bmt.1705531. Published Online First: Epub Date.

45. Yakoub-Agha I. Transplantations from HLA-identical siblings versus 10/10 HLA-matched unrelated donors. *Semin Hematol.* 2016;53(2):74–76. https://doi.org/10.1053/j.seminhematol.2016.01.013. Published Online First: Epub Date.

46. Yakoub-Agha I, Mesnil F, Kuentz M, et al. Allogeneic marrow stem-cell transplantation from human leukocyte antigen-identical siblings versus human leukocyte antigen-allelic-matched unrelated donors (10/10) in patients with standard-risk hematologic malignancy: a prospective study from the French Society of Bone Marrow Transplantation and Cell Therapy. *J Clin Oncol.* 2006;24(36):5695–5702. https://doi.org/10.1200/JCO.2006.08.0952. Published Online First: Epub Date.

47. Deeg HJ, Shulman HM, Anderson JE, et al. Allogeneic and syngeneic marrow transplantation for myelodysplastic syndrome in patients 55 to 66 years of age. *Blood.* 2000/2/15;95(4):1188–1194.

48. Koreth J, Biernacki M, Aldridge J, et al. Syngeneic donor hematopoietic stem cell transplantation is associated with high rates of engraftment syndrome. *Biol Blood Marrow Transplant.* 2011;17(3):421–428. https://doi.org/10.1016/j.bbmt.2010.09.013. Published Online First: Epub Date.

49. Kroger N, Brand R, van Biezen A, et al. Stem cell transplantation from identical twins in patients with myelodysplastic syndromes. *Bone Marrow Transplant.* 2005;35(1):37–43. https://doi.org/10.1038/sj.bmt.1704701. Published Online First: Epub Date.

50. Ciurea SO, Zhang MJ, Bacigalupo AA, et al. Haploidentical transplant with posttransplant cyclophosphamide vs matched unrelated donor transplant for acute myeloid leukemia. *Blood.* 2015;126(8):1033–1040. https://doi.org/10.1182/blood-2015-04-639831. Published Online First: Epub Date.

51. Kroger N, Zabelina T, Binder T, et al. HLA-mismatched unrelated donors as an alternative graft source for allogeneic stem cell transplantation after antithymocyte globulin-containing conditioning regimen. *Biol Blood Marrow Transplant.* 2009;15(4):454–462. https://doi.org/10.1016/j.bbmt.2009.01.002. Published Online First: Epub Date.

52. Robin M, Ruggeri A, Labopin M, et al. Comparison of unrelated cord blood and peripheral blood stem cell transplantation in adults with myelodysplastic syndrome after reduced-intensity conditioning regimen: a collaborative study from Eurocord (Cord blood Committee of Cellular Therapy & Immunobiology Working Party of EBMT) and Chronic Malignancies Working Party. *Biol Blood Marrow Transplant.* 2014;21(3):489–495. https://doi.org/10.1016/j.bbmt.2014.11.675. Published Online First: Epub Date.

53. Lee SJ, Klein J, Haagenson M, et al. High-resolution donor-recipient HLA matching contributes to the success of unrelated donor marrow transplantation. *Blood.* 2007;110(13):4576–4583. https://doi.org/10.1182/blood-2007-06-097386. Published Online First: Epub Date.

54. Anasetti C, Logan BR, Lee SJ, et al. Peripheral-blood stem cells versus bone marrow from unrelated donors. *N Engl J Med.* 2012;367(16):1487–1496. https://doi.org/10.1056/NEJMoa1203517. Published Online First: Epub Date.

55. Bensinger WI. Allogeneic transplantation: peripheral blood vs. bone marrow. *Curr Opin Oncol.* 2011;24(2):191–196. https://doi.org/10.1097/CCO.0b013e32834f5c27. Published Online First: Epub Date.

56. Blaise D, Kuentz M, Fortanier C, et al. Randomized trial of bone marrow versus lenograstim-primed blood cell allogeneic transplantation in patients with early-stage leukemia: a report from the Societe Francaise de Greffe de Moelle. *J Clin Oncol.* 2000;18(3):537–546. https://doi.org/10.1200/JCO.2000.18.3.537. Published Online First: Epub Date.

57. Friedrichs B, Tichelli A, Bacigalupo A, et al. Long-term outcome and late effects in patients transplanted with mobilised blood or bone marrow: a randomised trial. *Lancet Oncol.* 2010;11(4):331–338. https://doi.org/10.1016/S1470-2045(09)70352-3. Published Online First: Epub Date.

58. Mahmoud H, Fahmy O, Kamel A, Kamel M, El-Haddad A, El-Kadi D. Peripheral blood vs bone marrow as a source for allogeneic hematopoietic stem cell transplantation. *Bone Marrow Transplant.* 1999;24(4):355–358. https://doi.org/10.1038/sj.bmt.1701906. Published Online First: Epub Date.

59. Dulery R, Mohty M, Duhamel A, et al. Antithymocyte globulin before allogeneic stem cell transplantation for progressive myelodysplastic syndrome: a study from the French Society of Bone Marrow Transplantation and Cellular Therapy. *Biol Blood Marrow Transplant.* 2014;20(5):646–654. https://doi.org/10.1016/j.bbmt.2014.01.016. Published Online First: Epub Date.

60. Mohty M, Labopin M, Balere ML, et al. Antithymocyte globulins and chronic graft-vs-host disease after myeloablative allogeneic stem cell transplantation from HLA-matched unrelated donors: a report from the Societe Francaise de Greffe de Moelle et de Therapie Cellulaire. *Leukemia.* 2010;24(11):1867–1874. https://doi.org/10.1038/leu.2010.200. Published Online First: Epub Date.

61. Gomez E, Dulery R, Langlois C, et al. Bone marrow graft as a source of allogeneic hematopoietic stem cells in patients undergoing a reduced intensity conditioning regimen. *Bone Marrow Transplant.* 2014;49(12):1492–1497. https://doi.org/10.1038/bmt.2014.193. Published Online First: Epub Date.

62. Yakoub-Agha I, Saule P, Depil S, et al. Comparative analysis of naive and memory CD4+ and CD8+ T-cell subsets in bone marrow and G-CSF-mobilized peripheral blood stem cell allografts: impact of donor characteristics. *Exp Hematol.* 2007;35(6):861–871. https://doi.org/10.1016/j.exphem.2007.03.006. Published Online First: Epub Date.

63. Finke J, Bethge WA, Schmoor C, et al. Standard graft-versus-host disease prophylaxis with or without anti-T-cell globulin in haematopoietic cell transplantation from matched unrelated donors: a randomised, open-label, multicentre phase 3 trial. *Lancet Oncol.* 2009;10(9):855–864. https://doi.org/10.1016/S1470-2045(09)70225-6. Published Online First: Epub Date.

64. Guardiola P, Runde V, Bacigalupo A, et al. Retrospective comparison of bone marrow and granulocyte colony-stimulating factor-mobilized peripheral blood progenitor cells for allogeneic stem cell transplantation using HLA identical sibling donors in myelodysplastic syndromes. *Blood.* 2002;99(12):4370–4378.

65. del Canizo MC, Martinez C, Conde E, et al. Peripheral blood is safer than bone marrow as a source of hematopoietic progenitors in patients with myelodysplastic syndromes who receive an allogeneic transplantation. Results from the Spanish registry. *Bone Marrow Transplant.* 2003;32(10):987–992. https://doi.org/10.1038/sj.bmt.1704246. Published Online First: Epub Date.

66. Pascal L, Tucunduva L, Ruggeri A, et al. Impact of ATG-containing reduced-intensity conditioning after single- or double-unit allogeneic cord blood transplantation. *Blood*. 2015;126(8):1027–1032. https://doi.org/10.1182/blood-2014-09-599241. Published Online First: Epub Date.

67. Pascal L, Mohty M, Ruggeri A, et al. Impact of rabbit ATG-containing myeloablative conditioning regimens on the outcome of patients undergoing unrelated single-unit cord blood transplantation for hematological malignancies. *Bone Marrow Transplant*. 2014;50(1):45–50. https://doi.org/10.1038/bmt.2014.216. Published Online First: Epub Date.

68. Oosterveld M, Suciu S, Muus P, et al. Specific scoring systems to predict survival of patients with high-risk myelodysplastic syndrome (MDS) and de novo acute myeloid leukemia (AML) after intensive antileukemic treatment based on results of the EORTC-GIMEMA AML-10 and intergroup CRIANT studies. *Ann Hematol*. 2014;94(1):23–34. https://doi.org/10.1007/s00277-014-2177-y. Published Online First: Epub Date.

69. Fenaux P, Morel P, Rose C, Lai JL, Jouet JP, Bauters F. Prognostic factors in adult de novo myelodysplastic syndromes treated by intensive chemotherapy. *Br J Haematol*. 1991;77(4):497–501.

70. Itzykson R, Thepot S, Quesnel B, et al. Prognostic factors for response and overall survival in 282 patients with higher-risk myelodysplastic syndromes treated with azacitidine. *Blood*. 2010;117(2):403–411. https://doi.org/10.1182/blood-2010-06-289280. Published Online First: Epub Date.

71. Damaj G, Duhamel A, Robin M, et al. Impact of Azacitidine Before Allogeneic Stem-Cell Transplantation for Myelodysplastic Syndromes: a Study by the Societe Francaise de Greffe de Moelle et de Therapie-Cellulaire and the Groupe-Francophone des Myelodysplasies. *J Clin Oncol*. 2012. https://doi.org/10.1200/JCO.2012.44.3499. Published Online First: Epub Date.

72. Damaj G, Mohty M, Robin M, et al. Up-front allogeneic stem cell transplantation following reduced intensity/nonmyeloablative for patients with myelodysplastic syndrome. A Study By the Société Française de Greffe de Moelle et de Thérapie Cellulaire (SFGM-TC). *Biol Blood Marrow Transplant*. 2014.

73. Yakoub-Agha I, Deeg J. Are hypomethylating agents replacing induction-type chemotherapy before allogeneic stem cell transplantation in patients with myelodysplastic syndrome? *Biol Blood Marrow Transplant*. 2014;20(12):1885–1890. https://doi.org/10.1016/j.bbmt.2014.06.023. Published Online First: Epub Date.

74. Martino R, de Wreede L, Fiocco M, et al. Comparison of conditioning regimens of various intensities for allogeneic hematopoietic SCT using HLA-identical sibling donors in AML and MDS with <10% BM blasts: a report from EBMT. *Bone Marrow Transplant*. 2013;48(6):761–770. https://doi.org/10.1038/bmt.2012.236. Published Online First: Epub Date.

75. Ruutu T, Volin L, Beelen DW, et al. Reduced-toxicity conditioning with treosulfan and fludarabine in allogeneic hematopoietic stem cell transplantation for myelodysplastic syndromes: final results of an international prospective phase II trial. *Haematologica*. 2011;96(9):1344–1350. https://doi.org/10.3324/haematol.2011.043810. Published Online First: Epub Date.

76. Bolanos-Meade J, Fuchs EJ, Luznik L, et al. HLA-haploidentical bone marrow transplantation with post-transplant cyclophosphamide expands the donor pool for patients with sickle cell disease. *Blood*. 2012;120(22):4285–4291. https://doi.org/10.1182/blood-2012-07-438408. Published Online First: Epub Date.

77. Saure C, Schroeder T, Zohren F, et al. Upfront allogeneic blood stem cell transplantation for patients with high-risk myelodysplastic syndrome or secondary acute myeloid leukemia using a FLAMSA-based high-dose sequential conditioning regimen. *Biol Blood Marrow Transplant*. 2012;18(3):466–472. https://doi.org/10.1016/j.bbmt.2011.09.006. Published Online First: Epub Date.

78. Shimoni A, Hardan I, Shem-Tov N, et al. Allogeneic hematopoietic stem-cell transplantation in AML and MDS using myeloablative versus reduced-intensity conditioning: the role of dose intensity. *Leukemia*. 2006/2;20(2):322–328.

79. Scott BL, Pasquini MC, Logan BR, et al. Myeloablative versus reduced-intensity hematopoietic cell transplantation for acute myeloid leukemia and myelodysplastic syndromes. *J Clin Oncol*. 2017;35(11):1154–1161. https://doi.org/10.1200/JCO.2016.70.7091. Published Online First: Epub Date.

80. Maas F, Schaap N, Kolen S, et al. Quantification of donor and recipient hemopoietic cells by real-time PCR of single nucleotide polymorphisms. *Leukemia*. 2003;17(3):621–629. https://doi.org/10.1038/sj.leu.2402856. Published Online First: Epub Date.

81. Levenga H, Woestenenk R, Schattenberg AV, et al. Dynamics in chimerism of T cells and dendritic cells in relapsed CML patients and the influence on the induction of alloreactivity following donor lymphocyte infusion. *Bone Marrow Transplant*. 2007;40(6):585–592. https://doi.org/10.1038/sj.bmt.1705777. Published Online First: Epub Date.

82. Tang X, Alatrash G, Ning J, et al. Increasing chimerism after allogeneic stem cell transplantation is associated with longer survival time. *Biol Blood Marrow Transplant*. 2014;20(8):1139–1144. https://doi.org/10.1016/j.bbmt.2014.04.003. Published Online First: Epub Date.

83. Platzbecker U, Wermke M, Radke J, et al. Azacitidine for treatment of imminent relapse in MDS or AML patients after allogeneic HSCT: results of the RELAZA trial. *Leukemia*. 2012;26(3):381–389. https://doi.org/10.1038/leu.2011.234. Published Online First: Epub Date.

84. Dulery R, Nibourel O, Gauthier J, et al. Impact of Wilms' tumor 1 expression on outcome of patients undergoing allogeneic stem cell transplantation for AML. *Bone Marrow Transplant*. 2017;52(4):539–543. https://doi.org/10.1038/bmt.2016.318. Published Online First: Epub Date.

85. Krishnamurthy P, Potter VT, Barber LD, et al. Outcome of donor lymphocyte infusion after T cell-depleted allogeneic hematopoietic stem cell transplantation for acute myelogenous leukemia and myelodysplastic syndromes. *Biol Blood Marrow Transplant*. 2013;19(4):562–568. https://doi.org/10.1016/j.bbmt.2012.12.013. Published Online First: Epub Date.

86. Schaap N, Schattenberg A, Bar B, Preijers F, van de Wiel van Kemenade E, de Witte T. Induction of graft-versus-leukemia to prevent relapse after partially lymphocyte-depleted allogeneic bone marrow transplantation by pre-emptive donor leukocyte infusions. *Leukemia*. 2001;15(9):1339–1346.

87. Itzykson R, Thepot S, Eclache V, et al. Prognostic significance of monosomal karyotype in higher risk myelodysplastic syndrome treated with azacitidine. *Leukemia*. 2011;25(7):1207–1209. https://doi.org/10.1038/leu.2011.63. Published Online First: Epub Date.

88. Passweg JR, Baldomero H, Bregni M, et al. Hematopoietic SCT in Europe: data and trends in 2011. *Bone Marrow Transplant*. 2013;48(9):1161–1167. https://doi.org/10.1038/bmt.2013.51. Published Online First: Epub Date.

89. Guieze R, Damaj G, Pereira B, et al. Management of myelodysplastic syndrome relapsing after allogeneic hematopoietic stem cell transplantation: a study by the French society of bone marrow transplantation and cell therapies. *Biol Blood Marrow Transplant*. 2015;22(2):240–247. https://doi.org/10.1016/j.bbmt.2015.07.037. Published Online First: Epub Date.

90. Evens AM, Mehta J, Gordon LI. Rust and corrosion in hematopoietic stem cell transplantation: the problem of iron and oxidative stress. *Bone Marrow Transplant*. 2004/10;34(7):561–571.

91. Alessandrino EP, La Porta MG, Bacigalupo A, et al. Prognostic impact of pre-transplantation transfusion history and secondary iron overload in patients with myelodysplastic syndrome undergoing allogeneic stem cell transplantation: a GITMO study. *Haematologica*. 2010/3;95(3):476–484.

92. Armand P, Kim HT, Cutler CS, et al. Prognostic impact of elevated pretransplantation serum ferritin in patients undergoing myeloablative stem cell transplantation. *Blood*. 2007;109(10):4586–4588.

93. Rose C, Ernst O, Hecquet B, et al. Quantification by magnetic resonance imaging and liver consequences of posttransfusional iron overload alone in long term survivors after allogeneic hematopoietic stem cell transplantation (HSCT). *Haematologica*. 2007;92(6):850–853.

94. Bonkovsky HL, Rubin RB, Cable EE, Davidoff A, Rijcken TH, Stark DD. Hepatic iron concentration: noninvasive estimation by means of MR imaging techniques. *Radiology*. 1999;212(1):227–234. https://doi.org/10.1148/radiology.212.1.r99jl35227. Published Online First: Epub Date.

95. Kirk P, Roughton M, Porter JB, et al. Cardiac T2* magnetic resonance for prediction of cardiac complications in thalassemia major. *Circulation*. 2009;120(20):1961–1968. https://doi.org/10.1161/CIRCULATIONAHA.109.874487. Published Online First: Epub Date.

96. Lee JW, Kang HJ, Kim EK, Kim H, Shin HY, Ahn HS. Effect of iron overload and iron-chelating therapy on allogeneic hematopoietic SCT in children. *Bone Marrow Transplant*. 2009;44(12):793–797. https://doi.org/10.1038/bmt.2009.88. Published Online First: Epub Date.

97. Majhail NS, Lazarus HM, Burns LJ. A prospective study of iron overload management in allogeneic hematopoietic cell transplantation survivors. *Biol Blood Marrow Transplant*. 2010;16(6):832–837. https://doi.org/10.1016/j.bbmt.2010.01.004. Published Online First: Epub Date.

98. Sivgin S, Baldane S, Akyol G, et al. The oral iron chelator deferasirox might improve survival in allogeneic hematopoietic cell transplant (alloHSCT) recipients with transfusional iron overload. *Transfus Apheresis Sci*. 2013;49(2):295–301. https://doi.org/10.1016/j.transci.2013.07.004. Published Online First: Epub Date.

CHAPTER 14

Autologous Hematopoietic Stem Cell Transplantation for Non-Hodgkin Lymphoma

MUHAMMAD AYAZ MIR, MBBS, FACP • QAISER BASHIR, MD

INTRODUCTION

Non-Hodgkin Lymphomas (NHLs) include a very diverse group of nearly 70 subentities in updated World Health Organization (WHO) Classification of Lymphoid Tumors (Fig. 14.1). Spectrum includes low-grade small lymphocytic lymphoma (SLL) and follicular lymphoma (FL) which are indolent and may be observed for years without therapy to Burkitt's lymphoma, which may require therapy on the day of presentation. Therapeutic approach to these tumors is not thus uniform. Some are transplanted in the first complete remission (CR1), others in CR2 or beyond, and some may merit consideration of another chemo or immunotherapy instead of transplant even at relapse. NHL represents the second most common indication for autologous hematopoietic stem cell transplantation (auto-HSCT) after myeloma in the USA [~4100 performed in 2016: Center for Blood and Marrow Transplantation (CIBMTR) data, summary slide]. With a low treatment-related mortality (TRM) and ability to induce long-term durable remissions in a significant number of patients, auto-HSCT remains an attractive treatment option for NHL.

Following is a summary of clinical approach and evidence regarding auto-HSCT in major NHL subtypes.

DIFFUSE LARGE B CELL LYMPHOMA (DLBCL)

For the commonest NHL, R–CHOP (rituximab, cyclophosphamide, hydroxydaunorubicin, vincristine, prednisone) remains a standard of care for initial disease. However, a third of patients will have refractory/stable disease, early relapse (<1 year), or delayed relapse, despite 6–8 cycles of standard R–CHOP chemotherapy.[1]

Parma Study laid the foundation of auto-HSCT in relapsed NHL, showing 5-year event-free survival ([EFS] 46 versus 12%, $P=.001$) and overall survival ([OS] 53 versus 32%, $P=.038$) benefit, although numbers randomized to transplant versus conventional salvage were small (~50 patients each) and chemo-resistant patients were excluded.[2] Moreover, in Parma, rituximab was not a part of treatment arms, which is universally the case today.

Perfect salvage regimen before auto-HSCT is not well defined. R-ICE (rituximab, ifosfamide, carboplatin, and etoposide), which can be given as a fractionated outpatient regimen,[3] is at least as effective as R-DHAP (rituximab, dexamethasone, ara-C, and cisplatin) with overall response rate of >80% with both regimens (CORAL Study[4]). Platinum-based regimens such as R-gemcitabine-oxaliplatin appear to have a survival benefit based on retrospective data.[1] With any regimen, half of the patients will have adequate salvage, making them eligible for auto-HSCT, and of these, approximately half will relapse despite transplantation.[5]

Positron Emission Tomography (PET) scans before and after auto-HSCT if both negative (-pre/-post) ensure best prognosis as compared to +pre/- post or -pre/+ post groups.[6]

Double-hit lymphomas (DHLs) represent ~5% of DLBCL and have translocations of MYC gene with either Bcl-2 and/or Bcl-6 resulting in dismal prognosis. When present as proteins expressed on immunohistochemistry, the term double expresser lymphoma (DEL) is used, which still has a worse prognosis than non-DEL DLBCL. In a Southwestern Oncology Group study of CHOP +/- rituximab with or without auto-HSCT, transplant appeared to salvage some DEL but none of DHL patients. Best therapy for this subset thus remains controversial.[7,8]

Transplantation in CR1 as consolidation for those with high International Prognostic Index scores has been explored showing improvement (randomized after 5 R–CHOP to either 3 more R–CHOP or 1 additional R–CHOP and Auto HSCT) in progression-free

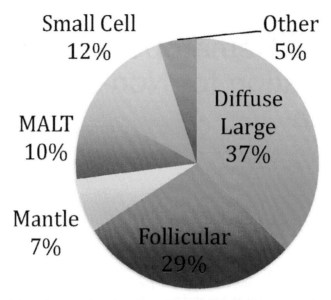

FIG. 14.1 Epidemiology of non-Hodgkin lymphoma Mucosa Associated Lymphoid Tissue (MALT). (WHO Classification 2008.)

survival [(PFS) 69% versus 55% at 2 years, $P = .005$] but not in OS in the auto-HSCT group.[9]

Mobilization can be performed using granulocyte colony-stimulating factor, chemotherapy such as cyclophosphamide, and adding plerixafor for heavily pretreated patients.[10]

Most well-studied conditioning regimen for auto-HSCT is BEAM with slight variations (Fig. 14.2: BCNU-Carmustine, Etoposide, Ara-C, and Melphalan). In general, TRM with this regimen is <5%, and auto-HSCT can be performed safely as an outpatient therapy, which may also be associated with some cost reduction as well ($17,000 saved per patient).[11] Shortages of carmustine have led to search for alternatives including BeEAM [12](bendamustine replacing carmustine) and FEAM (fortemustine replacing carmustine).[13]

Rituximab purging of graft and maintenance therapy after auto-HSCT have been studied in small series with encouraging results but is not the standard of care at this time.[14]

Transformed lymphoma (Richter's transformation) signifies evolution of an indolent lymphoma into an aggressive variant of DLBCL. Although some authorities advocate allogeneic rather than auto-HSCT in CR1, data on both sides are limited and retrospective.[15]

Secondary CNS involvement at onset or in relapsed DLBCL is ominous. Auto-HSCT with busulfan and thiotepa may offer survival benefit to a subset.[16]

Primary CNS lymphoma is histologically DLBCL in most cases (95%) and represents distinct challenges. Auto-HSCT with conditioning using CNS-penetrating drugs such as thiotepa and BCNU has resulted in 3-year OS >75%, which is remarkable for this aggressive disease, although all available prospective data to date are phase II only, due to rarity of the disease.[17]

Primary mediastinal lymphoma is a special subset of DLBCL confined to mediastinum with additional therapy (usually additional etoposide or radiation therapy) incorporated in the initial treatment. While chimeric antigen receptor T-cells therapy is FDA approved for relapsed refractory primary mediastinal lymphoma, conventional auto-HSCT has shown excellent results (85%–100% 3-year OS in CR1 and CR>1 and >40% in chemorefractory disease) and is commonly used for this entity.[18]

FOLLICULAR LYMPHOMA

Follicular lymphoma (FL) is the second most common NHL and represents the prototype of indolent lymphoma with a span of years without any chemoimmunotherapy in many cases. Despite mostly indolent course, about 2% of patients per year will transform to a more aggressive histology with poor prognosis. This means a substantial subset for a disease which may last 2 decades. FL International Prognostic Index

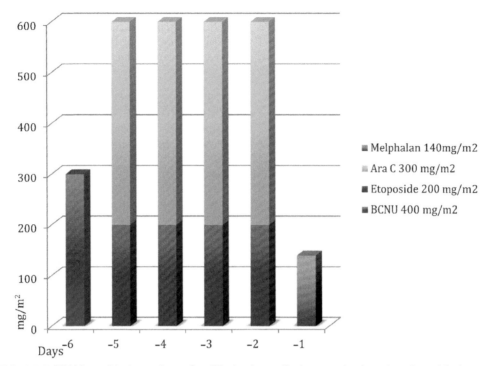

FIG. 14.2 BEAM conditioning regimen. Conditioning is usually done starting from day −6 to −1 in the manner shown (Ara C = Cytarbine, BCNU = Carmustine).

score and histologic tumor grade are prognostic but do not always guide initiation of therapy or proceeding to transplantation. Even when symptoms develop, options include radiotherapy or chemoimmunotherapy (such as rituximab-bendamustine, obinutuzumab, R–CVP (rituximab, cyclophosphamide, vincristine, and prednisone), and R–CHOP).

Relapsed disease merits consideration of a second period of observation of asymptomatic, small-molecular inhibitors including idelalisib, copanlisib (Phosphoinositide 3 Kinase (PIK)-αδ inhibitors), and ibritumomab (Yttrium-90 labeled, CD20 based radio-immunotherapy). Availability of these myriad options have pushed auto-HSCT further down in the algorithm for FL treatment, which never was an enthusiastic indication for transplant, invoking controversy for decades. Keeping this in mind, of ~10,000 cases of FL diagnosed per year in the USA, only 240 were reported by CIBMTR as having undergone auto-HSCT in a 10-year period, and referral for transplantation remained very low at < 3%.[19]

Auto-HSCT has been attempted at first and subsequent relapses, and unlike DLBCL, for which auto-HSCT is the standard of care in relapsed disease, for FL, appropriate timing is not well defined. Two relatively

less-contested indications for auto-HSCT in FL include early relapse (<12 months) [20] after initial therapy and transformed disease.[21] With blinding transplant versus no transplant being impossible, the only randomized open label trial (CUP study 1993-97 randomizing merely 89 patients across Europe to Chemo, Unpurged and Purged arms) to show PFS (26% vs. 58%–55% at 2 years) and OS (46% vs. 71%–77% at 4 years) benefit of auto-HSCT in relapsed FL was performed before rituximab was approved, making it of questionable relevance today.[22] Retrospective data attempting to show benefit of auto-HSCT have time and again demonstrated that exposure to rituximab and not transplant made the difference in outcomes.[23] Similar to aggressive lymphomas, auto-HSCT in CR1 (as initial consolidation in untreated disease almost certain to relapse) has been studied demonstrating PFS but no OS benefit in a summarized Cochrane Review of all five published trials meeting inclusion criteria.[24] Conventional conditioning regimens included total-body irradiation in the past, but increased risk of secondary myelodysplastic syndrome/acute myeloid leukemia has steered most centers to BEAM-like regimens as in other forms of NHL.[25] Rituximab purging of graft has not shown to be beneficial, but maintenance rituximab after auto-HSCT (3 monthly for 2 years) may prolong PFS without much impact on OS.[26] Relapsed patients after auto-HSCT should preferably be enrolled in clinical trials and may be considered for allogeneic HSCT when no other salvage options are available.

MANTLE CELL LYMPHOMA

Mantle cell lymphoma (MCL), arising from the mantle zone outside the follicles, is characterized by t11; 14 (Cyclin D1) and frequently involves gut, spleen, blood, and marrow. It presents a diverse clinical spectrum with a subset of patients on observation without therapy for years and other falling through multiple lines of chemotherapy within a few months. Presence of SOX-11 mutation, high MIPI score, and Ki-67 pronounces aggressive disease. Owing to rarity of the disease, clinical trial enrollment is encouraged in both initial and relapsed MCL.

Initial treatment may range from low-intensity regimens such as R-bendamustine to intermediate R-CHOP and high-intensity R-hyper CVAD/Nordic/Maxi-CHOP–like regimens although later approach has fallen out of favor in recent years (87% grade IV hematologic toxicity).[27] Ultimately it is not the initial regimen used but ability to achieve CR that impacts outcomes in MCL. R–CHOP as sole therapy is deemed inadequate and should be followed by auto-HSCT and/or rituximab maintenance.[28]

Most centers recommend, in absence of a randomized trial, auto-HSCT in CR1 particularly if less-intense induction therapy such R-CHOP is used (favored by retrospective data),[29] followed by rituximab maintenance for 2–4 years.[30] In elderly and frail individuals, a low/intermediate intensity regimen may be considered followed by rituximab maintenance only, without putting the patient through auto-HSCT.[27]

MARGINAL ZONE LYMPHOMA

Marginal zone lymphoma is mostly indolent. Data for auto-HSCT are scarce, and most recommendations are extrapolated from FL, considering auto-HSCT in CR2 and beyond.[31]

SMALL LYMPHOCYTIC LYMPHOMA/ CHRONIC LYMPHOCYTIC LEUKEMIA

With the advent of multiple novel agents (ibrutinib, idelalisib, obinutuzumab, and venetoclax), transplant for small lymphocytic lymphoma/chronic lymphocytic leukemia (SLL/CLL), even with p53 mutation, is becoming largely obsolete. One caveat, as mentioned previously, is Richter's transformation, for which both auto- and allogeneic-HSCT have been studied. With auto-HSCT, 3-year OS of ~60% and PFS of 45% may be expected.[15]

POSTTRANSPLANT LYMPHOPROLIFERATIVE DISORDER

Posttransplant lymphoproliferative disorder usually occurs in a triad of transplant, immunosuppression, and Epstein–Barr Virus activation. Depending on the degree of histologic transformation (early lesion, monomorphic, or polymorphic), therapy may range from decreasing immunosuppression, single-agent rituximab, or R–CHOP–like chemotherapy. Post-chemotherapy cytopenias may be challenging in this immunosuppressed population at high risk of transplanted organ dysfunction. Data regarding auto-transplant at relapsed disease are limited to case reports.[32]

PLASMABLASTIC LYMPHOMA

Plasmablastic lymphoma is an aggressive CD20-negative variant of DLBCL, sometimes associated with HIV and other immunocompromised states. It is characterized by early relapse despite aggressive treatments such as dose-adjusted Rituximab, Etoposide, Oncovin, Cyclophos, Hydroxydaunorubicin (R-EPOCH) with or without bortezomib with a median survival of 3–4 months. Expert consensus recommends auto-HSCT in CR1 along with institution of antiretroviral therapy when applicable.[33]

CONCLUSION

Auto-HSCT remains the standard of care in certain subtypes of NHL (relapsed DLBCL), is being displaced in others by novel targeted agents "ibs and mabs"(SLL), and remains controversial in some (FL). Maintenance therapy is emerging in several subtypes, e.g., MCL, and may eventually translate into OS benefit in addition to PFS benefit. Challenges such as DHLs and refractory/transformed disease await smarter answers.

REFERENCES

1. Filliatre-Clement L, Maucort-Boulch D, Bourbon E, et al. Refractory diffuse large B-cell lymphoma after first-line immune-CT: treatment options and outcomes. *Hematol Oncol.* May 2, 2018. [Epub ahead of print].
2. Philip T, Guglielmi C, Hegenbeek A, et al. Autologous bone Marrow transplantation as compared with salvage chemotherapy in relapses of chemotherapy-sensitive non-hodgkin's lymphoma. *N Eng J Med.* 1995;333:1540–1545.

3. George B, Benson W, Hertzberg MS, et al. A pilot study on the use of outpatient fractionated ifosfamide, carboplastin and etoposide (ICE) and pegfilgrastim as a salvage and mobilizing regimen for relapsed and refractory non-Hodgkin's and Hodgkin's lymphoma. *Bone Marrow Transpl.* 2012;47(7):1001–1002.

4. Gisselbrecht C, Glass B, Mounier N, et al. R-ICE versus R-DHAP in relapsed patients with CD20 diffuse large B-cell lymphoma (DLBCL) followed by autologous stem cell transplantation: CORAL study. *J Clin Onc.* 2009;27(15S): 8509–8509.

5. Gisselbrecht C, Van Den Neste E. How I manage patients with relapsed/refractory Diffuse large B Cell Lymphoma. *Br J Haematol.* May 29, 2018. https://doi.org/10.1111/bjh. 15412. [Epub ahead of print].

6. W1 Q, Zhao J, Xing Y, et al. Predictive value of [1^{8}F]fluoro-2-deoxy-D- glucose positron emission tomography for clinical outcome in patients with relapsed/refractory diffuse large B-cell lymphoma prior to and after autologous stem cell transplant. *Leuk Lymphoma.* 2014;55(2):276–282. https://doi.org/10.3109/10428194.2013.797974. Epub 2013 Jun 5.

7. Allen J, Ruano Mendez AL, Rybicki L, et al. Co-expression of MYC and BCL2 predicts poorer outcomes for relapsed/refractory diffuse large B-cell lymphoma with R-ICE and intent to transplant. *Ther Adv Hematol.* 2018;9(4):81–87. https://doi.org/10.1177/2040620718759249. Epub 2018 Mar 29.

8. Puvvada SD, Stiff PJ, Leblanc M, et al. Outcomes of MYC associated Lymphomas after R-CHOP with and without consolidative Autologous Stem Cell Transplant: subset analysis of randomized trial intergroup SWOP S9704. *Br J Haematol.* 2016;174(5):686–691.

9. Stiff PJ, Unger JM, Cook JR, et al. Autologous transplantation as consolidation for aggressive non-hodgkin's lymphoma. *N Engl J Med.* 31, 2013;369(18):1681–1690.

10. Clark RE, Bell J, Clark JO, et al. Plerixafor is superior to conventional chemotherapy for first-line stem cell mobilization and is effective even in heavily pretreated patients. *Blood Cancer J.* October 31, 2014;4:e255.

11. Reid RM, Baran A, Friedberg JW, et al. Outpatient administration of BEAM conditioning prior to autologous stem cell transplantation for lymphoma is safe, feasible and cost-effective. *Cancer Med.* 2016;5(11):3059–3067.

12. Chantepie SP, Garciaz S, Tchernonog E, et al. Bendamustine-based conditioning prior to autologous stem cell transplantation (ASCT): results of a French multicenter study of 474 patients for lymphoma study association (LYSA) centers. *Am J Hematol.* 2018;93(6):729–735.

13. Olivieri J, Mosna F, Pelosini M, et al. A comparison of the conditioning regimens BEAM and FEAM for autologous hematopoietic stem cell transplantation in lymphoma: an observational study on patients from Fondazione Italiana Linfomi (Fil). *Biol Blood Marrow Transpl.* 29, 2018;(18):30270:Pii S1083-8791.

14. W1 Z, Jiao L, Zhou DB, et al. Rituximab purging and maintenance therapy combined with autologous stem

cell transplantation in patients with diffuse large B-cell lymphoma. *Oncol Lett.* 2010;1(4):733–738. [Epub 2010 July 1].

15. Cwynarski K, van Biezen A, de Wreede L, et al. Autologous and Allogeneic stem cell transplantation for transformed chronic lymphocytic leukemia (Richter's Syndrome): a retrospective analysis of CLL working party and Lymphoma working party of EBMT. *J Clin Oncol.* 2012;30(18):2211.

16. Lee MY, Kim HS, Lee JY, et al. Efficacy and feasibility of autologous stem cell transplantation in patients with diffuse large B cell lymphoma with secondary central nervous system involvement. *Int J Hematol.* 2015;102(6):678–688.

17. Ferreri AJM, Illerhaus G. The role of autologous stem cell transplant in primary central nervous system lymphoma. *Blood.* March 2016;127(13):1642–1649.

18. Avivi I, Boumendil A, Finel H, et al. Autologous stem cell transplantation for primary medistinal B cell lymphoma: long-term outcome and role of post-transplant radiotherapy: a report from European Society of blood & Marrow transplantation. *Bone Marrow Transpl.* February 2018. https://doi.org/10.1038/s41409-017-0063-7.

19. Fenske TS. *Why is Stem Cell Transplant So Underused in Follicular Lymphoma.* The ASCO Post; July 25, 2013.

20. Casulo C, Friedberg JW, Ahn KW, et al. Autologous transplantation in follicular lymphoma with early therapy failure: a National LymphoCare/CIBMTR research analysis. *Biol Blood Marrow Transpl.* 2018;24(6):1163.

21. Kuruvilla J, MacDonald DA, Kourokis CT, et al. Salvage chemotherapy and autologous transplantation for transformed indolent lymphoma: a subset analysis of NCIC CTG LY12. *Blood.* 2015;126(6):733–738.

22. Schouten HC, Qian W, Kvayloy S, et al. High-dose therapy improves progression free survival and survival in Follicular non-Hodgkin's lymphoma: results from the randomized European CUP trial. *J Clin Oncol.* 2003;21(21):3918.

23. Sebban C, Brice P, Delarue R, et al. Impact of Rituximab and/or high-dose therapy with autotransplant at time of relapse in patients with follicular lymphoma: a GELA study. *J Clin Oncol.* 2008;26(21):3614.

24. Schaaf M, Reiser M, Borchmann P, et al. High dose therapy with autologous transplantation versus chemotherapy or immuno-chemotherapy for follicular lymphoma in adults. *Cochrane Database Syst Rev.* 2012;1:CD007678.

25. El-Najjar I, Boumendil A, Luan JJ, et al. The impact of total body irradiation on the outcome of patients with follicular lymphoma treated with autologous stem cell transplantation in the modern era: a retrospective study of the EBMT Lymphoma Working Party. *Ann Oncol.* 2014; 25(11):2224–2229.

26. Pettengell R, Schmitz N, Gisselbrecht C, et al. Rituximab purging and/or maintenance in patients undergoing autologous transplantation for relapsed follicular lymphoma: a prospective randomized trial from the Lymphoma Working party of the EBMT. *J Clin Oncol.* 2013;31(13):1624.

27. Vose JM. Mantle Cell Lymphoma: 2017 update on diagnosis, risk-stratification and clinical management. *Am J Hematol.* 2017;92:806–813.

28. LeCase AS, Vandergrift JL, Rodriguez MA, et al. Comparative Outcome of initial therapy for younger patients with mantle cell lymphoma: an analysis form the NCCN NHL Database. *Blood.* 2012;119:2093–2099.

29. Garcia-Noblejas A, Cannat-Ortiz J, Conde E, et al. Autologous stem cell transplantation (ASCT) in mantle cell lymphoma: a retrospective study of the Spanish Lymphoa group (GELTAMO). *Ann Hematol.* 2017;96(8):1323–1330.

30. Mei MG, Cao TM, Chen L, et al. Long-term results of high dose therapy and autologous stem cell transplantation for mantle cell lymphoma: effectiveness of maintenance rituximab. *Biol Blood Marrow Transpl.* 2017;23(11):1861-69.

31. Shimoni A. The role of stem cell transplant in the treatment of marginal zone lymphoma. *Best Pract Res Clin Haematol.* 2017;30(1–2):166–171.

32. Mlahotra B, Rahal AK, Farhoud H, et al. Treatment of recurrent post-transplant Lymphoproliferative disorder with autologous blood stem cell transplant. *Case Rep Transpl.* 2015;2015:801082.

33. Castillo JJ, Bibas M, Miranda RN. The biology and treatment of plasmablastic Lymhoma. *Blood.* 2014;125(15):2323–2330.

FURTHER READING

1. Hamadani M. Autologous hematopoietic stem cell transplantation: an update for clinicians by. *Ann Med.* 2014;46:619–632.

2. Lahoud OB, Sauter CS, Hamlin PA, et al. High-dose chemotherapy and autologous stem cell transplant in older patients with lymphoma. *Curr Oncol Rep.* 2015;17(9):42.

3. Krischbaum M, Frankel P, Popplewell L, et al. Phase II Study of Vorinostat for the treatment of relapsed or refractory indolent non-Hodgkin lymphoma and Mantle cell lymphoma. *J Clin Oncol.* 2011;29(9):1198–1203.

4. Alvarnas JC, Le Rademacher J, Wang Y, et al. Autologous hematopoietic stem cell transplantation for HIV-related lymphoma: results of the BMT-CTN 0803/AMC071 trial. *Blood.* 2016;128(8):1050–1058.

CHAPTER 15

Allogenic Transplant for Non-Hodgkin Lymphoma

RAVI KISHORE NARRA, MD • NIRAV N. SHAH, MD, MS

INTRODUCTION

Allogeneic hematopoietic stem cell transplant (allo-HCT) is a potentially curative treatment, involving infusion of hematopoietic stem cells collected from related donors, unrelated donors, or cord blood. Allo-HCT is defined as an episode of care starting with a preparative regimen and continuing through hematopoietic stem cell infusion and recovery.[1,2] Hematopoietic stem cell transplant involves the infusion of CD34-positive hematopoietic progenitor cells collected from bone marrow, peripheral blood, or cord blood.

In recent years, with introduction of novel biological agents in addition to traditional chemotherapeutic options and transplant, survival rates in patients diagnosed with non-Hodgkin lymphoma (NHL) have significantly improved with 5-year survival rates of about 71.4%.[3] In patients with high-risk and relapsed, refractory NHL, allo-HCT provides a potentially curative treatment option. An immune-mediated antitumor effect "graft-versus-lymphoma effect" (GVL) first reported in 1991[4] has since been a well-studied and established phenomenon.[5] A strong association and statistical correlation has been reported between the development of graft-versus-host disease (GVHD) and the induction of an antileukemic response.[5] Sustained complete remission (CR) after withdrawal of immune suppressions and donor lymphocyte infusion (DLI) past 100 days of allo transplant suggests a clinically relevant GVL effect.[6]

In many cases of high-risk NHL or NHL that has failed multiple lines of treatment, the only potentially curative treatment option, until recently, was allo-HCT. With advances in pretransplantation, peritransplantation, and posttransplantation care, allo-HCT can now be successfully applied to a wider population of patients, including those with advanced age. Although it is true that advanced age does increase the risk of transplantation-related complications and nonrelapse mortality (NRM), the widespread implementation of reduced-intensity (RI) and non-myeloablative conditioning has expanded the accessibility of this curative intent treatment to older patients. In this chapter we will first review the utility and outcomes of allo-HCT in patients with common forms of B-cell NHL with a focus on diffuse large B-cell lymphoma (DLBCL), follicular lymphoma (FL), and mantle cell lymphoma (MCL). These three lymphoma histologies accounted for 73% of allo-HCTs performed in patients aged above 60 years in the United States between 2010 and 2014 [1]. We will then discuss the role of allo-HCT in patients with mature T-cell lymphomas, a rarer and less common diagnosis encountered. Table 15.1 lists the American Society of Blood and Marrow Transplantation (ASBMT) current recommended indications and level of evidence for allo-HCT in NHL.[7] We will conclude with a review of data specifically supporting allo-HCT in elderly patients with NHL and discuss the future of allo-HCT in NHL. Finally, it is important to note that the role of allo-HCT in NHL will drastically evolve over the next decade. With the development of chimeric antigen receptor T-cell (CAR-T)–based therapies and the reported impressive response rates in patients with refractory B-cell NHL, it is quite possible that these genetically modified T-cell therapies may replace the role of allo-HCT in some forms of NHL in the near future.[8,9]

B-CELL LYMPHOMAS

Diffuse Large B-Cell Lymphoma

Overview of DLBCL

DLBCL is the most common form of aggressive B-cell NHL, encompassing several clinical-pathological entities. Although risk factors include HIV infection, solid organ transplantation, and autoimmune disorders, most of the cases are sporadic and occur predominantly in older individuals aged >60 years with no obvious predisposing factors. Overall, about 60% of those

Hematopoietic Cell Transplantation for Malignant Conditions. https://doi.org/10.1016/B978-0-323-56802-9.00015-8

TABLE 15.1
Indications for Allogeneic Transplant in NHL[7]

Diffuse large B-cell lymphoma	Recommendation		
CR1 (PET negative)	N	Relapse after autologous transplant	C
CR1 (PET positive)	N	**Burkitt's lymphoma**	
Primary refractory, sensitive	C	First remission	C
Primary refractory, resistant	C	First or greater relapse, sensitive	C
First relapse, sensitive	C	First or greater relapse, resistant	C
First relapse, resistant	C	Relapse after autologous transplant	C
Second or greater relapse	C	**T-cell lymphoma**	
Follicular lymphoma		CR1	C
CR1	N	Primary refractory, sensitive	C
Primary refractory, sensitive	S	Primary refractory, resistant	C
Primary refractory, resistant	S	First relapse, sensitive	C
First relapse, sensitive	S	First relapse, resistant	C
First relapse, resistant	S	Second or greater relapse	C
Second or greater relapse	S	Relapse after autologous transplant	C
Transformation to high-grade lymphoma	C	**Cutaneous T cell lymphoma**	
Relapse after autologous transplant	C	Relapse	C
Mantle cell lymphoma		Relapse after autologous transplant	C
CR1/PR1	C	**Lymphoplasmacytic lymphoma**	
Primary refractory, sensitive	S	CR1	N
Primary refractory, resistant	C	Primary refractory, sensitive	N
First relapse, sensitive	S	Primary refractory, resistant	R
First relapse, resistant	C	First or greater relapse, sensitive	R
Second or greater relapse	C	First or greater relapse, resistant	R
		Relapse after autologous transplant	C

Recommendation categories: Standard of care (S); Standard of care, clinical evidence available (C); Standard of care, rare indication (R); Developmental (D); Not generally recommended (N).
CR1, first CR; *NHL*, non-Hodgkin lymphoma; *PET*, positron emission tomography; *PR1*, first partial response.

diagnosed with DLBCL will be cured with combination chemoimmunotherapy without transplant. However, response-predicting tools such as National Comprehensive Cancer Network (NCCN) International Prognostic Index (NCCN-IPI) demonstrate a wide range of 5-year survival rates from as high as 96% in low-risk groups to as low as 38% in high-risk groups.[10,11]

Overall survival (OS) for DLBCL after anthracycline-based chemotherapy ranges from 35% to 60% based on subtype with improved OS in patients with germinal center B-cell–like DLBCL compared to those with an activated B-cell phenotype.[12] Translocation or overexpression of the MYC oncogene which is associated with negative

impact on survival is seen in 5%–16% of DLBCL. Bearing both MYC and BCL2 or BCL6 constitute double-hit lymphoma.[13] For high-risk disease subtypes, clinically defined by the NCCN-IPI[10] or biologically identified as "double-hit" and "triple-hit" lymphomas, standard frontline treatment options are less effective for providing long-lasting remission, and cure is difficult to achieve in the relapsed and refractory settings.[13,14] Auto-HCT has improved progression-free survival (PFS) and OS in chemosensitive patients with relapsed NHL. Early studies from 1990s showed a response rate of 84% with auto-HCT and only 44% with chemotherapy alone without auto-HCT. This correlated with improved 5-year OS of 53% with auto-HCT versus (vs.) 32% with continuation of conventional chemotherapy.[15] However, the Collaborative Trial in Relapsed Aggressive Lymphoma (CORAL) trial showed that only less than 25% of patients achieved long-term disease-free survival with auto-HCT, if relapsed within 1 year of diagnosis after frontline therapy.[16] Although auto-HCT remains the standard of care for chemosensitive relapsed, refractory DLBCL patients, better approaches are required for patients who relapse after auto-HCT.

ALLO-HCT FOR DLBCL

Allo-HCT provides the advantage of a tumor-free graft and the benefit of a potential GVL effect. This GVL effect has been well demonstrated by the fact that some patients who experience relapse after auto-HCT will attain cure with even a RI-conditioned allo-HCT. Further evidence of the GVL effect is through the use of DLI and/or withdrawal of immunosuppression after allo-HCT leading to cure in some cases.[6,17,18] A large retrospective analysis by the Center for International Blood and Marrow Transplant Research (CIBMTR) including 837 auto-HCTs and 79 allo-HCTs performed between 1995 and 2003 demonstrated higher transplant-related mortality (TRM), nonrelapse mortality (NRM), and overall mortality in the allo-HCT group, with no decrease in the risk of disease progression.[19] This analysis is limited by subject bias as those who underwent allo-HCT were more likely to have high-risk disease features, such as advanced-stage and resistant disease. Despite these limitations, outcomes with allo-HCT in DLBCL have demonstrated long-term OS in the 20%–50% range (Table 15.2). In the past, allo-HCT was performed with myeloablative (MA) conditioning to eliminate maximal tumor and permit engraftment by eliminating the host immune system. Such transplants increase the risk of NRM which remains a major barrier of successful allo-HCT. In recent years, less intensive preparative RI conditioning regimens have been used with increasing frequency. Retrospective comparisons between MA and RI conditioning show reduced NRM, at the expense of some increase in disease relapse, but producing long-term OS rates comparable with those for MA conditioning. In a CIBMTR analysis from Hamadani et al. among 533 patients with chemorefractory DLBCL or grade III FL, the intensity of conditioning did not impact PFS or OS. Although MA conditioning was associated with reduced risk of relapse, there was increased NRM in the MA cohort.[20,21] Most allo-HCTs for DLBCL are now performed using lower-intensity regimens, which also expands access for this procedure to selected fit older patients.[20] A summary of studies for allo-HCT adapted from the study by Fenske et al. involving at least 40 patients with DLBCL is listed in Table 15.2.[22]

Allo-HCT for DLBCL After Failed Auto-HCT

Approximately 30%–50% of DLBCL auto-HCT recipients ultimately will experience relapse or progression of DLBCL.[23] Owing to associated GVL effect in DLBCL, allo-HCT is a consideration in such patients after a failed previous auto-HCT.[24–27] The European Group for Blood and Marrow Transplantation (EBMT) reported on 101 patients from 1997 to 2006 who underwent allo-SCT after failure of auto-SCT in DLBCL. The 3-year PFS was 41.7% and OS was 53.8%. Worse outcomes were seen in those with early relapse (<12 months after auto-HCT) and those aged ≥45 years. PFS was not impacted by conditioning intensity despite increased NRM in MA-conditioned patients. This higher NRM was countered by higher relapse rates in RI patients.[24] In a more contemporary and larger analysis from the CIBMTR, 503 patients from 2000 to 2012 were identified as having an allo-HCT after failure from a prior auto-HCT for DLBCL. At 3 years after allo-HCT, NRM was 30%, with a progression/relapse rate of 38%. The PFS and OS at 3 years were 31% and 37%, respectively, which is an encouraging result given that the median survival typically seen in this population is in the 3- to 10-month range.[28,29] Factors contributing to a poorer OS were a Karnofsky performance score (KPS) < 80, chemoresistance, and MA conditioning. The authors also developed a prognostic model to estimate PFS in high-risk patients. KPS<80 (4 points), auto-HCT to allo-HCT interval < 1 year (2 points), and chemoresistance (5 points) were used to stratify patients into 4 groups from low risk to very high risk. Patients with low-risk disease had a predicted 3-year PFS of 40% compared with those in the very-high-risk group with a 3-year PFS of 6%.[26] For both studies mentioned previously a GVL effect was assumed as all had failed a prior auto-HCT, but subsequently a significant subset achieved a long-term remission with allo-HCT.

Summary: DLBCL

These data indicate that medically appropriate patients with DLBCL whose disease relapses after auto-HCT should consider allo-HCT as a potentially curative intent treatment. In this setting, patients should receive RI conditioning preferentially to lower NRM and ideally proceed in the setting of chemosensitive disease although a small portion of even chemorefractory patients can be cured.[21] Other potential indications for allo-HCT include patients in whom auto-HCT is not feasible, either by failure to obtain an adequate autologous graft for transplantation or coexistence of intrinsic bone marrow disease, particularly myelodysplastic syndrome and in DLBCL patients who have failed an auto-HCT. It should be

TABLE 15.2
Recent Studies Reporting Outcomes of Allo-HCT for DLBCL (>40 Patients)

Study	#. Of Patients	Previous Auto-HCT, %	Condition-ing (%)	Median Age, yr (Range)	NRM/TRM, % (yr)	Relapse, % (yr)	OS, % (yr)
Thomson et al., 2009[17]	48	69	RIC (100)	46 (23–64)	32 (4)	33 (4)	48 (4)
Sirvent et al., 2010[99]	68	79	RIC (100)	48 (17–66)	23 (1)	41 (2)	49 (2)
Lazarus et al., 2010[19]	79	0	MAC (100)	46 (21–59)	43 (3)	33 (3)	26 (3)
van Kampen et al., 2011[24]	101	100	MAC (37) RIC (63)	46 (18–66)	28 (3)	30 (3)	52 (3)
Rigacci et al., 2012[25]	165	100	MAC (30) RIC (70)	43 (16–65)	19–32 (2)	NR	39 (5)
Bacher et al., 2012[20]	396	32	MAC (42) RIC (58)	54 (18–66)	36–56 (5)	26–40 (5)	18–26 (5)
Hama-dani et al., 2013[21]	533	25	MAC (58) RIC (42)	46 (19–66) 53 (20–70)	53 (3)	28 (3)	19 (3)
Fenske et al., 2015[26]	503	100	MAC (25)	52 (19–72)	31 (5)	40 (5)	34 (5)

DLBCL, diffuse large B-cell lymphoma; *HCT*, hematopoietic cell transplantation; *MAC*, myeloablative conditioning; *NRM*, nonrelapse mortality; *OS*, overall survival; *RIC*, reduced-intensity conditioning; *TRM*, treatment-related mortality.
From Norbert Schmitz, Georg Lenz and Matthias Stelljes, Allogeneic hematopoietic stem cell transplantation for T-cell lymphomas, Blood 2018 132:245-253.

noted that the placement of allo-HCT in management of DLBCL has already been impacted by the recent FDA approvals of two commercial CAR-T products specifically for DLBCL. These studies have noted long-term PFS of 30%–40%, depending on the product, with lower NRM and decreased long-term toxicity due to the avoidance of GVHD.[9,30] With improvement in cellular targeted therapies, it is possible that allo-HCT is limited to only highly selected patients with DLBCL in the future.

FOLLICULAR LYMPHOMA
Overview of FL

FL is the most common subtype of indolent NHL, accounting for roughly 20% of all cases of NHL.[31]

Unlike patients with aggressive NHL, nearly all patients who complete induction therapy will relapse and require additional lines of therapy. Furthermore, although OS is prolonged for many patients, with standard therapies, FL remains incurable in many cases. The Follicular Lymphoma International Prognostic Index incorporates clinically based features and identifies a subgroup at high risk for early disease-related death.[32]

The Groupe d'Etude des Lymphomes Folliculaires (GELF) criteria are often used to identify patients who can be safely observed in comparison to those who would benefit from upfront treatment.[33] Front-line treatment options are based on tumor burden and presence of symptoms and ranges from single-agent rituximab to combination chemoimmunotherapy regimens.[31,34] There is no standard therapy for relapsed, refractory FL. More intensive treatments often are considered for patients with high-risk disease, especially those who relapse early after induction therapy as relapse within 2 years of initial therapy is associated with a 5-year OS of only 50%.[35] In this context, both auto-HCT and allo-HCT can provide long-term PFS in relapsed, refractory FL.

Multiple prospective studies have shown that auto-HCT in first remission of FL has a PFS benefit but not an OS benefit when compared to chemotherapy.[36–39] However, this lymphoma-specific survival benefit is offset by secondary malignancies and treatment-related toxicities such that auto-HCT is not recommended for consolidation of remission after first-line therapy for low-grade FL. In relapsed, refractory FL, auto-HCT is not considered a curative option. Although one study showed improved 2-year PFS and 4-year OS in auto-HCT recipients compared to standard chemotherapy,[40] a large majority of patients with FL relapse after auto-HCT.

Allo-HCT for Relapsed, Refractory FL: Prospective Studies

There are no randomized prospective trials or retrospective studies to support the application of allo-HCT as consolidation therapy for FL in first remission despite its incurability with conventional chemotherapy. However, there are several prospective studies reported using allo-HCT in patients with relapsed, refractory FL. The Cancer and Leukemia Group B (CALGB) conducted a phase II study to evaluate the efficacy of an RI-conditioned allo-HCT in patients with indolent B-cell malignancies. All patients received fludarabine/cyclophosphamide conditioning with a matched related donor and were required to have chemosensitive disease. Of the 16 patients with FL, the 3-year event-free survival (EFS) was 75%, and 3-year OS was 81%; 3 subjects relapsed.[41] MD Anderson conducted a Phase II study for relapsed FL patients receiving RI-conditioned allo-HCT with fludarabine, cyclophosphamide, and rituximab.[42] Among the 47 patients enrolled, the median 5-year PFS and OS were impressive at 83% and 85%, respectively, but 7 patients died, mostly related to infectious complications. Another report combined 2 prospective multicenter Spanish trials including 37 patients who received a fludarabine/melphalan RI conditioning regimen.[43] Outcomes were encouraging among patients in CR before allo-HCT with a 4-year OS as 71%, whereas for those with refractory or progressive disease the 4-year OS was 48% and 29%, respectively. The 4-year cumulative incidence of NRM was also exceedingly high in

those with progressive disease at 71%.[43] In a prospective study from the United Kingdom, 82 patients with relapsed/refractory FL underwent RI allo-HCT with fludarabine, melphalan, and alemtuzumab conditioning. Although patients had a median of four prior lines of therapy, the NRM at 4 years was only 15% with a relapse rate of 26%. The OS at 4 years was 76%. Of great interest were 13 patients who received escalating DLI for relapsed disease. Among these 13, 10 patients experienced remission, demonstrating the GVL effect associated with allo-HCT in FL.[44] Finally, another prospective multicenter study in 46 patients with FL coordinated by the Fred Hutchinson Cancer Research Center[45] reported a high (42%) rate of NRM, driven in large part by the use of mismatched unrelated allografts. The relapse rate at 3 years was low, at 14%.

Allo-HCT for Relapsed, Refractory FL: Retrospective Studies

There are several large database studies that have explored the use of allo-HCT among patients with FL. In an analysis from the NCCN lymphoma outcomes group, relapsed/refractory FL patients were stratified by transplant strategy. A total of 148 patients who underwent auto-HCT were compared with 48 patients who underwent allo-HCT. As expected, the 3-year NRM rates were significantly higher at 24% for allo-HCT versus 3% for auto-HCT. This correlated with poorer survival among the allo-HCT group (3-year OS 87% auto-HCT vs. 61% allo-HCT). However, patients in the allo-HCT group had more lines of treatment before transplant and were more likely to have resistant disease.[46] In contrast to these findings, the CIBMTR reported outcomes for patients with relapsed, refractory Grade 1–2 FL who underwent allo-HCT as first transplantation modality in comparison to auto-HCT. Similar to the prior study, the 5-year NRM was substantially higher in the allo-HCT group at 26% versus 5% ($P < .0001$). However, this finding is countered by the increased 5-year relapse/progression risk in auto-HCT at 54% versus only 20% ($P < .0001$) in the allo-HCT cohort. The 5-year PFS favored allo-HCT (41% auto-HCT vs. 58% allo-HCT, $P < .001$), whereas the 5-year OS trended toward auto-HCT (74% vs. 66%, $P = .05$). This was felt to be due to ongoing risk of relapse with auto-HCT and decreasing NRM over time with allo-HCT. Consistent with this finding were the results of a landmark analysis that demonstrated that OS was improved in the first 2 years after auto-HCT but that beyond 2 years it was associated with a worse OS.[47] The CIBMTR conducted a similar study with regard to Grade 3 FL, which is felt to have more aggressive clinical behavior than Grade 1–2 FL.

This study compared outcomes for first RI-conditioned allo-HCT (N = 61) versus first auto-HCT (N = 136) from 2000 to 2012 in relapsed FL. Findings were similar in this histology to other reports with transplant in FL with increased 5-year NRM (27% vs. 4%, P < .001) with allo-HCT but decreased 5-year relapse/progression with allo-HCT (20% vs. 61%, P < .001) in comparison to auto-HCT. Five-year OS was similar in the two groups at 59% for auto-HCT and 54% with allo-HCT. Using a 2-year landmark analysis, similar to the grade 1–2 FL study, OS was superior in the first 2 years after transplant with auto-HCT, whereas survival was superior beyond 2 years with allo-HCT.[48] A recently published study compared auto-HCT with either matched sibling donor (MSD) or matched unrelated donor (MUD) allo-HCT as the first transplant approach for patients with early treatment failure (relapse or progression within 2 years of chemoimmunotherapy). Although outcomes were comparable among the auto-HCT and MSD allo-HCT cohorts with an adjusted 5-year OS of 70% and 73%, respectively, outcomes after MUD allo-HCT were poorer (5-year OS 49%). This was largely driven by excess NRM in the patients who underwent MUD allo-HCT (5-year NRM: 34% MUD vs. 8% MSD vs. 6% auto-HCT). Consistent with other studies, relapse rates were lower with either form of allo-HCT (5-year relapse: MSD 31% and MUD 23% vs. auto-HCT 58%).[49] Finally, a retrospective study from Memorial Sloan Kettering compared outcomes for patients with relapsed/refractory FL undergoing auto-HCT versus allo-HCT in the post-rituximab era. In a subgroup analysis performed in patients with a remission duration of <12 months before salvage therapy, 3-year EFS was 42% with auto-HCT versus 80% with allo-HCT, suggesting that patients with a very short first remission (<1 year) may be better served with an allo-HCT approach.[50]

Summary: FL

Both auto-HCT and allo-HCT have improved long-term outcomes in patients with relapsed, refractory FL. Table 15.3 summarizes outcomes of several prospective and retrospective studies for allo-HCT in FL.[22] Owing to decreased NRM associated with auto-HCT, this is a reasonable consideration as second- or third-line therapy in those with chemosensitive disease. However, for patients with high-risk disease, allo-HCT has demonstrated decreased progression/relapse in comparison to auto-HCT and may be an appropriate consideration in select patients. For those who have failed auto-HCT, allo-HCT has demonstrated long-term PFS. With the increasing application of RI conditioning in allo-HCT and continued improvement in supportive care, NRM

rates likely will continue to decline for well-selected patients with FL who receive expert supportive care. As noted with patients with DLBCL, the advent and implementation of CAR-T therapies will also impact the current treatment algorithm for patients with FL. Although there is currently no FDA-approved product for FL, given encouraging outcomes, approvals are likely in the near future.[30]

MANTLE CELL LYMPHOMA

Overview of MCL and Nontransplantation Options for Frontline Therapy

MCL is characterized by CD5+CD23-mature follicular mantle B-cells with t(11;14)(q13;q32) translocation and cyclin D1 overexpression which is not typically expressed in normal lymphocytes.[51] MCL comprises ~6% of newly diagnosed cases of NHL and is generally considered incurable. The median age at diagnosis is in late 60s, with a 4:1 male predominance, and median survival is about 5 years. Combination chemoimmunotherapy as induction followed by auto-HCT in first remission have improved outcomes, although disease relapse eventually occurs in nearly all patients.[52] The MCL International Prognostic Index is a commonly used risk stratification score that classifies patients with MCL into low-, intermediate-, and high-risk groups, with median OS ranging from 29 months to > 5 years.[53] Although auto-HCT as part of frontline treatment is the current standard of care among fit patients with MCL, its role in relapsed refractory disease is less clear.[54] Initial retrospective studies in relapsed, refractory MCL, including an EBMT study,[55] have suggested that auto-HCT may have limited value in relapsed and refractory patients. However, recent data including from a large retrospective study from the CIBMTR have indicated that durable remissions in the 2- to 4-year range may be seen in selected patients with chemosensitive MCL.[56,57]

Allo-HCT for Relapsed, Refractory MCL

While allo-HCT represents a potentially curative option for patients with MCL, there are no prospective data to date assessing this approach in first remission. Owing to long remission with standard induction with consolidative auto-HCT, allo-HCT is generally reserved for patients with poor response to induction chemotherapy or those with relapsed, refractory disease.[54] Allo-HCT has demonstrated long-term efficacy in patients with relapsed, refractory MCL with 35%–45% of patients disease free at 3 years' posttransplantation (Table 15.4).[56,58–62] Although efficacy is impacted by chemosensitivity at transplant and performance status, allo-HCT has

TABLE 15.3
Studies Evaluating Allo-HCT in Relapsed/Refractory FL (>30 Patients)

Study	No. of Patients	Condition-ing (%)	Median Age, yr (Range)	TRM/NRM, % (yr)	Relapse % (yr)	OS, % (yr)	Comments
Rezvani et al., 2008[45]	46	RIC	54 (33–66)	42 (3)	14 (3)	52 (3)	Prospective
Hari et al., 2008[100]	208	MAC (58) RIC (42)	44 (27–70) 51 (27–700)	23 (1)	8–17 (3)	62–71 (3)	Retrospective (CIBMTR)
Thomson et al., 2010[44]	82	RIC	45 (26–65)	15 (4)	26 (4)	76 (4)	Prospective
Khouri et al., 2012[101]	47	RIC	53 (33–68)	15 (8)	4 (8)	85 (8)	Prospective; 45/47 MRD
Evens et al., 2013[46]	48	NR	50 (27–64)	24 (3)	16 (3)	61 (3)	Retrospective (NCCN)
Robinson et al., 2013[102]	149	RIC	51 (33–66)	22 (3)	20 (5)	67 (5)	Retrospective (EBMT)
Klyuchnikov et al., 2015[47]	268	RIC	52 (27–74)	26 (5)	20 (5)	66 (5)	Retrospective (CIBMTR); grade 1 and 2 FL
Klyuchnikov et al., 2015[48]	70	RIC	53 (36–64)	27 (5)	20 (5)	54 (5)	Retrospective (CIBMTR); grade 3 FL
Yano et al., 2015[103]	46	RIC	48 (34–66)	23 (5)	15 (5)	81 (5)	Retrospective (Japan)

CIBMTR, Center for International Blood and Marrow Transplant Research; EBMT, European Group for Blood and Marrow Transplantation; FL, follicular lymphoma; HCT, hematopoietic cell transplantation; MAC, myeloablative conditioning; MRD, matched related donor; NCCN, National Comprehensive Cancer Network; NRM, nonrelapse mortality; OS, overall survival; RIC, reduced-intensity conditioning; TRM, treatment-related mortality.
Adapted from Fenske TS, Hamadani M, Cohen JB, Costa LJ, Kahl B, Evens AM, Hamlin PA, Lazarus HM, Petersdorf E, Bredeson C, Allogeneic hematopoietic cell transplantation as curative therapy for patients with non-Hodgkin Lymphoma: increasingly successful application to older patients. Biol Blood Marrow Transplant. 2016. Permission Needed.

demonstrated a role even in chemorefractory patients. In a large analysis by the CIBMTR, Hamadani et al. evaluated allo-HCT outcomes for chemotherapy-unresponsive MCL patients. In this cohort of 202 patients, outcomes were stratified by intensity of conditioning (MA vs. RI). PFS and OS in the MA and RI groups were found to be similar at 20% versus 25% for PFS and 25% versus 30% for OS, respectively. There was no benefit to MA conditioning. The ability to demonstrate long-term disease control in 20%–25% of patients demonstrates the GVL effect in MCL with allo-HCT.[61] In a separate analysis also from the CIMBTR, the role of RIC allo-HCT was

evaluated as both an early and late transplant strategy. Early transplant was defined as one that occurred in first partial response (PR) or CR with no more than 2 lines of chemotherapy. For early RI-conditioned allo-HCT the 5-year PFS was 52% and 5-year OS was 62% which was statistically similar to patients who underwent early auto-HCT (5-year OS 61% and 5-year PFS 52%). However, as expected, NRM was significantly higher in the allo-HCT group (1-year NRM 25% vs. 3%, $P < .001$). For patients undergoing late allo-HCT, the 5-year PFS and OS was 24% and 31%, respectively. Although these outcomes are inferior to an early approach, they reflect

TABLE 15.4
Studies Evaluating Allo-HCT in Relapsed/Refractory MCL (>30 Patients)

Study	No. of Patients	Conditioning (%)	Median Age, yr, (Range)	TRM/NRM% (yr)	Relapse, % (yr)	OS, % (yr)
Maris et al., 2004[58]	33	RIC (100)	53 (33–70)	9 (2)	16 (2)	65 (2)
Cook et al., 2010[59]	70	RIC (100)	52 (25–69)	18 (3)	65 (5)	37 (5)
Le Gouill et al., 2012[60]	70	RIC (100)	56 (33–67)	32 (2)	18 (2)	53 (2)
Hamadani et al. 2013[61]	202	MAC (37) RIC (63)	54 (27–69)	38–43 (1)	32–33 (3)	25–30 (3)
Fenske et al., 2014[56]	88	RIC (100)	58 (26–75)	17 (1)	38 (5)	31 (5)
Krüger et al., 2014[62]	33	MAC (21) RIC (79)	59 (33–69)	24 (5)	15 (5)	73 (5)

HCT, hematopoietic cell transplantation; MAC, myeloablative conditioning; MCL, mantle cell lymphoma; NRM, nonrelapse mortality; OS, overall survival; RIC, reduced-intensity conditioning; TRM, treatment-related mortality.
Adapted from Fenske TS, Hamadani M, Cohen JB, Costa LJ, Kahl B, Evens AM, Hamlin PA, Lazarus HM, Petersdorf E, Bredeson C, Allogeneic hematopoietic cell transplantation as curative therapy for patients with non-Hodgkin Lymphoma: increasingly successful application to older patients. *Biol Blood Marrow Transplant.* 2016. Permission Needed.

outcomes with a more aggressive disease and demonstrate a potential cure with allo-HCT for patients who have failed prior therapies in MCL.[56] Finally, a French group evaluated outcomes for RI allo-HCT in patients with MCL who had failed an auto-HCT. Among the 106 patients, the 3-year TRM was estimated at 32%. However, the median OS for patients was nearly 61.8 months which is encouraging given the refractory nature of the patient population. Of great interest are the 8 patients in this cohort who received DLI for relapsed disease which resulted in a sustained response in 6 patients. This along with efficacy of allo-HCT after an auto-HCT demonstrates the GVL effect in MCL.[63]

Summary: MCL

Auto-HCT is not considered curative therapy for MCL, although the intensive induction and consolidation from auto-HCT may provide many patients with long-term remissions that can last 6–8 years or longer.[54] To date, allo-HCT remains the sole treatment option with curative potential,[64] although as noted for other B-cell malignancies, CAR-T cell approaches may be an alternative to allo-HCT in the future. With the use of RIC approach, properly selected patients with MCL who receive appropriate supportive care have a reasonable chance of being cured with allo-HCT.

ALLO-HCT IN OTHER RARE VARIANTS OF B-CELL NHL

There are limited data available on outcomes of allo-HCT in rare forms of B-cell NHL such as marginal zone lymphoma (MZL), Burkitt's lymphoma (BL), or mucosa-associated lymphoid tissue lymphoma. For MZL, the treatment approach and outcomes are similar to FL and auto-HCT, although not curative, can provide a durable remission. Allo-HCT can be considered as an upfront treatment option in young and fit patients rather than waiting until relapse after auto-HCT in select patients.[65] High-dose chemotherapy and auto-HCT are standard of therapy in relapsed, refractory aggressive lymphomas. Specific to BL, a CIMBTR analysis evaluated outcomes with allo-HCT after first CR (CR1), second, or later CR (CR2+), and for patients in non-CR. The 5-year PFS for CR1 was 50%, CR2+ 27% and non-CR 11%. The main cause of death was due to relapsed BL.[66] Though limited data are available, similar principles as those used in FL and DLBCL can be used to determine the appropriateness for allo-HCT in these rarer forms of indolent and aggressive B-cell NHL.

T-Cell Lymphomas

Mature T lymphomas consistent of a large spectrum of lymphoproliferative disorders with significant morphological and clinical heterogeneity. The 2017 WHO classification of lymphoid neoplasms identified >20 different T-cell entities.[67] T-cell neoplasms represent approximately 10%–15% of all cases of NHL,[68] and other than anaplastic lymphoma kinase (ALK) + anaplastic large cell lymphoma (ALCL), most T-cell neoplasm have a poor prognosis with a 3-year EFS that ranges from 36% to 67.5%, depending on histology.[69] The most common subtype of T-cell lymphoma is peripheral T-cell lymphoma not otherwise specified (PTCL-NOS) followed by angioimmunoblastic T-cell lymphoma (AITL).[70] Owing to the rarity of these diseases and the variability in presentation and response to treatment, there are limited data to guide the management of these conditions. Most patients are treated with induction chemotherapy consistent of combination cytotoxic agents (CHOP or CHOEP) with consideration of a frontline auto-HCT transplant in first remission as consolidation.[71] Allo-HCT is a tool often used in patients with high-risk or relapsed, refractory disease.[69] In the following sections we will review the outcomes with allo-HCT in patients with mature T-cell neoplasms.

Allogeneic Transplant in First Remission (Prospective Studies)

Two studies have prospectively evaluated if allo-HCT in the frontline setting would be a safe and efficacious option for patients with PTCL. In one Phase II study patients with PTCL-NOS, ALK- ALCL, or AITL, or enteropathy-associated T-cell lymphoma underwent induction chemotherapy followed by allo-HCT if they had a related or unrelated matched donor with chemosensitive disease (CR or PR). Of the 61 patients, 23 ultimately proceeded with allo-HCT, whereas 14 patients who did not have a donor underwent auto-HCT. The remaining patients did not make it to transplant, mostly due to early progression of disease. Four-year PFS was 69%, and 4-year OS was 69% for allo-HCT; this was not statistically different from patients who underwent auto-HCT (4-year PFS 70% and 4-year OS 92%).[72]

A second randomized prospective study compared outcomes with allo-HCT with auto-HCT in younger patients with PTCL. Patients were all treated with 4 cycles of cyclophosphamide, adriamyacin, vincristine, etoposide, prednisione (CHOEP) chemotherapy and were randomized at enrollment. Responding patient defined as (CR/PR/SD) received DHAP chemotherapy followed by stem cell collection in patients randomized to auto-HCT or to those without a suitable 10/10 human leukocyte antigen–matched donor. Similarly, patients randomized to allo-HCT with a suitable donor received MA conditioning with allo-HCT. After induction, 19 patients proceed with autologous transplant, and 13/28 patients randomized to allo-HCT received it. A proportion of 38% of patients did not proceed to transplantation due to early lymphoma progression. As a preplanned interim analysis did not demonstrate a survival benefit with allo-HCT and a low probability that the primary endpoint would be met, the study closed prematurely.[73]

With the limited prospective data as noted previously, at this time, allogeneic transplant in first remission is not a standard recommendation for most common forms of PTCL and should be approached in a case-by-case situation.[74]

RELAPSED/REFRACTORY T-CELL LYMPHOMA

PTCL-NOS, ALCL, and AITL

While allo-HCT is an accepted modality for the treatment option for patients with mature T-cell neoplasms, its use has been generally limited to patients with relapsed and refractory disease. As the frequency of PTCL remains low, most studies have combined analyses for PTCL-NOS, ALCL, and AITL, and thus outcomes for these three histologies will be reported in a collective fashion.[74]

The CIBMTR reported transplant outcomes for mature T-cell neoplasms between 1996 and 2006 and identified 126 patients with either PTCL-NOS, AITL, or ALCL who underwent allo-HCT and 115 patients who underwent auto-HCT. NRM was higher among allo-HCT recipients than auto-HCT recipients with no improvement in relapse/progression. However, allo-HCT patients were more heavily pretreated and more often had refractory disease than those undergoing auto-HCT. Despite this, the 3-year PFS and OS for allo-HCT were 36% and 47%, respectively. Of note, patients with ALCL had superior OS with auto-HCT that with allo-HCT in this analysis.[75] In a separate report from the Societe Francaise de Greffe de Moelle-Therapie Cellulaire (SFGM-TC) register, patients with aggressive T-cell lymphoma were retrospectively analyzed after receipt of an allo-HCT. Among the 77 identified patients, 55 had a diagnosis of PTCL, AITL, or ALCL. Sixteen of these patients had a prior autologous transplant, and 51% of patients were in a CR before allo-HCT. The 5-year OS by histology for PTCL, AITL, and ALCL were 63% (N = 27), 80% (N = 11), and 55% (N = 27), respectively. For the entire cohort, the 5-year TRM was 34%, and the 5-year OS was 57%.[76] Recently reports from a "real world" multicenter retrospective analysis of allo-HCT in mature T-cell neoplasms were presented in abstract form at the American Society of Hematology 2017 meeting. The 2-year PFS with allo-HCT for AITL, ALK-negative ALCL, and PTCL-NOS were 62%, 30%, and 55.8%, respectively.[77] Table 15.5 summarizes outcomes from several reported studies of allo-HCT for mature T-cell neoplasms.

TABLE 15.5
Outcomes With Allo-HCT in PTCL

References	Number of Patients	Histology	Median Age	NRM	GVHD	Relapse	PFS	OS
Smith, 2013[75]	126	PTCL-NOS 63, AITL 12, ALCL 51	38	MAC 34% at 3 years, RIC 27% at 3 years	NR	MAC 37% at 3 years, RIC 42% at 3 years	MAC 29% at 3 years, RIC 32% at 3 years	MAC 31% at 3 years, RIC 50% at 3 years
Le Gouill, 2008[76]	77	PTCL 27, AITL 11, ALCL 27 (8 ALK+), Other 12	41, 47, 26, 35	34% at 5 years	Acute 21% (Grade III/IV)	NR	58% at 5 years, 80% at 5 years, 48% at 5 years, NR	63% at 5 years, 80% at 5 years, 55% at 5 years, 33% at 5 years
Glass, 2011[104]	66	PTCL-NOS 23, AITL 12, ALCL 11, T-LBL 6, T-PLL 7, Other 7	NR	29% at 100 days	NR	NR	46% at 1 years	48% at 1 years
Dodero, 2012[105]	52	NOS; 23, AITL; 9, ALCL; 11	47	12% at 5 years	acute 22% (grade II-IV) chronic 27%	49% at 5 years	39% at 5 years, 44% at 5 years, 45% at 5 years, No difference by histology	45% at 5 years, 66% at 5 years, 54% at 5 years, No difference by histology
Jacobsen, 2011[106]	52	NOS; 20, AITL; 5, ALCL; 6, Other; 21	46	27% at 3 years	acute 21% (grade II-IV) chronic 27% (extensive)	43% at 3 years	30% at 3 years	41% at 3 years
Kyriakou, 2009[78]	45	AITL 45	48	25% at 5 years	acute 29% (grade II-IV) chronic 54%	20% at 3 years	53% at 3 years	64% at 3 years
Zain, 2011[107]	37	NOS; 8, AITL; 4, ALCL; 6 (3 ALK+), Other; 6, CTCL; 13	40 (50 for CTCL)	29% at 5 years	acute 51% chronic 62%	24% at 5 years	47% at 5 years	52% at 5 years
Delioukina, 2012[108]	27	NOS; 5, AITL; 3, ALCL; 2 (2 ALK+), CTCL; 11	50	22% at 2 years	acute 33% (grade II-IV) chronic 85%	30% at 2 years	47% at 2 years, No difference by histology	55% at 2 years, No difference by histology
Czajczynska, 2013[109]	24	PTCL-NOS 9, AITL 5, ALCL 4	53	2%	Acute 25% (Grade II-IV) Chronic 30%	25%	NR	42% at 3 years

AITL, angioimmunoblastic T-cell lymphoma; *ALCL*, anaplastic large cell lymphoma; *GVHD*, graft-versus-host disease; *HCT*, hematopoietic cell transplantation; *MAC*, myeloablative conditioning; *NOS*, not otherwise specified; *NRM*, nonrelapse mortality; *OS*, overall survival; *PFS*, progression-free survival; *PTCL*, peripheral T-cell lymphoma; *RIC*, reduced-intensity conditioning.

Permission needed from Schmitz N, Lenz G, Stelljes M. Allogeneic hematopoietic stem cell transplantation (HSCT) for T-cell lymphomas. *Blood*. 2018.

Of interest, in the aforementioned studies the outcomes for AITL with allo-HCT were superior than what was seen in other histologies. To further evaluate outcomes in this specific histology, the EBMT conducted a retrospective analysis of patients who underwent allo-HCT for AITL between January 1998 and December 2005. Among the 45 patients identified, 34 patients received ≥2 lines of systemic therapy before allo-HCT, and 11 had failed a prior auto-HCT, suggesting that this represented a high-risk group. Despite this, the 3-year PFS and OS were 53% and 64%, respectively, and were much higher than would be expected in such a refractory population. The cumulative incidence of NRM at 1 year was 25%, and patients with chemorefractory disease at the time of transplant and those with a poor performance status had an inferior PFS.[78]

The aforementioned data demonstrate that for a subset of patients with PTCL that allo-HCT provides a long-term remission despite relapse postautologous transplant or refractory disease. These long-term survivors with allo-HCT suggest that a GVL effect is present in patients with T-cell lymphoma. Supporting the presence of a GVL effect is the efficacy of a reduced-intensity/non-myeloablative allo-HCT in these patients. In both the CIBMTR analysis and the SFGM analysis, intensity of conditioning did not impact PFS or OS outcomes among transplanted patients. In conclusion, allo-HCT is a feasible option for appropriate patients with PTCL-NOS, AITL, and ALCL who have failed standard therapies and relapsed. For AITL, in particular, outcomes with allo-HCT seem to be superior than seen with the other histologies. Figures 15.1 and 15.2 highlight the 2017 consensus criteria recommendations from the ASBMT for allo-HCT in PTCL-NOS, ALK-negative ALCL, and AITL. Of note, recommendations for ALK+ALCL differ from ALK- ALCL given the overall improved responsiveness of that disease compared to other forms of PTCL (Figs. 15.1 and 15.2).[79,80]

Allogeneic Transplant for Natural Killer/T-Cell Lymphoma

Natural killer (NK)/T-cell lymphomas represent aggressive malignancies of NK cell origin. It generally presents in two forms, localized and disseminated. The localized form most commonly presents with an extranodal lesion involving the nasal tract and represents the majority of cases (~80%). Both are associated with Epstein–Barr virus infection and have a geographical predilection for Asian and South American populations.[81] The general approach to treatment for localized disease is combination chemoradiotherapy and for advanced-stage disease is L-asparaginase–containing regimens.[81]

Given the rarity of this disease, there are limited data on outcomes with allo-HCT. Consensus criteria for transplantation recommendations from ASBMT are seen in Figure 15.3. In one report from the Asia Lymphoma Study Group among 18 patients who underwent allo-HCT (14 myeloablative & 4 reduced intensity), the 5-year OS was 57%, and the 5-year EFS was 51%. Although patients in CR1 and CR2 had similar survival, all patients who proceeded with transplant with active disease died.[82] The CIBMTR reported on outcomes of 82 adult patients with extranodal NK/T-cell lymphoma who underwent allo-HCT from 2000 to 2014. Contrary to the prior mentioned study, remission status at the time of transplant (CR vs. PR vs. chemorefractory) did not impact relapse risk, PFS, or OS after transplant. Additionally, intensity of conditioning did not impact clinical outcomes. The 3-year PFS and OS were 28% and 34%, respectively. Although treatment failure and relapse remained the major cause of death, there were no relapses beyond 2 years, suggesting a GVL effect.[83]

Allogeneic Transplant for Cutaneous T-Cell Lymphoma (Mycosis Fungoides/Sezary Syndrome)

Cutaneous T-cell lymphomas (CTCL) are a heterogenous group of extranodal NHLs that are generally confined to the skin at diagnosis. Mycosis fungoides (MF) and Sézary dyndrome (SS) are the two most common forms of CTCL. While most patients with MF have an indolent clinical course that can be managed with a combination of oral and topical agents, patients with extensive nodal or visceral involvement are treated with systemic chemotherapy.[84] While response rates with chemotherapy are high, relapse is common, and in such patients, an allo-HCT is a consideration. The EBMT reported outcomes for relapsed, refractory MF/SS patients after allo-HCT from 1997 to 2007. Among the 60 identified patients, the 3-year OS was 54%, and 3-year PFS was 34%. Interestingly, patients who had RI conditioning had improved OS due to decreased NRM than those receiving MA conditioning without increased relapse. Twenty-one patients remained alive and relapse free after allo-HCT, suggesting that a GVL effect is present in CTCL. Further proving this effect was the efficacy of DLI in patients who experienced relapse. Among 17 patients who received DLI, 10 achieved a CR.[85] The French Study Group on Cutaneous Lymphomas and French Society of Bone Marrow Transplant

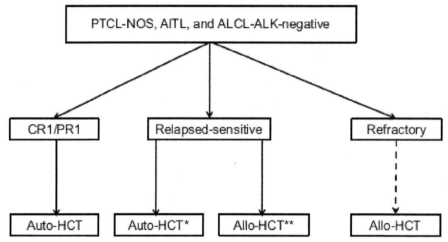

FIG. 15.1 Clinical practice guideline from ASBMT for PTCL-NOS, AITL, and ALCL-ALK-negative. *Dashed line* denotes a weak recommendation.[79] *AITL*, angioimmunoblastic T-cell lymphoma; *ALCL*, anaplastic large cell lymphoma; *ASBMT*, American Society of Blood and Marrow Transplantation; *PTCL-NOS*, peripheral T-cell lymphoma not otherwise specified.

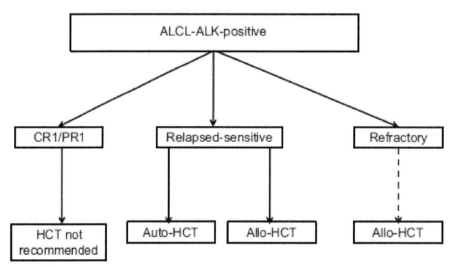

FIG. 15.2 Clinical practice guideline from ASBMT for ALK + ALCL. *Dashed line* denotes a weak recommendation.[79] *ALCL*, anaplastic large cell lymphoma; *ASBMT*, American Society of Blood and Marrow Transplantation.

reported their allo-HCT outcomes of 37 patients with advanced CTCL. The majority of patients had stage IV disease or nodal/visceral involvement with MF/SS who had failed prior therapies. After allo-HCT, the 2-year OS was 57%, and 2-year PFS was 31%. Patients who relapsed after allo-HCT could be salvaged with subsequent lines of therapies.[86] Finally, the CIBMTR reported on outcomes for allo-HCT for MF/SS from 2000 to 2009. Among the 129 patients identified, most subjects were multiply relapsed or had refractory disease, and 64% received non-myeloablative or RI conditioning. The 5-year PFS and OS were 17% and 32%, respectively. The 5-year NRM was 22%, and 5-year relapse was 61%.[87] These aforementioned studies demonstrate that

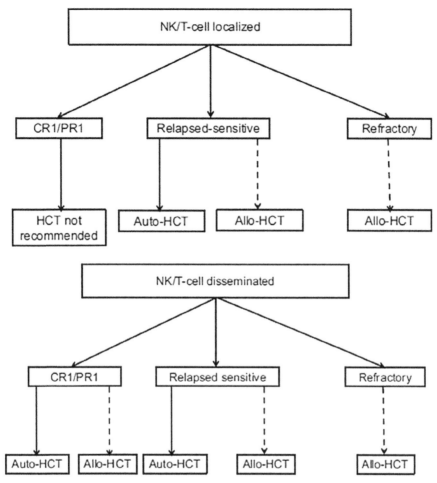

FIG. 15.3 Clinical practice guideline from ASBMT for localized and disseminated NK/T-cell lymphoma. *Dashed line* denotes a weak recommendation.[79] *ASBMT*, American Society of Blood and Marrow Transplantation; *NK*, natural killer.

for select patients with advanced MF/SS that allo-HCT can lead to long-term remission and improved OS. ASBMT practice guidelines for allo-HCT in MF/SS are shown in Fig. 15.4.

Allogeneic Transplant for Hepatosplenic T-Cell Lymphoma

Hepatosplenic T-cell lymphoma is an exceedingly rare and aggressive form of PTCL. It generally occurs in young male patients and presents with hepatosplenomegaly, thrombocytopenia, and systemic symptoms. Owing to rarity, there are limited data on allo-HCT outcomes available in this specific histology. In the largest available analysis published by the EMBT, 18

patients with hepatosplenic T-cell lymphoma who subsequently underwent allo-HCT were identified. Disease status at transplantation was CR (39%), PR (44%), or refractory disease (17%). The 3-year OS and PFS were 54% and 48%, respectively. The major cause of death in this cohort was NRM which occurred in 40% of patients at 3 years.[88] ASBMT transplant recommendations are shown in Fig. 15.5.

Allogeneic Transplant for Adult T-Cell Leukemia/Lymphoma

Adult T-cell leukemia/lymphoma (ATLL) is a form of mature T-cell neoplasm that develops in the context of an HTLV-I infection. Owing to geographic variance of

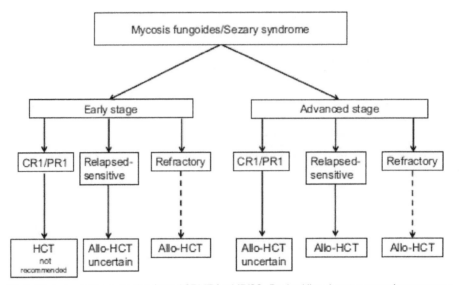

FIG. 15.4 Clinical practice guideline from ASBMT for MF/SS. *Dashed line* denotes a weak recommendation.[79] *ASBMT,* American Society of Blood and Marrow Transplantation; *MF,* Mycosis fungoides; *SS,* Sézary syndrome.

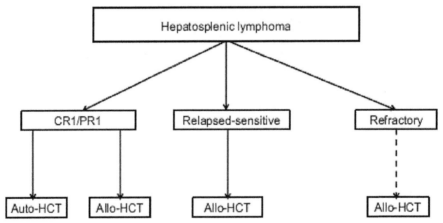

FIG. 15.5 Clinical practice guideline from ASBMT for hepatosplenic T-cell lymphoma. *Dashed line* denotes a weak recommendation.[79] *ASBMT,* American Society of Blood and Marrow Transplantation.

HTLV-1, Adult T-Cell Leukemia/Lymphoma (ATLL) is most common in patients from Japan, the Caribbean, South America, and certain areas of Africa. It is an aggressive disease for which transplantation is considered in the upfront setting.[89] Data for allo-HCT mostly stem from reports in Japan. In a retrospective analysis among 386 patients with ATLL who underwent allo-HCT, the 3-year OS was 33%. Male sex, older age, and less than a CR at transplant were related with poorer outcomes.[90] EBMT performed a similar analysis from their registry

data and identified 17 patients with ATLL who underwent allo-HCT and 4 patients who underwent auto-HCT. All patients who underwent auto-HCT died of relapsed disease. Among the allo-HCT patients, 6 remained alive while the remaining died due to relapse (8/11) or TRM (3/11) with a 3-year EFS and OS of 25.7%. Efficacy of allo-HCT is suggestive of a GVL effect in this disease. Supporting early allo-HCT was a recently published Markov decision analysis performed to determine the optimal timing and appropriateness of allo-HCT in ATLL. It

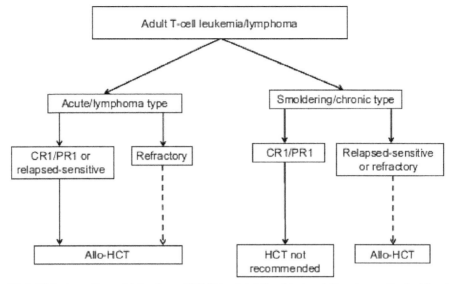

FIG. 15.6 Clinical practice guideline from ASBMT for Adult T-cell leukemia/lymphoma. *Dashed line* denotes a weak recommendation.[79] *ASBMT*, American Society of Blood and Marrow Transplantation.

determined that early, upfront allo-HCT was indicated in patients who met criteria for intermediate or high-risk disease.[91] This is in line with ASBMT consensus recommendations noted in Fig. 15.6.

Allogeneic Transplant for Rare Mature T-Cell Neoplasms

There are limited data for allo-HCT for patients with rare forms of PTCL such as enteropathy-associated T-cell lymphoma (EATL) and subcutaneous panniculitis–like T-cell lymphoma (SPTCL). EATL presents a complication of celiac disease and presents with weight loss, diarrhea, abdominal pain, and "B" symptoms. The general treatment approach is local debulking followed by standard induction chemotherapy and then consolidation with auto-HCT. Data for allo-HCT are limited to case reports, but the overall prognosis for relapsed disease is poor.[92,93] SPTCL is a rare form of skin lymphoma that infiltrates subcutaneous adipose tissue. The disease often follows an indolent course that can be managed with combination chemotherapy. For patients in first CR no further treatment is indicated.[79,94] For patients with relapsed disease, either auto-HCT or allo-HCT can be considered. Given the rarity of this disease, there are limited data for either approach.

Allogeneic Transplant in Older Patients

The application of allo-HCT has expanded with time to older patients due to improvements in supportive care

measure and the widespread application of both RI and non-myeloablative conditioning regimens. Tables 15.2–15.5 list numerous key studies of allo-HCT in DLBCL, FL, MCL, and PTCL, several of which include patients with age up to 70–75 years. McClune et al.[95] specifically analyzed outcomes among B and T-cell NHL patients after allo-HCT stratified by age. NRM at 1 year was higher in this older age group (34%) than in the two groups of younger populations of 40–54 years (22%) and 55–64 years (27%) but was not statistically significant. Relapse rates at 3 years were similar across all the 3 age groups (28%–33%). However, both PFS and OS at 3 years was slightly lower in the older cohorts. OS was 54% (40–54 years), 40% (55–64 years), and 39% (≥65 years), $P < .0001$. While this suggest worse outcomes in an older population, this study was limited by sample size with only 82 of the 1248 patients identified being ≥65 years of age.

A more contemporary study regarding allo-HCT outcomes specifically in elderly patients (age ≥65 years) with NHL was recently published. Similar to the prior study, this included both B- and T-cell NHL histologies. This CIBMTR analysis by Shah et al. compared outcomes in patients from an older cohort age ≥65 years to those aged 55–65 years. Among the identified patients (446 patients with age ≥65 and 1183 patients age 55–64 years), the multivariate analysis revealed no difference in the two cohorts in terms of relapse/progression, PFS, or OS. The 4-year PFS and OS

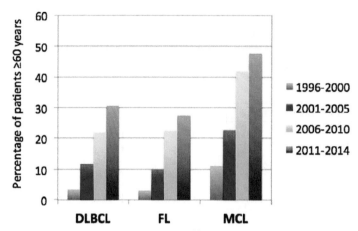

FIG. 15.7 Trends in allo-HCT for DLBCL, FL, and MCL.[22] *allo-HCT*, allogenic hematopoietic stem cell transplant; *DLBCL*, diffuse large B-cell lymphoma; *FL*, follicular lymphoma; *MCL*, mantle cell lymphoma. Adapted from Fenske TS, Hamadani M, Cohen JB, Costa LJ, Kahl B, Evens AM, Hamlin PA, Lazarus HM, Petersdorf E, Bredeson C, Allogeneic hematopoietic cell transplantation as curative therapy for patients with non-Hodgkin Lymphoma: increasingly successful application to older patients. Biol Blood Marrow Transplant. 2016. Permission Needed.

in the ≥65-year aged group were 42% and 46%, respectively. In a subset analysis of patients aged ≥70 years, the 4-year OS was 44% suggesting feasibility of transplant even in the extremes of age. These data strongly support that age alone should not be a determinant for allo-HCT eligibility in NHL but that allo-HCT consideration be based on individual patient characteristics, disease status, and evaluation of alternative treatment options.[96]

Future Directions in Allo-HCT for NHL

Owing to alternative donor transplants, milder conditioning regimens, and more novel agents to control and bridge patients to transplant, there has been an increasing utilization of allo-HCT in three of the more common forms of B-cell NHL (Fig. 15.7).[22] Recent studies have demonstrated that alternative donor transplantation (e.g., haploidentical transplant) in NHL compare favorably to those using matched unrelated donors.[97,98] However, the future of allo-HCT in B-cell NHL remains a significant question as CAR-T therapies gain wider acceptance and become more accessible throughout the international community. It is likely that increasing utilization of CAR-T cell treatments will lead to a decrease in the utilization of allo-HCT in the coming years, but until these therapies are widely available, allo-HCT offers patients a potential for long-term cure of their disease as outlined throughout this chapter. For patients with mature T-cell neoplasms there remains a lack of novel cellular therapies such that allo-HCT will continue to be a modality for long-term disease control in appropriate patients.

REFERENCES

1. LeMaistre CF, Farnia S, Crawford S, et al. Standardization of terminology for episodes of hematopoietic stem cell patient transplant care. *Biol Blood Marrow Transplant.* 2013;19(6):851–857.

2. Majhail NS, Giralt S, Bonagura A, et al. Guidelines for defining and implementing standard episode of care for hematopoietic stem cell transplantation within the context of clinical trials. *Biol Blood Marrow Transplant.* 2015;21(4):583–588.

3. Howlader NNA, Krapcho M, Miller D, et al., eds. *SEER Cancer Statistics Review, 1975–2014.* Bethesda, MD: National Cancer Institute; 2017. Available from: http://seer.cancer.gov/csr/1975_2014/.

4. Jones RJ, Ambinder RF, Piantadosi S, Santos GW. Evidence of a graft-versus-lymphoma effect associated with allogeneic bone marrow transplantation. *Blood.* 1991;77(3):649–653.

5. Butcher BW, Collins Jr RH. The graft-versus-lymphoma effect: clinical review and future opportunities. *Bone Marrow Transplant.* 2005;36:1.

6. Bishop MR, Dean RM, Steinberg SM, et al. Clinical evidence of a graft-versus-lymphoma effect against relapsed diffuse large B-cell lymphoma after allogeneic hematopoietic stem-cell transplantation. *Ann Oncol.* 2008;19(11):1935–1940.

7. Majhail NS, Farnia SH, Carpenter PA, et al. Indications for autologous and allogeneic hematopoietic cell transplantation: guidelines from the American Society for blood and marrow transplantation. *Biol Blood Marrow Transplant.* 2015;21(11):1863–1869.

8. Brudno JN, Kochenderfer JN. Chimeric antigen receptor T-cell therapies for lymphoma. *Nat Rev Clin Oncol.* 2017;15:31.

9. Neelapu SS, Locke FL, Bartlett NL, et al. Axicabtagene ciloleucel CAR T-cell therapy in refractory large B-cell lymphoma. *N Engl J Med.* 2017;377(26):2531–2544.

10. Zhou Z, Sehn LH, Rademaker AW, et al. An enhanced International Prognostic Index (NCCN-IPI) for patients with diffuse large B-cell lymphoma treated in the rituximab era. *Blood.* 2014;123(6):837–842.

11. Coiffier B, Lepage E, Brière J, et al. CHOP chemotherapy plus rituximab compared with CHOP alone in elderly patients with diffuse large-B-cell lymphoma. *Engl J Med.* 2002;346(4):235–242.

12. Rosenwald A, Wright G, Chan WC, et al. The use of molecular profiling to predict survival after chemotherapy for diffuse large-B-cell lymphoma. *Engl J Med.* 2002;346(25):1937–1947.

13. Yoon CC, Yasuhiro O, WJ R, Francesco T. A clinician's guide to double hit lymphomas. *Br J Haematol.* 2015;168(6):784–795.

14. Petrich AM, Gandhi M, Jovanovic B, et al. Impact of induction regimen and stem cell transplantation on outcomes in double-hit lymphoma: a multicenter retrospective analysis. *Blood.* 2014;124(15):2354–2361.

15. Philip T, Guglielmi C, Hagenbeek A, et al. Autologous bone marrow transplantation as compared with salvage chemotherapy in relapses of chemotherapy-sensitive non-Hodgkin's lymphoma. *Engl J Med.* 1995;333(23):1540–1545.

16. Gisselbrecht C, Glass B, Mounier N, et al. Salvage regimens with autologous transplantation for relapsed large B-cell lymphoma in the rituximab era. *J Clin Oncol.* 2010;28(27):4184–4190.

17. Thomson KJ, Morris EC, Bloor A, et al. Favorable long-term survival after reduced-intensity allogeneic transplantation for multiple-relapse aggressive non-Hodgkin's lymphoma. *J Clin Oncol.* 2009;27(3):426–432.

18. Klyuchnikov E, Bacher U, Kroll T, et al. Allogeneic hematopoietic cell transplantation for diffuse large B cell lymphoma: who, when and how? *Bone Marrow Transplant.* 2013;49:1.

19. Lazarus HM, Zhang MJ, Carreras J, et al. A comparison of HLA-identical sibling allogeneic versus autologous transplantation for diffuse large B cell lymphoma: a report from the CIBMTR. *Biol Blood Marrow Transplant.* 2010;16(1):35–45.

20. Bacher U, Klyuchnikov E, Le-Rademacher J, et al. Conditioning regimens for allo transplants for diffuse large B-cell lymphoma: myeloablative or reduced intensity? *Blood.* 2012;120(20):4256–4262.

21. Hamadani M, Saber W, Ahn KW, et al. Impact of pre-transplantation conditioning regimens on outcomes of allogeneic transplantation for chemotherapy-unresponsive diffuse large B cell lymphoma and grade III follicular lymphoma. *Biol Blood Marrow Transplant.* 2013;19(5):746–753.

22. Fenske TS, Hamadani M, Cohen JB, et al. Allogeneic hematopoietic cell transplantation as curative therapy for patients with non-Hodgkin lymphoma: increasingly successful application to older patients. *Biol Blood Marrow Transplant.* 2016.

23. Hamadani M, Hari PN, Zhang Y, et al. Early failure of frontline rituximab-containing chemo-immunotherapy in diffuse large B cell lymphoma does not predict futility of autologous hematopoietic cell transplantation. *Biol Blood Marrow Transplant.* 2014;20(11):1729–1736.

24. van Kampen RJ, Canals C, Schouten HC, et al. Allogeneic stem-cell transplantation as salvage therapy for patients with diffuse large B-cell non-Hodgkin's lymphoma relapsing after an autologous stem-cell transplantation: an analysis of the European Group for Blood and Marrow Transplantation Registry. *J Clin Oncol.* 2011;29(10):1342–1348.

25. Rigacci L, Puccini B, Dodero A, et al. Allogeneic hematopoietic stem cell transplantation in patients with diffuse large B cell lymphoma relapsed after autologous stem cell transplantation: a GITMO study. *Ann Hematol.* 2012;91(6):931–939.

26. Fenske TS, Ahn KW, Graff TM, et al. Allogeneic transplantation provides durable remission in a subset of DLBCL patients relapsing after autologous transplantation. *Br J Haematol.* 2016;174(2):235–248.

27. Kim JW, Kim SW, Tada K, et al. Allogeneic stem cell transplantation in patients with de novo diffuse large B-cell lymphoma who experienced relapse or progression after autologous stem cell transplantation: a Korea-Japan collaborative study. *Ann Hematol.* 2014;93(8):1345–1351.

28. Vose J, Bierman P, Anderson J, et al. Progressive disease after high-dose therapy and autologous transplantation for lymphoid malignancy: clinical course and patient follow-up. *Blood.* 1992;80(8):2142–2148.

29. Nagle SJ, Woo K, Schuster SJ, et al. Outcomes of patients with relapsed/refractory diffuse large B-cell lymphoma with progression of lymphoma after autologous stem cell transplantation in the rituximab era. *Am J Hematol.* 2013;88(10):890–894.

30. Schuster SJ, Svoboda J, Chong EA, et al. Chimeric antigen receptor T cells in refractory B-cell lymphomas. *N Engl J Med.* 2017;377(26):2545–2554.

31. Kahl BS, Yang DT. Follicular lymphoma: evolving therapeutic strategies. *Blood.* 2016;127(17):2055–2063.

32. Solal-Celigny P, Roy P, Colombat P, et al. Follicular lymphoma international prognostic index. *Blood.* 2004;104(5):1258–1265.

33. Brice P, Bastion Y, Lepage E, et al. Comparison in low-tumor-burden follicular lymphomas between an initial no-treatment policy, prednimustine, or interferon alfa: a randomized study from the Groupe d'Etude des Lymphomes Folliculaires. Groupe d'Etude des Lymphomes de l'Adulte. *J Clin Oncol.* 1997;15(3):1110–1117.

34. Kahl BS, Hong F, Williams ME, et al. Rituximab extended schedule or re-treatment trial for low-tumor burden follicular lymphoma: eastern cooperative oncology group protocol e4402. *J Clin Oncol.* 2014;32(28):3096–3102.

35. Casulo C, Byrtek M, Dawson KL, et al. Early relapse of follicular lymphoma after rituximab plus cyclophosphamide, doxorubicin, Vincristine, and Prednisone defines patients at high risk for death: an analysis from the national LymphoCare study. *J Clin Oncol.* 2015;33(23):2516–2522.

36. Lenz G, Dreyling M, Schiegnitz E, et al. Myeloablative radiochemotherapy followed by autologous stem cell transplantation in first remission prolongs progression-free survival in follicular lymphoma: results of a prospective, randomized trial of the German Low-Grade Lymphoma Study Group. *Blood.* 2004;104(9):2667–2674.

37. Deconinck E, Foussard C, Milpied N, et al. High-dose therapy followed by autologous purged stem-cell transplantation and doxorubicin-based chemotherapy in patients with advanced follicular lymphoma: a randomized multicenter study by GOELAMS. *Blood.* 2005;105(10):3817–3823.

38. Sebban C, Mounier N, Brousse N, et al. Standard chemotherapy with interferon compared with CHOP followed by high-dose therapy with autologous stem cell transplantation in untreated patients with advanced follicular lymphoma: the GELF-94 randomized study from the Groupe d'Etude des Lymphomes de l'Adulte (GELA). *Blood.* 2006;108(8):2540–2544.

39. Ladetto M, De Marco F, Benedetti F, et al. Prospective, multicenter randomized GITMO/IIL trial comparing intensive (R-HDS) versus conventional (CHOP-R) chemoimmunotherapy in high-risk follicular lymphoma at diagnosis: the superior disease control of R-HDS does not translate into an overall survival advantage. *Blood.* 2008;111(8):4004–4013.

40. Schouten HC, Qian W, Kvaloy S, et al. High-dose therapy improves progression-free survival and survival in relapsed follicular non-Hodgkin's lymphoma: results from the randomized European CUP trial. *J Clin Oncol.* 2003;21(21):3918–3927.

41. Shea T, Johnson J, Westervelt P, et al. Reduced intensity allogeneic transplantation provides high event-free and overall survival in patients with advanced indolent B cell malignancies: CALGB 109901. *Biol Blood Marrow Transplant.* 2011;17(9):1395–1403.

42. Khouri IF, McLaughlin P, Saliba RM, et al. Eight-year experience with allogeneic stem cell transplantation for relapsed follicular lymphoma after nonmyeloablative conditioning with fludarabine, cyclophosphamide, and rituximab. *Blood.* 2008;111(12):5530–5536.

43. Piñana JL, Martino R, Gayoso J, et al. Reduced intensity conditioning HLA identical sibling donor allogeneic stem cell transplantation for patients with follicular lymphoma: long-term follow-up from two prospective multicenter trials. *Haematologica.* 2010;95(7):1176–1182.

44. Thomson KJ, Morris EC, Milligan D, et al. T-Cell–Depleted reduced-intensity transplantation followed by donor leukocyte infusions to promote graft-versus-lymphoma activity results in excellent long-term survival in patients with multiply relapsed follicular lymphoma. *J Clin Oncol.* 2010;28(23):3695–3700.

45. Rezvani AR, Storer B, Maris M, et al. Nonmyeloablative allogeneic hematopoietic cell transplantation in relapsed, refractory, and transformed indolent non-Hodgkin's lymphoma. *J Clin Oncol.* 2008;26(2):211–217.

46. Evens AM, Vanderplas A, LaCasce AS, et al. Stem cell transplantation for follicular lymphoma relapsed/refractory after prior rituximab: a comprehensive analysis from the NCCN lymphoma outcomes project. *Cancer.* 2013;119(20):3662–3671.

47. Klyuchnikov E, Bacher U, Kroger NM, et al. Reduced-intensity allografting as first transplantation approach in relapsed/refractory grades one and two follicular lymphoma provides improved outcomes in long-term survivors. *Biol Blood Marrow Transplant.* 2015;21(12):2091–2099.

48. Klyuchnikov E, Bacher U, Woo Ahn K, et al. Long-term survival outcomes of reduced-intensity allogeneic or autologous transplantation in relapsed grade 3 follicular lymphoma. *Bone Marrow Transplant.* 2016;51(1):58–66.

49. Smith SM, Godfrey J, Ahn KW, et al. Autologous transplantation versus allogeneic transplantation in patients with follicular lymphoma experiencing early treatment failure. *Cancer.* 2018.

50. Lunning MA, Migliacci JC, Hilden P, et al. The potential benefit of allogeneic over autologous transplantation

in patients with very early relapsed and refractory follicular lymphoma with prior remission duration of ≤ 12 months. *Br J Haematol.* 2016;173(2):260–264.

51. Pérez-Galán P, Dreyling M, Wiestner A. Mantle cell lymphoma: biology, pathogenesis, and the molecular basis of treatment in the genomic era. *Blood.* 2011;117(1):26–38.

52. Vose JM. Mantle cell lymphoma: 2015 update on diagnosis, risk-stratification, and clinical management. *Am J Hematol.* 2015;90(8):739–745.

53. Hoster E, Dreyling M, Klapper W, et al. A new prognostic index (MIPI) for patients with advanced-stage mantle cell lymphoma. *Blood.* 2008;111(2):558–565.

54. Cheah CY, Seymour JF, Wang ML. Mantle cell lymphoma. *J Clin Oncol.* 2016.

55. Vandenberghe E, Ruiz de Elvira C, Loberiza FR, et al. Outcome of autologous transplantation for mantle cell lymphoma: a study by the European blood and bone marrow transplant and autologous blood and marrow transplant registries. *Br J Haematol.* 2003;120(5):793–800.

56. Fenske TS, Zhang M-J, Carreras J, et al. Autologous or reduced-intensity conditioning allogeneic hematopoietic cell transplantation for chemotherapy-sensitive mantle-cell lymphoma: analysis of transplantation timing and modality. *J Clin Oncol.* 2014;32(4):273–281.

57. Cassaday RD, Guthrie KA, Budde EL, et al. Specific features identify patients with relapsed or refractory mantle cell lymphoma benefitting from autologous hematopoietic cell transplantation. *Biol Blood Marrow Transplant.* 2013;19(9):1403–1406.

58. Maris MB, Sandmaier BM, Storer BE, et al. Allogeneic hematopoietic cell transplantation after fludarabine and 2 Gy total body irradiation for relapsed and refractory mantle cell lymphoma. *Blood.* 2004;104(12):3535–3542.

59. Cook G, Smith GM, Kirkland K, et al. Outcome following reduced-intensity allogeneic stem cell transplantation (RIC AlloSCT) for relapsed and refractory mantle cell lymphoma (MCL): a study of the British Society for blood and marrow transplantation. *Biol Blood Marrow Transplant.* 2010;16(10):1419–1427.

60. Le Gouill S, Kröger N, Dhedin N, et al. Reduced-intensity conditioning allogeneic stem cell transplantation for relapsed/refractory mantle cell lymphoma: a multicenter experience. *Ann Oncol.* 2012;23(10):2695–2703.

61. Hamadani M, Saber W, Ahn KW, et al. Allogeneic hematopoietic cell transplantation for chemotherapy-unresponsive mantle cell lymphoma: a cohort analysis from the CIBMTR. *Biol Blood Marrow Transplant.* 2013;19(4):625–631.

62. Kruger WH, Hirt C, Basara N, et al. Allogeneic stem cell transplantation for mantle cell lymphoma–final report from the prospective trials of the East German Study Group Haematology/Oncology (OSHO). *Ann Hematol.* 2014;93(9):1587–1597.

63. Tessoulin B, Ceballos P, Chevallier P, et al. Allogeneic stem cell transplantation for patients with mantle cell lymphoma who failed autologous stem cell transplantation: a national survey of the SFGM-TC. *Bone Marrow Transplant.* 2016;51:1184.

64. Cohen JB, Burns LJ, Bachanova V. Role of allogeneic stem cell transplantation in mantle cell lymphoma. *Eur J Haematol.* 2015;94(4):290–297.

65. Shimoni A. The role of stem-cell transplantation in the treatment of marginal zone lymphoma. *Best Pract Res Clin Haematol.* 2017;30(1):166–171.

66. Maramattom LV, Hari PN, Burns LJ, et al. Autologous and allogeneic transplantation for burkitt lymphoma outcomes and changes in utilization: a report from the center for international blood and marrow transplant research. *Biol Blood Marrow Transplant.* 2013;19(2):173–179.

67. Matutes E. The 2017 WHO update on mature T- and natural killer (NK) cell neoplasms. *Int J Lab Hematol.* 2018;40(Suppl 1):97–103.

68. Armitage JO. The aggressive peripheral T-cell lymphomas: 2017. *Am J Hematol.* 2017;92(7):706–715.

69. Schmitz N, Trumper L, Ziepert M, et al. Treatment and prognosis of mature T-cell and NK-cell lymphoma: an analysis of patients with T-cell lymphoma treated in studies of the German High-Grade Non-Hodgkin Lymphoma Study Group. *Blood.* 2010;116(18):3418–3425.

70. Vose J, Armitage J, Weisenburger D. International peripheral T-cell and natural killer/T-cell lymphoma study: pathology findings and clinical outcomes. *J Clin Oncol.* 2008;26(25):4124–4130.

71. Ellin F, Landstrom J, Jerkeman M, Relander T. Real-world data on prognostic factors and treatment in peripheral T-cell lymphomas: a study from the Swedish Lymphoma Registry. *Blood.* 2014;124(10):1570–1577.

72. Corradini P, Vitolo U, Rambaldi A, et al. Intensified chemo-immunotherapy with or without stem cell transplantation in newly diagnosed patients with peripheral T-cell lymphoma. *Leukemia.* 2014;28:1885.

73. Schmitz N, Nickelsen M, Altmann B, et al. Allogeneic or autologous transplantation as first-line therapy for younger patients with peripheral T-cell lymphoma: results of the interim analysis of the AATT trial. *J Clin Oncol.* 2015;33(suppl 15):8507.

74. Schmitz N, Lenz G, Stelljes M. Allogeneic hematopoietic stem cell transplantation (HSCT) for T-cell lymphomas. *Blood.* 2018.

75. Smith SM, Burns LJ, van Besien K, et al. Hematopoietic cell transplantation for systemic mature T-cell non-Hodgkin lymphoma. *J Clin Oncol.* 2013;31(25):3100–3109.

76. Le Gouill S, Milpied N, Buzyn A, et al. Graft-versus-lymphoma effect for aggressive T-cell lymphomas in adults: a study by the Societe Francaise de Greffe de Moelle et de Therapie Cellulaire. *J Clin Oncol.* 2008;26(14):2264–2271.

77. Mehta-Shah N, Teja S, Tao Y, et al. Successful treatment of mature T-cell lymphoma with allogeneic stem cell transplantation: the largest multicenter retrospective analysis. *Blood.* 2017;130(suppl 1):4597.

78. Kyriakou C, Canals C, Finke J, et al. Allogeneic stem cell transplantation is able to induce long-term remissions

in angioimmunoblastic T-cell lymphoma: a retrospective study from the lymphoma working party of the European group for blood and marrow transplantation. *J Clin Oncol.* 2009;27(24):3951–3958.

79. Kharfan-Dabaja MA, Kumar A, Ayala E, et al. Clinical practice recommendations on indication and timing of hematopoietic cell transplantation in mature T cell and NK/T cell lymphomas: an international collaborative effort on behalf of the guidelines Committee of the American Society for blood and marrow transplantation. *Biol Blood Marrow Transplant.* 2017;23(11):1826–1838.

80. Hapgood G, Savage KJ. The biology and management of systemic anaplastic large cell lymphoma. *Blood.* 2015;126(1):17–25.

81. Tse E, Kwong Y-L. The diagnosis and management of NK/T-cell lymphomas. *J Hematol Oncol.* 2017;10(1):85.

82. Tse E, Chan TS, Koh LP, et al. Allogeneic haematopoietic SCT for natural killer/T-cell lymphoma: a multicentre analysis from the Asia Lymphoma Study Group. *Bone Marrow Transplant.* 2014;49(7):902–906.

83. Kanate AS, DiGilio A, Ahn KW, et al. Allogeneic haematopoietic cell transplantation for extranodal natural killer/T-cell lymphoma, nasal type: a CIBMTR analysis. *Br J Haematol.* 2017.

84. Wilcox RA. Cutaneous T-cell lymphoma: 2016 update on diagnosis, risk-stratification, and management. *Am J Hematol.* 2016;91(1):151–165.

85. Duarte RF, Canals C, Onida F, et al. Allogeneic hematopoietic cell transplantation for patients with mycosis fungoides and Sezary syndrome: a retrospective analysis of the lymphoma working party of the European group for blood and marrow transplantation. *J Clin Oncol.* 2010;28(29):4492–4499.

86. de Masson A, Beylot-Barry M, Bouaziz JD, et al. Allogeneic stem cell transplantation for advanced cutaneous T-cell lymphomas: a study from the French society of bone marrow transplantation and French study group on cutaneous lymphomas. *Haematologica.* 2014;99(3):527–534.

87. Lechowicz MJ, Lazarus HM, Carreras J, et al. Allogeneic hematopoietic cell transplantation for mycosis fungoides and Sezary syndrome. *Bone Marrow Transplant.* 2014;49(11):1360–1365.

88. Tanase A, Schmitz N, Stein H, et al. Allogeneic and autologous stem cell transplantation for hepatosplenic T-cell lymphoma: a retrospective study of the EBMT Lymphoma Working Party. *Leukemia.* 2015;29(3):686–688.

89. Jabbour M, Tuncer H, Castillo J, et al. Hematopoietic SCT for adult T-cell leukemia/lymphoma: a review. *Bone Marrow Transplant.* 2011;46:1039.

90. Hishizawa M, Kanda J, Utsunomiya A, et al. Transplantation of allogeneic hematopoietic stem cells for adult T-cell leukemia: a nationwide retrospective study. *Blood.* 2010;116(8):1369–1376.

91. Fuji S, Kurosawa S, Inamoto Y, et al. Role of up-front allogeneic hematopoietic stem cell transplantation for patients with aggressive adult T-cell leukemia-lymphoma: a decision analysis. *Bone Marrow Transplant.* 2018.

92. Di Sabatino A, Biagi F, Gobbi PG, Corazza GR. How I treat enteropathy-associated T-cell lymphoma. *Blood.* 2012;119(11):2458–2468.

93. Nijeboer P, Malamut G, Mulder CJ, et al. Enteropathy-associated T-cell lymphoma: improving treatment strategies. *Dig Dis.* 2015;33(2):231–235.

94. Sugeeth MT, Narayanan G, Jayasudha AV, Nair RA. Subcutaneous panniculitis-like T-cell lymphoma. *Proc Bayl Univ Med Cent.* 2017;30(1):76–77.

95. McClune BL, Ahn KW, Wang HL, et al. Allotransplantation for patients age >/=40 years with non-Hodgkin lymphoma: encouraging progression-free survival. *Biol Blood Marrow Transplant.* 2014;20(7):960–968.

96. Shah NN, Ahn KW, Litovich C, et al. Outcomes of Medicare-age eligible NHL patients receiving RIC allogeneic transplantation: a CIBMTR analysis. *Blood Adv.* 2018;2(8):933–940.

97. Kanate AS, Mussetti A, Kharfan-Dabaja MA, et al. Reduced-intensity transplantation for lymphomas using haploidentical related donors vs HLA-matched unrelated donors. *Blood.* 2016;127(7):938–947.

98. Bachanova V, Burns LJ, Wang T, et al. Alternative donors extend transplantation for patients with lymphoma who lack an HLA matched donor. *Bone Marrow Transplant.* 2014;50:197.

99. Sirvent A, Dhedin N, Michallet M, et al. Low Nonrelapse Mortality and Prolonged Long-Term Survival after Reduced-Intensity Allogeneic Stem Cell Transplantation for Relapsed or Refractory Diffuse Large B Cell Lymphoma: report of the Société Française de Greffe de Moelle et de Thérapie Cellulaire. *Biol Blood Marrow Transplant.* 2010;16(1):78–85.

100. Hari P, Carreras J, Zhang MJ, et al. Allogeneic transplants in follicular lymphoma: higher risk of disease progression after reduced intensity compared to myeloablative conditioning. *Biol Blood and Marrow Transplant.* 2008;14(2):236–245.

101. Khouri IF, Saliba RM, Erwin WD, et al. Nonmyeloablative allogeneic transplantation with or without ^{90}yttrium ibritumomab tiuxetan is potentially curative for relapsed follicular lymphoma: 12-year results. *Blood.* 2012;119(26):6373–6378.

102. Robinson SP, Canals C, Luang JJ, et al. The outcome of reduced intensity allogeneic stem cell transplantation and autologous stem cell transplantation when performed as a first transplant strategy in relapsed follicular lymphoma: an analysis from the Lymphoma Working Party of the EBMT. *Bone Marrow Transplant.* 2013;48:1409.

103. Yano S, Mori T, Kanda Y, et al. Favorable survival after allogeneic stem cell transplantation with reduced-intensity conditioning regimens for relapsed/refractory follicular lymphoma. *Bone Marrow Transplant.* 2015;50:1299.

104. Glass BHJ, Jung W, et al. Allogeneic stem cell transplantation for patients with relapsed or chemorefractory

T-cell lymphoma: role of high intensity conditioning. *Ann Oncol.* 2011;22(suppl 4).

105. Dodero A, Spina F, Narni F, et al. Allogeneic transplantation following a reduced-intensity conditioning regimen in relapsed/refractory peripheral T-cell lymphomas: long-term remissions and response to donor lymphocyte infusions support the role of a graft-versus-lymphoma effect. *Leukemia.* 2012;26(3):520–526.

106. Jacobsen ED, Kim HT, Ho VT, et al. A large single-center experience with allogeneic stem-cell transplantation for peripheral T-cell non-Hodgkin lymphoma and advanced mycosis fungoides/Sezary syndrome. *Ann Oncol.* 2011;22(7):1608–1613.

107. Zain J, Palmer JM, Delioukina M, et al. Allogeneic hematopoietic cell transplant for peripheral T-cell non-Hodgkin lymphoma results in long-term disease control. *Leukemia Lymphoma.* 2011;52(8):1463–1473.

108. Delioukina M, Zain J, Palmer JM, Tsai N, Thomas S, Forman S. Reduced-intensity allogeneic hematopoietic cell transplantation using fludarabine-melphalan conditioning for treatment of mature T-cell lymphomas. *Bone Marrow Transplant.* 2012;47(1):65–72.

109. Czajczynska A, Gunther A, Repp R, et al. Allogeneic stem cell transplantation with BEAM and alemtuzumab conditioning immediately after remission induction has curative potential in advanced T-cell non-Hodgkin's lymphoma. *Biol Blood Marrow Transplant.* 2013;19(11):1632–1637.

Hematopoietic Stem Cell Transplantation for Hodgkin Lymphoma

SAIRAH AHMED, MD

Hodgkin lymphoma (HL) is an uncommon B-cell lymphoid malignancy composed of two distinct disease entities, the more commonly diagnosed classical HL and the rare nodular lymphocyte predominant HL. The disease has a bimodal distribution with an increased incidence in young adults as well as in patients aged 55 years and older. HL accounts for about 1% (7500 cases) annually of newly diagnosed cancer in the United States and is curable in the majority of patients using conventional chemotherapy and radiotherapy.[1,2] Currently, more than 80% of all newly diagnosed patients younger than 60 years are likely to be cured of their disease. However, some 20%–30% of patients will either be refractory to initial therapy or relapse after frontline therapy, with some proportion who are primary refractory (defined as progression of disease during induction treatment or within 90 days after end of treatment).[3,4] Many of these patients who fail initial therapy or relapse may be cured by high-dose therapy and autologous hematopoietic stem cell transplantation (auto-HSCT). Recurrence of HL ensues in 50% of patients after auto-HSCT,[5] and prognosis with relapse after an auto-HSCT is poor; however, allogeneic HSCT can induce long-term remissions in some patients although often with significant treatment-related mortality (TRM).

ROLE AUTOLOGOUS STEM CELL TRANSPLANTATION IN HL

High-dose chemotherapy and autologous stem cell transplantation is the standard of care for treatment of relapsed or refractory HL with chemosensitive disease. Two randomized trials testing multiagent chemotherapy compared with intensification with high-dose carmustine, etoposide, cytarabine, and melphalan (BEAM) have shown superior event-free survival for patients receiving the intensive chemotherapy supported by autologous stem cell transplantation.[6,7] The lack of overall survival benefit (OS) in the randomized trials is attributed to patients in the chemotherapy-only arms receiving HSCT at the time of second relapse. A prospective nonrandomized trial by the Groupe d'Étude des Lymphomes de l'Adulte (GELA) group revealed a 5-year OS rate of 71% in the transplant group, whereas only 32% OS in patients who did not undergo auto-HSCT and received chemotherapy alone.[8] A Cochrane systematic review and metaanalysis in 2013 demonstrated superior progression-free survival (PFS) for patients with relapsed or refractory disease who underwent auto-HSCT compared with conventional chemotherapy alone with a trend for improved OS.[9]

FACTORS THAT PREDICT RECURRENCE AFTER TRANSPLANTATION

Certain prognostic factors have been recognized to forecast failure after transplantation. The most important feature that predicts for success of transplant is the duration of remission (> or < than 12 months) after initial chemotherapy.[10,11]

Other prognostic factors include
- stage III/IV disease
- extranodal disease
- B symptoms
- bulky disease at diagnosis (>5 cm)
- anemia (hemoglobin <10 g/dL)
- disease status at the time of transplantation

The Center for International Blood and Marrow Transplant Research (CIBMTR) prognostic model is based on factors available at the time of transplantation and was developed based on the outcomes of 728 patients with relapsed/refractory HL who underwent an auto-HSCT. (The CIBMTR includes a voluntary working group of more than 450 transplantation centers worldwide that contribute detailed data on consecutive allogeneic and autologous hematopoietic cell

Hematopoietic Cell Transplantation for Malignant Conditions. https://doi.org/10.1016/B978-0-323-56802-9.00016-X

transplantations to a statistical center at the Medical College of Wisconsin in Milwaukee and the National Marrow Donor Program Coordinating Center in Minneapolis. Participating centers are required to report all transplants consecutively.) The multivariate model identified four major risk factors at the time of auto-HSCT with the following relative weights: Karnofsky performance score <90 and chemotherapy resistance at transplant were each assigned 1 point, whereas at least 3 chemotherapy regimens pre-HSCT and extranodal disease at auto-hsct were each assigned 2 points. Based on the total score summed for the 4 adverse risk factors, 3 risk groups were identified: low (score = 0), intermediate (score = 1 to 3), or high (score = 4 to 6). The 4-year PFS for the low-, intermediate-, and high-risk groups were 71%, 60%, and 42%, respectively.[12]

Refractory HL in contrast to relapsed disease has a disappointing prognosis and will be discussed further later in the chapter. There are various definitions of primary refractory disease, but all include patients with disease progression during frontline therapy; additionally, many also include patients with progressive disease within 90 days of completion of frontline therapy or patients failing to achieve a partial response to initial therapy. An Italian study reported that at 8 years the OS of patients whose initial complete response (CR) was longer than 12 months was 54%, whereas that in those in CR shorter than 12 months was 28%. However, in those patients who had primary induction failure the 8-year OS was 8%. Among patients who undergo auto-HSCT with primary refractory disease, long-term survival is as high as 48% at 10 years for those with chemosensitive disease to salvage second-line chemotherapy.[13]

Objectives of Salvage Chemotherapy Before Transplantation

The importance of a complete response to therapy before transplantation cannot be overstated. Attainment of a positron emission tomography (PET)–negative complete response (CR) has been shown to have a positive predictive value of 93% for PFS at 2 years and is a strong predictor for long-term survival after auto-hsct.[14] Nevertheless, patients who have a partial response or stable disease to salvage chemotherapy can still be cured with an autologous transplant although the risk of relapse is appreciably higher in these groups.

Minimizing disease burden before transplantation is achieved with salvage chemotherapy, radiotherapy, or targeted agents (e.g., brentuximab, vedotin, or nivolumab) or a combination of these. Commonly two cycles of salvage chemotherapy is given, and patients who do not attain a CR with initial salvage therapy often proceed to further salvage therapy before transplantation. Frequently used salvage regimens are ICE (ifosfamide, carboplatin, and etoposide), DHAP (dexamethasone, cytarabine, and cisplatin), and GDP (gemcitabine, dexamethasone, and cisplatin). There are no randomized trials that directly compare salvage chemotherapy for relapsed HL. Response rates for these regimens in various phase II studies range from 60% to 85%.[15]

Impact of Conditioning Regimen

The therapeutic rationale of high-dose therapy (HDT) with auto-HSCT relies on enhanced cytotoxicity through the delivery of myeloablative doses of chemotherapy or total-body irradiation (TBI). The principles of success for HDT are a steep dose-response curve using active synergistic cytotoxic agents that have a short half-life and primarily hematopoietic toxicity.

The goal of the preparative conditioning regimen is to eradicate remaining malignant cells that are present after the salvage chemotherapy. Peripheral blood progenitor cells are infused after the completion of the conditioning regimen to facilitate bone marrow recovery and "rescue" the hematopoietic system from myeloablative chemotherapy.

Different HDT regimens are associated with their own unique toxicities based on the individual agents or modalities used. For example, alkylating agents such as BCNU (carmustine) and TBI both have a higher risk of idiopathic pneumonia syndrome (IPS) which is a leading pulmonary toxicity after HDT.[16]

A prospective study to define the impact of conditioning regimens on overall outcomes for HL has not been conducted, and the choice of HDT regimen is predominantly based on institutional experience and preference as well as patient comorbidities. Several regimens are considered standard and routinely used for both HL and Non-Hodgkin Lymphoma (NHL),[17] and the most commonly used regimens are as follows:

BEAM (BCNU, etoposide, cytarabine, and melphalan); CBV (cyclophosphamide, BCNU, and etoposide [VP-16]) Busulfan and cyclophosphamide (BuCy) Busulfan, cyclophosphamide, and etoposide (BuCyE) TBI-containing treatment.

A recent CIBMTR retrospective registry study of more than 1000 HL patients from 1995 to 2008 who received an auto-HSCT revealed on multivariate analysis that patients who received BEAM had a superior OS compared with those who received all other regimens. In that analysis, factors associated with inferior OS for all patients included older age, male gender, body mass index <18.5, Karnofsy performance status KPS <90, chemoresistant disease, higher number of previous regimens of chemotherapy received, shorter time from diagnosis to auto-HSCT, and use of bone marrow.[18] In the same analysis the development of IPS was most common after CBV- or TBI-based regimens, and patients who developed IPS had much worse PFS and OS.

Poor-Risk HL and Autologous Transplant

Refractory HL is particularly difficult to treat with poor outcomes; nonetheless, the treatment of choice remains HDT and auto-HSCT given the high relapse rate with chemotherapy alone. Longo et al., reported a median survival of only 16 months in 51 patients treated with methotrexate, oncovin, procarbazine, and prednisone (MOPP) chemotherapy who never achieved a CR.[19] There is a paucity of prospective data to guide treatment decisions in this patient population, although the lack chemosensitive disease in both the primary refractory and the relapsed setting exhibits debatable benefit from HDT and auto-HSCT.

In a report of 75 consecutive patients with biopsy-confirmed primary refractory HL, patients received conventional-dose cytoreductive chemotherapy followed by HDT and auto-HSCT. At a median follow-up of 10 years for surviving patients, the event-free survival (EFS), PFS, and OS rates were 45%, 49%, and 48%, respectively. Only chemosensitivity to standard-dose second-line chemotherapy predicted for a better survival; thus responding patients had an EFS, PFS, and OS of 60%, 62%, and 66%, respectively, versus 19%, 23%, and 17% for patients who had a poor response to second-line chemotherapy.[13] In the review of available literature, results of autologous transplantation after induction therapy failure for HL demonstrate EFS in the range of 30%–42% at 5 years and OS in the range of 34%–60% at 5 years.[20-24]

Some groups have explored intensifying the conditioning regimen to improve efficacy of auto-HSCT in poor-risk HL patients. Nieto et al., have published using an all-alkylator construct of busulfan (Bu) and melphalan (Mel) which achieves a precise systemic exposure to busulfan through prospective pharmacokinetic monitoring and then building upon that with the addition of gemcitabine (Gem) and vorinostat (SAHA). The Gem-Bu-Mel combination exploits the synergy between gemcitabine and alkylating agents based on DNA damage repair inhibition, and the addition of SAHA, a histone deacetylase inhibitor, increases DNA damage response and apoptosis. In this group of patients the disease status at the time of transplant was less than CR, with 65% of patients having primary refractory disease and 17% having progressive disease at the time of auto-hsct; nevertheless, outcomes were remarkably good. At median follow-up of 36 (range, 3–72) months, EFS and OS were 57% and 82%, respectively, with manageable toxicity profile of mucositis and skin rash as well as the expected hematologic toxicity; however, for both trials the upper age limit was capped at 65 years due to increased risk of adverse side effects.[25,26] These are promising results from phase II trials and require confirmation with prospective phase III randomized clinical trials. The increased risk of pulmonary complications mandated that radiation near the lung fields was either performed 30 days before busulfan infusion or held until after completion of transplant with full recovery of counts.

Given these results, the preference would be to attempt HDT followed by autologous transplant in transplant-eligible patients with the qualification that chemosensitivity should be demonstrated even if a complete response is not attainable.

Table 16.1 summarizes the data regarding autologous transplants in HL.

Indications for Peritransplant Radiation

Peritransplant radiation is associated with improved local control although its influence on OS is unclear; however, the majority of HL recurrences after auto-HSCT occur at sites of prior disease involvement.[27-29] Historically, concerns about toxicity, including pneumonitis, has limited the adoption of peritransplantation radiation therapy as standard practice.[30,31] However, modern dosing, techniques, and timing of administration may be associated with substantially less toxicity. Several studies have shown that adjuvant radiation can control limited disease and may contribute to improved prognosis.[32] Mundt et al. evaluated 54 patients who received HDT and auto-HSCT for relapsed/refractory HL, 20 of whom received peritransplantation radiation. The majority of recurrences after transplantation occurred at sites of previous disease involvement, and radiation was found to be associated with a lower rate of disease recurrence at these sites ($P<.05$). Routinely bulky disease (>5 cm) was treated, and radiation was given either before or after transplantation. Another report using involved field radiation therapy (IFRT) before or after auto-HSCT in patients with relapsed or refractory HL reported that the use of IFRT was associated with an improved 3-year freedom from relapse (100% vs. 67%) and a trend toward improved survival.[32]

TABLE 16.1
Key Studies Using Autologous HSCT for Hodgkin Lymphoma

Study	N	Median Follow-Up (months)	Conditioning Regimen	PFS/DFS/EFS/ FFTF	Overall Survival	TRM
Linch et al.[6]	N=40	34	BEAM/HSCT vs. mini-BEAM	3-year EFS 53%	Not reached	10%
Lumley et al.[99]	N=42	33	BEAM/HSCT	2-year EFS 74%	2-year OS 81%	2%
Argiris et al.[100]	N=40	28	BEAM/HSCT	3-year PFS 69%	3-year OS 77%	3%
Schmitz et al.[7]	N=161	39	BEAM/HSCT vs. Dexa-BEAM	3-year FFTF 55%	3-year OS 68%	2%
Nieto et al.[26]	N=180 BEAM=57 GemBu-Mel=84	49 (BEAM) 36 (GemBuMel)	BEAM vs. GemBuMel	3-year EFS 39%: BEAM 57%: GemBuMel	3-year OS 59%: BEAM 82%: GemBuMel	0%
Chen et al.[18]	N=1012	NG	BEAM (n=316) CBV^{high} (n=224) CBV^{low}(n=283) BuCy (n=165) TBI-containing (n=24)	3-year PFS 62%: BEAM 60%: CBV^{low} 57%: CBV^{high} 51%: BuCy 43%: TBI	3-year OS 79%: BEAM 73%: CBV^{low} 68%: CBV^{high} 65%: BuCy 47%: TBI	4% at 1 year
Sellner et al.[101]	N=346	18	BEAM vs. TEAM	2.5-year PFS 49%: TEAM 62%: BEAM	2.5-year OS 77%: TEAM 77%: BEAM	1%
Nieto et al.[102]	N=21	15	GemBuMelSAHA	2-year EF 76%	2-year OS 95%	0%
Smith et al.[103]	N=82	72	Tandem Auto Cycle 1 – melphalan Cycle 2 - Etoposide/ Cytoxan+TBI or BCNU	2-year PFS 63% 5-year PFS 55%	2-year OS 91% 5-year OS 84%	0% at 1 year

BEAM, carmustine, etoposide, cytarabine, melphalan; *DFS*, disease-free survival; *EFS*, event-free survival; *GemBuMel*, gemcitabine, busulphan, melphalan; *NG*, not given; *NR*, not reached; *OS*, overall survival; *PFS*, progression-free survival; *TBI*, total-body irradiation; *TEAM*, thiotepa, etoposide, cytarabine, melphalan; *TRM*, treatment-related mortality.

Posttransplant Maintenance With Brentuximab Vedotin

Brentuximab Vedotin (BV) is an antibody-drug conjugate consisting of a recombinant chimeric IgG1 monoclonal antibody directed against CD30 that is covalently linked to monomethyl auristatin E (MMAE). On binding of the antibody to CD30 on the cell surface, the resulting MMAE-CD30 complex is internalized, and MMAE is proteolytically cleaved. Free MMAE acts as an antimicrotubule agent and leads to apoptosis in cells that have internalized MMAE, for example, CD30-expressing cells such as Reed–Sternberg cells.[33] BV has demonstrated impressive activity in patients with relapsed or refractory HL after autologous HSCT with overall response rates reported up to 75%.[34] The

Aethera trial was a single multicenter randomized trial that showed a significant prolongation of PFS when BV was used as maintenance after autologous HSCT in a select group of high-risk HL patients.[35] In this trial, 329 brentuximab-naïve patients with relapsed or refractory HL who underwent auto-hsct were randomly assigned to BV maintenance therapy or placebo. Intravenous BV was started 30–45 days after transplantation and administered every 3 weeks for up to 16 cycles. All patients were at high risk for relapse based on the following factors: (1) refractory to frontline therapy, (2) had relapsed <12 months after initial therapy, and (3) relapsed at a later time point with extranodal disease. Brentuximab maintenance resulted in significantly improved PFS (median 43 vs. 24 months); however, OS was not impacted likely because crossover was allowed. Based on this trial the FDA has approved BV for post–auto-HSCT maintenance for HL.

ALLOGENEIC HEMATOPOIETIC TRANSPLANTATION IN HL

Recurrence of HL develops in 50% of patients after auto-HSCT[5] and prognosis after relapse after an autologous transplant is poor. In a study of HL patients who failed auto-HSCT, the median time to progression after the next therapy was only 3.8 months, and the median survival after auto-HSCT failure was 26 months.[36] Allogeneic hematopoietic stem cell transplantation (allo-HSCT) can induce long-term remissions in a select group of patients and has been used in this setting since early 1980s.[37] Relapse and TRM, most commonly due to graft-versus-host disease and infections, are key obstacles in the success of allo-HSCT in HL. The efficacy of allo-HSCT is the result of the combination of a tumor-free graft, cytoreduction produced by high doses of chemotherapy with or without radiation, as well as the immune-mediated graft-versus-lymphoma effect.[38] The microenvironment of HL lesions is known to be potently immunosuppressive through mechanisms including galectin-1 expression, transforming growth factor β expression, programmed death 1 (PD-1) expression, and generation of regulatory T cell populations.[39–42]

The graft-versus-tumor effect has been well documented in hematologic malignancies[43,44]; however, it has been more difficult to document graft-versus-lymphoma effect in HL. The existence of a graft-versus-lymphoma effect was first suggested by Jones et al.,[38] in which outcomes in that study revealed significantly lower relapse rate among allograft recipients than among autologous HSCT recipients in HL and NHL, although a statistically meaningful difference in EFS between the two groups was not appreciated given the higher TRM associated with allogeneic transplantation. A graft-versus-lymphoma effect is most convincingly demonstrated by the durable resolution of residual or progressive disease after allograft in response to withdrawal of immunosuppression or donor lymphocyte infusion (DLI) administration.[45] There are multiple studies, which suggest that a durable graft-versus-lymphoma effect is closely associated with the development of GVHD.[46–48] Responses to donor lymphocyte infusions (DLIs) are often viewed as the gold standard to establish a graft-versus-HL effect. DLI response rates (complete plus partial responses) reported in the literature in patients not receiving concomitant salvage chemotherapy are in the range of 30%–40%.[49–51]

In a recent metaanalysis that included 1850 patients receiving an allogeneic HSCT for relapsed HL, the pooled estimates for 3-year relapse-free survival and OS were 31% (25–37) and 50% (41–58), respectively. In metaregression, accrual initiation year in 2000 or later was associated with 5%–10% lower nonrelapse mortality (NRM) and relapse rates and 15%–20% higher relapse-free survival and OS than earlier studies.[52] This corresponds with the advent of reduced-intensity conditioning regimens and the associated decrease in TRM as myeloablative regimens that have been essentially abandoned for allo-HSCT in HL.

Myeloablative Versus Reduced-Intensity Conditioning Regimens for HL

Myeloablative chemoradiotherapy and allogeneic transplantation for relapsed HL after autotransplant previously carried a prohibitively high TRM. A European analysis comparing auto-HSCT with allo-HSCT in HL revealed 4-year actuarial probability of OS and PFS of 25% and 15% with NRM in the range of 48%. TRM at 4 years was significantly higher for allo-BMT patients, and interestingly, having chemosensitive disease at the time of transplantation had a 4-year actuarial probability of survival was 30% after allo-HSCT and 64% after auto-HSCT which was mainly due to a higher TRM.[53] The International Bone Marrow Transplant Registry reported on 114 patients with lymphoma who underwent myeloablative allogeneic transplants reported a rate of disease progression at 3 years of 52% and TRM of 22%. There was no difference in TRM, PFS, or OS between patients with HL and other lymphoma subtypes.[54] Although some of the poor results after myeloablative conditioning could be explained by the very poor-risk features of many individuals included in these early trials, the high NRM prevents myeloablative conditioning from being widely used.

The advent of reduced-intensity conditioning regimens allowed the achievement of engraftment and induction of graft-versus-malignancy effect without the morbidity and mortality associated with myeloablative conditioning regimens in patients with relapsed and refractory HL.[55,56] These regimens rely on donor immune–mediated graft-versus-lymphoma effect rather than cytoreduction through a myeloablative regimen, consequently disease status and chemosensitivity at the time of transplant impact the realization of long-term survival profoundly. Several published reports have validated this approach with reduction in TRM down to 15%.[5,57]

Sureda et al. reported on a prospective study by the Grupo Español de.

Linfomas/Trasplante de Médula Osea (GEL/TAMO) and the European Group for Blood and Marrow Transplantation (EBMT) in which 92 patients with relapsed HL and matched related or unrelated donor were treated with salvage chemotherapy followed by reduced-intensity allogeneic transplantation.

Seventy-eight patients proceeded to allograft using fludarabine and melphalan for conditioning, and the NRM rate was 8% at 100 days and 15% at 1 year. Relapse was the major cause of failure. The PFS rate was 48% at 1 year and 24% at 4 years, and the OS rate was 71% at 1 year and 43% at 4 years. Chronic GVHD (cGVHD) was associated with a lower incidence of relapse. Patients allografted in complete response had a significantly better outcome.[5] Factors that predict outcomes for RIC allografts in HL were assessed in a retrospective analysis of 285 patients on behalf of the Lymphoma Working Party of the EBMT. Eighty percent of patients had received a prior autologous stem cell transplantation, and 25% had refractory disease at transplantation. NRM was associated with chemo-refractory disease, poor performance status, age >45, and transplantation before 2002. For patients with no risk factors, the 3-year NRM rate was 12.5% compared to 46.2% for patients with 2 or more risk factors. The use of an unrelated donor had no adverse effect on the NRM. The development of cGVHD was associated with a lower relapse rate, and disease progression rate at one and 5 years was 41% and 58.7%, respectively, and was associated with chemorefractory disease and extent of prior therapy. Donor lymphocyte infusions were administered to 64 patients for active disease of whom 32% showed a clinical response. PFS and OS were both associated with performance status and disease status at transplantation. Patients with neither risk factor had a 3-year PFS and OS of 42% and 56%, respectively, compared to 8% and 25% for patients with one or more risk factors. Relapse within 6 months of a prior autologous transplant was associated with a higher relapse rate and a lower PFS.[55]

ALTERNATIVE DONOR ALLOGENEIC TRANSPLANTATION IN HL

Alternative donor transplantation is increasingly used for high-risk lymphoma[58] patients as donor availability is a potential barrier for patients who are candidates for allogeneic HSCT but lack an adequately HLA-matched donor.[59] T-cell replete–related donor haploidentical HSCT (haplo-hsct) and umbilical cord blood (UCB)

HSCT are increasingly used in patients with hematological malignancies without an HLA-identical sibling or matched unrelated donor (MUD).[60,61] T-cell replete haplo-hsct have been transformed with recent advances in GVHD prophylaxis such as administration of cyclophosphamide early after transplantation, when the graft and host T cells recognize each other as foreign. These T cells generate bidirectional alloreactivity leading to high rates of TRM but posttransplant cyclophosphamide (PT-Cy) targets alloreactive T-cells, and decreases the risk of GVHD and graft rejection.[62] Several retrospective reports and a recent systematic review limited to patients with HL suggest higher median PFS rates for patients with haplo-hsct than for those with matched transplants.[56,63–65]

Majhail et al. recently compared UCB to matched sibling donors for 21 adults with advanced HL, and their results revealed comparable outcomes for reduced-intensity conditioning between the two groups in terms of acute and chronic GVHD, day 100 TRM, and PFS[66] although with small numbers of patients. The EBMT recently retrospectively compared the outcomes of patients with HL who received posttransplantation cyclophosphamide–based haploidentical allogeneic hematopoietic cell transplantation with the outcome of patients who received conventional HLA-matched sibling donor and HLA-matched unrelated donor.

A total of 709 adult patients with HL were evaluated with a median follow-up of survivors of 29 months. No differences were observed between groups in the incidence of acute GVHD, and haplo-hsct was associated with a lower risk of chronic GVHD (26%) compared with MUD (41%; $P = 0.04$). NRM at 1 year was comparable as was 2-year cumulative incidence of relapse or progression. On multivariate analysis, haplo-hsct was comparable to sibling allograft NRM and higher in MUD while risk of relapse was lower in both haplo-hsct and MUD allografts than sibling donor. There were no significant differences in OS or PFS between all donors, whereas the rate of extensive chronic GVHD and relapse-free survival was significantly better for haplo-hsct than sibling donors and similar to MUD. These results will need to be validated in a prospective trial but validate previous reports that haplo-hsct may be the graft of choice when a fully matched sibling donor is unavailable.[67]

Use of Donor Lymphocyte Infusions in HL

Patients who relapse after allo-HSCT have a particularly poor prognosis with limited therapeutic options. As mentioned in the EBMT study previously, DLI has been used augment the graft-versus-lymphoma effect in patients who progress after allo-hsct. In that study the overall response rate was 40%. Other investigators have also reported on DLI as treatment for relapse after allograft with overall response rates of 37%; however, all of those treated developed GVHD.[68] The largest body of data regarding the efficacy of DLI in patients with HL comes from the UK cooperative group trial. Seventy-six consecutive patients with relapsed/refractory HL underwent allo-HSCT following an RIC consisting of fludarabine, melphalan, and high-dose alemtuzumab as a means of in vivo T-cell depletion. DLI was effective in reverting mixed to complete donor chimerism in 86% of the patients. Durable response to DLI was observed in 79% of patients treated for relapse, while the DLI-related mortality at 3 years was 7%, and it was mainly attributed to GVHD.[69] More recently in small studies brentuximab vedotin (BV) has been administered in conjunction with DLI in hopes of exploiting the immune-modulating effect produced by BV and selectively targeting lymphoma cells.[70,71] Interestingly, patients who were previously refractory to BV (when administered after auto-HSCT) responded to retreatment with BV after allo-HSCT, and a subgroup of patients remain in continuous CR. DLI-associated GVHD occurred in most patients, and GVHD required immunosuppression, and in all cases, GVHD resolved after a short course of low-dose steroids, implying that an anti-GVHD modulating effect could be induced by the concurrent administration of BV.[71]

COMPLICATIONS ASSOCIATED WITH TRANSPLANTATION SPECIFIC TO HL

Transplant recipients are at risk of developing therapy-related complications that may present years after treatment; however, there are particular issues that are more prevalent in patients who have had transplantation for HL due to the predilection of specific preceding therapies.

Idiopathic Pneumonia Syndrome After Autologous Transplant

Idiopathic pneumonia syndrome (IPS) is characterized by the signs and symptoms of pneumonia associated with widespread alveolar injury in the absence of a lower respiratory tract infection and has been reported in 4%–28% of patients after an auto-HSCT.[72–75] The incidence of IPS appears to be higher after TBI-containing regimens than after using chemotherapeutic agents only.[73] Bilgrami et al.[76] retrospectively reviewed 271 patients receiving busulfan-containing myeloablative chemotherapy before an auto-HSCT without radiation and found a trend toward increased incidence of IPS, although not statistically significant. Wong et al.[77] also retrospectively reviewed the incidence of IPS in patients receiving cyclophosphamide, carmustine, and thiotepa followed by auto-HSCT for high-risk breast cancer and reported a 12% incidence, with median onset at 3 months after transplant. Carmustine-related IPS appears to be dose dependent with doses greater than $1500 \, mg/m^2$ leading to a profound increase in incidence of interstitial pneumonitis and pulmonary fibrosis.[78,79]

The median time to onset is 63 days with a range of 7–336 days.[80] Risk factors include prior mediastinal irradiation, a BCNU dose >1000 mg, and age less than 54 years.[81] Prompt initiation of steroids often results in clinical resolution.[77]

Secondary Malignancy

The second most common cause of late death after an auto-HCT, after disease relapse, is secondary malignancy. Reports for treatment-related myelodysplastic syndrome (t-MDS) or acute myeloid leukemia (t-AML) are as high as 8%–14% of patients who received high-dose chemotherapy with an auto-HSCT.[82] The majority of patients with t-MDS/AML have complex karyotypes, and the observed cytogenetic changes are often characteristic of known chemotherapy-induced damage by alkylating agents and topoisomerase II inhibitors.[82–84] Abnormalities of chromosomes 5 and/or 7 are the hallmark of t-MDS/t-AML after alkylating agent therapy,[85] typically occurring a median of 5 years after exposure with antecedent cytopenias and a poor prognosis.[86] In contrast, patients developing t-AML after therapy with topoisomerase II inhibitors rarely present with MDS, occurring after a shorter latency period (2–3 years), and have a more favorable response to induction chemotherapy but continue to have a poorer prognosis than de novo AML.[87]

Other known risk factors predicting increased risk of t-MDS/AML are older age at transplant[88,89] and exposure to radiation treatment before or during transplant.[84,90,91] Although most deaths from secondary malignancy are from a hematologic origin, there is also a significant risk for solid tumors, especially with extended follow-up.[92] Tarella et al.[91] reviewed 1347 lymphoma patients after auto-HSCT and reported a cumulative incidence of solid tumors of 2.5% at 5 years and 6.7% at 10 years. Patients had a median survival of 3.8 years after the diagnosis of a solid tumor, the most frequently occurring malignancies being lung, gastrointestinal tract, skin, breast, head and neck, and bladder cancers. Table 16.2 summarizes the most recent evidence regarding treatment related malignancy after autologous transplantation.

Table 16.2
Evidence Regarding Treatment-Related Malignancy After Autologous Transplantation

Author	N	Conditioning	Incidence/Risk	Predictive Factors (Adverse unless Otherwise Noted)
Krishnan et al.[89]	N = 612 HL = 218 NHL = 394 1986 to 1998	TBI/VP16/Cyclophospha- mide Cyclophosphamide/BCNU/ vincristine	Risk: 6 yrs: 8.6% ± 2.1% HL: 8.1% NHL: 9.1%	Priming with VP-16 for stem cell collection
Del Canizo et al.[93]	N = 1411 AML = 557 NHL = 308 HL = 225 MM = 189 CML = 37 Solid tu- mors = 95	Variable including: TBI + cyclophosphamide BCNU, VP-16, ARA-C, melphalan Cyclophosphamide/BCNU/ vincristine	Incidence HL: 2.7% NHL: 1.6% MM: 0.5% AML: 0.2% Cumulative incidence at 5 yrs: 3.1%	
Darrington et al.[90]	N = 511 patients HL = 249 NHL = 262 4/1983 to 12/1991	HL: Cyclophosphamide, etoposide, and carmus- tine NHL: TBI + alkylating agents (melphalan or cyclophos- phamide)	Incidence: HL: 5 yrs: 4% 7 yrs: 10% NHL: 5 yrs: 4% 7 yrs: 8% RISK: at 5 years HL: 11% NHL: 12%	Age ≥ 40 yrs at transplant TBI-containing regimen
Metayer et al.[84]	N = 2739 NHL = 1784 HL = 955 1989–1995	Variable TBI + cyclophosphamide TBI + VP16 ± cyclophospha- mide VP16 ± cyclophospha- mide ± other drugs	Incidence: 7 yrs: 3.7% NHL: 3.9% HL: 3.3% Risk: at 7 yrs NHL: 8.9% HL: 7.1%	Intensity of pretransplant therapy TBI doses 13.2 Gy
Bhatia et al.[92] *data collected for pts surviv-ing 2 yrs after transplant	N = 854 AML = 158 ALL = 59 NHL = 392 HL = 245 1981 to 1998	TBI = 575 Cyclophosphamide = 828 Busulfan = 33 VP16 = 635 BCNU = 234	Incidence: 4.6% hematologic Risk: for second tumor 12-fold higher than gen- eral population	
Kalaycio et al.[94]	N = 526 NHL = 405 HL = 121 1/1993 to 12/2001	Oral busulfan 1 mg/kg × 14 doses Etoposide 50–60 mg/ kg cyclophosphamide 60 mg/kg	Incidence: 10 yrs: 6.8%	≥ 5 days apheresis Prior radiation ≥ 4 prior chemotherapy regimens
Tarella et al.[91]	N = 1347 NHL = 1113 HL = 234 1985 to 2005	hd-mitoxantrone/melpha- lan BEAM (BCNU, etoposide, cytarabine, melphalan) TBI = 79 pts Rituximab = 523	Incidence for hematologic 5 yrs: 3.09% 10 yrs: 4.52% 15 yrs: 6.80% Incidence for solid tumors 5 yrs: 2.54% 10 yrs: 6.79% 15 yrs: 9.14%	Hematologic: male sex second harvest peripheral blood progenitor cells Solid tumor: advanced age consolidation RT after transplant *rituximab addition* **protective**

HL, Hodgkin lymphoma; NHL, non-Hodgkin lymphoma; TBI, total-body irradiation.

GVHD in Association With Checkpoint Inhibition

The PD-1 pathway serves as a checkpoint to limit T-cell–mediated immune responses. Blocking the PD-1 receptor on T cells results in T-cell activation and proliferation and can induce a potent immunotherapeutic antitumor effect. The therapeutic efficacy of monoclonal antibodies (mAbs) targeting the PD-1 receptor in classical Hodgkin lymphoma has been demonstrated in recent publications.[95] One retrospective study of 19 patients with hematologic malignancies treated with a PD-1 inhibitor (nivolumab or pembrolizumab) and subsequently treated with reduced-intensity conditioning allogeneic transplantation has been reported with a higher-than-expected rate of severe complications, including fatal early acute GVHD and venoocclusive disease.[96] PD-1 blockade after transplant for relapsed disease has also been reported in retrospective studies with conflicting findings in terms of the risk of GVHD induction or exacerbation as well as risk factors for onset of PD-1–provoked GVHD.[97] In one analysis 17 of 31 (55%) patients developed treatment-emergent GVHD after initiation of anti–PD-1, and of those, only 2 of 17 patients achieved complete response to GVHD treatment, and 14 of 17 required ≥2 systemic therapies. PD-1 toxicity independent of allo-HSCT has been reported with dermatologic and hepatic toxicity although rarely, and the clinical and histologic differences between GVHD and anti–PD-1 toxicity are not clearly defined.[98] Prospective data are needed to better define the correlation between PD-2 inhibition and GVHD.

In conclusion, both autologous and allogeneic hematopoietic stem cell transplantation play an important part in the treatment and cure of HL. High-dose chemotherapy and autologous hematopoietic cell transplantation should be considered as the treatment of choice for patients with primary refractory disease (i.e., induction failure) and relapse after frontline conventional therapy, and subsequently for a select group of patients, allogeneic transplant can confer long-term disease control. Conditioning therapy should be tailored to disease state and comorbidity status to minimize toxicity; furthermore, as novel agents advance into clinical practice, unique complications will emerge requiring effective management.

REFERENCES

1. Horning SJ, Hoppe RT, Breslin S, Bartlett NL, Brown BW, Rosenberg SA. Stanford V and radiotherapy for locally extensive and advanced Hodgkin's disease: mature results of a prospective clinical trial. *J Clin Oncol.* 2002;20:630–637.
2. Diehl V, Franklin J, Pfreundschuh M, et al. Standard and increased-dose BEACOPP chemotherapy compared with COPP-ABVD for advanced Hodgkin's disease. *N Engl J Med.* 2003;348:2386–2395.
3. Connors JM. State-of-the-art therapeutics: Hodgkin's lymphoma. *J Clinl Oncol.* 2005;23:6400–6408.
4. von Tresckow B, Engert A. The role of autologous transplantation in Hodgkin lymphoma. *Curr Hematol Malig Rep.* 2011;6:172–179.
5. Sureda A, Canals C, Arranz R, et al. Allogeneic stem cell transplantation after reduced intensity conditioning in patients with relapsed or refractory Hodgkin's lymphoma. Results of the HDR-ALLO study - a prospective clinical trial by the Grupo Espanol de Linfomas/Trasplante de Medula Osea (GEL/TAMO) and the Lymphoma Working Party of the European Group for Blood and Marrow Transplantation. *Haematologica.* 2012;97:310–317.
6. Linch DC, Winfield D, Goldstone AH, et al. Dose intensification with autologous bone-marrow transplantation in relapsed and resistant Hodgkin's disease: results of a BNLI randomised trial. *Lancet.* 1993;341:1051–1054.
7. Schmitz N, Pfistner B, Sextro M, et al. Aggressive conventional chemotherapy compared with high-dose chemotherapy with autologous haemopoietic stem-cell transplantation for relapsed chemosensitive Hodgkin's disease: a randomised trial. *Lancet.* 2002;359:2065–2071.
8. Ferme C, Mounier N, Divine M, et al. Intensive salvage therapy with high-dose chemotherapy for patients with advanced Hodgkin's disease in relapse or failure after initial chemotherapy: results of the Groupe d'Etudes des Lymphomes de l'Adulte H89 Trial. *J Clin Oncol.* 2002;20:467–475.
9. Rancea M, Monsef I, von Tresckow B, Engert A, Skoetz N. High-dose chemotherapy followed by autologous stem cell transplantation for patients with relapsed/refractory Hodgkin lymphoma. *Cochrane Database Syst Rev.* 2013:CD009411.
10. Lazarus HM, Loberiza Jr FR, Zhang MJ, et al. Autotransplants for Hodgkin's disease in first relapse or second remission: a report from the autologous blood and marrow transplant registry (ABMTR). *Bone Marrow Transpl.* 2001;27:387–396.
11. Sureda A, Constans M, Iriondo A, et al. Prognostic factors affecting long-term outcome after stem cell transplantation in Hodgkin's lymphoma autografted after a first relapse. *Ann Oncol.* 2005;16:625–633.
12. Hahn T, McCarthy PL, Carreras J, et al. Simplified validated prognostic model for progression-free survival after autologous transplantation for hodgkin lymphoma. *Biol Blood Marrow Transpl.* 2013;19:1740–1744.
13. Moskowitz CH, Kewalramani T, Nimer SD, Gonzalez M, Zelenetz AD, Yahalom J. Effectiveness of high dose chemoradiotherapy and autologous stem cell transplantation for patients with biopsy-proven primary refractory Hodgkin's disease. *Br J Haematol.* 2004;124:645–652.

14. Castagna L, Bramanti S, Balzarotti M, et al. Predictive value of early 18F-fluorodeoxyglucose positron emission tomography (FDG-PET) during salvage chemotherapy in relapsing/refractory Hodgkin lymphoma (HL) treated with high-dose chemotherapy. *Br J Haematol.* 2009;145:369–372.

15. Wannesson L, Bargetzi M, Cairoli A, et al. Autotransplant for Hodgkin lymphoma after failure of upfront BEA-COPP escalated (bleomycin, etoposide, doxorubicin, cyclophosphamide, vincristine, procarbazine and prednisone). *Leuk Lymphoma.* 2013;54:36–40.

16. Afessa B, Abdulai RM, Kremers WK, Hogan WJ, Litzow MR, Peters SG. Risk factors and outcome of pulmonary complications after autologous hematopoietic stem cell transplant. *Chest.* 2012;141:442–450.

17. Fernandez HF, Escalon MP, Pereira D, Lazarus HM. Autotransplant conditioning regimens for aggressive lymphoma: are we on the right road? *Bone Marrow Transpl.* 2007;40:505–513.

18. Chen YB, Lane AA, Logan B, et al. Impact of conditioning regimen on outcomes for patients with lymphoma undergoing high-dose therapy with autologous hematopoietic cell transplantation. *Biol Blood Marrow Transpl.* 2015;21:1046–1053.

19. Longo DL, Duffey PL, Young RC, et al. Conventional-dose salvage combination chemotherapy in patients relapsing with Hodgkin's disease after combination chemotherapy: the low probability for cure. *J Clin Oncol.* 1992;10:210–218.

20. Sweetenham JW. Following aggressive B-cell lymphoma. *Blood.* 2015;125:3673–3674.

21. Chopra R, McMillan AK, Linch DC, et al. The place of high-dose BEAM therapy and autologous bone marrow transplantation in poor-risk Hodgkin's disease. A single-center eight-year study of 155 patients. *Blood.* 1993;81:1137–1145.

22. Reece DE, Barnett MJ, Shepherd JD, et al. High-dose cyclophosphamide, carmustine (BCNU), and etoposide (VP16-213) with or without cisplatin (CBV +/- P) and autologous transplantation for patients with Hodgkin's disease who fail to enter a complete response after combination chemotherapy. *Blood.* 1995;86:451–456.

23. Yahalom J, Gulati SC, Toia M, et al. Accelerated hyperfractionated total-lymphoid irradiation, high-dose chemotherapy, and autologous bone marrow transplantation for refractory and relapsing patients with Hodgkin's disease. *J Clin Oncol.* 1993;11:1062–1070.

24. Gianni AM, Siena S, Bregni M, et al. High-dose sequential chemo-radiotherapy with peripheral blood progenitor cell support for relapsed or refractory Hodgkin's disease–a 6-year update. *Ann Oncol.* 1993;4:889–891.

25. Nieto Y, Valdez BC, Thall PF, et al. Vorinostat combined with high-dose gemcitabine, busulfan, and melphalan with autologous stem cell transplantation in patients with refractory lymphomas. *Biol Blood Marrow Transpl.* 2015;21:1914–1920.

26. Nieto Y, Popat U, Anderlini P, et al. Autologous stem cell transplantation for refractory or poor-risk relapsed Hodgkin's lymphoma: effect of the specific high-dose chemotherapy regimen on outcome. *Biol Blood Marrow Transpl.* 2013;19:410–417.

27. Phillips GL, Wolff SN, Herzig RH, et al. Treatment of progressive Hodgkin's disease with intensive chemoradiotherapy and autologous bone marrow transplantation. *Blood.* 1989;73:2086–2092.

28. Mundt AJ, Sibley G, Williams S, Hallahan D, Nautiyal J, Weichselbaum RR. Patterns of failure following high-dose chemotherapy and autologous bone marrow transplantation with involved field radiotherapy for relapsed/refractory Hodgkin's disease. *Int J Radiat Oncol Biol Phys.* 1995;33:261–270.

29. Biswas T, Culakova E, Friedberg JW, et al. Involved field radiation therapy following high dose chemotherapy and autologous stem cell transplant benefits local control and survival in refractory or recurrent Hodgkin lymphoma. *Radiother Oncol.* 2012;103:367–372.

30. Kahn S, Flowers C, Xu Z, Esiashvili N. Does the addition of involved field radiotherapy to high-dose chemotherapy and stem cell transplantation improve outcomes for patients with relapsed/refractory Hodgkin lymphoma? *Int J Radiat Oncol Biol Phys.* 2011;81:175–180.

31. Tsang RW, Gospodarowicz MK, Sutcliffe SB, Crump M, Keating A. Thoracic radiation therapy before autologous bone marrow transplantation in relapsed or refractory Hodgkin's disease. PMH Lymphoma Group, and the Toronto Autologous BMT Group. *Eur J Cancer.* 1999;35:73–78.

32. Poen JC, Hoppe RT, Horning SJ. High-dose therapy and autologous bone marrow transplantation for relapsed/refractory Hodgkin's disease: the impact of involved field radiotherapy on patterns of failure and survival. *Int J Radiat Oncol Biol Phys.* 1996;36:3–12.

33. Younes A, Bartlett NL, Leonard JP, et al. Brentuximab vedotin (SGN-35) for relapsed CD30-positive lymphomas. *N Engl J Med.* 2010;363:1812–1821.

34. Younes A, Gopal AK, Smith SE, et al. Results of a pivotal phase II study of brentuximab vedotin for patients with relapsed or refractory Hodgkin's lymphoma. *J Clin Oncol.* 2012;30:2183–2189.

35. Moskowitz CH, Nademanee A, Masszi T, et al. Brentuximab vedotin as consolidation therapy after autologous stem-cell transplantation in patients with Hodgkin's lymphoma at risk of relapse or progression (AETHERA): a randomised, double-blind, placebo-controlled, phase 3 trial. *Lancet.* 2015;385:1853–1862.

36. Kewalramani T, Nimer SD, Zelenetz AD, et al. Progressive disease following autologous transplantation in patients with chemosensitive relapsed or primary refractory Hodgkin's disease or aggressive non-Hodgkin's lymphoma. *Bone Marrow Transpl.* 2003;32:673–679.

37. Appelbaum FR, Sullivan KM, Thomas ED, et al. Allogeneic marrow transplantation in the treatment of MOPP-resistant Hodgkin's disease. *J Clin Oncol.* 1985;3:1490–1494.

38. Jones RJ, Ambinder RF, Piantadosi S, Santos GW. Evidence of a graft-versus-lymphoma effect associated with allogeneic bone marrow transplantation. *Blood.* 1991;77:649–653.

39. Gandhi MK, Moll G, Smith C, et al. Galectin-1 mediated suppression of Epstein-Barr virus specific T-cell immunity in classic Hodgkin lymphoma. *Blood.* 2007;110:1326–1329.

40. Newcom SR, Gu L. Transforming growth factor beta 1 messenger RNA in Reed-Sternberg cells in nodular sclerosing Hodgkin's disease. *J Clin Pathol.* 1995;48:160–163.

41. Ma Y, Visser L, Blokzijl T, et al. The CD4+CD26- T-cell population in classical Hodgkin's lymphoma displays a distinctive regulatory T-cell profile. *Lab Investig A J Tech Methods Pathol.* 2008;88:482–490.

42. Yamamoto R, Nishikori M, Kitawaki T, et al. PD-1-PD-1 ligand interaction contributes to immunosuppressive microenvironment of Hodgkin lymphoma. *Blood.* 2008;111:3220–3224.

43. Weiden PL, Flournoy N, Thomas ED, et al. Antileukemic effect of graft-versus-host disease in human recipients of allogeneic-marrow grafts. *N Engl J Med.* 1979;300:1068–1073.

44. Horowitz MM, Gale RP, Sondel PM, et al. Graft-versus-leukemia reactions after bone marrow transplantation. *Blood.* 1990;75:555–562.

45. Grigg A, Ritchie D. Graft-versus-lymphoma effects: clinical review, policy proposals, and immunobiology. *Biol Blood Marrow Transpl.* 2004;10:579–590.

46. Branson K, Chopra R, Kottaridis PD, et al. Role of nonmyeloablative allogeneic stem-cell transplantation after failure of autologous transplantation in patients with lymphoproliferative malignancies. *J Clin Oncol.* 2002;20:4022–4031.

47. Mohty M, Bay JO, Faucher C, et al. Graft-versus-host disease following allogeneic transplantation from HLA-identical sibling with antithymocyte globulin-based reduced-intensity preparative regimen. *Blood.* 2003;102:470–476.

48. Izutsu K, Kanda Y, Ohno H, et al. Unrelated bone marrow transplantation for non-Hodgkin lymphoma: a study from the Japan Marrow Donor Program. *Blood.* 2004;103:1955–1960.

49. Peggs KS, Hunter A, Chopra R, et al. Clinical evidence of a graft-versus-Hodgkin's-lymphoma effect after reduced-intensity allogeneic transplantation. *Lancet.* 2005;365:1934–1941.

50. Anderlini P, Swanston N, Rashid A, Bueso-Ramos C, Macapinlac HA, Champlin RE. Evidence of a graft-versus-Hodgkin lymphoma effect in the setting of extensive bone marrow involvement. *Biol Blood Marrow Transpl.* 2008;14:478–480.

51. Anderlini P, Acholonu SA, Okoroji GJ, et al. Donor leukocyte infusions in relapsed Hodgkin's lymphoma following allogeneic stem cell transplantation: CD3+ cell dose, GVHD and disease response. *Bone Marrow Transpl.* 2004;34:511–514.

52. Rashidi A, Ebadi M, Cashen AF. Allogeneic hematopoietic stem cell transplantation in Hodgkin lymphoma: a systematic review and meta-analysis. *Bone Marrow Transpl.* 2016;51:521–528.

53. Milpied N, Fielding AK, Pearce RM, Ernst P, Goldstone AH. Allogeneic bone marrow transplant is not better than autologous transplant for patients with relapsed Hodgkin's disease. European Group for Blood and Bone Marrow Transplantation. *J Clin Oncol.* 1996;14:1291–1296.

54. Freytes CO, Loberiza FR, Rizzo JD, et al. Myeloablative allogeneic hematopoietic stem cell transplantation in patients who experience relapse after autologous stem cell transplantation for lymphoma: a report of the International Bone Marrow Transplant Registry. *Blood.* 2004;104:3797–3803.

55. Robinson SP, Sureda A, Canals C, et al. Reduced intensity conditioning allogeneic stem cell transplantation for Hodgkin's lymphoma: identification of prognostic factors predicting outcome. *Haematologica.* 2009;94:230–238.

56. Burroughs LM, O'Donnell PV, Sandmaier BM, et al. Comparison of outcomes of HLA-matched related, unrelated, or HLA-haploidentical related hematopoietic cell transplantation following nonmyeloablative conditioning for relapsed or refractory Hodgkin lymphoma. *Biol Blood Marrow Transpl.* 2008;14:1279–1287.

57. Anderlini P, Saliba R, Acholonu S, et al. Fludarabine-melphalan as a preparative regimen for reduced-intensity conditioning allogeneic stem cell transplantation in relapsed and refractory Hodgkin's lymphoma: the updated M.D. Anderson Cancer Center experience. *Haematologica.* 2008;93:257–264.

58. Bachanova V, Burns LJ, Wang T, et al. Alternative donors extend transplantation for patients with lymphoma who lack an HLA matched donor. *Bone Marrow Transpl.* 2015;50:197–203.

59. Anasetti C, Aversa F, Brunstein CG. Back to the future: mismatched unrelated donor, haploidentical related donor, or unrelated umbilical cord blood transplantation? *Biol Blood Marrow Transpl.* 2012;18:S161–S165.

60. Kanakry CG, Fuchs EJ, Luznik L. Modern approaches to HLA-haploidentical blood or marrow transplantation. *Nat Rev Clin Oncol.* 2016;13:132.

61. Ciurea SO, Zhang MJ, Bacigalupo AA, et al. Haploidentical transplant with posttransplant cyclophosphamide vs matched unrelated donor transplant for acute myeloid leukemia. *Blood.* 2015;126:1033–1040.

62. Luznik L, O'Donnell PV, Symons HJ, et al. HLA-haploidentical bone marrow transplantation for hematologic malignancies using nonmyeloablative conditioning and high-dose, posttransplantation cyclophosphamide. *Biol Blood Marrow Transpl.* 2008;14:641–650.

63. Baron F, Storb R, Storer BE, et al. Factors associated with outcomes in allogeneic hematopoietic cell transplantation with nonmyeloablative conditioning after failed myeloablative hematopoietic cell transplantation. *J Clin Oncol.* 2006;24:4150–4157.

64. Feinstein LC, Sandmaier BM, Maloney DG, et al. Allografting after nonmyeloablative conditioning as a treatment after a failed conventional hematopoietic cell transplant. *Biol Blood Marrow Transpl.* 2003;9:266–272.

65. Messer M, Steinzen A, Vervolgyi E, et al. Unrelated and alternative donor allogeneic stem cell transplant in patients with relapsed or refractory Hodgkin lymphoma: a systematic review. *Leuk Lymphoma.* 2014;55:296–306.

66. Majhail NS, Weisdorf DJ, Wagner JE, Defor TE, Brunstein CG, Burns LJ. Comparable results of umbilical cord blood and HLA-matched sibling donor hematopoietic stem cell transplantation after reduced-intensity preparative regimen for advanced Hodgkin lymphoma. *Blood.* 2006;107: 3804–3807.

67. Martinez C, Gayoso J, Canals C, et al. Post-transplantation cyclophosphamide-based haploidentical transplantation as alternative to matched sibling or unrelated donor transplantation for hodgkin lymphoma: a registry study of the lymphoma working party of the European Society for Blood and Marrow Transplantation. *J Clin Oncol*2017: JCO2017726869.

68. Anderlini P, Saliba R, Acholonu S, et al. Donor leukocyte infusions in recurrent Hodgkin lymphoma following allogeneic stem cell transplant: 10-year experience at the M. D. Anderson Cancer Center. *Leuk Lymphoma.* 2012;53:1239–1241.

69. Peggs KS, Kayani I, Edwards N, et al. Donor lymphocyte infusions modulate relapse risk in mixed chimeras and induce durable salvage in relapsed patients after T-cell-depleted allogeneic transplantation for Hodgkin's lymphoma. *J Clin Oncol.* 2011;29:971–978.

70. Theurich S, Malcher J, Wennhold K, et al. Brentuximab vedotin combined with donor lymphocyte infusions for early relapse of Hodgkin lymphoma after allogeneic stem-cell transplantation induces tumor-specific immunity and sustained clinical remission. *J Clin Oncol.* 2013;31:e59–e63.

71. Tsirigotis P, Danylesko I, Gkirkas K, et al. Brentuximab vedotin in combination with or without donor lymphocyte infusion for patients with Hodgkin lymphoma after allogeneic stem cell transplantation. *Bone Marrow Transpl.* 2016;51:1313–1317.

72. Ballester OF, Agaliotis DP, Hiemenz JW, et al. Phase I-II study of high-dose busulfan and cyclophosphamide followed by autologous peripheral blood stem cell transplantation for hematological malignancies: toxicities and hematopoietic recovery. *Bone Marrow Transpl.* 1996;18:9–14.

73. Carlson K, Backlund L, Smedmyr B, Oberg G, Simonsson B. Pulmonary function and complications subsequent to autologous bone marrow transplantation. *Bone Marrow Transpl.* 1994;14:805–811.

74. Wingard JR, Sostrin MB, Vriesendorp HM, et al. Interstitial pneumonitis following autologous bone marrow transplantation. *Transplantation.* 1988;46:61–65.

75. Pecego R, Hill R, Appelbaum FR, et al. Interstitial pneumonitis following autologous bone marrow transplantation. *Transplantation.* 1986;42:515–517.

76. Bilgrami SF, Metersky ML, McNally D, et al. Idiopathic pneumonia syndrome following myeloablative chemotherapy and autologous transplantation. *Ann Pharmacother.* 2001;35:196–201.

77. Wong R, Rondon G, Saliba RM, et al. Idiopathic pneumonia syndrome after high-dose chemotherapy and autologous hematopoietic stem cell transplantation for high-risk breast cancer. *Bone Marrow Transpl.* 2003;31:1157–1163.

78. Clark JG, Hansen JA, Hertz MI, Parkman R, Jensen L, Peavy HH. NHLBI workshop summary. Idiopathic pneumonia syndrome after bone marrow transplantation. *Am Rev Respir Dis.* 1993;147:1601–1606.

79. Aronin PA, Mahaley Jr MS, Rudnick SA, et al. Prediction of BCNU pulmonary toxicity in patients with malignant gliomas: an assessment of risk factors. *N Engl J Med.* 1980;303:183–188.

80. Panoskaltsis-Mortari A, Griese M, Madtes DK, et al. An official American Thoracic Society research statement: noninfectious lung injury after hematopoietic stem cell transplantation: idiopathic pneumonia syndrome. *Am J Respir Crit Care Med.* 2011;183:1262–1279.

81. Lane AA, Armand P, Feng Y, et al. Risk factors for development of pneumonitis after high-dose chemotherapy with cyclophosphamide, BCNU and etoposide followed by autologous stem cell transplant. *Leuk Lymphoma.* 2012;53:1130–1136.

82. Armitage JO, Carbone PP, Connors JM, Levine A, Bennett JM, Kroll S. Treatment-related myelodysplasia and acute leukemia in non-Hodgkin's lymphoma patients. *J Clin Oncol.* 2003;21:897–906.

83. Borthakur G, Estey AE. Therapy-related acute myelogenous leukemia and myelodysplastic syndrome. *Curr Oncol Rep.* 2007;9:373–377.

84. Metayer C, Curtis RE, Vose J, et al. Myelodysplastic syndrome and acute myeloid leukemia after autotransplantation for lymphoma: a multicenter case-control study. *Blood.* 2003;101:2015–2023.

85. Smith SM, Le Beau MM, Huo D, et al. Clinical-cytogenetic associations in 306 patients with therapy-related myelodysplasia and myeloid leukemia: the University of Chicago series. *Blood.* 2003;102:43–52.

86. Qian Z, Joslin JM, Tennant TR, et al. Cytogenetic and genetic pathways in therapy-related acute myeloid leukemia. *Chem Biol Interact.* 2010;184:50–57.

87. Pedersen-Bjergaard J, Philip P. Balanced translocations involving chromosome bands 11q23 and 21q22 are highly characteristic of myelodysplasia and leukemia following therapy with cytostatic agents targeting at DNA-topoisomerase II. *Blood.* 1991;78:1147–1148.

88. Bhatia S, Ramsay NK, Steinbuch M, et al. Malignant neoplasms following bone marrow transplantation. *Blood.* 1996;87:3633–3639.

89. Krishnan A, Bhatia S, Slovak ML, et al. Predictors of therapy-related leukemia and myelodysplasia following autologous transplantation for lymphoma: an assessment of risk factors. *Blood.* 2000;95:1588–1593.

90. Darrington DL, Vose JM, Anderson JR, et al. Incidence and characterization of secondary myelodysplastic syndrome and acute myelogenous leukemia following high-dose chemoradiotherapy and autologous stem-cell transplantation for lymphoid malignancies. *J Clin Oncol.* 1994;12:2527–2534.
91. Tarella C, Passera R, Magni M, et al. Risk factors for the development of secondary malignancy after high-dose chemotherapy and autograft, with or without rituximab: a 20-year retrospective follow-up study in patients with lymphoma. *J Clin Oncol.* 2011;29:814–824.
92. Bhatia S, Robison LL, Francisco L, et al. Late mortality in survivors of autologous hematopoietic-cell transplantation: report from the Bone Marrow Transplant Survivor Study. *Blood.* 2005;105:4215–4222.
93. Del Canizo M, Amigo M, Hernandez JM, et al. Incidence and characterization of secondary myelodysplastic syndromes following autologous transplantation. *Haematologica.* 2000;85:403–409.
94. Kalaycio M, Rybicki L, Pohlman B, et al. Risk factors before autologous stem-cell transplantation for lymphoma predict for secondary myelodysplasia and acute myelogenous leukemia. *J Clin Oncol.* 2006;24:3604–3610.
95. Borchmann S, von Tresckow B. Novel agents in classical Hodgkin lymphoma. *Leuk Lymphoma.* 2017;58:2275–2286.
96. Merryman RW, Kim HT, Zinzani PL, et al. Safety and efficacy of allogeneic hematopoietic stem cell transplant after PD-1 blockade in relapsed/refractory lymphoma. *Blood.* 2017;129:1380–1388.
97. Herbaux C, Gauthier J, Brice P, et al. Efficacy and tolerability of nivolumab after allogeneic transplantation for relapsed Hodgkin lymphoma. *Blood.* 2017;129:2471–2478.
98. Haverkos BM, Abbott D, Hamadani M, et al. PD-1 blockade for relapsed lymphoma post-allogeneic hematopoietic cell transplant: high response rate but frequent GVHD. *Blood.* 2017;130:221–228.
99. Lumley MA, Milligan DW, Knechtli CJ, Long SG, Billingham LJ, McDonald DF. High lactate dehydrogenase level is associated with an adverse outlook in autografting for Hodgkin's disease. *Bone Marrow Transpl.* 1996;17:383–388.
100. Argiris A, Seropian S, Cooper DL. High-dose BEAM chemotherapy with autologous peripheral blood progenitor-cell transplantation for unselected patients with primary refractory or relapsed Hodgkin's disease. *Ann Oncol.* 2000;11:665–672.
101. Sellner L, Boumendil A, Finel H, et al. Thiotepa-based high-dose therapy for autologous stem cell transplantation in lymphoma: a retrospective study from the EBMT. *Bone Marrow Transpl.* 2016;51:212–218.
102. Nieto Y, Valdez BC, Thall PF, et al. Double epigenetic modulation of high-dose chemotherapy with azacitidine and vorinostat for patients with refractory or poor-risk relapsed lymphoma. *Cancer.* 2016;122:2680–2688.
103. Smith EP, Li H, Friedberg JW, et al. Tandem Autologous Hematopoietic Cell Transplantation for Patients with Primary Progressive or Recurrent Hodgkin Lymphoma: A SWOG and Blood and Marrow Transplant Clinical Trials Network Phase II Trial (SWOG S0410/BMT CTN 0703). *Biol Blood Marrow Transplant.* 2018;24:700–707.

Hematopoietic Cell Transplantation in Patients With Multiple Myeloma

MOHAMMED JUNAID HUSSAIN, MD • SAAD ZAFAR USMANI, MD FACP

AUTOLOGOUS STEM CELL TRANSPLANT: THE STANDARD OF CARE IN MULTIPLE MYELOMA

Several prospective, randomized clinical trials have been performed to define the role of high-dose melphalan (HDM) and autologous hematopoietic cell transplant (AHCT), as a component of front-line therapy for MM patients in the 1980s.[1-4] Two studies, the Intergroupe Francophone du Myélome 90 (IFM 90) and Medical Research Council VII (MRC VII), reported the superiority of HDM and AHCT with respect to response rate, progression-free survival (PFS), and overall survival (OS), leading to the widespread use of HDM and AHCT for patients up to the age of 65 years.[5,6] In the IFM 90 study the complete response (CR) was lower for those receiving standard-dose chemotherapy (SDT) than those receiving HDM/AHCT (5% vs. 22%), as was the very good partial response (VGPR; 9% vs. 16%). The median event-free survival (EFS) was 18 months for those assigned to SDT and 27 months for those assigned to HDM/AHCT. The 5-year EFS was 10% with SDT and 28% with HDM/AHCT ($P = .03$), and 5-year OS was 12% with SDT and 52% with HDM/AHCT ($P = .01$). For patients aged 60 years or less the 5-year OS was lower with SDT than with HDM/AHCT: 18% versus 70% ($P = .02$). Only 9% of patients in the conventional-dose chemotherapy (CCT) arm received HDM/AHCT as salvage therapy. The MRC VII trial randomly assigned 401 patients to HDT or HDM/AHCT. Compared with HDT, HDM/AHCT produced higher CR rates (8% vs. 44%; $P < .001$) and improved median OS (42.3 vs. 54.1 months; $P = .03$) and PFS (19.6 months vs. 31.6 months; $P < .001$). Only 15% of patients assigned to HDT received salvage HDM/AHCT. However, other phase III studies failed to demonstrate the improvement in OS seen with HDM/AHCT in the IFM and MRC studies, in part owing to differences in study design, choice of SDT, and differences in the rate of salvage SCT for patients assigned to HDT. Nonetheless, most these studies confirmed a notable improvement in depth of response and PFS/EFS with HDM/AHCT. Thus HDM/AHCT became an important standard of care for younger patients with multiple myeloma (MM). Results of several randomized studies comparing SDT versus HDM[5-9] are summarized in Table 17.1.

AUTOLOGOUS STEM CELL TRANSPLANT IN THE ERA OF NOVEL AGENTS

Because majority of the trials supporting the use of HDM/AHCT were conducted before the development of novel agents, highly effective, newer agents (lenalidomide, bortezomib, and carfilzomib) have become available for patients with MM. Treatment with these agents has resulted in complete response rates that mimic those previously only achievable with AHCT. Even with the availability of these agents, two large randomized trials demonstrated a survival benefit from AHCT. Exposure to lenalidomide should be limited to 4–6 cycles because it compromises stem cell mobilization.

A randomized phase III study of 402 patients compared melphalan at a dose of 200 mg/m^2 followed by autologous stem cell transplantation with melphalan-prednisone-lenalidomide (MPR) and compared lenalidomide maintenance therapy with no maintenance therapy in patients with newly diagnosed MM.[10] The median follow-up period was 51.2 months. Both PFS and OS were significantly longer with HDM/AHCT than with MPR [median PFS, 43.0 months vs. 22.4 months; hazard ratio (HR), 0.44; $P < .001$; 4-year OS, 81.6% vs. 65.3%; HR, 0.55; $P = .02$]. Median PFS was significantly longer with lenalidomide maintenance, then with no maintenance (41.9 months vs. 21.6 months; HR, 0.47; $P < .001$), but 3-year OS was not significantly prolonged (88.0% vs. 79.2%; HR, 0.64; $P = .14$).

Hematopoietic Cell Transplantation for Malignant Conditions. https://doi.org/10.1016/B978-0-323-56802-9.00017-1

TABLE 17.1
Randomized Clinical Trials Comparing HDM/AHCT to Conventional Chemotherapy

Study	Therapy	Patients (n)	CR (%)	EFS (Median Months)	OS (Median Months)
Attal et al.[5]	Conventional	100	5	18	37
	High-dose	100	22	27	52
Fermand et al.[6]	Conventional	96	-	18.7	50.4
	High-dose	94	-	24.3	55.3
Blade et al.[7]	Conventional	83	11	34.3	66.9
	High-dose	81	30	42.5	67.4
Child et al.[8]	Conventional	200	8.5	19.6	42.3
	High-dose	201	44	31.6	54.8
Barlogie et al.[9]	Conventional	255	15	21	53
	High-dose	261	17	25	58

CR, complete response; *EFS*, event-free survival; *HDM/AHCT*, high-dose melphalan-autologous hematopoietic cell transplant; *OS*, overall survival.

Another randomized, multicenter, phase III trial enrolled 389 patients with newly diagnosed MM, aged 65 years or less. Patients underwent induction with lenalidomide (25 mg, days 1–21) and dexamethasone (40 mg, days 1, 8, 15, and 22) and subsequent chemotherapy with cyclophosphamide (3 g/m^2), followed by granulocyte colony-stimulating factor for stem cell mobilization and collection. They were randomly assigned to tandem AHCT with HDM (200 mg/m^2) or 6 cycles of cyclophosphamide, lenalidomide, and dexamethasone (CRD) [cyclophosphamide 300 mg/m^2, days 1, 8, and 15, dexamethasone 40 mg, days 1, 8, 15, and 22 and lenalidomide 25 mg, days 1–21].[11] A second randomization occurred after consolidation therapy, in which patients were assigned to maintenance therapy with lenalidomide (10 mg, days 1–21) or lenalidomide/prednisone (len + prednisone 50 mg, every other day). Median follow-up was 52·0 months. PFS during consolidation was significantly shorter with chemotherapy plus lenalidomide, compared with HDM and AHCT (median 28·6 months vs. 43·3 months; HR for the first 24 months 2·51; $P < .0001$). For the entire study population, the median PFS was 24.2, 27.6, 37.6, and 31.5 months for patients receiving CRD with lenalidomide/prednisone maintenance therapy, CRD with lenalidomide maintenance therapy, HDM/AHCT with lenalidomide/prednisone maintenance therapy, and HDM/AHCT with lenalidomide maintenance therapy, respectively, whereas the 4-year OS was 68%, 76%, 77%, and 75%.

The role of HDM/AHCT in the context of bortezomib-based induction and consolidation therapy has been evaluated in prospective studies as well. The EMN02/HOVON 95 MM study is a phase III trial, in which patients with newly diagnosed MM were randomly assigned to early HDM/AHCT (single vs. tandem) versus four cycles of bortezomib, melphalan, and prednisone (VMP) consolidation after induction therapy with 4 cycles of cyclophosphamide, bortezomib, and dexamethasone (VCD).[12] Patients underwent a second randomization, consisting of consolidation therapy with lenalidomide, bortezomib, and dexamethasone (RVD) or no consolidation therapy after HDM/AHCT or VMP. All patients received lenalidomide maintenance. The median follow-up from the first randomization was 24 months. The rate of VGPR or better was higher in the HDM/AHCT arm than in the VMP arm (85.5% vs. 73.8%; $P < .001$). Importantly, patients assigned to HDM/AHCT had a 24% reduction in the risk of disease progression or death, with a median PFS that had not been reached versus 44 months for those assigned to HDM/AHCT and VMP, respectively, and a 3-year PFS of 66.1% and 57.5% for those assigned to HDM/AHCT and VMP, respectively (HR, 0.73; $P = .003$). The improvement in PFS was seen for those with revised International Staging System (ISS) stage III disease (HR, 0.52; $P = .008$) and high-risk cytogenetics (t [4; 14], del[17p], del[1p], gain 1q; HR, 0.72; $P = .028$). However, the difference in the 3-year PFS for those receiving VMP and single HDM/AHCT did not reach statistical significance (3-year PFS, 57.5% vs. 63.0%, respectively; HR, 0.81; $P = .06$). In addition, the OS was similar between the HDM/AHCT and VMP arms, with early follow-up.

If transplant eligible, AHCT can be performed earlier after completion of induction therapy or delayed as salvage treatment option for relapsed disease. A statistically significant improvement in PFS with early AHCT was seen in a recently published prospective, open-label phase III trial led by the Intergroupe Francophone du Myelome (IFM) and the Dana-Farber Cancer Institute, addressing the early versus delayed AHCT, in patients with newly diagnosed MM with symptomatic and measurable disease.[13] Patients underwent induction therapy with an immunomodulatory drug and a proteasome inhibitor. After 3 cycles of lenalidomide, bortezomib, and dexamethasone (RVD) and subsequent stem cell collection, patients assigned to the delayed-HDM/AHCT arm received an additional 5 cycles of RVD followed by lenalidomide maintenance therapy, whereas those in the early HDM/AHCT group directly underwent HDM/AHCT, followed by 2 cycles of RVD consolidation therapy after HDM/AHCT and then lenalidomide maintenance therapy. This trial showed that early transplant was associated with a higher rate of complete response (59 vs. 48%; $P = .003$), a lower rate of minimal residual disease (65 vs. 79%; $P < .001$), and a longer median PFS (50 vs. 36 months; HR 0.65; $P < .001$). OS at 4 years did not differ significantly between the transplantation group and the RVD-alone group (81% and 82%, respectively). Results should be interpreted with caution because the trial was not powered to detect an effect on OS.

Carfilzomib, lenalidomide, and dexamethasone (KRD) therapy has been shown to be a highly effective induction strategy for the treatment of newly diagnosed MM.[14] Zimmerman et al. conducted a single-arm, phase II study evaluating HDM/AHCT as part of consolidation therapy for patients treated with KRD induction therapy.[15] Patients were treated with 4 cycles of KRD, HDM/AHCT, 4 cycles of KRD consolidation therapy, 10 cycles of KRD maintenance therapy, and subsequent lenalidomide monotherapy. Seventy-five patients were enrolled, 36% of whom had high-risk cytogenetics. The rate of VGPR or better increased from 77% to 98% from the end of induction therapy to the end of HDM/AHCT, whereas the rate of CR or better increased from 12% to 26%, and the rate of stringent CR increased from 8% to 20%. By the end of KRD maintenance therapy, the rate of stringent CR was an unprecedented 82%.

A similar open-label, single-arm, phase II study was conducted at 10 IFM transplant centers where 66 patients with symptomatic newly diagnosed MM received four 28-day induction cycles of KRd, followed by stem cell collection.[16] All pts proceeded to HDM (200 mg/m²) followed by AHCT. Two months after hematological recovery, pts rece ived four 28-day consolidation cycles of KRd, followed by 1 year of lenalidomide maintenance (10 mg, D1-21). Among 42 evaluable pts, 27 were in stringent complete response (sCR). Overall response rate (ORR) was 97.5%, including 23.5% VGPR, 69% CR or better, and 32 of 36 pts (89%) were MRD negative by flow. For pts tested by next-generation sequencing, 13 of 22 (59%) were MRD negative. Median PFS was not reached.

These prospective studies further reinforce the pivotal role of HDM/AHCT with an induction strategy comprising of a proteasome inhibitor or an immunomodulatory drug that not only improves the depth of response and PFS when used as consolidation therapy for MM but also translates into a survival benefit. Therefore HDM/AHCT remains an important standard of care in managing patients with MM.

AUTOLOGOUS HEMATOPOEITIC CELL TRANSPLANT AS PART OF FIRST-LINE OR SECOND-LINE THERAPY

In the last decade the major advances in the management of MM have been the introduction of the novel agents such as thalidomide, bortezomib, and lenalidomide into the therapeutic armamentarium. These novel agents have markedly improved the rate of CR both before and after AHCT, without substantially increasing toxicity, which has important implications, as the achievement of high-quality responses is a significant prognostic factor for outcome. Not only an induction treatment comprising new drugs significantly increased the rates of high-quality responses and improved survival outcomes, but the manageable toxicity profiles of these agents make them suitable for long-term treatment. The burning questions remains if HDM/AHCT can be deferred until disease progression? This was addressed in a multicenter, sequential, randomized trial to assess the optimal timing of HDM/AHCT by Fermand et al.[17] Among 202 enrolled patients who were up to 56 years old, 185 were randomly assigned to receive high-dose therapy and autologous hematopoietic cell transplant (HDT/AHCT) (early HDT group, n = 91) or a CCT regimen (late HDT group, n = 94). All patients underwent hematopoietic cell collection at the beginning of the study. Seventy four of 81 eligible patients in the delayed-HDM/AHCT arm underwent salvage HDT/AHCT at progression. Although the median EFS was 39 months in the early-HDT/AHCT arm compared with 13 months for those assigned to delayed HDT/AHCT, the median OS was 64.6 and 64.0 months, respectively ($P = .92$). Average time without symptoms, treatment, and treatment toxicity (TWiSTT) were 27.8 and 22.3 months for those assigned to early versus late HDT/AHCT, respectively.

Although this study suggests that AHCT can be performed as part of first-line or second-line therapy, it remains unclear whether this is the case with the application of more effective induction and nontransplant consolidation therapies consisting of a proteasome inhibitor, corticosteroids, and either an immunomodulatory or an alkylating agent. For now, given that most published studies demonstrating the benefit of HDM/AHCT in MM incorporated high-dose therapy (HDT) as a part of first-line treatment, the standard approach for a transplant-eligible, newly diagnosed MM patient, treated outside of a clinical trial, should be early HDM/AHCT. Considering the clear clinical benefit seen with the use of delayed HDM/AHCT, postponement of HDM/AHCT until second-line therapy is reasonable, especially for healthier, younger patients with lower-risk disease, who are more likely to remain good candidates for high-dose therapy at relapse. Any decision to defer HDM/AHCT must be made after discussing with the patient thoroughly, delineating the risks and benefits of the both approaches. Hematopoietic cells should be collected after initial induction therapy to minimize the risk of unsuccessful mobilization at relapse, if possible. Lastly, patients who defer HDM/AHCT should be offered high-dose therapy (HDT) for first relapse after a course of initial cytoreductive salvage therapy, given that there are no phase III studies demonstrating the value of an initial HDM/AHCT, beyond second-line therapy.

SINGLE VERSUS TANDEM AUTOLOGOUS HEMATOPOIETIC CELL TRANSPLANT

Tandem or double autologous transplant means that two autologous transplants are performed within a period of no more than 6 months. The feasibility, safety, and clinical efficacy of tandem HDM/AHCT was first evaluated in the 1980s by the French researchers.[18] Researchers at the Myeloma Institute for Research and Therapy at the University of Arkansas for Medical Sciences further worked on this approach, incorporating tandem HDM/AHCT into the framework of their total therapy treatment(TTT) approaches and achieving durable responses for many of their patients.[19-22] To better understand the additional value of the second HDM/

AHCT, Attal et al. conducted a phase III study comparing single HDM/AHCT (melphalan 140 mg/m^2 + total-body irradiation) with tandem HDM/AHCT (AHCT 1: melphalan 140 mg/m^2; AHCT 2: melphalan 140 mg/m^2 + total-body irradiation) in patients with newly diagnosed MM, who were younger than 60 years.[23] After induction therapy with 3–4 cycles of infusional vincristine and doxorubicin with pulse dexamethasone (VAD), 85% of patients assigned to single HDM/AHCT successfully underwent the planned high-dose therapy (HDT), whereas 88% of patients assigned to tandem HDM/AHCT underwent the first HDM/AHCT, and 78% underwent the second HDM/AHCT. Twenty-two percent of those receiving single HDM/AHCT underwent transplant as salvage therapy at relapse, in contrast to 26% of those assigned to tandem HDM/AHCT. The median EFS for those assigned to single HDM/AHCT was 25 months, whereas the median EFS for the tandem HDM/AHCT group was 30 months ($P = .03$). The median OS was 48 months versus 58 months ($P = .01$), and the 7-year OS was 21% versus 42%, respectively. In subset analysis, patients who did not have at least a VGPR after the first HDM/AHCT benefitted the most from the second HDM/AHCT, with a 7-year OS of 43%, compared with 11% for those undergoing single HDM/AHCT. There was no survival advantage demonstrated for the patients who had at least a VGPR after their first HDM/AHCT.

Cavo et al. conducted a study, in which patients were randomly assigned to either single HDM/AHCT (melphalan 200 mg/m^2) or tandem HDM/AHCT (AHCT 1: Melphalan 200 mg/m^2; AHCT 2: Melphalan 120 mg/m^2 + Busulfan 12 mg/kg), after an initial 4 cycles of VAD induction therapy.[24] Eighty-five percent of patients assigned to single HDM/AHCT successfully underwent the therapy, whereas 90% of those assigned to tandem HDM/AHCT received the first AHCT, and 65% received the second AHCT. Thirty-three percent of those assigned to single HDM/AHCT underwent AHCT as a salvage therapy at relapse, in contrast to 10% of those undergoing tandem HDM/AHCT. The median EFS was improved for those assigned to the tandem HDM/AHCT arm of the study (35 months vs. 23 months; $P = .001$). However, no OS advantage was demonstrated (median OS, 65 months vs. 71 months; $P = .90$; 7-year OS, 46% vs. 43%). Patients who did not achieve a near CR benefitted the most from a tandem HDM/AHCT strategy, achieving a median EFS of 42 months versus 22 months ($P < .001$) and a trend toward improved OS (7-year OS, 60% vs. 47%; $P = .10$).

The relevance of these findings to current practice remain unclear because the clinical trials comparing single to tandem HDM/AHCT were performed before the availability of novel agents. A retrospective analysis was performed on four phase III studies in which single or tandem HDM/AHCT therapy was pursued after bortezomib-based induction therapy.[25] The choice of single versus tandem HDM/AHCT was determined by the center at which the patient was treated. The median PFS was 38 versus 50 months for those receiving single or tandem HDM/AHCT, respectively (HR, 0.72; $P<.001$), whereas the 5-year OS was 63% versus 75% ($P = .002$). For those with high-risk cytogenetics (t [4; 14] and/or del[17p]) who had not entered a CR with induction therapy, the median PFS was 42 versus 21 months (HR, 0.41; $P = .006$) and the 5-year OS was 70% versus 17% (HR, 0.22; $P<.001$) in favor of a tandem HDM/AHCT approach.

To address whether a second HDM/AHCT is beneficial in the context of currently available induction therapies based on immunomodulatory drugs and proteasome inhibitors, the Blood and Marrow Transplant Clinical Trials Network (BMT CTN) undertook a prospective phase III study, designed to compare long-term outcomes among patients randomized on the BMT CTN 0702 protocol (NCT01109004), "A Trial of Single Autologous Transplant with or without Consolidation Therapy versus Tandem Autologous Transplant with Lenalidomide Maintenance, for Patients with Multiple Myeloma". It is hypothesized that use of novel antimyeloma agents will improve long-term PFS after high-dose melphalan followed by autologous hematopoietic cell transplantation (HCT), as compared to a second autologous transplantation. Until these data mature, it is advisable to collect enough hematopoietic cells for 2 AHCTs and consider a tandem HDM/AHCT strategy for high-risk patients who achieve further cytoreduction of disease with their initial HDM/AHCT without excessive toxicity.

THE ROLE OF SALVAGE AUTOLOGOUS HEMATOPOIETIC CELL TRANSPLANT IN MM

Survival outcomes are similar, regardless of whether high-dose therapy is used as part of first-line or second-line treatment, and patients with relapsed MM have considerable options for salvage treatment. For transplant-eligible, HDM-naive patients with first disease progression, salvage HDM/AHCT therefore remains a standard of care. However, for patients whose disease progresses after an initial HDM/AHCT, the role of repeat HDM/AHCT as part of salvage therapy remains less clear. Results of the retrospective

analyses of salvage HDM/AHCT in relapsed MM are summarized in Table 17.2,[26–33] and several conclusions can be drawn.

First, salvage HDM/AHCT is feasible, with non-relapse mortality rates that are acceptably low. Second, several factors consistently emerge that are predictive of outcomes with salvage HDM/AHCT. Specifically, a shorter PFS, measured from the time of the first HDM/AHCT, is universally associated with shorter PFS and OS, with a second transplant in multivariate analysis. Finally, several studies revealed age to be a predictor of OS with salvage HDM/AHCT, thus indicating that frailer patients should not be considered for such an approach. The American Society for Blood and Marrow Transplantation, the European Society for Blood and Marrow Transplantation, the BMT CTN, and the International Myeloma Working Group recently published consensus guidelines on the use of salvage HDM/AHCT in relapsed MM.[34] The consensus committee agreed on the following guideline statements:

1. In transplant-eligible patients, relapsing after primary therapy that did not include an HDM/AHCT, salvage HDM/AHCT should be considered standard.
2. HDM/AHCT should be considered appropriate therapy for any patients relapsing after primary therapy that includes an HDM/AHCT with initial remission duration of more than 18 months.
3. HDM/AHCT can be used as a bridging strategy to allogeneic HCT.
4. The role of postsalvage HDM/AHCT maintenance needs to be explored in the context of well-designed prospective trials that should include new agents such as monoclonal antibodies, immune-modulating agents, and oral proteasome inhibitors.
5. HDM/AHCT consolidation should be explored as a strategy to develop novel conditioning regimens or post-HDM/AHCT strategies in patients with short remission (less than 18 months).

The Myeloma X Relapse trial compared conventional chemotherapy (CCT) at relapse with HDM/AHCT.[26] Patients with disease progression, at least 18 months from their initial HDM/AHCT (later reduced to 12 months), underwent initial cytoreductive therapy with 2–4 cycles of bortezomib, doxorubicin, and dexamethasone (PAD) induction therapy, followed by peripheral blood hematopoietic cell collection (if not already available). Ninety-four percent of the registered patients were bortezomib naïve, and none had received lenalidomide as part of first-line therapy. Patients with adequate hematopoietic cells for a second AHCT were randomly assigned to

TABLE 17.2
HDM/AHCT in Salvage Setting

Study	Results	Factors Associated With PFS and OS
Cook[26] 2011	• 4-y OS: 32% for HDM/AHCT, 22% for CCT - Median OS for patients with RD > 18 mo: 3.9 y for HDM/AHCT, 1.8 y for CCT	• RD > 18 mo, younger age associated with improved OS
Yhim[27] 2013	• Median PFS: 18 mo for HDM/AHCT, 9.1 mo for CCT - Median OS: 55.5 mo for HDM/AHCT, 25.4 mo for CCT	• CCT, RD < 18 mo, ISS stage III disease associated with worse OS
Fenk[28] 2011	• Median EFS: 14 mo • Median OS: 52 mo	• RD > 12 mo
Jimenez-Zepeda[29] 2012	• RD ≤ 24 mo • Median PFS: 9.83 mo, median OS: 28.47 mo - RD > 24 mo • Median PFS: 17.3 mo, median OS: 71.3 mo	• RD > 24 mo associated with improved PFS and OS
Lemieux[30] 2013	• Median PFS: 18 mo • Median OS: 4 y	• Inferior PFS: RD < 24 mo, <VGPR with salvage treatment, no maintenance therapy • Inferior OS: Age >60 y, RD < 24 mo
Michaelis [31] 2013	• Median PFS: 18 mo (3-y PFS: 13%) • 3-y OS: 46%	• RD ≥ 36 mo, 3-y OS: 58% • RD < 36 mo, 3-y OS: 42%
Olin[32] 2009	• Median PFS: 8.5 mo • Median OS: 20.7 mo	• RD ≤ 12 mo, ≥5 prior lines of therapy associated with worse OS
Shah[33] 2012	• Median PFS: 12.3 mo - Median OS: 31.7 mo	• Shorter RD, ↑ number of prior lines of therapy associated with worse OS

AHCT, autologous stem cell transplant; *AHCT 1*, initial autologous stem cell transplant; *AHCT 2*, salvage autologous stem cell transplant; *CCT*, conventional chemotherapy; *EFS*, event-free survival; *HDM*, high-dose melphalan; *ISS*, International Staging System; *mo*, month/months; *OS*, overall survival; *PFS*, progression-free survival; *RD*, remission duration; *TTP*, time to progression; *VGPR*, very good partial response; *y*, year/years.

treatment with HDM (200 mg/m^2)/AHCT or cyclophosphamide $(400 \text{ mg}^{-2}$ once weekly for 12 weeks). Of the 293 patients who underwent PAD induction therapy, 174 had adequate numbers of hematopoietic cells to pursue a second AHCT. The rate of VGPR or better was 47% for patients assigned to cyclophosphamide, and 60% for patients assigned to HDM/AHCT $(P = .0036)$. The rate of stringent CR was 22% versus 39% $(P = .021)$. Importantly the median time to progression was 11 months for those assigned to cyclophosphamide, versus 19 months for those assigned to HDM/AHCT (HR, 0.36; $P < .0001$). In addition, the median time to progression was 11 months for those assigned to cyclophosphamide, versus 24 months for those assigned to HDM/AHCT among those with a remission duration of more than 24 months with the first HDM/AHCT (HR, 0.35; $P < .0001$). For those with a remission duration after the initial HDM/AHCT of 12–24 months, the median time to progression was 9 months with cyclophosphamide and 13 months

with HDM/AHCT (HR, 0.37; $P < .0037$). There was a trend toward better OS for those assigned to HDM/AHCT, with a 3-year OS of 62.9% for those assigned to cyclophosphamide versus 80.3% for those assigned to HDM/AHCT, but this did not reach statistical significance (HR, 0.62; $P = .19$). Although the results of this study are important, the sample size was small, and the comparator arm of weekly cyclophosphamide would not be considered a standard nontransplant salvage therapy in the current era of treating MM.

In this era of personalized medicine, decisions should be made on a case-by-case basis, considering the duration of response to the first HDM/AHCT, the application of consolidation and maintenance therapy after HDM/AHCT, and toxicities associated with the initial HDM/AHCT. In addition, the salvage HDM/AHCT represents a promising area for studying novel conditioning strategies, as well as consolidation and maintenance therapies, to maximize the benefit of this therapeutic strategy.

ALLOGENEIC HEMATOPOIETIC CELL TRANSPLANTATION FOR MM

Allogeneic hematopoietic cell transplant (Allo-HCT) offers the potential of harnessing an immunologic graft-versus-myeloma effect along with a tumor-free graft, capable of controlling residual disease and offering the potential for cure. However, the role of Allo-HCT in MM remains limited, given an elderly patient population, other comorbid conditions and complications associated with acute and chronic graft-versus-host disease (GVHD). In addition, the perturbed immune system due to the disease is worsened by posttransplant immunosuppression, resulting in a high transplant-related mortality rate with standard myeloablative conditioning regimens. Traditional myeloablative conditioning and its associated toxicities have given way to more tolerable reduced-intensity conditioning regimens. In addition, marked improvements have been made over the past decade and the supportive care and HLA typing. A retrospective case-matched analysis suggested that Allo-HCT is associated with significantly higher early mortality rates than AHCT. The main reason for the poorer survival in Allo-HCT patients was higher transplant-related mortality (41% v 13% for AHCT, $P = .0001$), which was not compensated for by a lower rate of relapse and progression.[35]

Published prospective trials on the use of an allograft in the setting of relapsed multiple MM are very few. In a prospective multicenter European Society for Blood and Marrow Transplantation (EBMT) trial, Kroger et al. investigated the role of allografting from unrelated donors in 49 patients who relapsed after a previous autograft.[36] Conditioning regimen consisted of melphalan (140 mg/m^2), fludarabine (90 mg/m^2), and antithymocyte globulin Fresenius (60 mg/kg BW). The median time for leukocyte and platelet engraftments were 15 and 19 days, respectively. Grade II–IV acute GVHD occurred in 25% and 35% of the patients experienced chronic GVHD. The ORR was 95% including 46% complete remissions. Cumulative incidence of 1-year transplant-related mortality was 25% and was significantly lower in transplants from fully HLA-matched donors, as compared with mismatched donors (10% vs. 53%, $P = .001$). After a median follow-up of 43 months, the 5-year PFS and OS were 20% and 26%, respectively, and were significantly better in patients who achieved posttransplant CR (41% vs. 7%, $P = .04$, and 56% vs. 16%, $P = .02$).

The expert committee agreed on the following guideline statements regarding the role of Allo-HCT in relapsed myeloma:

1. Allo-HCT should be considered appropriate therapy for any eligible patient with early relapse (less than 24 months) after primary therapy that included an autologous HCT or with high-risk features (i.e., cytogenetics, extramedullary disease, plasma cell leukemia, or high lactate dehydrogenase (LDH)) if they responded favorably to salvage therapy before allogeneic HCT.
2. Whenever possible, Allo-HCT should be performed in the context of a clinical trial.
3. The role of post-Allo-HCT maintenance therapy needs to be further explored.
4. Prospective randomized trials need to be performed to define the role of salvage Allo-HCT in patients with MM relapsing after primary therapy.

CONCLUSIONS

The recent advances in therapy for MM have dramatically improved the outcomes for most patients with MM. Although HDM/AHCT is still considered a valuable tool for tumor reduction and remission consolidation in MM, the discussion will likely continue regarding the magnitude of benefit associated with using this strategy in the era of novel agents and the optimal timing of AHCT in the modern myeloma therapy. There is no doubt that HDM/AHCT leads to improvements in depth of response and PFS in the context of the best currently available therapies. Moving forward, it will be prudent to identify patient subsets who are more likely to benefit from early HDM/AHCT, as well as those who may not require such an intervention at all. Detection of MRD by flow cytometry and next-generation sequencing has emerged as a powerful tool in the monitoring of response depth in MM. Similarly, recommendations regarding the optimal candidates for a second HDM/AHCT will need to be updated and will increasingly account for the application of continuous therapy after first HDM/AHCT, be it consolidation therapy or maintenance therapy. Novel conditioning and post-AHCT consolidation and maintenance strategies will need to be studied if salvage HDM/AHCT is to remain a viable therapeutic option in the future. With the emergence and potential incorporation of monoclonal antibodies in induction therapies, it will be important to reassess the role and timing of HDM/AHCT to maximize the benefit of this tested and proven therapeutic modality. In the era of immune oncology, it is imperative that we continually challenge established treatment paradigms.

REFERENCES

1. McElwain TJ, Powles RL. High-dose intravenous melphalan for plasma-cell leukaemia and myeloma. *Lancet.* 1983;2(8354):822–824.
2. Barlogie B, Hall R, Zander A, Dicke K, Alexanian R. High-dose melphalan with autologous bone marrow transplantation for multiple myeloma. *Blood.* 1986; 67(5):1298–1301.
3. Barlogie B, Alexanian R, Dicke KA, et al. High-dose chemoradiotherapy and autologous bone marrow transplantation for resistant multiple myeloma. *Blood.* 1987;70(3):869–872.
4. Selby PJ, McElwain TJ, Nandi AC, et al. Multiple myeloma treated with high dose intravenous melphalan. *Br J Haematol.* 1987;66(1):55–62.
5. Attal M, Harousseau JL, Stoppa AM, et al. A prospective, randomized trial of autologous bone marrow transplantation and chemotherapy in multiple myeloma. Intergroupe Français du Myélome. *N Engl J Med.* 1996;335(2):91–97.
6. Fermand JP, Katsahian S, Divine M, et al. Group Myelome-Autogreffe. High-dose therapy and autologous blood stem-cell transplantation compared with conventional treatment in myeloma patients aged 55 to 65 years: long-term results of a randomized control trial from the Group Myelome-Autogreffe. *J Clin Oncol.* 2005;23(36):9227–9233.
7. Blade J, Surenda A, et al. High-dose therapy auto-transplantation/intensification vs continued conventional chemotherapy in multiple myeloma patients responding to initial treatment chemotherapy. Results of a prospective randomized trial from the Spanish Cooperative group PETHEMA. *Blood.* 2005;106(12):3755–3759.
8. Child JA, Morgan GJ, Davies FE, et al. High-dose chemotherapy with hematopoietic stem-cell rescue for multiple myeloma. *N Engl J Med.* 2003;348(19):1875–1883.
9. Barlogie B, Kyle RA, Anderson KC, et al. Standard chemotherapy compared with high-dose chemoradiotherapy for multiple myeloma: results of phase III US Intergroup Trial S9321. *J Clin Oncol.* 2006;24(6):929–936.
10. Palumbo A, Cavallo F, Gay F, et al. Autologous transplantation and maintenance therapy in multiple myeloma. *N Engl J Med.* 2014;371(10):895–905.
11. Gay F, Oliva S, Petrucci MT, et al. Chemotherapy plus lenalidomide versus autologous transplantation, followed by lenalidomide plus prednisone versus lenalidomide maintenance, in patients with multiple myeloma: a randomised, multicentre, phase 3 trial. *Lancet Oncol.* 2015;16(16):1617–1629.
12. Cavo M, Palumbo A, Zweegman S, et al. Upfront autologous stem cell transplantation (AHCT) versus novel agent-based therapy for multiple myeloma (MM): a randomized phase 3 study of the European Myeloma Network (EMN02/HO95 MM trial) [ASCO abstract 8000]. *J Clin Oncol.* 2016;34(15).
13. Michel A, Valerie L-C, Cyrille H, et al. Lenalidomide, bortezomib, and dexamethasone with transplantation for myeloma. *N Engl J Med.* 2017;376:1311–1320.
14. Jakubowiak AJ, Dytfeld D, Griffith KA, et al. A phase 1/2 study of carfilzomib in combination with lenalidomide and low-dose dexamethasone as a frontline treatment for multiple myeloma. *Blood.* 2012;120(9):1801–1809.
15. Zimmerman T, Griffith K, Jasielec J, et al. *Carfilzomib,lenalidomide and Dexamethasone (KRd) Combined with Autologous Stem Cell Transplant (AHCT) Shows Improved Efficacy Compared with Krd without AHCT in Newly Diagnosed Multiple Myeloma (NDMM).* Honolulu, HI: Oral abstract presented at: BMT Tandem Meetings 2016; February 18-22, 2016. Abstract 28.
16. Murielle R, Valerie L-C, Nelly R, et al. Frontline therapy with carfilzomib, lenalidomide, and dexamethasone (KRd) induction followed by autologous stem cell transplantation, Krd consolidation and lenalidomide maintenance in newly diagnosed multiple myeloma (NDMM) patients: primary results of the Intergroupe Francophone du MyéLome (IFM) KRd phase II study. *Blood.* 2016;128:1142.
17. Fermand JP, Ravaud P, Chevret S, et al. High-dose therapy and autologous peripheral blood stem cell transplantation in multiple myeloma: up-front or rescue treatment? Results of a multicenter sequential randomized clinical trial. *Blood.* 1998;92(9):3131–3136.
18. Harousseau JL, Milpied N, Laporte JP, et al. Double-intensive therapy in high- risk multiple myeloma. *Blood.* 1992;79(11):2827–2833.
19. Usmani SZ, Crowley J, Hoering A, et al. Improvement in long-term outcomes with successive total therapy trials for multiple myeloma: are patients now being cured? *Leukemia.* 2013;27(1):226–232.
20. Nair B, van Rhee F, Shaughnessy Jr JD, et al. Superior results of Total Therapy 3 (2003-33) in gene expression profiling-defined low-risk multiple myeloma confirmed in subsequent trial 2006-66 with VRD maintenance. *Blood.* 2010;115(21):4168–4173.
21. Barlogie B, Jagannath S, Desikan KR, et al. Total therapy with tandem transplants for newly diagnosed multiple myeloma. *Blood.* 1999;93(1):55–65.
22. Barlogie B, Tricot G, Rasmussen E, et al. Total therapy 2 without thalidomide in comparison with total therapy 1: role of intensified induction and posttransplantation consolidation therapies. *Blood.* 2006;107(7):2633–2638.
23. Attal M, Harousseau JL, Facon T, et al. InterGroupe Francophone du Myélome. Single versus double autologous stem-cell transplantation for multiple myeloma. *N Engl J Med.* 2003;349(26):2495–2502.
24. Cavo M, Tosi P, Zamagni E, et al. Prospective, randomized study of single compared with double autologous stem-cell transplantation for multiple myeloma: Bologna 96 clinical study. *J Clin Oncol.* 2007;25(17):2434–2441.

25. Cavo M, Salwender H, Rosiñol L, et al. Double vs single autologous stem cell transplantation after bortezomib-based induction regimens for multiple myeloma: an integrated analysis of patient-level data from phase European III studies [ASH abstract 767]. *Blood*. 2013;122(21).

26. Cook G, Williams C, Brown JM, et al. National Cancer Research Institute Haemato-oncology Clinical Studies Group. High-dose chemotherapy plus autologous stem-cell transplantation as consolidation therapy in patients with relapsed multiple myeloma after previous autologous stem-cell transplantation (NCRI Myeloma X Relapse [Intensive trial]): a randomised, open-label, phase 3 trial. *Lancet Oncol*. 2014;15(8):874–885.

27. Yhim HY, Kim K, Kim JS, et al. Matched-pair analysis to compare the outcomes of a second salvage auto-SCT to systemic chemotherapy alone in patients with multiple myeloma who relapsed after front-line auto-SCT. *Bone Marrow Transpl*. 2013;48(3):425–432.

28. Fenk R, Liese V, Neubauer F, et al. Predictive factors for successful salvage high-dose therapy in patients with multiple myeloma relapsing after autologous blood stem cell transplantation. *Leuk Lymphoma*. 2011;52(8):1455–1462.

29. Jimenez-Zepeda VH, Mikhael J, Winter A, et al. Second autologous stem cell transplantation as salvage therapy for multiple myeloma: impact on progression-free and overall survival. *Biol Blood Marrow Transpl*. 2012;18(5):773–779.

30. Lemieux E, Hulin C, Cailxlot D, et al. Autologous stem cell transplantation: an effective salvage therapy in multiple myeloma. *Biol Blood Marrow Transpl*. 2013;19(3):445–449.

31. Michaelis LC, Saad A, Zhong X, et al. Plasma cell Disorders working committee of the center for International blood and marrow transplant Research. Salvage second hematopoietic cell transplantation in myeloma. *Biol Blood Marrow Transpl*. 2013;19(5):760–766.

32. Olin RL, Vogl DT, Porter DL, et al. Second auto-SCT is safe and effective salvage therapy for relapsed multiple myeloma. *Bone Marrow Transpl*. 2009;43(5):417–422.

33. Shah N, Ahmed F, Bashir Q, et al. Durable remission with salvage second auto-transplants in patients with multiple myeloma. *Cancer*. 2012;118(14):3549–3555.

34. Giralt S, Garderet L, Durie B, et al. American Society of blood and marrow transplantation, European Society of blood and marrow transplantation, blood and marrow transplant clinical trials Network, and International myeloma working group consensus Conference on salvage hematopoietic cell transplantation in patients with relapsed multiple myeloma. *Biol Blood Marrow Transpl*. 2015;21(12):2039–2051.

35. Björkstrand BB, Ljungman P, Svensson H, et al. Allogeneic bone marrow transplantation versus autologous stem cell transplantation in multiple myeloma: a retrospective case-matched study from the European Group for Blood and Marrow Transplantation. *Blood*. 1996;88:4711.

36. Kröger N, Shimoni A, Schilling G, et al. Unrelated stem cell transplantation after reduced intensity conditioning for patients with multiple myeloma relapsing after autologous transplantation. *Br J Haematol*. 2010;148:323–331.

CHAPTER 18

Hematopoietic Cell Transplantation for Light-Chain Amyloidosis

ANITA D'SOUZA, MD, MS • PARAMESWARAN HARI, MD, MS

INTRODUCTION

Light-chain (AL) amyloidosis, also known as primary systemic amyloidosis, is a plasma cell clonal neoplasm associated with multiorgan dysfunction from insoluble fibril (amyloid) deposition.[1] The plasma cell clone, although similar to multiple myeloma, is usually with a lower plasma cell burden in AL amyloidosis. However, these plasma cells produce immunoglobulin light chains that misfold into insoluble fibrils. The resultant misfolded, insoluble fibrils deposit in various organs such as the heart, kidney, liver, and nerves among others, causing organ dysfunction.[2] This disease tends to have a progressive course due to uncontrolled tissue damage from extracellular amyloid deposition and can be rapidly fatal without treatment.[1] Treatment is directed at eliminating the underlying plasma cell clone and in turn the source of the amyloidogenic light chain, by the use of chemotherapy. In this chapter, we review the evidence and use of autologous hematopoietic cell transplantation (auto-HCT) in AL amyloidosis in the context of other treatment options.

History and Current Data of Transplantation for AL Amyloidosis

Since the late 1980s high-dose melphalan with auto-HCT has been used successfully to treat multiple myeloma.[3] The first report of the use of auto-HCT in AL amyloidosis was in 1993 with the use of busulfan and melphalan, followed by infusion of CD34+ cells from bone marrow and peripheral blood.[4] Although the patient died of complications, she nonetheless had full engraftment. Subsequently, a report from the Netherlands demonstrated a successful syngeneic allogeneic transplant using cyclophosphamide with total-body irradiation, followed by bone marrow transplantation. The patient had a hematologic and clinical response. The first report of a successful auto-HCT using high-dose melphalan was reported by Moreau et al. in 1996 and immediately thereafter followed by a report of

5 patients treated with high-dose melphalan at Boston University with success.[5,6] With further transplant experience in AL amyloidosis, it became apparent that there was a much higher morbidity and mortality seen among patients with AL amyloidosis than patients with MM. A transplant-related mortality (TRM) of as high as 43% was reported in this early transplant period.[7] In addition, a retrospective study from the Mayo Clinic suggested that patients who met transplant eligibility had good outcomes even with nontransplant therapies, thus showing the possibility of a selection bias in single-center nonrandomized studies.[8,9]

In the early 2000s larger transplant series from the Boston University, Mayo Clinic showed decreasing TRM of under 20% with refinements in the selection of patients to undergo transplant, along with hematologic responses in 30%–40% and organ responses ranging 44%–58%.

The much anticipated randomized phase III clinical trial comparing high-dose melphalan and auto-HCT with standard melphalan/dexamethasone oral chemotherapy was published in 2007 and failed to show a survival benefit for transplant compared with chemotherapy.[10] This study, although a commendable effort for a large multicenter trial in such a rare disease, was criticized for the high mortality (24%) in the transplant arm, 13 of 50 transplant-randomized patients not getting planned transplants, and the lowering of melphalan conditioning chemotherapy in a third of the transplanted patients. What was clear again was that carefully selected patients had good outcomes.

The identification of the N-terminal prohormone of brain natriuretic peptide (NT-pro-BNP) and troponin T as biomarkers of severity of amyloid cardiac involvement led to a simple risk staging system in 2004 and further refined in 2012 resulting in identification of AL patients who have early mortality of as high as 40% regardless of therapy.[11,12] It became clear that similar factors which help define the degree of cardiac

Hematopoietic Cell Transplantation for Malignant Conditions. https://doi.org/10.1016/B978-0-323-56802-9.00018-3

TABLE 18.1
Auto-HCT in AL Amyloidosis—Who, When, and How

A. Transplant eligibility factors for auto-HCT
1. Karnofsky Performance Score 80% or higher
2. Cardiac biomarkers: NT-pro-BNP < 5000, TnT < 0.06
3. Fewer than 3 organs involved with AL
4. Nonsevere autonomic neuropathy
5. Nonadvanced cardiac involvement (NYHA≤2, left ventricular ejection fraction ≥40%)

B. Conditioning therapy:
High-dose melphalan therapy has remained the standard of choice. Dose reductions in melphalan have been associated with lower PFS and increased relapse rate in the current era of novel triplet therapy.

AL amyloidosis, light-chain amyloidosis; *Auto-HCT*, autologous hematopoietic cell transplantation; *NT-pro-BNP*, N-terminal prohormone of brain natriuretic peptide; *PFS*, progression-free survival; *TnT*, troponin T. NYHA - New York Heart Association

AL involvement are also critical in patient selection for transplant and posttransplant AL outcomes.[13,14] Table 18.1 shows factors associated with a high risk of posttransplant mortality and poor survival in AL amyloidosis.

A large database analysis of all auto-HCT conducted in the US and Canada between 1995 and 2012 was then performed.[15] In this largest transplant series to date, which included over 1500 patients, a trend was seen for decreasing rates of early mortality after transplantation in more recent years, down to 5% at day 100 in 2007–12 versus 20% at day 100 in 1995–2000. Similarly, the 5-year predicted overall survival (OS) was 55% in 1995–2000 and had improved to 77% in 2007–12. Furthermore, this study showed that centers performing at least 4 AL amyloidosis transplants each year had better success in lowering early posttransplant mortality, thus emphasizing the need for center experience in this rare disease.

Mobilization and Collection of CD34+ Cells

Although mobilization of hematopoietic progenitor cells (HPCs) is generally associated with minimal morbidity, this is not true for most AL amyloidosis patients. Chemotherapy-based mobilization in AL amyloidosis has largely been abandoned because of the high risk of cardiac events, infections, bleeding complications, and mortality. Granulocyte colony–stimulating factor (G-CSF)-based mobilization

has become the standard method in AL amyloidosis.[16] Even with this approach, significant morbidity, including deaths, has been reported during or immediately after G-CSF–based mobilization in AL amyloidosis patients. Complications during G-CSF–induced HPC mobilization in AL amyloidosis patients (especially with cardiac involvement) have included fluid overload, splenic rupture, significant weight gain, cardiac arrhythmias, and cardiopulmonary decompensation (hypoxia, hypotension, and cardiopulmonary failure). The presence of concomitant autonomic dysfunction can further exacerbate blood pressure–related issues, making it difficult to maintain proper fluid balance. In fact, significant weight gain during HPC collection has been shown to be an independent predictor of peritransplant mortality. Mobilization failure rates, in otherwise transplantation-eligible AL amyloidosis patients, with a cytokine-only approach ranges from 5% to 10%. Patients have to be monitored closely, sometimes inpatient, during this period. Recently, success has been seen with the use of plerixafor in combination with G-CSF resulting in fewer days of exposure to G-CSF leading to lesser weight gain and no mobilization failures.[17] Patients with autonomic neuropathy and cardiac involvement can develop hypocalcemia and citrate toxicity from the use of citrate as an anticoagulant during apheresis; this risk is reduced by the use of heparin as anticoagulant during apheresis. A dose of CD34+ cells $\geq 5 \times 10^6$ cells/kg is targeted.

Do Patients Need Induction Chemotherapy Before Auto-HCT?

Most patients with AL amyloidosis have low plasma cell burden, and there are no prospective data to date showing a benefit to induction chemotherapy before autotransplant. Prospective studies using melphalan and prednisone induction before chemotherapy showed potential detriment from this approach owing to organ progression leading to transplant ineligibility as a result. However, bortezomib therapy is being studied in the setting of a clinical trial, and retrospective data of use of bortezomib and dexamethasone with/out cyclophosphamide appear to have good outcomes, allowing for some transplant-ineligible patients being converted to transplant eligible.[18] Again, one has to consider the possibility of selection bias with retrospective data, and induction therapy should be used with caution so that there is no further deterioration of organ function. Other approaches have included using induction chemotherapy in patients with >10% plasma cell clone. In the future, successful antifibrillary agents may need to be explored as pretransplant induction to induce organ responses and increase the safety of transplantation.[19]

Conditioning Chemotherapy

High-dose melphalan remains the standard of care for conditioning for AL. A risk-adapted approach was proposed based on creatinine clearance, number of organs involved with amyloidosis, and presence of cardiac involvement with adjustment of melphalan dose between 100 and 200 mg/m². It is noteworthy to point out that lowering the dose of melphalan < 140 mg/m² is associated with lower hematologic response as well as higher rate of hematologic relapse. A risk-adapted approach using lower doses of melphalan for conditioning in association with posttransplant consolidation using novel agents such as bortezomib for consolidation has considerable attraction.[20] Newer formulations of propylene glycol-free melphalan which have become available recently need to be studied in AL amyloidosis to evaluate safety and peritransplant complications.

Supportive Care During Transplant

In addition to refinements in selecting patients, improvement in supportive treatment during the peritransplant period is critical in lowering TRM in AL amyloidosis. Patients with AL amyloidosis are at an increased risk of becoming volume overloaded. Diuresis ought to be undertaken judiciously, as even mild intravascular depletion can induce cardiorenal syndrome. Diuresis is sometimes performed with albumin infusions to maintain euvolemia. Posttransplantation complications that may be unique and more amplified in AL patients include gastrointestinal bleeding, cardiac arrhythmias, and unresponsive hypotension in selected patients with AL amyloidosis. Patients can develop severe gastrointestinal bleeding from mucositis related to chemotherapy further compounded by AL amyloidosis–related bleeding diathesis.[21] Patients with orthostatic hypotension may need midodrine and fludrocortisone. However, fludrocortisone can cause resultant fluid retention. Table 18.2 describes various examples of supportive care that may be needed during the peritransplant period highlighting the need for a multidisciplinary team approach.

Posttransplant Consolidation

Day-100 hematologic responses to transplant showed that patients achieving a very good partial remission (VGPR) or better had excellent outcomes, whereas those with less VGPR had uniformly poor progression-free

and OS. Posttransplant consolidation based on day-100 response has been used in a risk-adapted chemotherapy approach. In this approach, patients with persistent clonal disease after transplantation receive further therapy with novel agents (thalidomide/dexamethasone, bortezomib/dexamethasone). This has been associated with low TRM and high overall hematologic and organ response rates.

Response to Treatment—Hematologic and Organ Responses

Hematologic response is measured using the serum and urine electrophoresis and immunofixation tests, and the free light-chain assay.[22] Noteworthy is the absence of bone marrow plasma cell clearance in response criteria (unlike with MM) as well as the importance of absolute reduction in the free light-chain excess (rather than the M-protein). Hematologic response correlates with organ response and OS. We recommend monoclonal protein studies in blood and urine (serum protein electrophoresis with immunofixation, free light chains) and organ amyloid measures such as cardiac (NT-pro-BNP, troponin T), renal (creatinine, 24-hour urine protein or urine protein-creatinine ratio), hepatic (alkaline phosphatase, liver span) at day 100 after transplantation, and every 3–6 months thereafter in the first year.[23] After that, depending on response, patients may continue to be seen at 3 monthly intervals or slightly less frequently. In patients with cardiac amyloidosis, we perform cardiac imaging with 2D echocardiogram with strain imaging or cardiac magnetic resonance at day 100 and 1 year after transplantation.

Role of Allogeneic Transplant in AL Amyloidosis

Allo-HCT is seldom used in most AL amyloidosis patients. There are individual case reports and small series suggesting a role for allogeneic transplant in AL amyloidosis. The largest data are reported from the European Group for Blood and Marrow Transplantation registry and describe 15 patients with allogeneic and 4 patients with syngeneic allogeneic transplant.[24] The TRM was high at 40%, with 7 long-term survivors at a median follow-up of 19 months.

Role of Solid Organ Transplant in AL Amyloidosis

The United Network for Organ Sharing data in both renal and cardiac transplant suggest poor outcomes in amyloidosis; however, there may be a role for organ transplant in AL amyloidosis. The danger is for

TABLE 18.2
Supportive Care During Peritransplant Period

	Helpful	Caution
Fluid retention and weight gain	Loop diuretics, Spironolactone Periodic thoracentesis may be needed	Fludrocortisone/salt tablets for hypotension
Heart failure	Diuretics Salt and fluid restriction	Rate-lowering calcium channel blockers Digoxin can bind to fibrils leading to digitalis toxicity Beta blockers may cause decompensation Afterload reduction (ACE-I, ARBs) poorly tolerated
Cardiac arrhythmias (atrial and ventricular, sudden cardiac death)	Amiodarone AV nodal ablation and pacemaker AICD in select patients	Rate-lowering calcium channel blockers, beta blockers, digoxin
Orthostatic hypotension	Waist-high elastic stockings Midodrine Salt tablets, fludrocortisone (can worsen fluid retention) Continuous noradrenalin infusion (for refractory hypotension)	
Neuropathic pain	Gabapentin Pregabalin Duloxetine Amitriptyline Nortriptyline Topical agents (lidocaine, TCA, ketamine)	
Nephrotic syndrome	Diuretics Low-dose ACE-I (if patient is not hypotensive)	
Renal failure	Dialysis Patients may need pretransplant midodrine (particularly in those with autonomic neuropathy)	
Gastroparesis causing nausea and vomiting	Antiemetics, metoclopramide	
Intestinal pseudo-obstruction	Neostigmine	
Diarrhea	Fiber supplements Bile salt–binding agents Loperamide Octreotide (in refractory cases)	
Malnutrition	Dietician consultation early Parenteral nutrition may be needed in those with severe steatorrhea	
Anticoagulation	May be needed in patients with cardiomyopathy and atrial fibrillation	Check factor X levels Higher risk of GI bleeding

ACE-I, Angiotensin Converting Enzyme Inhibitors; *ARB*, Angiotensin II Receptor Blockers; *TCA*, Tricyclic Anti Depressants; AICD, Automated implanted cardioverter defibrillator recurrence of the amyloid process in the transplanted organ, in the setting of an incurable underlying clonal disease. In select patients with amyloid cardiomyopathy, cardiac transplantation may be of benefit either after chemotherapy or with an adjuvant auto-HCT post-cardiac transplant.[25] This has been reported with varying success in the form of case reports and case series from around the world. Successful renal transplant has also been reported before or after autotransplant from high-volume specialized amyloid centers such as the National Amyloid Center in the UK, Mayo Clinic, and Boston University in small series.

Relapse and Retreatment after Transplant

In a series reported from the Mayo clinic, median time from auto-HCT to second-line therapy was 24.3 months and was instituted for a clinical suspicion of relapse or organ progression in 10%, hematologic progression in 23%, isolated organ progression in 32%, and combined hematologic and organ progression in 31%. Patients with organ progression at the time of second-line therapy had inferior survival. It is therefore critical to monitor both organ function and hematologic parameters (mainly dFLC or delta free light chain measured as the difference between involved and uninvolved light chains) after transplantation.

CONCLUSIONS

Melphalan and dexamethasone is the only chemotherapy regimen that has shown to be beneficial based on a randomized phase 3 clinical trial thus far with its superiority demonstrated even over auto-HCT. However, auto-HCT can induce deep hematologic responses and organ responses, as well as long-term survival. Patients with AL amyloidosis are at a much higher risk of complications and death in the peri-transplant period than those with MM and therefore need to be managed at centers with experience and expertise in performing these transplants.

In the last 15–20 years, multiple novel agents have revolutionized the treatment of multiple myeloma. These agents are being studied in patients with AL amyloidosis. Of these drugs, bortezomib has shown prompt (and deep) hematologic responses with organ improvement resulting in patients becoming transplant eligible in some instances. Daratumumab, an anti-CD38 monoclonal antibody, has shown very promising results in small series and is currently being tested prospectively in AL amyloidosis. Ultimately, there is a need for adjunctive amyloid-fibril–directed

therapies to complement chemotherapies. NEOD001 is an investigational monoclonal antibody that targets deposited aggregated amyloid that accumulates in organs of patients with AL amyloidosis.[26] It is reasonable to expect clinical trials incorporating newer antifibril agents to improve organ function before transplant and thus improve both the safety and organ responses after transplantation.

Contraindications for Auto-HCT

Absolute	• Cardiac biomarkers: NT-pro-BNP > 5000, TnT > 0.06 • Greater than three organs involved with AL • Severe autonomic neuropathy • Advanced cardiac involvement (NYHA > 2; LVEF ≥ 40%)
Relative	• Centers performing less than 4 auto-HCT in AL amyloid patients/year

Factors Associated With Prognosis in AL Amyloidosis

Early mortality
Cardiac troponin T [cTnT] > 0.01 ng/mL
N-terminal prohormone of brain natriuretic peptide [NT-pro-BNP] > 4200 pg/mL
Serum uric acid > 8 mg/dL

Plasma cell clone
Absolute measure of amyloidogenic light-chain burden (dFLC > 18 mg/dL)
Size of bone marrow plasma cells, >10%
B_2-microglobulin
Proliferation rate of plasma cells
Presence of plasma cells in the peripheral circulation
LDH
Organs involved with amyloidosis
Cardiac involvement
Number of organs involved with amyloidosis
Extent of organ involvement (e.g., presence of symptomatic heart failure, orthostatic hypotension, and so forth)
Weight loss
Severe autonomic neuropathy

AL Amyloidosis Staging System

Staging		
Thresholds	Categories	Survival (months)
NT-pro-BNP > 1800 pg/mL	I (0 factors)	94.1
Troponin T > 0.025	II (1 factor)	40.3
dFLC > 18 mg/mL	III (2 factors)	14
	IV (3 factors)	5.8

SELECTED READING

1. High-Dose Melphalan versus Melphalan plus Dexamethasone for AL Amyloidosis. *New England Journal of Medicine.* 2007; 357(11):1083–1093.
2. Consensus Guidelines for the conduct and reporting of clinical trials in systemic light-chain amyloidosis. *Leukemia.* 2012; 26(11):2317–2325.
3. Superior survival in primary systemic amyloidosis patients undergoing peripheral blood stem cell transplantation: a case-control study. *Blood.* 2004; 103(10):3960–3963.
4. Recent Improvements in Survival in primary Systemic Amyloidosis and the Importance of an Early Mortality Risk Score. *Mayo Clinic Proceedings.* 2011; 86(1):12–18.
5. Improved Outcomes After Autologous Hematopoietic Cell Transplantation for Light Chain Amyloidosis: A Center for International Blood and Marrow Transplant Research Study. *Journal of Clinical Oncology.* 2015; 33(32):3741–3749.

REFERENCES

1. Kyle RA, Gertz MA. Primary systemic amyloidosis: clinical and laboratory features in 474 cases. *Semin Hematol.* 1995;32(1):45–59.
2. Falk RH, Comenzo RL, Skinner M. The systemic amyloidoses. *N Engl J Med.* 1997;337(13):898–909. https://doi.org/10.1056/NEJM199709253371306. [published Online First: Epub Date].
3. McElwain TJ, Powles RL. High-dose intravenous melphalan for plasma-cell leukaemia and myeloma. *Lancet.* 1983;2(8354):822–824.
4. Majolino I, Marceno R, Pecoraro G, et al. High-dose therapy and autologous transplantation in amyloidosis-AL. *Haematologica.* 1993;78(1):68–71.
5. Comenzo RL, Vosburgh E, Simms RW, et al. Dose-intensive melphalan with blood stem cell support for the treatment of AL amyloidosis: one-year follow-up in five patients. *Blood.* 1996;88(7):2801–2806.
6. Moreau P, Milpied N, de Faucal P, et al. High-dose melphalan and autologous bone marrow transplantation for systemic AL amyloidosis with cardiac involvement. *Blood.* 1996;87(7):3063–3064.
7. Moreau P, Leblond V, Bourquelot P, et al. Prognostic factors for survival and response after high-dose therapy and autologous stem cell transplantation in systemic AL amyloidosis: a report on 21 patients. *Br J Haematol.* 1998;101(4):766–769.
8. Comenzo RL, Gertz MA. Autologous stem cell transplantation for primary systemic amyloidosis. *Blood.* 2002;99(12):4276–4282.
9. Palladini G, Perfetti V, Obici L, et al. Association of melphalan and high-dose dexamethasone is effective and well tolerated in patients with AL (primary) amyloidosis who are ineligible for stem cell transplantation. *Blood.* 2004;103(8):2936–2938. https://doi.org/10.1182/blood-2003-08-2788. [published Online First: Epub Date].
10. Jaccard A, Moreau P, Leblond V, et al. High-dose melphalan versus melphalan plus dexamethasone for AL amyloidosis. *N Engl J Med.* 2007;357(11):1083–1093. https://doi.org/10.1056/NEJMoa070484. [published Online First: Epub Date].
11. Palladini G, Campana C, Klersy C, et al. Serum N-terminal pro-brain natriuretic peptide is a sensitive marker of myocardial dysfunction in AL amyloidosis. *Circulation.* 2003;107(19):2440–2445. https://doi.org/10.1161/01.CIR.0000068314.02595.B2. [published Online First: Epub Date].
12. Dispenzieri A, Lacy MQ, Katzmann JA, et al. Absolute values of immunoglobulin free light chains are prognostic in patients with primary systemic amyloidosis undergoing peripheral blood stem cell transplantation. *Blood.* 2006;107(8):3378–3383. https://doi.org/10.1182/blood-2005-07-2922. [published Online First: Epub Date].
13. Migrino RQ, Mareedu RK, Eastwood D, Bowers M, Harmann L, Hari P. Left ventricular ejection time on echocardiography predicts long-term mortality in light chain amyloidosis. *J Am Soc Echocardiogr.* 2009;22(12):1396–1402. https://doi.org/10.1016/j.echo.2009.09.012. [published Online First: Epub Date].
14. Kumar S, Dispenzieri A, Lacy MQ, et al. Revised prognostic staging system for light chain amyloidosis incorporating cardiac biomarkers and serum free light chain measurements. *J Clin Oncol.* 2012;30(9):989–995. https://doi.org/10.1200/JCO.2011.38.5724. [published Online First: Epub Date].
15. D'Souza A, Dispenzieri A, Wirk B, et al. Improved outcomes after autologous hematopoietic cell transplantation for light chain amyloidosis: a center for international blood and marrow transplant Research study. *J Clin Oncol.* 2015;33(32):3741–3749. https://doi.org/10.1200/JCO.2015.62.4015. [published Online First: Epub Date].
16. Gertz MA, Lacy MQ, Dispenzieri A, et al. Stem cell transplantation for the management of primary systemic amyloidosis. *Am J Med.* 2002;113(7):549–555.
17. Dhakal B, D'Souza A, Arce-Lara C, et al. Superior efficacy but higher cost of plerixafor and abbreviated-course G-CSF for mobilizing hematopoietic progenitor cells (HPC) in AL amyloidosis. *Bone Marrow Transplant.* 2015;50(4):610–612. https://doi.org/10.1038/bmt.2014.318. [published Online First: Epub Date].
18. Kastritis E, Wechalekar AD, Dimopoulos MA, et al. Bortezomib with or without dexamethasone in primary systemic (light chain) amyloidosis. *J Clin Oncol.* 2010;28(6):1031–1037. https://doi.org/10.1200/JCO.2009.23.8220. [published Online First: Epub Date].

19. Gertz MA, Landau H, Comenzo RL, et al. First-in-Human phase I/II study of NEOD001 in patients with light chain amyloidosis and persistent organ dysfunction. *J Clin Oncol*. 2016;34(10):1097–1103. https://doi.org/10.1200/JCO.2015.63.6530. [published Online First: Epub Date].

20. Landau H, Smith M, Landry C, et al. Long-term event-free and overall survival after risk-adapted melphalan and SCT for systemic light chain amyloidosis. *Leukemia*. 2017;31(1):136–142. https://doi.org/10.1038/leu.2016.229. [published Online First: Epub Date].

21. Kumar S, Dispenzieri A, Lacy MQ, Litzow MR, Gertz MA. High incidence of gastrointestinal tract bleeding after autologous stem cell transplant for primary systemic amyloidosis. *Bone Marrow Transpl*. 2001;28(4):381–385. https://doi.org/10.1038/sj.bmt.1703155. [published Online First: Epub Date].

22. Palladini G, Dispenzieri A, Gertz MA, et al. New criteria for response to treatment in immunoglobulin light chain amyloidosis based on free light chain measurement and cardiac biomarkers: impact on survival outcomes. *J Clin Oncol*. 2012;30(36):4541–4549. https://doi.org/10.1200/JCO.2011.37.7614. [published Online First: Epub Date].

23. D'Souza A, Huang J, Hari P. New light chain amyloid response criteria help risk stratification of patients by day 100 after autologous hematopoietic cell transplantation. *Biol Blood Marrow Transplant*. 2016;22(4):768–770. https://doi.org/10.1016/j.bbmt.2015.12.021. [published Online First: Epub Date].

24. Schonland SO, Lokhorst H, Buzyn A, et al. Allogeneic and syngeneic hematopoietic cell transplantation in patients with amyloid light-chain amyloidosis: a report from the European Group for Blood and Marrow Transplantation. *Blood*. 2006;107(6):2578–2584. https://doi.org/10.1182/blood-2005-06-2462. [published Online First: Epub Date].

25. Gillmore JD, Goodman HJ, Lachmann HJ, et al. Sequential heart and autologous stem cell transplantation for systemic AL amyloidosis. *Blood*. 2006;107(3):1227–1229. https://doi.org/10.1182/blood-2005-08-3253. [published Online First: Epub Date].

26. Gertz MA, Landau HJ, Weiss BM. Organ response in patients with AL amyloidosis treated with NEOD001, an amyloid-directed monoclonal antibody. *Am J Hematol*. 2016;91(12):E506–E508. https://doi.org/10.1002/ajh.24563. [published Online First: Epub Date].

CHAPTER 19

Hematopoietic Stem Cell Transplantation for Rare Hematological Malignancies

SHUKAIB ARSLAN, MD • CHITRA HOSING, MD

INTRODUCTION

In this chapter, we describe the role of hematopoietic stem cell transplant (HSCT) for rare myeloid and lymphoid malignancies (Table 19.1). Owing to the rarity of these disorders, conducting prospective studies may not be possible. We review the literature on the feasibility of autologous HSCT (auto-HSCT) and allogeneic HSCT (allo-HSCT) in these rare disorders and summarize the recommendations based on currently available data.

SYSTEMIC MASTOCYTOSIS

Systemic mastocytosis (SM) is characterized by infiltration of the bone marrow and other organs by malignant mast cells. In the 2016 revision of WHO classification of myeloid neoplasms (Table 19.2), SM is subcategorized into indolent SM (*ISM*; absence of B and C findings), smoldering SM (*SSM*; B findings, no C findings), systemic mastocytosis with an associated hematological neoplasm (*SM-AHN*), aggressive SM (*ASM*; presence of one or more C findings) (Table 19.3), and mast cell leukemia (*MCL*), with >20% malignant mast cells on bone marrow aspirate (Table 19.4). Other forms of mastocytosis are cutaneous mastocytosis and mast cell sarcoma.[5]

Activating mutations in the KIT-gene are almost always present in the malignant mast cells. More than 90–95% of patients with SM have activating mutations in the KIT gene, where valine (V) replaces an aspartate (D) at position 816 of KIT gene (D816V). SM-AHN can have multiple other mutations like TET2, SRSF2, ASXL1, CBL, and RUNX1.[8] Patients with a mutation in one or more of these genes (especially SRSF2, ASXL1, or RUNX1) carry a worse prognosis compared with patients who only have the KIT D816V mutation. In chronic myelomonocytic leukemia (CMML) associated with SM (SM-CMML), neoplastic monocytes usually carry KIT D816V mutation. In other SM-AHNs such as acute myeloid leukemia (SM-AML), leukemic blast cells may lack KIT D816V mutation even when the mast cells carry KIT D816V. Patients with SM-AHN seem to do poorly as compared to patients with respective hematological malignancy alone. A particular association between SM and t(8;21) has been reported.[9,10]

Diagnostic evaluation for SM requires serum tryptase level, immunohistochemistry analysis (Tryptase, CD 117/KIT, CD2, CD25, and CD30), flow cytometry, and KIT mutation analysis. Serum tryptase level is the most useful blood marker to assess response to cytoreductive therapy.

Patients with ISM have a life expectancy comparable to the general population; disease progression to ASM may occur, but it is a rare event. However, in some patients, transformation to SM-AHN or ASM may occur. Median overall survival for ASM, SM-AHN, and MCL is given in Table 19.4.

Tyrosine kinase inhibitors have been studied for SM treatment.[11] Imatinib may have activity in a small minority of SM patients who lack D816V mutation. Dasatinib appears to have some activity (33%–50% overall response rate [ORR]).[12] Midostaurin is a multikinase inhibitor which inhibits both nonmutant KIT and D816V. In an international, multicenter, single-group, open-label, phase 2 study of the efficacy and safety of midostaurin treatment in patients with advanced SM, midostaurin had ORR of 60% (major response, 45%; partial response, 15%) in the primary efficacy population and 46% in the intention-to-treat population. Median duration of response (DOR) was 24.1 months, and median overall survival (OS) was 28.7 months in primary-efficacy population and 33.9 months in intention-to-treat population.[13] Midostaurin is approved by the Food and Drug Administration (FDA) for the treatment of advanced SM.

Hematopoietic Cell Transplantation for Malignant Conditions. https://doi.org/10.1016/B978-0-323-56802-9.00019-5

Nakamura et al. reported outcome of three patients with advanced SM in a prospective study published in 2006.[14] All patients underwent reduced-intensity conditioning (RIC) and HSCT from human leukocyte antigen (HLA)-matched sibling donors (MRDs). These patients included one each with ASM, SM-AHN (MDS), and MCL. All patients achieved complete donor T-cell chimerism with evidence of graft-versus-mast cell (GvMC) effect.

However, no durable remissions were noted, and all patients relapsed. The longest DOR was 39 months in patient with SM-AHN who achieved partial remission (PR). The patient with MCL developed severe symptoms from mediator release on day +3, and acute graft versus host disease (GVHD) with progressive disease. Patient with ASM had only a brief PR. No transplant-related mortality (TRM) was reported. Authors concluded that mast cell degranulation might be triggered during conditioning and engraftment, and although GvMC effect was observed with RIC transplant, a sustained remission was not achieved.[14]

Usten et al. reported outcome of allo-HSCT in 57 patients with advanced SM in a retrospective, multicenter analysis published in 2014.[15] Of these 57 patients, 38 had SM-AHN, seven had ASM, and 12 had MCL. Median age was 46 years (range, 11–67). Donors were HLA-identical (34), unrelated (17), umbilical cord (2), haploidentical (1), or unknown (3). Thirty-six patients received myeloablative conditioning (MAC), and 21 received RIC. ORR was 70%, with complete remission (CR) in 28%. Twenty-one percent had stable disease, and 9% had primary refractory disease. The OS at 3 years was 57% for all patients, 74% for SM-AHN, 43% for ASM, and 17% for MCL. The strongest risk factor for inferior OS was MCL. Survival was also lower in patients receiving RIC than MAC and in patients with progressive disease at transplant.

Usten et al. published a consensus opinion on allo-HSCT in advanced SM in 2016. The recommendation is that patients with SM-AHN should be evaluated for allo-HSCT when indicated for AHN component or when SM component presents with or progresses to advanced SM. Allo-HSCT is not recommended for ISM/SSM or for low-risk AHN-like low-risk MDS, low-risk MPN (CMML-1), chronic eosinophilic leukemia with

TABLE 19.1
Rare Myeloid and Lymphoid Hematological Malignancies[1–4]

Hematological Malignancies	Annual Incidence in the United States
Rare myeloid malignancies:	
Systemic mastocytosis	5–10 per 1000,000
Langerhans cell histiocytosis	0.5–5.4 per 1,000,000
Hypereosinophilic syndrome (myeloproliferative)	0.35 per 1000,000
Chronic myelomonocytic leukemia	3 per 1000,000
Rare lymphoid malignancies:	
Primary central nervous system (CNS) lymphoma	1 per 100,000
Adult T-cell leukemia/lymphoma	0.04 per 100,000
Natural killer cell leukemia/lymphoma	0.49 per 100,000
Cutaneous T-cell lymphoma	0.64 per 100,000
Blastic plasmacytoid dendritic cell neoplasm	—
Hepatosplenic T-cell lymphoma	—
Subcutaneous panniculitic T-cell lymphoma	—

TABLE 19.2
SM is Defined by the Presence of Either One Major and One Minor Criterion or three Minor Criteria[6,7]

WHO Diagnostic Criteria for Systemic Mastocytosis

Major Criterion:
Multifocal, dense infiltrates of mast cells (≥15 mast cells in aggregates) in sections of bone marrow and/or other extracutaneous organ(s)

Minor Criteria:
1. >25% of mast cells are spindle/atypically shaped cells in bone marrow or other extracutaneous organs or >25% of mast cells in bone marrow aspirate are immature or atypical
2. *KIT* point mutation at codon 816 in bone marrow, blood, or other extracutaneous organ(s).
3. Mast cells express CD2 and/or CD25
4. Serum tryptase level persistently >20 ng/mL

WHO, World Health Organization.

platelet-derived growth factor receptor A (PDGFRA) rearrangement, or favorable-risk CLL. Allo-HSCT is recommended for acute MCL as front-line therapy. In patients with chronic myeloid leukemia, evaluation for allo-HSCT is recommended on progression on midostaurin, progression to advanced SM including acute MCL, or if there is evidence of organ dysfunction and/or fibrosis. All patients with ASM should be evaluated for allo-HSCT after careful differentiation from ISM and SSM. Treatment-related hematological complications including persistent pancytopenia in patients with advanced SM may be treated with allo-HSCT. Aggressive induction chemotherapy (±midostaurin)

for remission induction and debulking before allo-HSCT is recommended. For patients with acute MCL and myelomastocytic leukemia, HLA typing, donor search, and discussion about allo-HSCT should be initiated as soon as diagnosis is made. Use of interferon-alpha before allo-HSCT should be avoided as it may be associated with an increased risk of acute GVHD. MAC may be associated with better survival than RIC and is recommended whenever possible. Mast cell degranulation during induction chemotherapy and conditioning with release of mediators may cause varying degrees of reactions; epinephrine should be kept available at the bedside, and EpiPen should be provided to the

---

TABLE 19.3
B and C Findings[7]

B Findings	C Findings
Indication of high mast cell burden:	Indication of organ damage due to infiltration of malignant mast cells:
1. Serum tryptase level >200 ng/mL	1. Cytopenia(s): ANC < 1000/μL or hemoglobin < 10 g/dL or platelets < 100,000/μL
2. Hypercellular marrow with loss of fat cells, discrete signs of dysmyelopoiesis without substantial cytopenias, or WHO criteria for an MDS or MPN	2. Hepatomegaly with ascites and/or impaired liver function
3. Organomegaly: palpable hepatomegaly, splenomegaly, or lymphadenopathy (on CT or ultrasound) greater than 2 cm without impaired organ function	3. Palpable splenomegaly with hypersplenism
	4. Malabsorption with hypo-albuminemia and weight loss
	5. Skeletal lesions: large-sized osteolytic lesion(s) or severe osteoporosis causing pathologic fractures
	6. Life-threatening organopathy in other organ systems that is definitively caused by an infiltration of the tissue by neoplastic mast cells

ANC, absolute neutrophil count; CT, computed tomography; MDS, myelodysplastic syndrome; MPN, myeloproliferative neoplasms; WHO, World Health Organization.

TABLE 19.4
Forms of Advanced Systemic Mastocytosis

Type of Advanced SM	% of SM	Diagnostic Criteria	Median Overall Survival
ASM	5–10	Meets criteria for SM. One or more C findings. No associated clonal hematologic malignancy/disorder. No evidence of mast cell leukemia.	3.5 years
SM-AHN	20–30	Meets criteria for SM as well as for an associated hematologic neoplasm	2 years
MCL	1	Meets criteria for SM. Bone marrow aspirate smears show **20% or more** mast cells or >10% immature mast cells in the peripheral blood. Bone marrow biopsy: high-grade involvement **(>50%)** of the medullary space with sheets of atypical mast cells.	2–6 months

ASM, aggressive systemic mastocytosis; MCL, mast cell leukemia; SM-AHN, systemic mastocytosis with an associated hematological neoplasm.

patients for outpatient use. Prophylactic therapy with H1 and H2 blockers with or without corticosteroids should be standardized during induction and conditioning. Progression of advanced SM occurs in 20% of patients after allo-HSCT; donor lymphocyte infusions (DLIs) may be given for disease progression. Midostaurin maintenance after HSCT may be used in high-risk patients, although data are lacking. Disease burden and response should be monitored with frequent serum tryptase level assessment.[16]

Allo-HSCT remains the only chance to induce durable remission in patients with advanced SM. Adequate debulking should be performed in sensitive disease cases, and cytoreduction should be attempted in relapsed/refractory disease before HSCT.

LANGERHANS CELL HISTIOCYTOSIS

Langerhans cell histiocytosis (LCH) is a group of disorders characterized by a clonal Langerhans cell proliferation, most recently described as a myeloid neoplasm.[17,18] This group of disorders is mostly recognized in infants and young children but can also present in adults. It may present as a single system Langerhans cell histiocytosis (SS-LCH) or multisystem Langerhans cell histiocytosis (MS-LCH). Well-recognized prognostic factors include age (<2 years and >65 years), extent of organ system involvement (SS-LCH vs. MS-LCH), organ dysfunction, and response to initial treatment.[1] Organ systems usually affected by this disorder include skin, bone marrow, skeleton, liver, spleen, and lungs. Some patients may develop secondary hemophagocytic lymphohistiocytosis (HLH). Involvement of bone marrow may cause cytopenias; involvement of liver may cause coagulopathy and portal hypertension with thrombocytopenia; and involvement of the gastrointestinal tract (GI) may cause malabsorption with protein-calorie malnutrition with increased risk of sepsis and death.[19] A comprehensive multisystemic evaluation is recommended at the time of diagnosis to evaluate the extent of organ system involvement.[20]

A classic histopathological feature of LCH is presence of lesional Langerhans cells with macrophages, multinucleated giant cells, T lymphocytes, and eosinophils. A definitive diagnosis is based on the histopathological findings of at least one of the following: (1) positivity for Langerin (CD 207 or CD1a) or (2) the presence of Birbeck granules on electron microscopy. Gene mutations commonly found in this disorder include activating BRAF mutations, ARAF mutations, and somatic MAP2K1 mutations in BRAF-negative patients.[19]

In pediatric age group, 20% of all MS-LCH fall under low risk with no "risk organ" involvement including liver, spleen, lungs, bone marrow, and central nervous system. These patients have an excellent prognosis. Eighty percent of all MS-LCH fall under high risk with one or more 'risk organ' involvement and have a dismal prognosis.[20] A unifocal involvement in SS-LCH could be observed or treated by excision with or without radiation treatment. SS-LCH with multifocal involvement, SS-LCH with critical anatomical sites involvement, and MS-LCH require treatment with systemic therapy. Systemic therapy usually involves a single agent (e.g., cytarabine) except in cases of aggressive presentation.[21]

Kudo et al. reported outcome of 15 children with refractory LCH who underwent allo-HSCT at various institutions in Japan. MAC and RIC were used in 10 and 5 patients, respectively. Ten patients received cord blood graft. There were 11 long-term survivors. Median 10-year OS rate was 73% for all patients and 55% for high-risk group.[22]

The French Langerhans cell study group reported outcomes of eight patients with refractory MS-LCH undergoing HSCT. Out of the three patients who underwent auto-HSCT, two patients died of relapse, and one was alive in CR 7 years later. Of the five patients who underwent MAC allo-HSCT, three died of treatment toxicity, only two patients were alive and in CR, 21 months and 12 years later.[23]

Steiner et al. reported the outcomes of RIC allo-HSCT in nine children with high-risk LCH. Donors included matched siblings and matched unrelated, mismatched unrelated, and haploidentical parents. Three patients undergoing haploidentical HSCT underwent a second transplant for graft failure. Seven out of nine patients were alive without evidence of disease at 390-day median follow-up.[24]

In 2015, Veys et al. analyzed the data from Center for International Blood and Marrow Transplant Research (CIBMTR) and European Society for Blood and Marrow Transplantation (EBMT) for patients who received transplant for refractory MS-LCH between 1990 and 2013. Between 1990 and 1999, 18 patients received MAC HSCT and two patients received RIC HSCT. Between 2000 and 2013, 41 patients received MAC HSCT, and 26 patients received RIC HSCT. They concluded that because of better supportive care, 75% of the patients survived after the year 2000 compared with 28% in the earlier cohort. Relapse rates were slightly higher with RIC than with MAC. This may be explained by inclusion of higher risk LCH patients in RIC HSCT group. Four out of six patients, who relapsed after RIC transplant, obtained a remission with chemotherapy.[19]

TABLE 19.5
Subgroups of CMML Based on Blast Percentage in Peripheral Blood and Bone Marrow

CMML Subgroup	Blasts in Peripheral Blood	Blasts in Bone Marrow
CMML–0	<2%	<5%
CMML–1	2%–4%	5%–9%
CMML–2	5%–19%	10%–19%

CMML–2 is diagnosed with 5%–19% blasts in peripheral blood, 10%–19% blasts in bone marrow, or when any Auer rods are present.

Based on poor prognosis of refractory MS-LCH, allo-HSCT should be considered early in the disease course especially in patients who have available donors. Auto-HSCT may be an option for patients without acceptable donors. In case of allo-HSCT, increased relapse rate is noted with RIC as compared with MAC. Alternative donor transplant may be an option for patients with refractory MS-LCH who do not have HLA matched donors available.

CHRONIC MYELOMONOCYTIC LEUKEMIA

Chronic myelomonocytic leukemia (CMML) is a clonal stem cell disorder that is characterized by peripheral blood monocytosis. Median age at diagnosis is 65–75 years with a male predominance. Overall prognosis is poor with median survival of only 12 months.[1]

According to 2016 revision of WHO classification, a diagnosis of CMML requires both the presence of persistent peripheral blood monocytosis (≥1000/dL) and monocytes accounting for ≥10% of the white blood cell differential count. CMML is further subdivided into proliferative type (CMML–MP; WBC ≥ 13,000/dL) and dysplastic type (CMML-MD; WBC < 13,000/dL) based on the differences related to aberrancies in the RAS/ (mitogen-activated protein kinase (MAPK) signaling pathways.[5] Blast percentage has a critical prognostic value (Table 19.5).

BCR-ABL1 rearrangement should be excluded in all cases. PDGFRA, platelet-derived growth factor receptor B (PDGFRB), fibroblast growth factor receptor 1 (FGFR1) rearrangements, or Pericentriolar material 1–Janus Kinase 2 (PCM1-JAK2) fusions should be excluded if eosinophilia is present.[5] Cytogenetic abnormalities are present in only 25%–30% of the patients, and among these, the most common being trisomy 8, loss of Y chromosome, monosomy 7, and complex karyotype. Somatic mutations are almost always present; most

TABLE 19.6
Variables and Scores Used for Predicting Likelihood of Survival and Leukemic Transformation in the Individual Patient With CMML Obtained by CPSS

	VARIABLE SCORES		
Variables	0	1	2
WHO subtype	CMML-1 blasts: 2%–4% in PB, and 5%–9% in BM	CMML-2 blasts: 5%–19% in PB and 10%–19% in BM or presence of Auer rods	–
FAB subtype	CMML-MD: WBC < 13,000/dL	CMML-MP: WBC ≥ 13,000/dL	
CMML-specific cytogenetic risk stratification	Low	Intermediate	High
RBC transfusion dependency	No	Yes	–

CMML-specific cytogenetic risk stratification: Low, normal and isolated–Y; intermediate, other abnormalities; high, trisomy 8, chromosome 7 abnormalities, and complex karyotype.
RBC transfusion dependency was defined as requiring 1 unit of RBCs every 8 weeks over a period of 4 months.[27]
BM, bone marrow; *CMML*, chronic myelomonocytic leukemia; *CMML-MD*, chronic myelomonocytic leukemia–dysplastic type; *CMML-MP*, chronic myelomonocytic leukemia–proliferative type; *CPSS*, CMML-specific prognostic scoring system; *FAB*, French-American-British; *PB*, peripheral blood; *RBC*, red blood cell; *WBC*, white blood cell; *WHO*, World Health Organization.

frequent ones are TET2, SRSF2, and ASXL1.[4] Other mutations found in CMML include RUNX1 (frequent thrombocytopenia), DNMT3A, SETBP1, NRAS (mostly in CMML-MP), KRAS, and CBL.[25]

CMML is incurable with conventional chemotherapy, and allo-HSCT is a potentially curative therapy, although offered to relatively small number of patients as most patients are over 70 years of age at diagnosis.[25]

In 2017, Liu et al. reported outcomes of allo-HSCT from CIBMTR data in patients with CMML from 2001 to 2012. Median age at HSCT was 57 years. Sixty-seven percent of patients had CMML-1, and 25% patients had CMML-2. Donor type was as follows: (1) MRD, 35%; (2) matched unrelated donor (MUD), 45%; (3) partially matched unrelated, 15%; and (4) mismatched unrelated (MMUD), 2%. Fifty percent patients received MAC, and 48% patients received RIC. CMML-specific prognostic scoring system (CPSS) (Table 19.6), Karnofsky performance status (KPS), and graft source were significant predictors of survival. Patients with intermediate-2/high-risk disease had a nearly twofold increased risk of death after relapse compared with those with low/intermediate-1 CPSS scores. One-year, 3-year, and 5-year survival rates for low/intermediate-1 risk subjects were 61%, 48%, and 44% and those for intermediate-2/high-risk subjects were 38%, 32%, and 19%, respectively. Authors concluded that higher CPSS score at the time of HSCT, lower KPS, and bone marrow graft were associated with inferior survival after HSCT.[26]

In 2015, Symeonidis et al. reported that achievement of CR predicted outcome of allo-HSCT in patients with CMML in a study of Chronic Malignancies Working Party of the EBMT. They reported outcome of allo-HSCT in 513 patients with CMML (including patients with secondary acute myelogenous leukemia [AML]). The median age of patients was 53 years. For transplant conditioning, 52.4% patients received MAC, 47.6% patients received RIC HSCT, 53.8% patients received MRD, 20.7% patients received MUD, and 23.8% patients received MMUD HSCT. At the time of HSCT, 26.2% patients were in CR, 46.4% patients had relapsed/refractory disease, and 27.4% patients were untreated. CMML subgroups included as follows: 39.9% with CMML-MD, 60.1% with CMML-MP, 40.7% with CMML-1, and 15% with CMML-2. The study included 44.3% patients with secondary AML. Grades 2–4 acute GVHD was reported in 33% cases, and chronic GVHD was reported in 24%. A 4-year estimated relapse-free survival was 27%, and OS was 33%. Patients undergoing HSCT in CR had lower probability of nonrelapse death and longer relapse-free OS. Only significant prognostic factor for survival was the presence of CR at HSCT.[28]

In 2016 Kongtim et al. reported outcomes of 83 patients with CMML who received allo-HSCT at a single institution. Median age at transplant was 57 years. Out of these 83 patients, 47 patients had CMML-1/2, and 36 patients had CMML with progression to AML. Seventy-eight patients had received induction therapy before HSCT. This included 37 patients who received hypo-methylating agents, and 41 received cytotoxic chemotherapy. The incidence of relapse at 3 years after HSCT for patients receiving hypomethylating agent was 22%, which was significantly lower than that for patients who received other agents (35%). This lower relapse rate resulted in significantly higher 3-year PFS rate in patients receiving hypomethylating agents (43%) than that in those treated with other agents (27%). These data supported the use of hypomethylating agents before allo-HSCT for patients with CMML to achieve morphologic remission and improve PFS for these patients.[29]

Allo-HSCT should be considered early in the management of patients with CMML who have suitable donors. Improved outcomes with RIC in older age group with other conditions enforce the need of exploring this option for more elderly patients with CMML. Comorbidity is a strong predictor of outcome and should be taken into account for selection of patients for this treatment modality. Patients with lower CPSS score and higher KPS should be referred early for HSCT evaluation. Use of hypomethylating agents for remission induction should be preferred over the use of other agents before HSCT.

HYPEREOSINOPHILIC SYNDROME

Hypereosinophilic syndrome (HES) is a group of heterogeneous disorders and is characterized by eosinophilia with a tendency to cause organ damage, most commonly endomyocardial fibrosis, leading to cardiac dysfunction, which is one of the leading causes of morbidity and mortality. Eosinophilia is usually defined by peripheral blood eosinophil count of >1500/dL. HES has myeloid and lymphoid variants. In 2016 revision of WHO classification of myeloid neoplasms, eosinophilia-related disorders associated with specific molecular genetic changes are included in the classification (Table 19.7).[5]

The outcomes of allo-HSCT for HES are limited to only few case reports. Cooper at al. summarized 13 of such case reports in 2005. Out of these 13 cases, nine patients underwent MRD HSCT, and four patients underwent MUD HSCT. Majority of the cases underwent MAC, and only a few patients received RIC. Disease-free survival of up to 6 years was described in one patient.[31]

In 2014, Fathi et al. described a case of idiopathic HES, with gastrointestinal and cardiac involvement, who received MUD-HSCT with RIC. Alemtuzumab was administered with conditioning chemotherapy to deplete eosinophils and to provide added protection against GVHD.[30]

Eosinophilia can recur in a few cases even after obtaining 100% bone marrow and peripheral blood donor chimerism.[31] This usually resolves spontaneously. Abnormal T cells may persist in lymphoid organs, as suggested by high interleukin-5 levels detected in some patients and may lead to eosinophilia, which resolves after complete donor chimerism is achieved in lymphoid organs.

Chockalingham et al., in 1999, reported a case of refractory HES with cardiac dysfunction who had improvement in cardiac function after allo-HSCT.[32]

TABLE 19.7

Molecular Genetic Abnormalities in Myeloid/Lymphoid Neoplasms Associated With Eosinophilia, Their Presentation, and Treatment[5,30]

Disease	Presentation	Genetics	Treatment
PDGFRA	Eosinophilia; increased serum tryptase level; increased marrow mast cells	Cryptic deletion at 4q12; FIP1L1–PDGFRA, at least 66 other partners	Responds to TKI
PDGFRB	Eosinophilia; monocytosis	T(5;15) (q32;p13.2) ETV6-PDG-FRB, at least 25 other partners	Responds to TKI
FGFR 1	Eosinophilia; often presents with T-ALL or AML	Translocations of 8p11.2; FGFR 1—various partners	Poor prognosis; do not respond to TKI
PCM1–JAK2	Eosinophilia; rarely presents with T-LBL or B-ALL Bone marrow shows left shifted erythroid predominance and lymphoid aggregates	T(8;9) (p22;p24.1) PCM1–JAK2	May respond to JAK2 inhibitors
CEL-NOS	Persistent eosinophilia with evidence of a clonal myeloid proliferation (abnormal karyotype, increased blasts, or morphologic dysplasia)	No rearrangements of PDGF RA, PDGF RB, FGFR1, or BCR-ABL 1	

CEL-NOS, chronic eosinophilic leukemia not otherwise specified; *FGFR1*, fibroblast growth factor receptor 1; *JAK2*, Janus Kinase 2; *PCM1*, pericentriolar material 1; *PDGFRA*, platelet-derived growth factor receptor A; *PDGFRB*, platelet-derived growth factor receptor B; *TKI*, tyrosine kinase inhibitors.

Bergua et al. describe the case of resolution of left and right ventricular thrombosis secondary to HES with RIC allo-HSCT.[33]

Although responsiveness of FIP1L1-PDGFR rearrangement–positive cases to imatinib therapy is superior, PDGFRA/B rearrangement–negative cases usually do not respond well to imatinib treatment. As prognosis of PDGFR A/B rearrangement–negative patients who develop organ dysfunction is poor, allo-HSCT should be considered in suitable patients who have early signs of organ damage and have failed standard therapy.[1]

PRIMARY CENTRAL NERVOUS SYSTEM LYMPHOMA

Primary central nervous system lymphoma (PCNSL) is a rare form of non-Hodgkin's lymphoma (NHL) accounting for 1%–2% of all NHL cases and 4% of primary CNS tumors.[1,34] It is an aggressive malignancy, with a median survival, if untreated, of approximately 3 months. The incidence is increasing in both immunocompetent and immunocompromised individuals. PCNSL is usually found as unifocal or multifocal periventricular parenchymal masses. Ocular involvement, at the time of diagnosis, may be present in 10%–20% of the patients. Median age at diagnosis is 60 years. On histology, over 90% of

PCNSLs are diffuse large B cell lymphomas (DLBCL), and 2%–4% are of T-cell origin. PCNSLs tend to be Epstein-Barr virus (EBV) positive in immunocompromised patients; in contrast, EBV has no role in the pathogenesis of PCNSLs in immunocompetent patients.[1]

Whole brain irradiation (WBRT) is associated with quick response but with significant toxicity including neurotoxicity and leukoencephalopathy. Combination immune-chemotherapy regimens that use agents such as high-dose methotrexate, Ara-C, thioTEPA, ifosfamide, mitoxantrone, and vincristine with or without rituximab are used for induction treatment with good responses. Neurotoxicity resulting from chemotherapy and WBRT is one of the leading causes of morbidity in survivors especially in elderly people who comprise a major subset of population with this diagnosis (>60% are diagnosed at age >60 years). Studies of auto-HSCT either as consolidation treatment or in relapsed setting have shown good responses. This strategy has helped to reduce the use of WBRT, thus minimizing morbidity with neurotoxicity.[1,34]

In 2017 Atilla et al. reported outcomes of 13 PCNSL patients analyzed in a retrospective manner. Mean age was 51.6 years. Nine patients underwent auto-HSCT. Conditioning regimen for auto-HSCT included cyclophosphamide, etoposide, and carmustine. Eighty-nine percent of the patients who underwent HSCT remained in CR on follow-up. One patient, who relapsed, underwent allo-HSCT.[34]

In 2016, Cho H et al. retrospectively analyzed the role of upfront auto-HSCT in 66 high-risk (International Extranodal Lymphoma Study Group (IELSG) prognostic score ≥ 2) younger (<65 years) patients with PCNSL who achieved at least a PR after initial high-dose methotrexate–based chemotherapy. Nineteen patients received upfront auto-HSCT. These patients had significantly better OS and PFS than patients who did not receive an upfront auto-HSCT. Authors concluded that upfront auto-HSCT consolidation might especially be beneficial for high-risk PCNSL patients.[35]

In 2015, Madle et al. retrospectively analyzed outcome of 81 PCNSL patients and concluded that rituximab treatment, auto-HSCT, and age were independent prognostic factors for OS in the first-line treatment of PCNSL. Among patients treated with rituximab (n = 27), 3-year OS was 77.8%, in contrast to 39.9% in patients treated without rituximab (n = 52). Among younger patients (≤60 years, n = 28), 3-year OS was 78.2% as compared with 38.7% in older patients (>60 years, n = 51). The 3-year OS in patients who received high-dose therapy and auto-HSCT was 85.2% as compared with 35.2% in patients who did not receive HSCT.[36]

Some studies have used a response-adapted WBRT approach in patients with PCNSL using WBRT only in patients who fail to achieve CR after auto-HSCT. In 2011, Yoon et al. reported outcomes of 11 patients with PCNSL who underwent auto-HSCT with conditioning regimen consisting of busulfan, cyclophosphamide, and etoposide. Two patients failed to achieve CR after HSCT and underwent WBRT. Six patients relapsed. Median PFS was 15 months, with 2-year PFS of 30.3% and OS of 88.9%.[37]

In 2011, Kiefer et al. reported outcomes of long-term follow-up of high-dose chemotherapy with auto-HSCT and response-adapted WBRT for 23 patients with newly diagnosed PCNSL. Patients refractory to induction or without CR after auto-HSCT received WBRT. On long-term follow-up, eight patients were alive with a median follow-up of 116.9 months. Only one of nine irradiated patients was still alive with severe neurologic deficit. Ten-year OS of 35% with excellent neurocognitive functioning was found in patients who did not receive WBRT.

High-dose chemotherapy with auto-HSCT has been studied as salvage therapy for patients with relapsed or refractory PCNSL. In 2012, Soussain et al. retrospectively analyzed the outcome of 79 patients with relapsed/refractory PCNSL with a median age of 52.4 years who received auto-HSCT with conditioning consisting of busulfan, cyclophosphamide, and thioTEPA. With a median follow-up of 56 months, 5-year OS was 51%, and 5-year EFS was 37.8% in the whole population. A 5-year OS was 62%, and 5-year EFS was 43.7% among patients who were chemosensitive to salvage therapy.[38]

In 2017, Kasenda et al. reported outcomes of prospective multicenter trial using high-dose chemotherapy, followed by auto-HSCT for 39 patients with relapsed or refractory PCNSL with a median age of 57 years. Conditioning regimen consisted of rituximab, carmustine, and thioTEPA. Patients, who did not achieve CR after auto-HSCT, underwent WBRT. Twenty-two patients responded to induction treatment, and 32 patients underwent auto-HSCT. CR was achieved by 56.4% of patients after auto-HSCT. Median PFS on the study was 12.4 months. Median OS was not reached. A 2-year PFS rate was 46.0%, and a 2-year OS rate was 56.4%. Four treatment-related deaths were reported. Authors concluded that thioTEPA-based auto-HSCT is an effective treatment option in eligible patients with relapsed or refractory PCNSL.[39]

High-dose immune-chemotherapy with auto-HSCT carries a low treatment-related mortality, at least in patients younger than 65 years, and should be offered as frontline therapy to eligible patients with chemosensitive PCNSL.[1] A reduced dose of WBRT can be offered after HSCT with little short-term neurotoxicity, though it is not clear if high-dose chemotherapy will allow for complete elimination of WBRT. Full-dose WBRT should be reserved for patients only with incomplete response or persistent disease after auto-HSCT. Use of conditioning regimen with agents that have better CNS penetration, such as busulfan and thioTEPA, seems to be superior to conventional lymphoma regimens such as BEAM (carmustine, etoposide, Ara–C, melphalan). Auto-HSCT may have a role as salvage treatment for patients with relapsed/refractory PCNSL after initial high-dose chemoradiotherapy, although neurotoxicity appears to be high in this setting.[1] Use of rituximab in high-dose induction immune-chemotherapy has shown to improve outcomes.

ADULT T-CELL LEUKEMIA/LYMPHOMA

Adult T-cell leukemia/lymphoma (ATLL) refers to a clinicopathological syndrome which is characterized by presence of leukemic cells with typical flower-like nuclei in blood, lymph nodes, and skin lesions; an elevated serum LDH; hypercalcemia; and organ involvement including GI tract, lungs, CNS, reticuloendothelial system.[1] It is specifically associated with infection with human T-cell lymphotropic virus type I (HTLV-1) which is endemic in parts of Japan, Africa, Middle East, and South America. The classification divides this heterogeneous disease into subgroups: (1) acute, (2) lymphoma, (3) chronic, and (4) smoldering types; the chronic subtype is further segregated into favorable and unfavorable types based on serum LDH, BUN, and serum albumin levels. ATLL can be broadly subdivided into two categories: (1) indolent and (2) aggressive types. Indolent ATLL includes favorable chronic and smoldering types, and aggressive type includes acute, lymphoma, and unfavorable chronic types. The Ann Arbor staging system (I–II vs. III–IV), Eastern Cooperative Oncology Group (ECOC) performance status (0–1 vs. 2–4), age, serum albumin, and soluble interleukin-2 receptor (sIL-2R) are identified as independent prognostic factors in patients with acute and lymphoma ATLL. Treatment for indolent-type ATLL includes observation with watchful waiting, interferon-alpha, and zidovudine and skin-directed therapy including topical steroids, radiation, and UV light. Treatment of aggressive-type ATLL or progression of indolent ATLL to aggressive ATLL includes induction with multi-agent chemotherapy ± immunotherapy with mogamulizumab, an antibody to chemokine receptor 4. Induction therapy is followed by consolidation with allo-HSCT with MAC or RIC.[40]

Several studies have reviewed the outcomes of HSCT in patients with aggressive-type ATLL. Results of auto-HSCT in ATLL are not satisfactory, so most of the studies evaluated the role of allo-HSCT.

In 2017, Fuji et al. attempted to develop a modified prognostic index for patients with aggressive ATLL, 70 years or younger, for risk-adapted management strategies including allo-HSCT. A total of 1792 patients aged <70 years, diagnosed with aggressive ATLL, who received intensive first-line chemotherapy were included in the study. Five independent adverse prognostic factors including acute type, poor performance status, sIL-2R levels (>5000 U/mL), high adjusted calcium levels (≥12 mg/dL), and high C-reactive protein levels (≥2.5 mg/dL) were used to segregate patients into low-, intermediate-, and high-risk groups. Median OS for the respective risk groups was 626, 322, and 197 days. In the intermediate- and high-risk groups, patients who received HSCT had significantly better OS than patients who did not undergo HSCT. Authors concluded that patients with aggressive ATLL who are younger than 70 years should be evaluated for allo-HSCT if they fall into intermediate- and high-risk groups.[41]

In 2007, Okamura et al. reported outcomes of a prospective study of allo-HSCT with RIC in elderly patients with ATLL (>50 years). Fourteen patients achieved complete donor chimerism. OS was 35% at 5 years. The HTLV-1 proviral load became undetectable in 8 out of 15 patients. This suggested graft-versus-leukemia and graft-versus-virus effect. This study indicated that RIC allo-HSCT is a feasible option to achieve long-term survival in elderly patients with aggressive ATLL.[42]

In 2005, Fukushima et al. reported outcomes of 40 patients with acute or lymphoma-type ATLL who underwent allo-HSCT at seven institutions in Japan between 1997 and 2002. Thirty-nine patients received MAC. Donors included Matched related donors (MRD) in 27 patients, Mismatched related donors (MMRD) in five patients, and matched unrelated donors (MUD) in eight patients. All evaluable patients entered CR after allo-HSCT. The estimated 3-year OS was 45.3%. The estimated 3-year relapse-free survival was 33.8%, and disease relapse was 39.3%. Three out of 10 patients who relapsed achieved remission by reduction in immunosuppression suggestive of GVL effect.[43]

In 2012, Ishida et al. reported outcomes of 586 patients who underwent allo-HSCT at several institutions in Japan. The 3-year OS was 36%. The 3-year OS rates were 39% for MAC and 34% for RIC. In a multivariate analysis, poor prognostic features for OS included older age, male gender, active disease, poor performance status, and use of unrelated donors. There was no significant difference in OS between MAC and RIC. Of the 174 patients who received cord blood grafts, the 3-year OS was only 21%. For patients not in CR at the time of allo-HSCT, a higher sIL-2R level was associated with poor outcome.[44]

ATLL patients who relapse after allo-HSCT or have progressive disease have a high mortality rate and present a serious therapeutic challenge. In 2013 Itonaga et al. reported outcomes of 35 patients with relapsed or progressive disease after allo-HSCT. CR was achieved in seven patients by either withdrawing immunosuppression or by use of DLI in combination with cytoreductive therapy. DLI-induced remissions were durable with the 3-year OS of 19.3%. This suggests that strategies to augment GVL effect are likely to improve HSCT outcomes.[45]

There has been an interesting observation of viral clearance after allo-HSCT from seropositive or seronegative donors. This, probably, is mediated by donor-derived cytotoxic T-cell response to viral epitopes resulting in viral clearance.[1] Donor-derived ATLL has been reported. Its precise incidence is not known. It is not clear if HTLV-1 seronegative unrelated donors should be preferred over seropositive matched siblings.

There is a concern that pretransplant mogamulizumab increases the risk of severe and steroid-refractory GVHD after HSCT increasing nonrelapse mortality. This seems to be secondary to effects of mogamulizumab on immune reconstitution after allo-HSCT. Mogamulizumab depletes regulatory T cells for few months after HSCT which may increase the risk of GVHD.[46]

Allo-HSCT is the only treatment modality currently available which offers long-term survival in patients with aggressive ATLL. Risk stratification seems to be important in patients with aggressive ATLL to select patients for frontline evaluation for allo-HSCT. Patients aged <70 years who fall in intermediate- or high-risk group should be offered allo-HSCT. Allo-HSCT with RIC should be considered for elderly patients. There seems to be no significant difference between RIC and MAC allo-HSCT. If disease relapse occurs after allo-HSCT, withdrawal of immunosuppression and/or DLI should be considered.

NK CELL NEOPLASMS

NK cell neoplasms include extra-nodal NK/T-cell lymphoma, nasal type, and aggressive NK cell leukemia. NK/T-cell lymphomas almost exclusively arise in extra-nodal sites and are more common in Asian and South American population. They may involve skin and GI tract and testes in 20% of cases. Involvement of peripheral blood is frequently found, which is referred to as aggressive NK cell leukemia/lymphoma. The absence of EBV excludes the diagnosis of NK/T-cell lymphoma. However, EBV is required, but not adequate for the diagnosis. Either CD 56 or cytotoxic molecules (granzyme B, perforin, TIA 1) must be present. Deletion of chromosome 6q is common. Most common somatic gene mutations identified in NK/T-cell lymphoma include DDX3X, JAK3, STAT3, STAT5B, TP53, or K-RAS. Aggressive NK-cell leukemia/lymphoma is a very rare NK/T-cell malignancy. It usually presents with fever, lymphadenopathy, rash, hepatosplenomegaly, elevated ferritin level, and pancytopenia. Hemophagocytosis is often found. There is usually high expression of multidrug-resistant P-glycoprotein on NK lymphoma cells, rendering these malignancies resistant to chemotherapy. Treatment for stage I/II NK/T-cell lymphoma include radiotherapy and/or chemotherapy. Combination chemotherapy using non-anthracycline agents is the standard of care for management of newly diagnosed advanced stage NK/T-cell lymphoma. Patients with relapsed disease or systemic disease at presentation have a poorer outcome.[1,47] Aggressive NK cell leukemia (ANKL) as a median survival of only 2 months.[48]

The role of both auto- and allo-HSCT has been evaluated in the management of NK/T-cell lymphomas and has been reported in case reports and small retrospective studies.

In 2015, Yhim et al. retrospectively analyzed outcomes of 62 patients with NK/T-cell lymphoma who received auto-HSCT after initial chemotherapy. Median age was 45.5 years. Thirty-one patients in the advanced stage, and 61.3% patients were in CR at the time of auto-HSCT. After auto-HSCT, 78.3% of all patients achieved a CR (65.5% for advanced stage, and 90.3% for early stage disease). With a median follow-up of 43.3 months, the 3-year OS and PFS were 60% and 52.4%, respectively. For early stage disease, the 3-year OS and PFS were 67.6% and 64.5%, respectively, and for advanced stage disease, OS and PFS were 52.3% and 40.1%, respectively. Radiotherapy was an independent prognostic factor for reduced progression and survival in patients with limited disease, and anthracycline-based chemotherapy was a poor prognostic factor for progression in patients with advanced disease. Authors concluded that upfront auto-ASCT is an active treatment for patients with extra-nodal NK/T-cell lymphoma responding to initial therapy.[49]

In 2009, Kwong et al. reported an analysis of 57 patients. There was no benefit of auto-HSCT in cases of relapsed/refractory NK cell lymphomas.[50]

EBV DNA level in peripheral blood has been shown to be a marker of disease burden and may prove to be useful in Monitoring response to chemotherapy and selecting Patients for Auto-HSCT in CR1.[1]

In 2005, Murashige et al. reported outcomes on 28 patients with NK cell neoplasms who underwent allo-HSCT. Of these 28 patients, 22 patients had extra-nodal NK/T-cell lymphoma, three patients had blastic NK cell lymphoma, and three patients had ANKL. Twelve patients were chemosensitive, and 16 were chemotherapy refractory. Twenty-two patients received MRD HSCT. Conditioning regimen was MAC in 23 patients and RIC in five patients. With a median follow-up of 34 months, the 2-year PFS and OS were 34% and 40%, respectively. Patients who did not relapse within 10 months after allo-HSCT remained free of disease. In a multivariate analysis, stem cell source, age, and diagnosis significantly affected PFS.[51]

In 2017, Hamadani et al. reported outcome of 21 patients with ANKL who underwent allo-HSCT using CIBMTR database. Median age was 45 years. Sixty-seven percent of patients were in CR at the time of allo-HSCT. The 2-year estimates of non-relapse mortality (NRM), relapse/progression, PFS, and OS were 21%, 59%, 20%, and 24%, respectively. The 2-year PFS of patients in CR at the time of allo-HSCT was significantly better than that of patients with active disease at transplant (30% vs. 0%); the 2-year OS was 38% and 0%, respectively. This study concluded that allo-HSCT could provide durable disease control in a subset of patients with ANKL. CR at the time of HSCT appears to be a strong predictor of survival after allo-HSCT.[48]

Results of allo-HSCT seem to be better when L-asparaginase-containing regimens are used. In 2014, Tse et al. reported the outcome of 18 patients with NK cell lymphoma who underwent allo-HSCT. At the time of transplant, nine patients were in CR 1, seven in CR 2, one in PR, and 1 with progressive disease. Fourteen patients received MAC, and four patients received RIC. With a median follow-up of 20.5 months, the 5-year OS was 57%, and 5-year DFS was 1%. The use of SMILE regimen (steroid [dexamethasone], methotrexate, ifosfamide, L-asparaginase, and etoposide) pretransplant was the most important positive prognostic indicator, resulting in significantly superior OS and PFS. CR 1 and CR 2 patients had similar survivals, but all patients who were not transplanted in remission died. Type of conditioning regimen did not affect survival. Authors concluded that although allo-HSCT leads to a reasonable survival for NK/T-cell lymphoma patients, results need to be compared with those in patients receiving L-asparaginase-containing regimens. Circulating EBV DNA may be used to identify high-risk patients who may benefit from allo-HSCT.[52]

Based on the aforementioned data, for extra-nodal NK/T-cell lymphoma with advanced-stage disease, auto-HSCT should be considered as consolidation therapy for patients in CR after chemotherapy. Auto-HSCT has no role in refractory nasal-type extra-nodal NK/T-cell lymphoma or ANKL, and these patients should be strongly considered and evaluated for allo-HSCT. In cases of systemic NK cell malignancies, major obstacle to allo-HSCT seems to be comorbidity from cytokine release from paraneoplastic phenomenon along with hepatic dysfunction. There is an evidence of GVL effect. Monitoring EBV DNA in peripheral blood may help with the selection of patients for HSCT as well as monitoring of minimal residual disease after HSCT.[1]

BLASTIC PLASMACYTOID DENDRITIC CELL NEOPLASM

Blastic plasmacytoid dendritic cell neoplasm (BPDCN), a rare hematological malignancy, is derived from precursors of plasmacytoid dendritic cells, usually involves skin and bone marrow and has a very aggressive clinical course, with a median survival of only a few month. Bone marrow involvement may cause cytopenias. Patients may also present with leptomeningeal involvement, lymphadenopathy, and splenomegaly. Circulating tumor cells can be detected by flow cytometry. Neoplastic cells express CD4, CD43, CD45RA, and CD56, as well as plasmacytoid dendritic cell-associated antigens CD 123 (IL3RA), BDCA–2, TCL 1, and CTLA1. Cytogenetic abnormalities are usually detected in BPDCN

and include deletions on chromosomes 5q21 or 5q34, 12p13, 13q13–q 21, 6q23, 15q, and 9. Genetic alterations may involve following genes: (1) RB1, (2) LATS2, (3) CDKN1B, (4) CDKN2A, and (5) TP53. Patients with isolated cutaneous disease undergo treatment with surgical resection, focal radiation therapy, and systemic steroids. These therapies may be initially effective, but there is high rate of relapse with no significant long-term benefit. Systemic approaches are recommended. Patients are usually treated with induction chemotherapy regimens that are used for acute leukemias.[53]

Because BPDCN blasts over express CD 123 which is an interleukin-3 receptor (IL3R), the activity of SL-401(diptheria toxin fused to IL3), was evaluated in BPDCN patients in a phase 1-2 study. Eleven patients were treated with a single course of SL-401 for up to 5 doses. Three patients who had initial responses to SL-401 received a second course in relapse. Seven of 9 evaluable (78%) BPDCN patients had major responses including 5 CRs and 2 PRs after a single course of SL-401.[53a]

In 2013, Pagano et al. reported a series of 43 patients with BPDCN treated at 28 Italian centers. Forty-one patients received an induction therapy; 60% patients received AML-type regimen, and 35% patients received acute lymphoblastic leukemia (ALL)-type regimen. Fourteen percent of patients underwent allo-HSCT. Patients were treated with ALL regimens had a significantly higher CR rate and OS than dose treated with an AML regimen. The median OS of allo-HSCT recipients was 22.7 months, and these patients had a significant survival advantage on the patients who did not undergo HSCT.[54]

In 2013, Roos-Weil et al. reported outcomes of 39 patients with BPDCN who underwent auto-HSCT or allo-HSCT from EBMT Registry. Thirty-four patients underwent allo-HSCT, and five patients underwent auto-HSCT. MAC was used in 74% of the patients. Fifty-six percent patients on allo-HSCT arm received HSCT in CR1. The 3-year cumulative incidence of relapse, DFS, and OS was 32%, 33%, and 41%, respectively. By univariate comparison, CR1 at allo-HSCT favorably influenced survival, whereas age, donor source, and chronic GVHD had no significant impact. The authors concluded that high-dose therapy followed by allo-HSCT from related or unrelated donors could provide durable remissions even in elderly patients with BPDCN.[55]

In 2015, Aoki et al. reported outcomes of 25 patients with BPDCN who underwent auto-HSCT or allo-HSCT. Fourteen patients received allo-HSCT, whereas 11 received auto-HSCT. Median age at HSCT was 58 years. All 11 patients who underwent auto-HSCT were in CR1. With a median follow-up of 53.5 months, the OS rates at 4 years for patients who underwent auto-HSCT and allo-HSCT were 82% and 53%, respectively, and PFS rates were 73% and 48%, respectively. The authors concluded that auto-HSCT in CR1 provides long-term remission in BPDCN patients, and RIC and MAC allo-HSCT results are comparable.[56]

Based on the aforementioned data, allo-HSCT performed in CR 1 offers the best chance of long-term survival. Relapse rates are high in patients undergoing HSCT with active disease. Auto-HSCT may be an option in selected patients for consolidation in CR 1.

HEPATOSPLENIC T-CELL LYMPHOMA

Hepatosplenic T-cell lymphoma (HSTCL) is a rare but aggressive T-cell lymphoma which involves sinusoids of liver, red pulp of spleen, and sinuses of the bone marrow causing marked hepatosplenomegaly and cytopenias. Most cases are of gamma/delta T-cell type.

Gamma/delta T-cell–type HSTCL is usually described in patients who are on immunosuppressive therapy for inflammatory bowel disease or solid organ transplantation and patients with rheumatological disorders treated with TNF-alpha inhibitors. Cytogenetic abnormalities include isochromosome 17 and trisomy 8. Neoplastic T cells are usually CD4 and CD8 negative. HSTCL is usually chemotherapy refractory.[57]

In 2015, Rashidi et al. retrospectively analyzed the outcome of 54 patients with HSTCL from Europe and North America. Median age was 34 years. Gamma/delta subtype was present in 87% of the patients. The disease was stage IV at diagnosis in 93% of the patients. The disease status at the time of allo-HSCT was CR in 41%, PR in 43%, and progressive disease in 16% of the patients. The donor was MRD in 53%, MUD in 33%, haploidentical in 8%, and cord blood in 6%. Seventy percent patients received MAC, and 30% patients received RIC. Overall, 35% of the 44 patients with known outcome relapsed at a median of 4 months after HSCT. There were no relapses reported 1.5 years after HSCT. The median RFS and OS were 18 and 68 months, respectively. The estimated 3-year RFS and OS were 42% and 56%, respectively. The authors concluded that as many as 40% of the patients with HSTCL who underwent allo-HSCT have durable RFS. Active disease at the time of HSCT did not predict poorer outcomes.[57]

In 2014, Tanase et al. reported results of 76 patients with HSTCL from EBMT lymphoma working party who underwent allo- or auto-HSCT. The final analysis was available for 25 patients. Out of these, 18 patients underwent allo-HSCT, and seven underwent auto-HSCT. With a median follow-up of 36 months, two patients relapsed after allo-HSCT, resulting in a 3-year PFS of 48%. Five patients relapsed and subsequently died after auto-HSCT. The authors concluded that GVL

effect resulting from allo-HSCT could lead to long-term survival in a subset of patients with HSTCL.[58]

Upfront allo-HSCT seems to be the treatment of choice in patients with HSTCL, preferably after inducing remission with chemotherapy or antibody-based therapy.

SUBCUTANEOUS PANNICULITIC T-CELL LYMPHOMA

Subcutaneous panniculitic T-cell lymphoma (SPTCL) mostly affects young adults, usually, presents with subcutaneous nodules. Patients may have a hemophagocytic syndrome. The panniculitic T-cell lymphomas (TCLs) consists of two distinct subtypes, alpha-beta subcutaneous panniculitis-like TCL and gamma-delta cutaneous TCL with pannicular involvement.[59]

There are individual case reports for both auto-HSCT and allo-HSCT for SPTCL.

Gibson et al. reported outcome of 14 patients who underwent HSCT. Four patients had alpha-beta subtype, and 10 patients had gamma-delta subtype. Seven patients underwent allo-HSCT, of which four are alive at 7.8, 6.9, 6.2, and 0.25 years. Two patients underwent auto-HSCT, and both are alive at median follow-up of 1.91 years.[59]

Ghobriel et al. reported outcomes on 21 patients with SPTCL. Median age at diagnosis was 42 years. HSCT was performed in five patients (three auto-HSCT and two allo-HSCT). Patients treated aggressively with HSCT appear to have an improved OS.[60]

It is reasonable to perform auto-HSCT as consolidation in CR1 or at chemosensitive relapse in patients with SPTCL. Allo-HSCT is reserved for primary refractory disease or relapsed cases and for patients who have poor prognostic factors such as extensive bone marrow involvement.

CUTANEOUS T-CELL LYMPHOMAS

Mycosis fungoides (MF), a malignancy of CD4 positive T cells, is the most common form of cutaneous T-cell lymphomas (CTCLs). It usually starts with a patch or a plaque on skin and has very slow progression. In advanced stages, patients may develop skin tumors and involvement of lymph nodes and visceral organs. The usual treatment for early stage MF includes retinoids, extracorporeal photopheresis, monoclonal antibodies, interferon-alpha, and chemotherapy. In spite of therapy with these modalities, MF usually progresses to more advanced stages.

Sezary syndrome (SS) is an aggressive variant of CTCL/leukemia. This entity usually presents as erythroderma, circulating leukemic T cells, and lymphadenopathy. It shows rapid progression and fatal course without treatment.

In 2008, Duarte et al. reported outcomes of 20 patients with CTCL who were treated with auto-HSCT. A CR rate of 90% was obtained. But, 1-year OS was only 50%, and time to progression was 2.3 months. [61]

In 2014, Duarte et al. reported long-term outcomes of 60 patients with CTCL who underwent allo-HSCT at EBMT centers. There were 36 patients with MF and 24 with SS. The 1- and 3-year OS was 66% and 54%, and PFS was 42% and 32%, respectively. RIC resulted in significantly reduced NRM compared with MAC. T-cell depletion increased relapse risk. The OS was 44% and PFS was 30% at 7 years. Relapse/progression was reported in 45% of patients. The median time to relapse was 3.8 months, and only two relapses were recorded beyond 2 years after HSCT.[62]

In 2014, Shiratori et al. reported outcomes of RIC allo-HSCT in nine patients with advanced CTCL. With a median follow-up of 954 days, the estimated 3-year OS was 85.7% with no NRM. Five patients relapsed, and this was managed by tapering immunosuppressive or by giving DLI. The authors concluded that with allo-HSCT, GVL, and down-staging from advanced stage to early stage improves the prognosis of advanced-stage CTCL.[63]

In 2015, Hosing et al. reported a prospective case series of 47 patients with CTCL who underwent allo-HSCT after failure of standard therapy between 2001 and 2013. At 4 years, OS and PFS were 51% and 26%, respectively. There was no statistical difference in the OS in patients who had MF alone, SS, and MF with large cell transformation. PFS at 4 years was superior in patients who had SS versus those who did not (52.4% vs. 9.9%). The cumulative NRM was 16.7% at 2 years. Authors concluded that allo-HSCT might result in long-term remissions in a subset of patients with advanced CTCL. Although post-HSCT relapse rates are high, many patients respond to immunomodulation and achieve durable remissions.[64]

For patients with MF and SS, allo-HSCT should be recommended. RIC regimens seem to be better tolerated and result in lower NRM. There is evidence of potent GVL effect, and cases of relapse can be treated with withdrawal of immunosuppression or DLI. For patients with mycosis fungoides, allo-HSCT should be considered after failure of two or three initial therapies, at least in patients aged <60 years. Auto-HSCT seems to have no role in the management of CTCL.

REFERENCES

1. Pullarkat V, Forman S. Hematopoietic cell transplantation for rare hematologic malignancies. In: Forman S, Negrin R, Antin J, Appelbaum F, eds. *Thomas' Hematopoietic Cell Transplantation*. 5th ed. Vol. 2. John Wiley & Sons, Ltd; 2016:804–815.

2. Wang SS, Vose JM. Epidemiology and prognosis of T-cell lymphoma. In: *T-Cell Lymphomas*. 2013:25–39.

3. Chihara D, Ito H, Katanoda K, et al. Increase in incidence of adult T-cell leukemia/lymphoma in non-endemic areas of Japan and the United States. *Cancer Sci.* 2012;103(10):1857–1860.

4. Sanz GF. A lot to learn about allogeneic hematopoietic cell transplantation for chronic myelomonocytic leukemia. *Biol Blood Marrow Transplant.* 2017;23(5):713–714.

5. Swerdlow S, Campo E, Pileri S, Harris N. The 2016 revision of the World Health Organization classification of lymphoid neoplasms. *Blood.* 2016;127(20):2375–2390.

6. Johnson MR, Verstovsek S, Jorgensen JL, et al. Utility of the World Heath Organization classification criteria for the diagnosis of systemic mastocytosis in bone marrow. *Mod Pathol.* 2009;22(1):50–57.

7. Horny HP, Sotlar K, Valent P. Mastocytosis: state of the art. *Pathobiology.* 2007;74(2):121–132.

8. Schwaab J, Schnittger S, Sotlar K, et al. Comprehensive mutational profiling in advanced systemic mastocytosis. *Blood.* 2013;122(14):2460–2466.

9. Pullarkat VA, Bueso-Ramos C, Lai R, et al. Systemic mastocytosis with associated clonal hematological non-mast-cell lineage disease: analysis of clinicopathologic features and activating c-kit mutations. *Am J Hematol.* 2003;73(1):12–17.

10. Sperr WR, Drach J, Hauswirth AW, et al. Myelomastocytic leukemia: evidence for the origin of mast cells from the leukemic clone and eradication by allogeneic stem cell transplantation. *Clin Cancer Res.* 2005;11(19 Pt 1):6787–6792.

11. Vega-Ruiz A, Cortes JE, Sever M, et al. Phase II study of imatinib mesylate as therapy for patients with systemic mastocytosis. *Leuk Res.* 2009;33(11):1481–1484.

12. Shah N, Lee F, Luo R, Jiang Y, Donker M, Akin C. Dasatinib (BMS-354825) inhibits KITD816V, an imatinib-resistant activating mutation that triggers neoplastic growth in most patients with systemic mastocytosis. *Blood.* 2006.

13. Gotlib J, Kluin-Nelemans HC, George TI, et al. Efficacy and safety of midostaurin in advanced systemic mastocytosis. *N Engl J Med.* 2016;374(26):2530–2541.

14. Nakamura R, Chakrabarti S, Akin C, et al. A pilot study of nonmyeloablative allogeneic hematopoietic stem cell transplant for advanced systemic mastocytosis. *Bone Marrow Transplant.* 2006;37(4):353–358.

15. Ustun C, Reiter A, Scott BL, et al. Hematopoietic stem-cell transplantation for advanced systemic mastocytosis. *J Clin Oncol.* 2014;32(29):3264–3274.

16. Ustun C, Gotlib J, Popat U, et al. Consensus opinion on allogeneic hematopoietic cell transplantation in advanced systemic mastocytosis. *Biol Blood Marrow Transplant.* 2016;22(8):1348–1356.

17. Badalian-Very G, Vergilio JA, Degar BA, Rodriguez-Galindo C, Rollins BJ. Recent advances in the understanding of Langerhans cell histiocytosis. *Br J Haematol.* 2012;156(2):163–172.

18. Berres ML, Merad M, Allen CE. Progress in understanding the pathogenesis of Langerhans cell histiocytosis: back to Histiocytosis X? *Br J Haematol.* 2015;169(1):3–13.

19. Veys PA, Nanduri V, Baker KS, et al. Haematopoietic stem cell transplantation for refractory Langerhans cell histiocytosis: outcome by intensity of conditioning. *Br J Haematol.* 2015;169(5):711–718.

20. Cruz-Chacon A, Mathews J, Ayala E. Transplantation in rare lymphoproliferative and histiocytic disorders. *Cancer Control.* 2014;21(4):335–342.

21. Derenzini E, Fina MP, Stefoni V, et al. MACOP-B regimen in the treatment of adult Langerhans cell histiocytosis: experience on seven patients. *Ann Oncol.* 2010;21(6): 1173–1178.

22. Kudo K, Ohga S, Morimoto A, et al. Improved outcome of refractory Langerhans cell histiocytosis in children with hematopoietic stem cell transplantation in Japan. *Bone Marrow Transplant.* 2010;45(5):901–906.

23. Akkari V, Donadieu J, Piguet C, et al. Hematopoietic stem cell transplantation in patients with severe Langerhans cell histiocytosis and hematological dysfunction: experience of the French Langerhans Cell Study Group. *Bone Marrow Transplant.* 2003;31(12):1097–1103.

24. Steiner M, Matthes-Martin S, Attarbaschi A, et al. Improved outcome of treatment-resistant high-risk Langerhans cell histiocytosis after allogeneic stem cell transplantation with reduced-intensity conditioning. *Bone Marrow Transplant.* 2005;36(3):215–225.

25. Solary E, Itzykson R. How I treat chronic myelomonocytic leukemia. *Blood.* 2017;130(2):126–136.

26. Liu HD, Ahn KW, Hu ZH, et al. Allogeneic hematopoietic cell transplantation for adult chronic myelomonocytic leukemia. *Biol Blood Marrow Transplant.* 2017;23(5):767–775.

27. Such E, Germing U, Malcovati L, et al. Development and validation of a prognostic scoring system for patients with chronic myelomonocytic leukemia. *Blood.* 2013;121(15):3005–3015.

28. Symeonidis A, van Biezen A, de Wreede L, et al. Achievement of complete remission predicts outcome of allogeneic haematopoietic stem cell transplantation in patients with chronic myelomonocytic leukaemia. A study of the Chronic Malignancies Working Party of the European Group for Blood and Marrow Transplantation. *Br J Haematol.* 2015.

29. Kongtim P, Popat U, Jimenez A, et al. Treatment with hypomethylating agents before allogeneic stem cell transplant improves progression-free survival for patients with chronic myelomonocytic leukemia. *Biol Blood Marrow Transplant.* 2016;22(1):47–53.

30. Fathi AT, Dec Jr GW, Richter JM, et al. Case records of the Massachusetts General Hospital. Case 7-2014. A 27-year-old man with diarrhea, fatigue, and eosinophilia. *N Engl J Med.* 2014;370(9):861–872.

31. Cooper MA, Akard LP, Thompson JM, Dugan MJ, Jansen J. Hypereosinophilic syndrome: long-term remission following allogeneic stem cell transplant in spite of transient eosinophilia post-transplant. *Am J Hematol.* 2005;78(1):33–36.

32. Chockalingam A, Jalil A, Shadduck R, Lister J. Allogeneic peripheral blood stem cell transplantation for hypereosinophilic syndrome with severe cardiac dysfunction. *Bone Marrow Transplant.* 1999;23:1093–1094.

33. Bergua JM, Prieto-Pliego E, Roman-Barbera A, et al. Resolution of left and right ventricular thrombosis secondary to hypereosinophilic syndrome (lymphoproliferative variant) with reduced intensity conditioning allogenic stem cell transplantation. *Ann Hematol.* 2008;87(11):937–938.

34. Atilla PA, Atilla E, Bozdag SC, et al. Treatment with methotrexate, rituximab, and cytosine arabinoside followed by autologous stem cell transplantation in primary central nervous system lymphoma: a single-center experience. *Hematol Oncol Stem Cel Ther.* 2017.

35. Cho H, Chang JH, Kim YR, et al. The role of upfront autologous stem cell transplantation in high-risk younger patients with primary central nervous system lymphoma. *Br J Haematol.* 2016;174(3):444–453.

36. Madle M, Kramer I, Lehners N, et al. The influence of rituximab, high-dose therapy followed by autologous stem cell transplantation, and age in patients with primary CNS lymphoma. *Ann Hematol.* 2015;94(11):1853–1857.

37. Yoon DH, Lee DH, Choi DR, et al. Feasibility of BU, CY and etoposide (BUCYE), and auto-SCT in patients with newly diagnosed primary CNS lymphoma: a single-center experience. *Bone Marrow Transplant.* 2011;46(1):105–109.

38. Soussain C, Choquet S, Fourme E, et al. Intensive chemotherapy with thiotepa, busulfan and cyclophosphamide and hematopoietic stem cell rescue in relapsed or refractory primary central nervous system lymphoma and intraocular lymphoma: a retrospective study of 79 cases. *Haematologica.* 2012;97(11):1751–1756.

39. Kasenda B, Ihorst G, Schroers R, et al. High-dose chemotherapy with autologous haematopoietic stem cell support for relapsed or refractory primary CNS lymphoma: a prospective multicentre trial by the German Cooperative PCNSL study group. *Leukemia.* 2017.

40. Katsuya H, Ishitsuka K. Treatment advances and prognosis for patients with adult T-cell leukemia-lymphoma. *J Clinical Experimental Hematopathol.* 2017;57(2):1–11.

41. Fuji S, Yamaguchi T, Inoue Y, et al. Development of a modified prognostic index for patients with aggressive adult T-cell leukemia-lymphoma aged 70 years or younger: possible risk-adapted management strategies including allogeneic transplantation. *Haematologica.* 2017;102(7):1258–1265.

42. Okamura J, Uike N, Utsunomiya A, Tanosaki R. Allogeneic stem cell transplantation for adult T-cell leukemia/lymphoma. *Int J Hematol.* 2007;86(2):118–125.

43. Fukushima T, Miyazaki Y, Honda S, et al. Allogeneic hematopoietic stem cell transplantation provides sustained long-term survival for patients with adult T-cell leukemia/lymphoma. *Leukemia.* 2005;19(5):829–834.

44. Ishida T, Hishizawa M, Kato K, et al. Allogeneic hematopoietic stem cell transplantation for adult T-cell leukemia-lymphoma with special emphasis on preconditioning regimen: a nationwide retrospective study. *Blood.* 2012;120(8):1734–1741.

45. Itonaga H, Tsushima H, Taguchi J, et al. Treatment of relapsed adult T-cell leukemia/lymphoma after allogeneic hematopoietic stem cell transplantation: the Nagasaki Transplant Group experience. *Blood.* 2013;121(1):219–225.

46. Fuji S, Shindo T. Friend or foe? Mogamulizumab in allogeneic hematopoietic stem cell transplantation for adult T-cell leukemia/lymphoma. *Stem Cel Investig.* 2016;3:70.

47. Tse E, Kwong YL. The diagnosis and management of NK/T-cell lymphomas. *J Hematol Oncol.* 2017;10(1):85.

48. Hamadani M, Kanate AS, DiGilio A, et al. Allogeneic hematopoietic cell transplantation for aggressive NK cell leukemia. A center for international blood and marrow transplant Research analysis. *Biol Blood Marrow Transplant.* 2017;23(5):853–856.

49. Yhim HY, Kim JS, Mun YC, et al. Clinical outcomes and prognostic factors of up-front autologous stem cell transplantation in patients with extranodal natural killer/T cell lymphoma. *Biol Blood Marrow Transplant.* 2015;21(9):1597–1604.

50. Kwong YL. High-dose chemotherapy and hematopoietic SCT in the management of natural killer-cell malignancies. *Bone Marrow Transplant.* 2009;44(11):709–714.

51. Murashige N, Kami M, Kishi Y, et al. Allogeneic haematopoietic stem cell transplantation as a promising treatment for natural killer-cell neoplasms. *Br J Haematol.* 2005;130(4):561–567.

52. Tse E, Chan TS, Koh LP, et al. Allogeneic haematopoietic SCT for natural killer/T-cell lymphoma: a multicentre analysis from the Asia Lymphoma Study Group. *Bone Marrow Transplant.* 2014;49(7):902–906.

53. Pagano L, Valentini CG, Grammatico S, Pulsoni A. Blastic plasmacytoid dendritic cell neoplasm: diagnostic criteria and therapeutical approaches. *Br J Haematol.* 2016;174(2):188–202.

53a. Frankel AE, Woo JH, Ahn C, et al. Activity of SL-401, a targeted therapy directed to interleukin-3 receptor, in blastic plasmacytoid dendritic cell neoplasm patients. *Blood.* 2014;124(3):385–392.

54. Pagano L, Valentini CG, Pulsoni A, et al. Blastic plasmacytoid dendritic cell neoplasm with leukemic presentation: an Italian multicenter study. *Haematologica.* 2013;98(2):239–246.

55. Roos-Weil D, Dietrich S, Boumendil A, et al. Stem cell transplantation can provide durable disease control in blastic plasmacytoid dendritic cell neoplasm: a retrospective study from the European Group for Blood and Marrow Transplantation. *Blood.* 2013;121(3):440–446.

56. Aoki T, Suzuki R, Kuwatsuka Y, et al. Long-term survival following autologous and allogeneic stem cell transplantation for blastic plasmacytoid dendritic cell neoplasm. *Blood.* 2015;125(23):3559–3562.

57. Rashidi A, Cashen AF. Outcomes of allogeneic stem cell transplantation in hepatosplenic T-cell lymphoma. *Blood Cancer J.* 2015;5:e318.

58. Tanase A, Schmitz N, Stein H, et al. Allogeneic and autologous stem cell transplantation for hepatosplenic T-cell lymphoma: a retrospective study of the EBMT Lymphoma Working Party. *Leukemia.* 2015;29(3):686–688.

59. Gibson JF, Alpdogan O, Subtil A, et al. Hematopoietic stem cell transplantation for primary cutaneous gamma delta T-cell lymphoma and refractory subcutaneous panniculitis-like T-cell lymphoma. *J Am Acad Dermatol.* 2015;72(6):1010–1015. e1015.

60. Ghobrial IM, Weenig RH, Pittlekow MR, et al. Clinical outcome of patients with subcutaneous panniculitis-like T-cell lymphoma. *Leuk Lymphoma.* 2005;46(5):703–708.

61. Duarte RF, Schmitz N, Servitje O, Sureda A. Haematopoietic stem cell transplantation for patients with primary cutaneous T-cell lymphoma. *Bone Marrow Transplant.* 2008;41(7):597–604.

62. Duarte RF, Boumendil A, Onida F, et al. Long-term outcome of allogeneic hematopoietic cell transplantation for patients with mycosis fungoides and Sezary syndrome: a European society for blood and marrow transplantation lymphoma working party extended analysis. *J Clin Oncol.* 2014;32(29):3347–3348.

63. Shiratori S, Fujimoto K, Nishimura M, et al. Allogeneic hematopoietic stem cell transplantation following reduced-intensity conditioning for mycosis fungoides and Sezary syndrome. *Hematol Oncol.* 2016;34(1):9–16.

64. Hosing C, Bassett R, Dabaja B, et al. Allogeneic stem-cell transplantation in patients with cutaneous lymphoma: updated results from a single institution. *Ann Oncol.* 2015;26(12):2490–2495.

CHAPTER 20

Hematopoietic Cell Transplantation for Germ Cell Tumors and Other Adult Solid Tumors

LAUREN VELTRI, MD • YAGO NIETO, MD, PHD

GERM CELL TUMORS

Testicular GCT is the most common malignancy in young men between the ages of 20 and 35 years. GCTs are considered highly curable, even in patients with advanced disease.[1] The prognosis of newly diagnosed tumors depends on their International Germ Cell Consensus Classification (IGCCCG) risk stratification.[2] Frontline standard-dose chemotherapy (SDC) with bleomycin/etoposide/cisplatin (BEP) yields 90% long-term EFS rates in advanced-disease good-risk patients, 80% EFS for intermediate-risk, and 50% EFS for poor-risk patients.[2] In patients with relapsed disease, the best approach for salvage therapy remains unsettled. Salvage SDC with vinblastine/ifosfamide/cisplatin (VeIP) or etoposide/ifosfamide/cisplatin (VIP)[3–5] or with paclitaxel/ifosfamide/cisplatin (TIP)[6] results in CR rates of 50%–60% and long-term EFS of 20%–30%.

In the mid-1980s investigators at Indiana University pioneered the use of tandem cycles of HDC with carboplatin and etoposide (CE) with ASCT as salvage therapy for refractory GCTs. In their initial trials, patients in second relapse experienced long-term EFS rates of 15%,[7–9] whereas those transplanted in first relapse had long-term EFS of 39%.[10] This group has subsequently updated their results in successive patient cohorts. Einhorn et al. retrospectively reviewed 184 patients with relapsed, metastatic GCT treated with tandem CE between 1996 and 2004.[11] Most patients (73%) were transplanted at the time of first relapse, and 27% patients at second or later relapse. With a median follow-up of 4 years, EFS for patients in the first relapse was 70% and 45% for those in second or later relapse. The outcome was similar in patients with seminoma and nonseminoma histologies. Those excellent results partly reflected patient selection

as no patients with late relapses or primary mediastinal tumors were included, and around one-third of the patients had good prognosis features predictive of favorable outcomes with SDC alone. More recently, Adra et al. from the Indiana group retrospectively reported on a subsequent cohort of 364 patients transplanted with tandem CE between 2004 and 2014.[12] As in their prior report, most patients (83%) were in first relapse and had better outcomes than patients transplanted in second or later relapse (2-year EFS of 63% and 49%, respectively).

Several investigators have tested the addition of a third drug to the CE backbone. Motzer et al. at Memorial Sloan Kettering Cancer Center (MSKCC) evaluated 58 refractory GCT patients treated with high-dose carboplatin, etoposide, and cyclophosphamide (CEC).[13] The EFS was 21% with a median follow-up of 28 months. Siegert et al. treated 74 patients with recurrent disease with two SDC cycles followed by one cycle of HDC with ifosfamide/carboplatin/etoposide (ICE), with 50% 2-year EFS rates among patients with sensitive tumors, but only 4% EFS in those with refractory disease. Margolin et al. reported a 45% EFS rate after tandem cycles of ICE in 20 patients with relapsed and cisplatin-sensitive tumors.[14] These investigators subsequently treated 31 relapsed patients with sequential cycles of HDC with paclitaxel/carboplatin/etoposide and ICE.[15] At median follow-up of 5 years, 12 (39%) patients remained free of disease. Rick et al. treated 80 patients, most with cisplatin-sensitive disease, with 3–4 cycles of SDC followed by one cycle of high-dose carboplatin/etoposide/thiotepa.[16] At median follow-up of 3 years, the EFS rate was 26%. Overall, high-dose triplets achieve 40%–50% EFS rate in patients with cisplatin-sensitive tumors, and 4%–20% in those with refractory disease.[13,17]

Hematopoietic Cell Transplantation for Malignant Conditions. https://doi.org/10.1016/B978-0-323-56802-9.00020-1

Predictive Models of Outcome for Patients with Relapsed GCT Receiving HDC (Table 20.1)

Beyer et al. reported in 1996 an influential prognostic model based on their analysis of 283 relapsed/refractory patients treated with HDC with CE.[18] This model included the following independent adverse predictors: refractoriness to cisplatin (progression within 4 weeks after treatment with cisplatin), absolute refractoriness to cisplatin (no response), primary mediastinal tumor, high B-HCG >1000 U/L after relapse, and progressive disease at the time of HDC. A prognostic score based on these variables allocated patients to good-, intermediate-, and poor-risk groups, with respective 2-year EFS of 51%, 27%, and 5%. The Beyer model, initially developed on patients treated between 1984 and 1993 mostly with a single course of HDC, was subsequently validated in patients with cisplatin-refractory disease

treated with tandem cycles of ICE, where the groups with good, intermediate and poor risk had 62%, 13%, and 0% EFS rates, respectively.[19]

Einhorn et al. developed a different prognostic model based on their experience at Indiana with tandem CE, mostly with patients in first relapse.[11] Patients with primary mediastinal tumors were not included. Three independent adverse prognostic factors were identified: an IGCCCG poor-risk classification at initial diagnosis, cisplatin-refractory disease, and administration of HDC as third-line or later treatment. Patients in the low-, intermediate-, and high-risk categories had EFS rates of approximately 80%, 60%, and 40%, respectively.

A large analysis by the International Prognostic Factor Study Group (IPFSG) included 1594 patients treated after 1990 with HDC (N = 821) or SDC (N = 773) as first salvage therapy.[20] Among patients receiving HDC,

TABLE 20.1
Prognostic Models for HDC for NSGCT

MODEL		FACTOR	Points	2-year EFS
Beyer	Variables	Progressive disease before HDC	1	
		Mediastinal primary tumor	1	
		Cisplatin-refractory disease (relapse within 4 weeks of completion of 1st line chemotherapy)	1	
		Absolute cisplatin-refractory disease (PD as best response to prior therapy)	2	
		B-HCG > 1000 IU/L before HDC	2	
	Stratification	**Low risk**	0	51%
		Intermediate risk	1–2	27%
		High risk	>2	5%
Indiana	Variables	HDC at third-line or subsequent line of treatment	3	
		Refractory disease before HDC (relapse within 4 weeks of completion of 1st line chemotherapy)	2	
		High-risk IGCCCG stage	2	
	Stratification	**Low risk**	0	80%
		Intermediate risk	2–3	60%
		High risk	>3	40%

TABLE 20.1
Prognostic Models for HDC for NSGCT—cont'd

MODEL		FACTOR		Points	2-year EFS
Interna-tional Prog-nostic Factors Study Group	Variables	Histology	Seminoma	−1	
			Nonseminoma	0	
		Primary tumor site	Mediastinal	3	
			Retroperitoneal	1	
			Gonadal	0	
		Response to 1st-line che-motherapy	CR/PRm-	0	
			PRm+/SD	1	
			PD	2	
		Progression-free interval following 1st line chemo-therapy	>3 months	0	
			≤3 months	1	
		AFP at salvage	Normal	0	
			≤1000	1	
			>1000	2	
		B-HCG at salvage	≤1000	0	
			>1000	1	
		Liver/brain/bone metas-tases	No	0	
			Yes	1	
	Stratification	**Very low risk (semino-ma+low risk)**		−1	92%
		Low risk		0	64%
		Intermediate risk		1–2	53%
		High risk		3–4	33%
		Very high risk		>4	22%

EFS, event-free survival; *HDC*, high-dose chemotherapy; *IGCCCG*, International Germ Cell Consensus Classification; *PD*, programmed death.

half of them received a single cycle, and the other half received tandem cycles. Seven factors were found to be independent predictors of outcome, both after SDC or HDC: primary tumor site (mediastinal vs. retroperitoneal vs. gonadal), response to first-line therapy, length of prior progression-free interval, Alfa Feto Protein (AFP) at sal-vage, B-HCG at salvage, and presence of nonpulmonary visceral metastases. A composite score based on these factors assigned patients to a very-low-(only seminoma), low-, intermediate-, high-, or very-high-risk categories. Within each prognostic category, PFS at 2 years was sig-nificantly superior after HDC compared to SDC, which translated into improved OS (Table 20.2). This model is applicable to patients receiving either SDC or HDC at the time of first recurrence, a setting in which it seems more robust than the other two models. In contrast, both the Beyer and the Indiana models are applicable to patients in second or later relapses. The patient populations that served to develop the IPFSG and Beyer models received either one (50% and 91% of the patients, respectively) or tandem HDC cycles (50% and 9%, respectively). In con-trast, all patients in the Indiana study received tandem cycles, which better reflects the common US practice. The Beyer score seems better capable than the Indiana model of detecting a very poor prognosis subset of patients, for which novel approaches are needed.

Novel HDC Approaches to Relapsed GCT

Feldman et al. at the MSKCC tested the use of 3 cycles of HDC and reported encouraging results in 107 patients

TABLE 20.2
EFS and OS Rates in Patients Treated With HDC or SDC (International Prognostic Factors Study Group)

		2-year EFS	P Value	5-year OS	P Value
All patients (N = 1594)	SDC	28%	<0.001	41%	<0.001
	HDC	50%		53%	
Very low risk (N = 76)	SDC	58%	<0.001	64%	<0.01
	HDC	92%		89%	
Low risk (N = 257)	SDC	40%	<0.001	66%	0.98
	HDC	64%		64%	
Intermediate risk (N = 646)	SDC	32%	<0.001	45%	<0.001
	HDC	53%		58%	
High risk (N = 351)	SDC	17%	<0.001	23%	<0.005
	HDC	33%		35%	
Very high risk (N = 105)	SDC	2%	<0.001	3%	<0.001
	HDc	22%		27%	

EFS, event-free survival; *HDC*, high-dose chemotherapy; *OS*, overall survival; *SDC*, standard-dose chemotherapy.

with relapsed disease and unfavorable prognostic features (incomplete response to first-line therapy, second relapse or later, or extragonadal primary site). Of them, 76% were transplanted at first relapse, 20% at second relapse, and 4% at third or later relapse; 74% were cisplatin refractory and 2% absolute cisplatin refractory. These patients received two biweekly cycles of paclitaxel/ifosfamide followed by high-dose CE x 3 (TI-CE), with 47% EFS at 5 years.[21] The EFS rates in patients in first relapse and second or later relapses were 55% and 23%, respectively. Five of 21 patients with primary mediastinal tumors remained in CR. These results have prompted an ongoing international randomized phase III trial comparing 3 cycles of HDC (TI-CE) to SDC with 4 cycles of TIP in patients in first relapse.[22]

Lotz and French collaborators have also pioneered the use of 3 cycles of HDC in their sequential multicentric studies. In the TAXIF I trial these investigators treated 45 patients, most of them pretreated with a median 2 regimens of chemotherapy and half of them cisplatin refractory, with 2 cycles of epirubicin/paclitaxel followed by 3 cycles of HDC (cyclophosphamide/paclitaxel in the first ASCT, followed by ICE for the second and third ASCT). The 3-year EFS and OS rates were 23.5%. In their continuation study TAXIF II, Selle et al. treated 45 nonrefractory patients, most of them treated with 2 prior lines of therapy, in a similar fashion, except for the use of thiotepa/paclitaxel in the first ASCT, followed again by ICE in the next two ASCT. [23] At median follow-up

of 26 months, the 2-year EFS and OS rates of this better prognosis group were 50% and 66%, respectively.

Our group at MD Anderson Cancer Center focused on very poor prognosis patients for the development of more potent HDC seeking new synergistic interactions and incorporating novel agents with different targets. Vascular endothelial growth factor (VEGF) expression plays an essential role in tumor development, angiogenesis, and metastasis in GCTs.[24,25] Bevacizumab, an anti-VEGF monoclonal antibody, has been shown to decrease tumor perfusion and interstitial fluid pressure leading to increased access of the cytotoxic agents into the malignant tumor.[26] To evaluate the potential synergy between bevacizumab and chemotherapy, we conducted a phase II trial of tandem cycles of bevacizumab-HDC in patients with intermediate-risk or high-risk relapse (Beyer model).[27] In our initial report, 42 patients with heavily pretreated tumors (median 3 prior relapses and 4 prior lines of chemotherapy), 40% cisplatin refractory and 47% absolute cisplatin refractory, received bevacizumab, gemcitabine, docetaxel, melphalan, and carboplatin (first ASCT) followed by bevacizumab and ICE (second ASCT). At a median follow-up of 46 months, the EFS and OS rates were 56%, and OS was 58% for the entire cohort. The EFS and OS rates for the Beyer intermediate-risk group were 60% and 75%, respectively; for the Beyer high-risk group, those rates were 46% and 48%, respectively. These results clearly exceeded the expected outcomes in this very poor prognosis population.

We subsequently evaluated the omission of bevacizumab from their HDC strategy, attempting to ameliorate the prominent mucositis previously seen in the first cohort. We reported an update of our trial at ASCO 2017 in a second cohort of 28 patients, which was comparable to the prior cohort for all prognostic factors, including prior exposure to chemotherapy, number of prior relapses, resistance to cisplatin and overall risk according to either the Beyer or the IPFSG models.[28] The omission of bevacizumab made HDC better tolerated with less mucositis. At median follow-up of this second cohort of 26 months, the EFS and OS rates were 71% and 74%, respectively. The EFS rates in the Beyer intermediate-risk and high-risk subgroups were 56% and 80%, respectively. These encouraging results in the non-bevacizumab cohort are likely to result from a synergistic interaction between gemcitabine and the other agents based on DNA damage repair inhibition through suppression of nucleotide excision repair (NER), a major mechanism of cisplatin resistance in GCT cells.[29] It is also apparent that the addition of bevacizumab to HDC increases toxicity without significantly improving antitumor activity.

One or More Cycles of HDC?

Most experts believe that at least two HDC cycles should be administered as part of the ASCT. Lorch et al. randomized 216 patients with relapsed or refractory GCTs to one cycle of SDC with VIP followed by three sequential cycles of HDC with CE versus three cycles of VIP followed by one cycle of high-dose carboplatin, etoposide, and cyclophosphamide.[30] Enrollment in the trial was stopped prematurely after recruitment of 216 patients due to excessive TRM of 14% in the single HDC arm. No statistically significant differences in survival were found between the two treatment arms. Sequential HDC was better tolerated and resulted in fewer treatment-related deaths (4% vs. 16%, respectively) with the deaths predominantly being related to cardiotoxicity or sepsis.

A retrospective analysis was performed by the IPFSG on the outcomes of 1594 patients with recurrent or refractory GCT after SDC versus HDC.[31] With a median follow-up of 5 years, the 2-year PFS for SDC, single-course HDC and sequential HDC was 27.8%, 44.1% and 55%, respectively. The 5-year OS rates were 40.8% for SDC and 53.2% for HDC (HR 0.65). While the optimal number of HDC cycles is unknown as there have been no formal comparisons, the best results are seen with two or three HDC cycles, which constitutes the common practice in the US.

Randomized Trials of HDC in the Salvage Setting

Retrospective matched pair comparisons of HDC versus SDC for patients in first relapse have suggested a large benefit from transplant.[31,32] Pico et al. of the EBMT conducted the only randomized trial to date comparing HDC to SDC in relapsed patients. These investigators randomized 280 relapsed patients to receive three cycles of SDC followed by one more cycle (SDC arm) or a single course of high-dose CEC with ASCT (HDC arm).[33] At median follow-up of 45 months, no differences in EFS (35% vs. 42%, P = .16) or OS (53% in both arms) were apparent. This trial has been criticized because of a 30% drop-out rate in the HDC arm, a higher than expected treatment-related mortality in both study arms (3% and 7%, respectively) and the use of a single rather than sequential cycles of HDC.

In summary, there is no consensus yet as to whether HDC should be considered for all patients at the time of first relapse. Results of tandem cycles of HDC as salvage treatment appear superior to those expected with SDC, which have prompted many to consider HDC the standard salvage treatment,[34] despite the absence of evidence of benefit from randomized studies. It is possible that more than one cycle of HDC is necessary to achieve a favorable outcome and that a single cycle, as administered in the European randomized study, may not be sufficient to improve results. Of note, in the IPFSG analysis, the 2-year DFS rates of patients receiving sequential HDC cycles appeared superior to those receiving a single high-dose cycle (55% *v* 44%, P < .001). The randomized phase III TIGER trial is underway addressing this important question, comparing TI-CE, with 3 cycles of HDC, to SDC (TIP x 4).[22]

First-Line High-Dose Chemotherapy for Poor-Risk Non Seminomatous Germ Cell Tumors (NSGCT)

The value of upfront HDC for GCTs with poor risk-features has been evaluated. Motzer et al. used high-dose CEC (carboplatin, etoposide, and cyclophosphamide) for patients with poor-risk tumors receiving SDC and those with prolonged clearance of elevated serum two markers after two cycles of a cisplatin-containing SDC regimen.[35] They reported a 57% CR rate and 50% EFS at median follow-up of 30 months. When compared to their prior experience with SDC alone in this patient population, early intervention with HDC resulted in superior OS. Schmoll et al. evaluated patients with poor-risk disease who received one cycle of SDC followed by three cycles of HDC with VIP (etoposide, ifosfamide, and cisplatin).[36] After 4-year median follow-up, the EFS rate was 69%. A matched-pair analysis was performed in patients with poor-risk GCT who received sequential HDC with VIP in patients treated with SDC, and results suggested that HDC led to improvement in PFS and OS.[37]

Three randomized trials have evaluated the role of HDC as first-line therapy in patients with poor-risk characteristics. A European randomized trial conducted in the 1980s failed to show a therapeutic benefit for HDC in 115 untreated poor-risk patients, who were randomized to receive 3–4 cycles of SDC or two cycles followed by one cycle of a stem cell–supported high-dose cisplatin-containing regimen.[38] Patients randomized to the transplant arm received less total cisplatin than those on the standard-dose arm, as well as an HDC regimen that can be considered substandard by present criteria.

A second European study compared the efficacy of four cycles of SDC with VIP to one cycle of standard-dose VIP followed by three cycles of high-dose VIP in patients with poor-risk GCTs.[39] Owing to slow accrual, the study closed prematurely with 137 patients enrolled instead of the goal 222 patients. The CR rates (44.6% vs. 33.3%, $P = .18$), 2-year EFS (45% vs. 58%, $P = .06$), and 2-year OS (66% vs. 73%, $P > .1$) did not differ.

In a US Intergroup trial, Motzer et al. randomized 219 patients with newly diagnosed, intermediate- or poor-risk GCTs to either four cycles of standard BEP or two cycles of BEP followed by two cycles of HDC with CEC.[40] The 1-year CR rates were 52% and 48%, respectively ($P = .53$). There were no significant differences in EFS ($P = .4$) or OS ($P = .9$). A planned subset analysis according to early tumor marker clearance suggested a significant benefit of HDC among those patients experiencing a slow marker decline (61% vs. 34% 1-year EFS, $P = .03$), in contrast with similar outcomes in both arms in the group of patients with a satisfactory marker drop ($P = .5$). Given the small size of this subset analysis, these provocative observations are not robust enough to allow firm conclusions.

In summary, the current data available from randomized trials do not support a standard role for HDC in frontline treatment of GCT. Further clarity in its role as part of salvage treatment in first relapse awaits completion of the ongoing randomized TIGER trial. Finally, HDC is widely accepted as an established treatment for patients in second or later relapse.

BREAST CANCER

The benefit of HDC and ASCT in patients with breast cancer became controversial almost since its inception.[41] In the late 1980s, after in vitro and retrospective

observations of a clear dose response to treatment, phase II trials were published using HDC in both high-risk primary breast cancer (HRPBC) and metastatic breast cancer (MBC). The results showed improved complete response (CR) rates and PFS outcomes compared to those expected with SDC, which inspired several randomized phase III trials.

High-Dose Chemotherapy in HRPBC

Initial nonrandomized studies with HDC in patients with HRPBC by Peters et al. at Duke University[42] and by Gianni's group at the National Tumor Institute in Milan[43] sparked enthusiasm by demonstrating encouraging long-term PFS rates of 72% and 57%, respectively, in patients with ≥10 axillary lymph nodes. These trials led to a significant increase in the number of transplantations performed in the 1990s and also prompted subsequent randomized phase III trials.

Fifteen randomized trials of HDC with ASCT for HRPBC were conducted.[44] All patients had gross axillary lymph node involvement at the time of surgery (≥4 positive nodes and, in many trials, ≥10 positive nodes). The chemotherapeutic induction agents and HDC regimens varied among trials. While some trials showed EFS benefit, only two had OS benefit. A metaanalysis of all 15 randomized trials with a total of 6210 patients was reported.[45] With a median follow-up of 6 years, a significant benefit in EFS was present (HR 0.87, $P < .001$), but there was no difference in OS (HR 0.94, $P = .13$). In this metaanalysis, subgroup analyses did not identify any HRPBC subgroup with a significant improvement in survival with HDC.

Metastatic Breast Cancer

The initial prospective trials in MBC with HDC evaluated patients with refractory,[46,47] untreated,[48] and responsive disease[49] and consistently demonstrated the highest response rates reported in MBC and improved long-term disease control compared to prior treatment with SDC. Those initial studies led to eight randomized trials comparing HDC with SDC in chemosensitive MBC.[44] Six of them demonstrated an EFS advantage for HDC, but only one showed OS benefit. A metaanalysis of these trials showed a statistically significant improvement in PFS (median 11 vs. 8 months, hazard ratio (HR) of 0.76, $P < .001$), however, with no statistically significant OS benefit (median 2.16 vs. 2.02 years; $P = .08$).[45]

In conclusion, randomized trials in the MBC and HRPBC settings have shown improvement in PFS; however, they have largely failed to show OS benefit with many of them not powered to show overall benefit. The metaanalyses did detect a statistically significant 13% decrease in the risk of relapse in HRPBC and a 24% decrease in the risk of progression in MBC. While there are still populations that may benefit from HDC, such as those with inflammatory breast cancer[50] or with oligometastatic disease,[51] HDC has been largely abandoned for breast cancer.

Autologous Transplantation in Other Solid Tumors

HDC has been evaluated in other chemosensitive solid tumors in adults, including ovarian cancer, small-cell lung cancer, melanoma, malignant gliomas, and sarcomas. Most of those studies were small and failed to show a survival benefit.[52]

Allogeneic Stem Cell Transplantation for Solid Tumors

Allogeneic SCT provides an immune graft-versus-tumor (GVT) effect, which has been well described in hematologic malignancies, but whose efficacy (or even existence) has not been as defined in solid tumors. Owing to the high toxicity associated with high-dose myeloablative conditioning regimens, this approach has largely used reduced-intensity chemotherapy, which is less toxic, while still allowing enough immunosuppression to allow allogeneic stem cell engraftment.

Renal cell carcinoma (RCC) is the solid tumor on which allogeneic SCT has been most studied. Investigators at the NCI published the first series of 19 patients with cytokine-refractory, clear-cell RCC treated with an NMA allo-HSCT with fludarabine and cyclophosphamide conditioning from an HLA-identical sibling donor.[53] Response was seen in 53% patients at a median of 4 months after transplantation. Reponses were attributed to GVT based on the delayed response, occurrence after withdrawal of immunosuppression and common association with graft-versus-host-disease (GVHD). Other investigators reported similar results.[54,55] Taken together, the available data indicate that this approach is seriously limited by the common need to elicit GVHD to induce tumor responses. In consequence, allogeneic SCT for RCC remains experimental. As new agents have become available for RCC including VEGF inhibitors and immune checkpoint blockers, any possible future role of allogeneic SCT will need to be evaluated in combination with targeted therapies.

REFERENCES

1. Hanna NH, Einhorn LH. Testicular cancer–discoveries and updates. *N Engl J Med.* 2014;371(21):2005–2016.
2. International germ cell consensus classification: a prognostic factor-based staging system for metastatic germ cell cancers. International germ cell cancer collaborative group. *J Clin Oncol.* 1997;15:594–603.
3. Loehrer Sr PJ, Lauer R, Roth BJ, Williams SD, Kalasinski LA, Einhorn LH. Salvage therapy in recurrent germ cell cancer: ifosfamide and cisplatin plus either vinblastine or etoposide. *Ann Intern Med.* 1988;109:540–546.
4. Loehrer Sr PJ, Gonin R, Nichols CR, Weathers T, Einhorn LH. Vinblastine plus ifosfamide plus cisplatin as initial salvage therapy in recurrent germ cell tumor. *J Clin Oncol.* 1998;16:2500–2504.
5. Loehrer Sr PJ, Einhorn LH, Williams SD. VP-16 plus ifosfamide plus cisplatin as salvage therapy in refractory germ cell cancer. *J Clin Oncol.* 1986;4:528–536.
6. Kondagunta GV, Bacik J, Donadio A, et al. Combination of paclitaxel, ifosfamide, and cisplatin is an effective second-line therapy for patients with relapsed testicular germ cell tumors. *J Clin Oncol.* 2005;23:6549–6555.
7. Nichols CR, Tricot G, Williams SD, et al. Dose-intensive chemotherapy in refractory germ cell cancer–a phase I/II trial of high-dose carboplatin and etoposide with autologous bone marrow transplantation. *J Clin Oncol.* 1989;7:932–939.
8. Nichols CR, Andersen J, Lazarus HM, et al. High-dose carboplatin and etoposide with autologous bone marrow transplantation in refractory germ cell cancer: an Eastern Cooperative Oncology Group protocol. *J Clin Oncol.* 1992;10:558–563.
9. Broun ER, Nichols CR, Gize G, et al. Tandem high dose chemotherapy with autologous bone marrow transplantation for initial relapse of testicular germ cell cancer. *Cancer.* 1997;79:1605–1610.
10. Broun ER, Nichols CR, Turns M, et al. Early salvage therapy for germ cell cancer using high dose chemotherapy with autologous bone marrow support. *Cancer.* 1994;73:1716–1720.
11. Einhorn LH, Williams SD, Chamness A, Brames MJ, Perkins SM, Abonour R. High-dose chemotherapy and stem-cell rescue for metastatic germ-cell tumors. *N Engl J Med.* 2007;357:340–348.
12. Adra N, Abonour R, Althouse SK, Albany C, Hanna NH, Einhorn LH. High-dose chemotherapy and autologous peripheral-blood stem-cell transplantation for relapsed metastatic germ cell tumors: the Indiana University experience. *J Clin Oncol.* 2017;35:1096–1102.
13. Motzer RJ, Mazumdar M, Bosl GJ, et al. High-dose carboplatin, etoposide, and cyclophosphamide for patients with refractory germ cell tumors: treatment results and prognostic factors for survival and toxicity. *J Clin Oncol.* 1996;14:1098–1105.
14. Margolin K, Doroshow JH, Ahn C, et al. Treatment of germ cell cancer with two cycles of high-dose ifosfamide, carboplatin, and etoposide with autologous stem-cell support. *J Clin Oncol.* 1996;14:2631–2637.
15. Margolin KA, Doroshow JH, Frankel P, et al. Paclitaxel-based high-dose chemotherapy with autologous stem-cell rescue for relapsed germ cell cancer. *Biol Blood Marrow Transpl.* 2005;11:903–911.

16. Rick O, Bokemeyer C, Beyer J, et al. Salvage treatment with paclitaxel, ifosfamide, and cisplatin plus high-dose carboplatin, etoposide, and thiotepa followed by autologous stem-cell rescue in patients with relapsed or refractory germ cell cancer. *J Clin Oncol.* 2001;19:81–88.

17. Siegert W, Beyer J, Strohscheer I, et al. High-dose treatment with carboplatin, etoposide and ifosfamide followed by autologous stem-cell transplantation in relapsed or refractory germ cell cancer: a phase I/II study. *J Clin Oncol.* 1994;12:1223–1231.

18. Beyer J, Kramar A, Mandanas R, et al. High-dose chemotherapy as salvage treatment in germ cell tumors: a multivariate analysis of prognostic variables. *J Clin Oncol.* 1996;14:2638–2645.

19. Lotz J-P, Bui B, Gomez F, et al. Sequential high-dose chemotherapy protocol for relapsed poor prognosis germ cell tumors combining two mobilization and cytoreductive treatments followed by three high-dose chemotherapy regimens supported by autologous stem cell transplantation. Results of the phase II multicentric TAXIF trial. *Ann Oncol.* 2005;16:411–418.

20. The International Prognostic Factors Study Group. Prognostic factors in patients with metastatic germ cell tumors who experienced treatment failure with cisplatin-based first-line chemotherapy. *J Clin Oncol.* 2011;28:4906–4911.

21. Feldman DR, Sheinfeld J, Bajorin DF, et al. TI-CE high-dose chemotherapy for patients with previously treated germ cell tumors; Results and prognostic factor analysis. *J Clin Oncol.* 2010;28:1706–1713.

22. Feldman DR, Huddart R, Hall E, Beyer J, Powles T. Is high dose therapy superior to conventional dose therapy as initial treatment for relapsed germ cell tumors? The TIGER Trial. *J Cancer.* 2011;2:374–377.

23. Selle F, Wittnebel S, Biron P, et al. A phase II trial of high-dose chemotherapy (HDCT) supported by hematopoetic stem-cell transplantation (HSCT) in germ-cell tumors (GCTs) patients failing cisplatin-based chemotherapy: the Multicentric TAXIF II study. *Ann Oncol.* 2014;25:1775–1782.

24. Fukuda S, Shirahama T, Imazono Y, et al. Expression of vascular endothelial growth factor in patients with testicular germ cell tumors as an indicator of metastatic disease. *Cancer.* 1999;85:1323–1330.

25. Bentas W, Beecken WD, Glienke W, Binder J, Schuldes H. Serum levels of basic fibroblast growth factor reflect disseminated disease in patients with testicular germ cell tumors. *Urol Res.* 2003;30:390–393.

26. Willett CG, Boucher Y, di Tomaso E, et al. Direct evidence that the VEGF-specific antibody bevacizumab has antivascular effects in human rectal cancer. *Nat Med.* 2004;10:145–147.

27. Nieto Y, Tu SM, Bassett R, et al. Bevacizumab/high-dose chemotherapy with autologous stem-cell transplant for poor-risk relapsed or refractory germ-cell tumors. *Ann Oncol.* 2015;26:2125–2132.

28. Nieto Y, Tu S-M, Campbell MT, et al. Infusional gemcitabine + docetaxel/melphalan/carboplatin (GemDMC) ± bevacizumab (BEV) as an effective high-dose chemotherapy (HDC) regimen for refractory of poor-risk relapsed germ-cell tumors (GCT). *J Clin Oncol.* 2017;35. suppl; abstr 4519.

29. Usanova S, Piée-Staffa A, Sied U, et al. Cisplatin sensitivity of testis tumour cells is due to deficiency in interstrand-crosslink repair and low ERCC1-XPF expression. *Mol Cancer.* 2010;9:248.

30. Lorch A, Kollmannsberger C, Hartmann JT, et al. Single versus sequential high-dose chemotherapy in patients with relapsed or refractory germ cell tumors: a prospective randomized multicenter trial of the German Testicular Cancer Study Group. *J Clin Oncol.* 2007;25:2778–2784.

31. Lorch A, Bascoul-Mollevi C, Kramar A, et al. Conventional-dose versus high-dose chemotherapy as first salvage treatment in male patients with metastatic germ cell tumors: evidence from a large international database. *J Clin Oncol.* 2011;29:2178–2184.

32. Beyer J, Stenning S, Gerl A, Fossa S, Siegert W. High-dose versus conventional-dose chemotherapy as first-salvage treatment in patients with non-seminomatous germ-cell tumors: a matched-pair analysis. *Ann Oncol.* 2001;13:599–605.

33. Pico J-L, Rosti G, Kramar A, et al. A randomized trial of high-dose chemotherapy in the salvage treatment of patients failing first-line platinum chemotherapy for advanced germ cell tumors. *Ann Oncol.* 2005;16:1152–1159.

34. Einhorn LH. Curing metastatic testicular cancer. *PNAS.* 2002;99:4592–4595.

35. Motzer RJ, Mazumdar M, Bajorin DF, Bosl GJ, Lyn P, Vlamis V. High-dose carboplatin, etoposide, and cyclophosphamide with autologous bone marrow transplantation in first-line therapy for patients with poor-risk germ cell tumors. *J Clin Oncol.* 1997;15:2546–2552.

36. Schmoll HJ, Kollmannsberger C, Metzner B, et al. Long-term results of first-line sequential high-dose etoposide, ifosfamide, and cisplatin chemotherapy plus autologous stem cell support for patients with advanced metastatic germ cell cancer: an extended phase I/II study of the German Testicular Cancer Study Group. *J Clin Oncol.* 2003;21:4083–4091.

37. Bokemeyer C, Kollmannsberger C, Meisner C, et al. First-line high-dose chemotherapy compared with standard-dose PEB/VIP chemotherapy in patients with advanced germ cell tumors: a multivariate and matched-pair analysis. *J Clin Oncol.* 1999;17:3450–3456.

38. Chevreau C, Droz JP, Pico JL, et al. Early intensified chemotherapy with autologous bone marrow transplantation in first line treatment of poor risk non-seminomatous germ cell tumors. *Eur Urol.* 1993;23:213–218.

39. Daugaard G, Skoneczna A, Aass N, et al. A randomized phase III study comparing standard dose BEP with sequential high-dose cisplatin, etoposide, ifosfamide (VIP) plus stem cell support in males with poor prognosis germ cell cancer (GCC): an intergroup study of EORTC, GTCSG, and Grupo Germinal. *Ann Oncol.* 2010;22:1054–1061.

40. Motzer RJ, Nichols CJ, Margolin KA, et al. Phase III trial of conventional-dose chemotherapy with or without high-dose chemotherapy and autologous hematopoietic stem-cell rescue as first-line treatment for patients with poor prognosis metastatic germ cell tumors. *J Clin Oncol.* 2007;25:247–256.
41. Nieto Y, Champlin RE, Wingard JR, et al. Status of high-dose chemotherapy for breast cancer: a review. *Biol Blood Marrow Transpl.* 2000;6:476–495.
42. Peters WP, Ross M, Vredenburgh JJ, et al. High-dose chemotherapy and autologous bone marrow support as consolidation after standard-dose adjuvant therapy for high-risk primary breast cancer. *J Clin Oncol.* 1993;11:1132–1143.
43. Gianni AM, Siena S, Bregni M, et al. Efficacy, toxicity, and applicability of high-dose sequential chemotherapy as adjuvant treatment in operable breast cancer with 10 or more involved axillary nodes: five-year results. *J Clin Oncol.* 1997;15:2312–2321.
44. Nieto Y. The verdict is not in yet. Analysis of the randomized trials of high-dose chemotherapy for breast cancer. *Haematologica.* 2003;88:201–211.
45. Berry DA, Ueno NT, Johnson MM, et al. High-dose chemotherapy with autologous hematopoietic stem-cell transplantation in metastatic breast cancer: overview of six randomized trials. *J Clin Oncol.* 2011;29:3224–3231.
46. Peters WP, Eder JP, Henner WD, et al. High-dose combination alkylating agents with autologous bone marrow support: a Phase 1 trial. *J Clin Oncol.* 1986;4:646–654.
47. Eder JP, Antman K, Peters W, et al. High-dose combination alkylating agent chemotherapy with autologous bone marrow support for metastatic breast cancer. *J Clin Oncol.* 1986;4:1592–1597.
48. Peters WP, Shpall EJ, Jones RB, et al. High-dose combination alkylating agents with bone marrow support as initial treatment for metastatic breast cancer. *J Clin Oncol.* 1988;6:1368–1376.
49. Antman K, Ayash L, Elias A, et al. A phase II study of high-dose cyclophosphamide, thiotepa, and carboplatin with autologous marrow support in women with measurable advanced breast cancer responding to standard-dose therapy. *J Clin Oncol.* 1992;10:102–110.
50. Cagnoni PJ, Nieto Y, Shpall EJ, et al. High-dose chemotherapy with autologous hematopoietic progenitor-cell support as part of combined modality therapy in patients with inflammatory breast cancer. *J Clin Oncol.* 1998;16:1661–1668.
51. Nieto Y, Nawaz S, Jones RB, et al. Prognostic model for relapse after high-dose chemotherapy with autologous stem-cell transplantation for stage IV oligometastatic breast cancer. *J Clin Oncol.* 2002;20:707–718.
52. Nieto Y, Jones RB, Shpall EJ. Stem-cell transplantation for the treatment of advanced solid tumors. *Springer Semin Immunopathol.* 2004;26:31–56.
53. Childs R, Chernoff A, Contentin N, et al. Regression of metastatic renal-cell carcinoma after nonmyeloablative allogeneic peripheral-blood stem-cell transplantation. *N Engl J Med.* 2000;343:750–758.
54. Bregni M, Bernardi M, Servida P, et al. Long-term follow-up of metastatic renal cancer patients undergoing reduced-intensity allografting. *Bone Marrow Transpl.* 2009;44: 237–242.
55. Barkholt L, Bregni M, Remberger M, et al. Allogeneic haematopoietic stem cell transplantation for metastatic renal carcinoma in Europe. *Ann Oncol.* 2006;17:1134–1140.

CHAPTER 21

Hematopoietic Cell Transplantation for Pediatric Solid Tumors

MIRA A. KOHORST, MD • SHAKILA P. KHAN, MD

HEMATOPOIETIC CELL TRANSPLANTATION FOR PEDIATRIC SOLID TUMORS

Autologous hematopoietic cell transplant (AHCT) in pediatrics is performed in selected pediatric solid tumors. It helps dose intensification of chemotherapy to eradicate the malignancy, and also in cases of tandem transplants, it reduces the period of recovery in between transplant cycles. There is no concern for rejection or graft-versus-host disease as patients are getting their own hematopoietic cells, and the recovery of peripheral counts is more rapid because of use of peripheral blood hematopoietic cells. The two most common solid tumors treated with high-dose chemotherapy (HDCT), followed by autologous hematopoietic cell rescue (AHCR), are neuroblastoma stage IV and high-risk medulloblastoma. Transplant is also used for other central nervous system (CNS) embryonal tumors and as salvage therapy for recurrent germ cell tumors (GCTs). Its role in metastatic and relapsed Ewing's sarcoma is debatable. In this chapter, we will present the current recommendation for transplant in these solid tumors.

Neuroblastoma

Neuroblastoma is the most common extracranial solid tumor in children with an incidence of 10.5 per million children less than 15 years of age. Risk stratification is assessed based on clinical and pathological criteria and has prognostic significance.[1] Outcomes for low- and intermediate-risk neuroblastoma have improved significantly with treatment, but most patients present with high-risk metastatic disease. Outcomes in these patients have improved with multimodal therapy comprised of chemotherapy, surgery, radiation, HDCT/AHCR, and biological and immunotherapy, but disease relapse is still a major issue. Long-term disease-free survival is 40%–50%.[2]

The role of AHCT for high-risk neuroblastoma has been studied for several years, and there are a number of prospective and retrospective studies indicating the benefit of transplant.[3] The Children's Oncology Group (COG) study 3891 was a phase III study that randomized patients to receive continuation chemotherapy versus HDCT/AHCR using purged bone marrow, followed by a second randomization between no further treatment or 13-Cis retinoic acid for 6 months. Results showed that event-free survival (EFS) was better in patients who received the transplant versus the ones who received chemotherapy, and patients who were randomized to the retinoic acid had better outcomes. EFS in the group who received AHCT and retinoic acid was 38%. This study established transplant, followed by retinoic acid as standard of care.[4]

After this, there have been multiple studies looking at dose intensification of chemotherapy, use of non–total-body irradiation (TBI)-based regimens and use of peripheral hematopoietic cells instead of bone marrow for rapid recovery to improve survival in this group of patients.[5,6] Use of TBI in young children is concerning because of late effects. Carboplatin, etoposide, and melphalan (CEM) are considered the standard conditioning regimen for patient with high-risk neuroblastoma. Studies from Europe suggest that busulfan with melphalan (BuMel) may have less toxicity than CEM. A retrospective review at a single institution compared CEM with BuMel. Sinusoidal obstruction was higher and more prolonged in the busulfan group. Pulmonary hypertension was also seen in the busulfan group but not in the group receiving CEM. Nephrotoxicity, transfusions, and pain management due to mucositis was increased in the CEM group.[7] COG 3891 established CEM as standard conditioning regimen. There are ongoing studies not published yet trying to answer this question.

Another concern is presence of tumor cells in the bone marrow in all patients and the question of purging the bone marrow before infusion to reduce toxicity. COG 3891 did use purged bone marrow cells using antitumor monoclonal antibody, followed by magnetic depletion, and evidence suggested that process may be important.[8] With the advent of peripheral blood stem cell (PBSC) collection, CD 34 selection may have fewer tumor cells. It is not clear if purging is required with PBSC.[9] COG A3973 was a phase III comparison of purged versus unpurged PBSC. Data presented at the American Society of Clinical Oncology (ASCO) meeting showed no difference in outcome between purged versus unpurged PBSC.[10,11]

COG study ANBL 0032 was a phase III randomized study of addition of chimeric anti-GD2 antibody in high-risk neuroblastoma after myeloablative therapy and AHCR. The patients were randomized to receive chimeric antibody with granulocyte-macrophage colony-stimulating factor or interleukin 2 with 13-cisretinoic acid versus retinoic acid alone. At a median follow-up of 2.1 years, EFS was significantly higher in the immunotherapy arm, 66% compared with 46%, and because interim monitoring boundary for large early benefit was met, the randomization was stopped, and the recommendation was to treat all patients with high-risk neuroblastoma with immunotherapy and retinoic acid after HDCT/AHCR and radiation.[12]

Another phase III study, COG ANBL 0532, looked at further intensification of chemotherapy, and randomization was between single versus tandem transplant after induction chemotherapy. The single transplant used CEM, and the tandem transplant used thiotepa and cyclophosphamide for the first transplant, followed by a modified regimen of CEM with lower doses for the second transplant. Total patients enrolled were 652. There were 27 patients who did not have N Myc amplification and were nonrandomly assigned to receive single transplant regimen. After that randomization, patients entered a second trial with anti-GD2 (also known as Ch 14.18 or dinutuximab) immunotherapy with or without isotretinoin. This group was evaluated to determine whether tandem transplant provided additional benefit to the immunotherapy. Results were presented at a plenary session at the 2016 ASCO meeting. The 3-year EFS was 61.4% in the tandem group versus 48.4% in the single transplant arm. Overall survival (OS) was not statistically, significantly different. The benefit of the tandem transplant was sustained in the immunotherapy group with a 3-year EFS of 73.7% compared with 56%, and an OS of 83.7% versus 74.4%, which was statistically significant. Treatment-related mortality was 2.6% both in induction and consolidation, but rates of mucosal, infectious, and liver toxicities were similar in the two arms.[13]

The role of metaiodobenzylguanidine (MIBG) alone or as part of conditioning is being studied currently.

MIBG conjugated with radioactive iodine can be used for imaging (^{123}I) and treatment (^{131}I) for neuroblastoma. High-dose ^{131}I MIBG has been shown to have an excellent response rate in relapsed neuroblastoma patients whose tumors were MIBG avid. These patients do require PBSC support for bone marrow recovery. A pilot study which incorporated MIBG (12 mCi/kg) with CEM conditioning followed by AHCR showed response in 5 of 6 patients with metastatic disease and 3 of 4 with localized disease.[14] This was followed by the neuroblastoma consortium, New Approaches to Neuroblastoma Therapy (NANT) study which used the same dose with CEM for patients with refractory disease and showed a complete or partial response rate of 27%. Major grade III toxicities were mucositis and hepatic with high incidence of sinusoidal obstructive syndrome.[15] There have been a number of phase I and II studies from Europe and the United States showing the feasibility of this approach in MIBG avid nonresponsive or progressive disease. The NANT consortium used vincristine and irinotecan as a transplant regimen with ^{131}I MIBG with less oral and hepatic toxicity.[16] This option is being looked at in the next COG phase III trial.

The role of allogeneic hematopoietic cell transplantation is not clear in neuroblastoma. The Center for Blood and Marrow Transplantation did a retrospective review of 143 allogeneic BMT for neuroblastoma from 1990 to 2007. Patients were separated in two groups depending on if they had an autotransplant before. Patients who were in complete remission (CR) or good partial response had lower relapse rates. There was an advantage with lower relapse rates and survival in the allogeneic patients who did not receive an autotransplant before, but outcomes overall were poor. There was no benefit for an allogeneic transplant after auto-BMT.[17] Prospective trials would be needed to answer this question.

At this time the standard treatment for neuroblastoma in the United States is induction chemotherapy with six cycles, PBSC collection after cycle 2 or 3, surgery after cycle 5, consolidation therapy with tandem transplants, radiation therapy, and then immunotherapy followed by 6 cycles of 13-Cisretinoic acid.

CNS Tumors

CNS tumors are the most common pediatric solid tumors and account for 20%–25% of all childhood malignancies.[18] The estimated incidence of CNS tumors is 5.6 cases per 100,000 person-years for patients aged ≤19 years. In the United States the 10-year survival rate for all CNS tumors is 70%, and they are the leading cause of cancer death in children of age range 0–14 years.[19]

Management generally requires multimodal therapy with surgery, chemotherapy, and/or radiation. Tumors that are more chemosensitive and demonstrate a clear dose-dependent response may benefit from high-dose myeloablative chemotherapy with AHCR.[20] HDCT may help overcome drug-resistance mechanisms as well as the blood-brain barrier. An escalation in chemotherapy may also help reduce and/or delay radiotherapy and improve neurocognitive outcomes. Furthermore, the efficacy of radiotherapy may improve with smaller tumor burden.[21]

Encouraging results have been seen in patients with medulloblastoma,[22-25] supratentorial primitive neuro-ectodermal tumors (PNETs; now termed CNS embryonal tumors, not otherwise specified (NOS)),[26-28] and atypical teratoid/rhabdoid tumors (AT/RTs).[29-35] HDCT with AHCR has been attempted in other high-risk brain tumors such as high-grade gliomas without as much success.[36-38] Patients have the greatest benefit if they have had a good response to standard chemotherapy with minimal residual disease at the time of transplant.[37]

Medulloblastoma and CNS Embryonal Tumors, NOS

Medulloblastoma is the most common malignant brain tumor of childhood and accounts for 15%–20% of all CNS tumors.[21] CNS embryonal tumors, NOS (formerly primitive neuroectodermal tumors [PNETs]), are much more rare, accounting for 2%–3% of childhood brain tumors, and are often included in studies with high-risk medulloblastoma.[39-41] Treatment for medulloblastoma depends on risk stratification, which is determined by degree of resection, dissemination, and age. Children with high-risk disease, defined by ≥1.5 cm^2 of postoperative residual tumor or evidence of disseminated/metastatic disease, and children with recurrent disease are often treated with HDCT/AHCR.[21]

Many groups have studied the role of autologous hematopoietic transplant in high-risk and relapsed medulloblastoma, as well as CNS embryonal tumors, NOS. One of the first studies by Strother et al. included 19 patients with metastatic medulloblastoma treated with topotecan, followed by craniospinal radiation and four cycles of high-dose cyclophosphamide, cisplatin, and vincristine with AHCR. The 2-year progression-free survival (PFS) for this group was 73.7%.[42] As a continuation of this study, the St. Jude Medulloblastoma (SJMB)-96 trial included 48 patients with high-risk medulloblastoma and PNET, who received risk-adapted craniospinal radiation with boost to the tumor bed, followed by 4 cycles of HDCT with cisplatin, cyclophosphamide, and vincristine and subsequent AHCR. The

5-year EFS for all high-risk patients was 70%. For those with metastatic disease, the 5-year EFS was 66%.[23] This is compared to the previous 5-year survival rates of less than 55% for children with high-risk disease.[43-45]

Other preparative regimens for HDCT/AHCR have been used both before and after radiotherapy in a variety of small retrospective and prospective studies. Dhodapkar et al. reported 9 patients with metastatic medulloblastoma or PNET treated with high-dose cyclophosphamide with cisplatin, vincristine, etoposide, and high-dose methotrexate with AHCR for 2–3 cycles before radiation. Seven out of nine patients remained tumor free at a median follow-up of 27 months.[46] Another study including 21 patients with high-risk or disseminated medulloblastoma were treated with intensified induction chemotherapy and a single myeloablative chemotherapy cycle (carboplatin, thiotepa, and etoposide) with AHCR. This was followed by radiotherapy for all patients older than 6 years and for patients with evidence of residual disease if aged less than 6 years. The 3-year EFS and OS were 49% and 60%, respectively.[47] Gandola et al. studied 33 patients with metastatic medulloblastoma treated with postoperative induction chemotherapy, hyperfractionated accelerated radiotherapy, and consolidation chemotherapy with 2 courses of myeloablative chemotherapy with AHCR for those who had persistent disease before radiotherapy and maintenance chemotherapy for those with no persistent disease. The 5-year EFS, PFS, and OS were 70%, 72%, and 73%, respectively.[48] Dufour et al. described the results of tandem HDCT/AHCR in 24 children aged >5 years with newly diagnosed high-risk medulloblastoma or supratentorial PNETs. They were treated with conventional chemotherapy, followed by two courses of high-dose thiotepa with AHCR followed by craniospinal radiotherapy. The 5-year EFS and OS was 65% and 74%, respectively. For those with metastatic disease, the 5-year EFS and OS was 72% and 83%, respectively.[25]

In infants and young children, HDCT can be used to either delay or exclude radiotherapy due to the unacceptable toxicity profile in this age group. Berthold et al. assessed high-dose busulfan and thiotepa with AHCR, followed by radiotherapy in 19 children aged <5 years with classical or incompletely resected medulloblastoma. The 3-year EFS and OS were 68% and 84%, respectively. However, 6 out of 19 patients developed sinusoidal obstruction syndrome.[24] Another study in young children aged <3 years with malignant brain tumors (Children's Cancer Group, CCG-99,703) assessed the feasibility, tolerability, and response rate of HDCT/AHCR using 3 cycles of high-dose thiotepa and carboplatin after induction therapy without radiotherapy. The patient cohort represented many different histologic groups including medulloblastoma (n = 36), PNET (n = 17), ependymoma (n = 21), AT/RTs (n = 8), and other (n = 10) for a total of 92 patients. Five-year EFS and OS were 43.9% and 63.6%, respectively, with 2.6% toxic death rate during consolidation (HDCT/AHCR). This study had significantly better survival rates than the previous study, CCG-9921, which used standard-dose chemotherapy without myeloablative consolidation chemotherapy or radiotherapy in children aged <3 years (5-year EFS, 26%; OS, 43%).[49]

For patients with relapsed medulloblastoma or PNET, Gajjar and Pizer compiled the results from 8 HDCT/AHCR studies which revealed 35 out of 159 disease-free survivors (22.0%). Among those who had a relapse after radiotherapy, there were even fewer survivors (17.3%). They concluded that the role for HDCT/AHCR is less clear in relapsed disease.[50]

Atypical Teratoid/Rhabdoid Tumor

AT/RTs are the most common malignant CNS tumor in infants aged <6 months. In the first year of life, AT/RTs comprise 40%–50% of all embryonal CNS tumors. The majority of these tumors have genomic alterations in *SMARCB1*.[29] The prognosis for these tumors is very poor, which may in part be related to the inability to give aggressive radiotherapy without significant late effects.[31] Many groups have investigated the role of HDCT/AHCR in AT/RTs.

A retrospective review performed by Hilden et al. evaluated 42 patients with AT/RT, of which 13 patients received HDCT/AHCR. A conditioning regimen of carboplatin and thiotepa was used in the majority of patients. The median EFS for those receiving HDCT/AHCR was 10 months, and median OS was 21.5 months from the time of diagnosis. Of the 13 patients, 6 had no evidence of disease, 6 died of disease, and there was 1 toxic death by the end of the study.[51]

Tekautz et al. reported the results from the SJMB-96 study which contained 9 patients aged >3 years with AT/RT, 7 of which underwent HDCT/AHCR with cyclophosphamide, cisplatin, and vincristine after craniospinal radiation. The 2-year EFS and OS were 78% and 89%, respectively. This survival rate was significantly higher than that of younger children aged <3 years who received conventional chemotherapy without radiation (2-year EFS 11% and OS 8%). These authors concluded that patients have better outcomes with a combination of radiation and tandem HDCT/AHCR.[52]

In 2008 Gardner et al. reported the results of the Head Start I (HS I) and Head Start II (HS II) trials

which included a total of 13 patients with AT/RT. Chemotherapy included five cycles of cisplatin, vincristine, cyclophosphamide, and etoposide with high-dose methotrexate added in HS II. Consolidation for both regimens included HDCT with carboplatin, thiotepa, and etoposide, followed by AHCR. The 3-year EFS for the patients receiving HS II was 43% compared with 0% in HS I, suggesting a potential role for high-dose methotrexate. Of note, both regimens had significant toxicities during induction chemotherapy with every patient having at least one episode of bacterial infection including one fatal case of *Staphylococcus aureus* meningitis.[53]

In another retrospective review of the Canadian Pediatric Brain Tumor Consortium experience, a cohort of 50 patients with AT/RT was studied. Fourteen underwent HDCT/AHCR using three rounds of carboplatin and thiotepa, and four received carboplatin, thiotepa, and etoposide. Nine of the 18 patients are alive with a median survival of 40.8 months and 2-year OS of 48%. In those who did not receive HDCT, the 2-year OS was significantly less at 27% (P = .036).[35]

A phase I/II prospective study using tandem HDCT/ASCR for very young children (<3 years old) with malignant brain tumors was conducted by the Korean Society of Pediatric Neuro-Oncology. Nine patients with AT/RT were on this study, 6 of which received two cycles of tandem HDCT/AHCR with the first cycle comprised of carboplatin, thiotepa, and etoposide, and the second cycle comprised of cyclophosphamide and melphalan. At the end of the therapy, four patients had no evidence of disease. Five of nine patients relapsed or had progression during induction chemotherapy requiring radiotherapy. Four of the patients who received radiotherapy were alive at the end of this study. The authors suggested considering early administration of radiotherapy before HDCT/AHCR to improve outcomes after these therapies, even in this young age group.[34]

Zaky et al. conducted the Head Start III trial in which 19 patients with newly diagnosed AT/RT were treated with 5 cycles of induction chemotherapy (cisplatin, vincristine, etoposide, cyclophosphamide, and high-dose methotrexate), followed by consolidation with one cycle of HDCT/AHCR (carboplatin, thiotepa, etoposide) and radiation depending on age. Only 3 proceeded to consolidation, and of those, one had no evidence of disease, one was alive with disease, and one died of disease. Again, this Head Start regimen demonstrated significant toxicity with five toxic deaths.[33]

A retrospective study from the European Rhabdoid Registry assessed the outcome of children with AT/RT who underwent HDCT/AHCR with carboplatin and thiotepa. The 2-year EFS and OS were 29% and 50%, respectively.[30]

Slavc et al. reported the results of the Medical University of Vienna (MUV)-AT/RT prospective study which included 9 patients treated with three 9-week courses of induction chemotherapy including intrathecal chemotherapy (liposomal cytarabine and etoposide). This was followed by consolidation HDCT/AHCR with carboplatin, thiotepa, and etoposide. Finally, all patients received focal radiotherapy. The 5-year EFS and OS for this cohort were 88.9% and 100%, respectively. They compared these results to those of 13 patients who were treated on various other protocols and had a 5-year EFS and OS of 28.8%. No toxic deaths or unexpected toxicities were reported on the MUV-ATRT regimen, though hearing loss was present in 5 out of 9 patients. These remarkable results require further verification with larger studies but do suggest a potential role for both radiotherapy and intrathecal chemotherapy in addition to HDCT/AHCR in AT/RT.[32]

A prospective study of 13 patients (5 children aged less than 3 years and 8 children older than 3 years) with AT/RT was performed by Sung et al. Of the 13 patients, 10 were able to proceed to HDCT/AHCR with carboplatin, thiotepa, and etoposide for the first regimen and with cyclophosphamide and melphalan for the second. All five of the younger patients died secondary to disease progression. Four of the eight older patients remain progression free with a median follow-up of 64 months. One of the key differences between the younger and older groups was the use of radiotherapy in the older patients. Therefore the authors propose that early administration of radiotherapy should be considered even in young patients, balancing the risk of progression with the risk of neurotoxicity.[31]

The most recent COG study, ACNS0333, used induction chemotherapy (including high-dose methotrexate), followed by focal radiotherapy in children as young as 6 months, followed by three cycles of HDCT/AHCR with thiotepa and carboplatin. The 2-year EFS and OS for the entire 65-patient cohort were 42% and 53%, respectively. For those aged <3 years, the 2-year EFS and OS were 39% and 48%, respectively, which was deemed significantly better than historic controls ($P < .025$).[54] A common trend among most AT/RT studies has been that both HDCT/AHCR and early radiotherapy, regardless of young age, are important for improving survival. Despite this, survival remains poor, and more targeted approaches are currently being evaluated.

High-Grade Glioma

High-grade gliomas (WHO grade III and IV) have a very poor prognosis and no universal consensus on standard care in the pediatric setting. Numerous treatment approaches have been used in children, including HDCT/AHCR. Lee et al. performed a retrospective review of 30 pediatric patients with high-grade gliomas, of which 13 underwent 2 cycles of HDCT/AHCR with carboplatin, thiotepa, and etoposide, followed by cyclophosphamide/melphalan. For those who achieved complete or partial remission before HDCT/AHCR, OS was higher with HDCT/AHCR than that in the previous 5 years (no HDCT/AHCR; $P = .029$). Three-year EFS and OS were 23.7% and 31.5%, respectively. There was no improved survival for patients who started HDCT/AHCR with progressed tumors. There was one death due to sinusoidal obstructive syndrome, otherwise acceptable toxicity aside from neutropenic fever.[36]

Durable remissions were seen in 5 out of 27 patients with high-grade gliomas who received HDCT/AHCR with thiotepa and etoposide regimens in the setting of minimal residual tumor burden compared with none of 56 who received conventional chemotherapy in a study by Finlay et al.[37] Another group assessed a regimen of induction chemotherapy, HDCT/AHCR with thiotepa, and focal radiotherapy which demonstrated a 4-year PFS and OS of 43% and 46%, respectively.[38] However, an earlier study by Heideman et al. did not demonstrate any benefit of HDCT/AHCR over conventional chemotherapy.[55] Overall, there is not enough evidence to suggest HDCT/AHCR as the standard of care, though it does warrant further investigation.

Germ Cell Tumors

GCTs are malignancies which arise from the primordial germ cells of the embryo which eventually develop into gonads. They originate from the yolk sac. GCTs represent approximately 2%–3% of all pediatric malignancies. Common sites are the gonads and coccyx, but they can arise from extragonadal sites such as mediastinum, brain, and retroperitoneum. GCTs are classified into different categories based on histological findings. Malignant germinomas that are in the gonads, dysgerminoma in ovary, and seminoma in testis are comprised of immature germ cells. Teratomas arise from the three germ layers and can be benign or malignant. Yolk cell tumors are epithelial neoplasms, and mixed GCTs are combinations of the aforementioned cell types. Tumor markers alpha fetoprotein and beta-human chorionic gonadotropin, when present, are of prognostic significance and help monitor response to treatment and relapse. Many CNS tumors are not biopsied, and diagnosis is based on markers.[56]

Surgery plays an important role in extracranial GCTs but not in intracranial GCTs. Radiation therapy is an integral part of the treatment for intracranial germ cell but not for extracranial tumors. Dose and field of radiation has been reduced to minimize risk of late effects.[57] Conventional treatment with cisplatin-based chemotherapy has a very high cure rate of about 80% in children with gonadal tumors. Extragonadal tumors have a higher risk of recurrence after treatment than gonadal tumors. Similarly intracranial GCTs have a higher recurrence rate. Carboplatin is considered the standard platinum agent for intracranial GCTs, whereas cisplatin is considered the standard for extracranial tumors.[58] Patients with relapsed disease can still be salvaged by second-line chemotherapy.

The international germ cell cancer collaborative group recommended stratification into low-, intermediate-, and high-risk groups. Indication for HDCT/AHCR is variable depending on the number of recurrences and location of the tumor. Most of the data are from adult patients, and there have been no randomized trials in the pediatric setting to answer these questions. HDCT with AHCR is the treatment of choice in patients who have failed standard salvage therapy or have refractory disease. There is no standard in pediatrics of optimal conditioning regimen and number of transplants, one versus tandem. For extragonadal GCT, a phase II trial of 107 relapsed patients who received chemotherapy with ifosfamide and paclitaxel and then received HDCT/AHCR had an improved EFS of 47% and OS of 52%.[59] The European Group for Blood and Marrow Transplantation reviewed 23 children with extragonadal GCT who received HDCT/AHCR. Locations were intracranial, sacrococcyx, retroperitoneum, and mediastinum. One had germinoma, and rest were nongerminomatous. Nine patients were in first relapse, and 14 patients were in second or third relapse. There were no deaths due to toxicity. Patients received chemotherapy before coming for transplant and had chemosensitive disease. Conditioning mostly included carboplatin, etoposide, and cyclophosphamide in seven patients, carboplatin and etoposide with or without thiotepa in 10, and others received different combinations including melphalan. Nineteen received PBSC, nine had bone marrow, and one had both. A total of 70% achieved a CR, and 48% are disease free at the median follow-up of 66 months. Patients with extracranial disease did better than those with intracranial disease.[60]

Agarwal et al. published a report on 37 high-risk GCT patients who received HDCT/AHCR. Pediatric patients were included in this study. Twenty patients had gonadal disease, 10 had extragonadal tumors, and three had intracranial tumors. Twenty-nine patients received salvage chemotherapy before transplant. All patients received the same conditioning with etoposide, carboplatin, and cyclophosphamide, followed by one infusion of peripheral hematopoietic stem cells collected after mobilization with cyclophosphamide. Outcomes were not different in patients who received salvage chemotherapy versus those who did not. They reported a 3-year OS of 57% and a 3-year EFS of 49%. Treatment-related mortality was 3%. Patients with seminomas seemed to have a better outcome than patients without seminomas.[61]

HDCT with AHCR is not used upfront for intracranial GCTs. It is indicated as a salvage therapy for refractory or nonresponsive nongerminomatous GCTs and germinoma. Results are variable because of selection of patients and conditioning used. The role of transplant in intracranial GCTs is not clear.

The role of single versus tandem transplants in GCT is also not fully understood. There is an ongoing current phase III study (TIGER study) which is a randomized trial comparing chemotherapy to tandem transplant in refractory or recurrent GCTs to answer this question.

Sarcomas

Sarcomas comprise 10%–15% of all childhood malignancies.[62] Overall prognosis has improved with advances in chemotherapy combinations, radiotherapy, and aggressive surgery for local control. Nevertheless, the prognosis of children with metastatic or recurrent sarcomas remains dismal. Therefore, HDCT with autologous hematopoietic stem cell rescue has been explored in this setting.

Ewing Sarcoma

For Ewing sarcoma, there have been mixed results with HDCT/AHCR, with some studies demonstrating a benefit, others demonstrating no benefit, and many with a concern of toxicity. The most widely used preparative regimen in previous studies has been busulfan/melphalan (BuMel). An early study by Meyers et al. evaluated patients with metastatic Ewing sarcoma to the bone and/or bone marrow and revealed no benefit of HDCT/AHCR when using a regimen of melphalan, etoposide, and TBI. The 2-year EFS was 24%, and there were 3 toxic deaths with this regimen.[63] Oberlin et al. reported a potential benefit of HDCT/AHCR (BuMel) for patients with lung-only or bone metastases with 5-year EFS of 53% and 36% for these two groups, respectively.[64] However, similar survival was being achieved with conventional chemotherapy with whole-lung irradiation for lung metastases.[65] Luksch et al. evaluated HDCT/AHCR (BuMel) with whole-lung radiation in patients with lung-only metastases or a single-bone metastasis. The 5-year EFS was 43%, but there was significant toxicity with one toxic death, one secondary malignancy resulting in death, and 12 episodes of sinusoidal obstructive syndrome.[66] Drabko et al. performed a retrospective analysis on pediatric patients with high risk or relapsed Ewing sarcoma and reported an advantage in relapse-free survival with HDCT/AHCR (BuMel) (0.27 vs. 0.66; P = .008) and in OS (0.31 vs. 0.71; P = .007).[67]

These mixed results led to a randomized prospective study, EURO-EWING 99, which evaluated pediatric patients with either high-risk localized Ewing sarcoma or lung-only metastatic Ewing sarcoma. Patients with lung-only metastases were randomized to consolidation with HDCT/AHCR (BuMel) versus conventional chemotherapy with vincristine, actinomycin, and ifosfamide (VAI) plus whole-lung irradiation. The BuMel arm had a 3-year EFS of 55.7% compared with 50.3% in the conventional arm, and it also had a 3-year OS of 55.9% compared with 51.5% (neither were statistically significant). The BuMel group had 3 toxic deaths, compared with 0 in the conventional arm, and more severe acute toxicities.[68] The patients with high-risk localized Ewing sarcoma, defined as poor histologic response or large tumor size >200 mL, were randomized to consolidation treatment with HDCT/AHCR (BuMel) or conventional chemotherapy with VAI. The 3-year EFS for the BuMel arm was 66.9% compared with 53.1% in the conventional arm, and the 3-year OS was 77.8% compared with 69.9% (both statistically significant). There were 2 toxic deaths in the BuMel group as well as more severe acute toxicities, however.[69] These results suggest a possible benefit in high-risk localized disease, but not in lung-only metastatic disease.

The role of HDCT/AHCR is unclear in relapsed Ewing sarcoma. Some studies suggest potential benefit in certain subgroups, such as those who achieved complete or partial remission before HDCT/AHCR,[70] but no consistent benefit has been demonstrated, and morbidity from toxicity is high.[70-73]

Osteosarcoma

Patients with osteosarcoma have a survival rate of 60%–70%, but this is much lower for patients with poor tumor necrosis <90% (35%–45%), metastases (24%), and relapsed disease (18%).[74-76] Many studies have evaluated the role of HDCT/AHCR in these poor prognosis groups, the vast majority of which have

demonstrated no benefit.[77-82] The French Society of Pediatric Oncology has retrospectively analyzed the role of HDCT/AHCR with thiotepa in patients with relapsed or refractory osteosarcoma and found a radiological response rate of 31% and a 5-year OS of 31%. Given the feasibility, safety, and potential benefit of this regimen, the French group currently has a randomized study underway to compare this treatment to conventional chemotherapy in relapsed osteosarcoma.[83] Another retrospective review demonstrated possible benefit with HDCT/AHCR using melphalan, etoposide, and carboplatin in high-risk osteosarcoma, with an EFS and OS of 67.4% and 78.3%, respectively, at a short median follow-up of 31 months. This study was limited by small sample size (19 patients) and short follow-up time.[84] Overall, HDCT/AHCR does not seem like a promising option in osteosarcoma.

Rhabdomyosarcoma

Rhabdomyosarcoma is the most common soft tissue sarcoma of childhood and accounts for 3% of all childhood malignancies. For all patients with rhabdomyosarcoma, the OS is around 70% at 5 years.[85] However, for those with metastatic rhabdomyosarcoma, the survival is dismal. A Cochrane review of HDCT/AHCR was evaluated in patients with metastatic rhabdomyosarcoma and identified 3 nonrandomized controlled trials. In the transplant groups, 3-year OS ranged from 22% to 53% compared with 18%–55% in the control groups. A meta-analysis on OS demonstrated no difference between the treatment groups.[86,87] Prospective randomized controlled trials are lacking in this patient population.

Nonrhabdomyosarcoma Soft Tissue Sarcomas

Nonrhabdomyosarcoma soft tissue sarcomas represent a heterogeneous group of rare malignant soft tissue solid tumors excluding rhabdomyosarcoma. HDCT with AHCR has been evaluated in patients with high-risk tumors or metastatic disease. A recent Cochrane review was performed on these tumor types and only identified one randomized controlled trial with 87 patients receiving HDCT/AHCR versus conventional chemotherapy. The 3-year OS was 32.7% for the HDCT/AHCR arm compared with 49.4% in the standard-dose chemotherapy arm, though this was not statistically significant (hazard ratio was 1.26 with 95% confidence interval of 0.70–2.29, P = .44). For those with a complete response before the treatment, there was a higher OS in both the groups, favoring standard chemotherapy (83.9% compared with 42.8%). There are limited data on HDCT/AHCR in nonrhabdomyosarcoma soft tissue sarcomas; however, this study has shown no survival advantage.[88,89]

Wilms Tumor

The OS rates for children with Wilms tumor have improved significantly with multimodal therapy and are currently around 90%. However, approximately 15% will relapse, and relapsed Wilms tumor survival rates are poor with only 50% surviving past 4 years.[90] HDCT with AHCR has been evaluated in relapsed Wilms tumor. Ha et al. performed a retrospective analysis of 19 publications on this topic and did not find any difference in EFS or OS. However, for patients with very high risk, group III, recurrent Wilms, there was some benefit identified for the HDCT group (hazard ratio for EFS was 0.5, 95% confidence interval was 0.31 to 0.81), and they recommended a randomized controlled trial for this group alone. Of note, a higher rate of serious toxicities was seen in the HDCT/AHCR group.[91] Data were also analyzed from the Center for International Blood and Marrow Transplantation Research between 1990 and 2013 for patients with relapsed Wilms tumor who underwent HDCT/AHCR. The 5-year EFS and OS were 36% and 45%, respectively. The authors concluded that this was a well-tolerated treatment regimen with outcomes similar to those previously reported and that a randomized trial comparing HDCT/AHCR to conventional chemotherapy is needed.[90]

REFERENCES

1. Cheung NV, Heller G. Chemotherapy dose intensity correlates strongly with response, median survival, and median progression-free survival in metastatic neuroblastoma. *J Clin Oncol.* 1991;9(6):1050–1058.
2. Matthay KK, O'Leary MC, Ramsay NK, et al. Role of myeloablative therapy in improved outcome for high risk neuroblastoma: review of recent Children's Cancer Group results. *Eur J Cancer.* 1995;31A(4):572–575.
3. Dini G, Philip T, Hartmann O, et al. Bone marrow transplantation for neuroblastoma: a review of 509 cases. EBMT Group. *Bone Marrow Transplant.* 1989;4(suppl 4):42–46.
4. Matthay KK, Villablanca JG, Seeger RC, et al. Treatment of high-risk neuroblastoma with intensive chemotherapy, radiotherapy, autologous bone marrow transplantation, and 13-cis-retinoic acid. Children's Cancer Group. *N Engl J Med.* 1999;341(16):1165–1173.
5. Grupp SA, Stern JW, Bunin N, et al. Tandem high-dose therapy in rapid sequence for children with high-risk neuroblastoma. *J Clin Oncol.* 2000;18(13):2567–2575.
6. Kletzel M, Katzenstein HM, Haut PR, et al. Treatment of high-risk neuroblastoma with triple-tandem high-dose therapy and stem-cell rescue: results of the Chicago Pilot II Study. *J Clin Oncol.* 2002;20(9):2284–2292.
7. Desai AV, Heneghan MB, Li Y, et al. Toxicities of busulfan/melphalan versus carboplatin/etoposide/melphalan for high-dose chemotherapy with stem cell rescue for high-risk neuroblastoma. *Bone Marrow Transplant.* 2016;51(9):1204–1210.
8. Seeger RC, Vo DD, Ugelstad J, Reynolds CP. Removal of neuroblastoma cells from bone marrow with monoclonal antibodies and magnetic immunobeads. *Prog Clin Biol Res.* 1986;211:285–293.
9. Voigt A, Hafer R, Gruhn B, Zintl F. Expression of CD34 and other haematopoietic antigens on neuroblastoma cells: consequences for autologous bone marrow and peripheral blood stem cell transplantation. *J Neuroimmunol.* 1997;78(1–2):117–126.
10. Kreissman SG, Villablanca JG, Seeger RC, et al. A randomized phase III trial of myeloablative autologous peripheral blood stem cell (PBSC) transplant (ASCT) for high-risk neuroblastoma (HR-NB) employing immunomagnetic purged (P) versus unpurged (UP) PBSC: a Children's Oncology Group study. *J Clin Oncol.* 2008;26(15).
11. Fish JD, Grupp SA. Stem cell transplantation for neuroblastoma. *Bone Marrow Transplant.* 2008;41(2):159–165.
12. Yu AL, Gilman AL, Ozkaynak MF, et al. Anti-GD2 antibody with GM-CSF, Interleukin-2, and isotretinoin for neuroblastoma. *New Engl J Med.* 2010;363(14):1324–1334.
13. Park JRKS, London WB, et al. A phase 3 randomized clinical trial of tandem myeloablative autologous stem cell transplant using peripheral blood stem cell as consolidation therapy for high-risk neuroblastoma: a Children's Oncology Group study. *2016 ASCO Annu Meet.* 2016; Abstract LBA3.
14. Yanik GA, Levine JE, Matthay KK, et al. Pilot study of iodine-131-metaiodobenzylguanidine in combination with myeloablative chemotherapy and autologous stem-cell support for the treatment of neuroblastoma. *J Clin Oncol.* 2002;20(8):2142–2149.
15. Matthay KK, Tan JC, Villablanca JG, et al. Phase I dose escalation of iodine-131-metaiodobenzylguanidine with myeloablative chemotherapy and autologous stem-cell transplantation in refractory neuroblastoma: a new approaches to Neuroblastoma Therapy Consortium Study. *J Clin Oncol.* 2006;24(3):500–506.
16. DuBois SG, Mody R, Naranjo A, et al. MIBG avidity correlates with clinical features, tumor biology, and outcomes in neuroblastoma: a report from the Children's Oncology Group. *Pediatr Blood Cancer.* 2017;64(11).
17. Hale GA, Arora M, Ahn KW, et al. Allogeneic hematopoietic cell transplantation for neuroblastoma: the CIBMTR experience. *Bone Marrow Transplant.* 2013;48(8):1056–1064.
18. Linabery AM, Ross JA. Trends in childhood cancer incidence in the U.S. (1992–2004). *Cancer.* 2008;112(2):416–432.

19. Ostrom QT, Gittleman H, Fulop J, et al. CBTRUS statistical report: primary brain and central nervous system tumors diagnosed in the United States in 2008-2012. *Neuro Oncol.* 2015;17(suppl 4):iv1–iv62.
20. Ziegler DS, Cohn RJ, McCowage G, et al. Efficacy of vincristine and etoposide with escalating cyclophosphamide in poor-prognosis pediatric brain tumors. *Neuro Oncol.* 2006;8(1):53–59.
21. Massimino M, Biassoni V, Gandola L, et al. Childhood medulloblastoma. *Crit Rev Oncol Hematol.* 2016;105:35–51.
22. Ridola V, Grill J, Doz F, et al. High-dose chemotherapy with autologous stem cell rescue followed by posterior fossa irradiation for local medulloblastoma recurrence or progression after conventional chemotherapy. *Cancer.* 2007;110(1):156–163.
23. Gajjar A, Chintagumpala M, Ashley D, et al. Risk-adapted craniospinal radiotherapy followed by high-dose chemotherapy and stem-cell rescue in children with newly diagnosed medulloblastoma (St Jude Medulloblastoma-96): long-term results from a prospective, multicentre trial. *Lancet Oncol.* 2006;7(10):813–820.
24. Bergthold G, El Kababri M, Varlet P, et al. High-dose busulfan-thiotepa with autologous stem cell transplantation followed by posterior fossa irradiation in young children with classical or incompletely resected medulloblastoma. *Pediatr Blood Cancer.* 2014;61(5):907–912.
25. Dufour C, Kieffer V, Varlet P, et al. Tandem high-dose chemotherapy and autologous stem cell rescue in children with newly diagnosed high-risk medulloblastoma or supratentorial primitive neuro-ectodermic tumors. *Pediatr Blood Cancer.* 2014;61(8):1398–1402.
26. Chintagumpala M, Hassall T, Palmer S, et al. A pilot study of risk-adapted radiotherapy and chemotherapy in patients with supratentorial PNET. *Neuro Oncol.* 2009;11(1):33–40.
27. Sung KW, Yoo KH, Cho EJ, et al. High-dose chemotherapy and autologous stem cell rescue in children with newly diagnosed high-risk or relapsed medulloblastoma or supratentorial primitive neuroectodermal tumor. *Pediatr Blood Cancer.* 2007;48(4):408–415.
28. Fangusaro J, Finlay J, Sposto R, et al. Intensive chemotherapy followed by consolidative myeloablative chemotherapy with autologous hematopoietic cell rescue (AuHCR) in young children with newly diagnosed supratentorial primitive neuroectodermal tumors (sPNETs): report of the Head Start I and II experience. *Pediatr Blood Cancer.* 2008;50(2):312–318.
29. Fruhwald MC, Biegel JA, Bourdeaut F, Roberts CW, Chi SN. Atypical teratoid/rhabdoid tumors-current concepts, advances in biology, and potential future therapies. *Neuro Oncol.* 2016;18(6):764–778.
30. Benesch M, Bartelheim K, Fleischhack G, et al. High-dose chemotherapy (HDCT) with auto-SCT in children with atypical teratoid/rhabdoid tumors (AT/RT): a report from the European Rhabdoid Registry (EU-RHAB). *Bone Marrow Transplant.* 2014;49(3):370–375.
31. Sung KW, Lim DH, Yi ES, et al. Tandem high-dose chemotherapy and autologous stem cell transplantation for atypical teratoid/rhabdoid tumor. *Cancer Res Treat.* 2016;48(4):1408–1419.
32. Slavc I, Chocholous M, Leiss U, et al. Atypical teratoid rhabdoid tumor: improved long-term survival with an intensive multimodal therapy and delayed radiotherapy. The Medical University of Vienna Experience 1992–2012. *Cancer Med.* 2014;3(1):91–100.
33. Zaky W, Dhall G, Ji L, et al. Intensive induction chemotherapy followed by myeloablative chemotherapy with autologous hematopoietic progenitor cell rescue for young children newly-diagnosed with central nervous system atypical teratoid/rhabdoid tumors: the Head Start III experience. *Pediatr Blood Cancer.* 2014;61(1):95–101.
34. Park ES, Sung KW, Baek HJ, et al. Tandem high-dose chemotherapy and autologous stem cell transplantation in young children with atypical teratoid/rhabdoid tumor of the central nervous system. *J Korean Med Sci.* 2012;27(2):135–140.
35. Lafay-Cousin L, Hawkins C, Carret AS, et al. Central nervous system atypical teratoid rhabdoid tumours: the Canadian Paediatric Brain Tumour Consortium experience. *Eur J Cancer.* 2012;48(3):353–359.
36. Lee JW, Lim DH, Sung KW, et al. Tandem high-dose chemotherapy and autologous stem cell transplantation for high-grade gliomas in children and adolescents. *J Korean Med Sci.* 2017;32(2):195–203.
37. Finlay JL, Dhall G, Boyett JM, et al. Myeloablative chemotherapy with autologous bone marrow rescue in children and adolescents with recurrent malignant astrocytoma: outcome compared with conventional chemotherapy: a report from the Children's Oncology Group. *Pediatr Blood Cancer.* 2008;51(6):806–811.
38. Massimino M, Gandola L, Luksch R, et al. Sequential chemotherapy, high-dose thiotepa, circulating progenitor cell rescue, and radiotherapy for childhood high-grade glioma. *Neuro Oncol.* 2005;7(1):41–48.
39. Gaffney CC, Sloane JP, Bradley NJ, Bloom HJ. Primitive neuroectodermal tumours of the cerebrum. Pathology and treatment. *J Neurooncol.* 1985;3(1):23–33.
40. Gurney JG, Wall DA, Jukich PJ, Davis FG. The contribution of nonmalignant tumors to CNS tumor incidence rates among children in the United States. *Cancer Causes Control.* 1999;10(2):101–105.
41. McNeil DE, Cote TR, Clegg L, Rorke LB. Incidence and trends in pediatric malignancies medulloblastoma/primitive neuroectodermal tumor: a SEER update. Surveillance Epidemiology and End Results. *Med Pediatr Oncol.* 2002;39(3):190–194.
42. Strother D, Ashley D, Kellie SJ, et al. Feasibility of four consecutive high-dose chemotherapy cycles with stem-cell rescue for patients with newly diagnosed medulloblastoma or supratentorial primitive neuroectodermal tumor after craniospinal radiotherapy: results of a collaborative study. *J Clin Oncol.* 2001;19(10):2696–2704.

43. Zeltzer PM, Boyett JM, Finlay JL, et al. Metastasis stage, adjuvant treatment, and residual tumor are prognostic factors for medulloblastoma in children: conclusions from the Children's Cancer Group 921 randomized phase III study. *J Clin Oncol.* 1999;17(3):832–845.

44. Taylor RE, Bailey CC, Robinson KJ, et al. Outcome for patients with metastatic (M2-3) medulloblastoma treated with SIOP/UKCCSG PNET-3 chemotherapy. *Eur J Cancer.* 2005;41(5):727–734.

45. Kortmann RD, Kuhl J, Timmermann B, et al. Postoperative neoadjuvant chemotherapy before radiotherapy as compared to immediate radiotherapy followed by maintenance chemotherapy in the treatment of medulloblastoma in childhood: results of the German prospective randomized trial HIT '91. *Int J Radiat Oncol Biol Phys.* 2000;46(2):269–279.

46. Dhodapkar K, Dunkel IJ, Gardner S, Sapp M, Thoron L, Finlay J. Preliminary results of dose intensive preirradiation chemotherapy in patients older than 10 years of age with high risk medulloblastoma and supratentorial primitive neuroectodermal tumors. *Med Pediatr Oncol.* 2002;38(1):47–48.

47. Chi SN, Gardner SL, Levy AS, et al. Feasibility and response to induction chemotherapy intensified with high-dose methotrexate for young children with newly diagnosed high-risk disseminated medulloblastoma. *J Clin Oncol.* 2004;22(24):4881–4887.

48. Gandola L, Massimino M, Cefalo G, et al. Hyperfractionated accelerated radiotherapy in the Milan strategy for metastatic medulloblastoma. *J Clin Oncol.* 2009;27(4):566–571.

49. Cohen BH, Geyer JR, Miller DC, et al. Pilot study of intensive chemotherapy with peripheral hematopoietic cell support for children less than 3 Years of age with malignant brain tumors, the CCG-99703 phase I/II study. A report from the children's Oncology group. *Pediatr Neurol.* 2015;53(1):31–46.

50. Gajjar A, Pizer B. Role of high-dose chemotherapy for recurrent medulloblastoma and other CNS primitive neuroectodermal tumors. *Pediatr Blood Cancer.* 2010;54(4):649–651.

51. Hilden JM, Meerbaum S, Burger P, et al. Central nervous system atypical teratoid/rhabdoid tumor: results of therapy in children enrolled in a registry. *J Clin Oncol.* 2004;22(14):2877–2884.

52. Tekautz TM, Fuller CE, Blaney S, et al. Atypical teratoid/rhabdoid tumors (ATRT): improved survival in children 3 years of age and older with radiation therapy and high-dose alkylator-based chemotherapy. *J Clin Oncol.* 2005;23(7):1491–1499.

53. Gardner SL, Asgharzadeh S, Green A, Horn B, McCowage G, Finlay J. Intensive induction chemotherapy followed by high dose chemotherapy with autologous hematopoietic progenitor cell rescue in young children newly diagnosed with central nervous system atypical teratoid rhabdoid tumors. *Pediatr Blood Cancer.* 2008;51(2):235–240.

54. Reddy A, Strother D, Judkins A, et al. Treatment of atypical teratoid rhabdoid tumors (Atrt) of the central nervous system with surgery, intensive chemotherapy, and 3-D conformal radiation (Acns0333). A report from the children's Oncology group. *Neuro Oncol.* 2016;18:2.

55. Heideman RL, Douglass EC, Krance RA, et al. High-dose chemotherapy and autologous bone marrow rescue followed by interstitial and external-beam radiotherapy in newly diagnosed pediatric malignant gliomas. *J Clin Oncol.* 1993;11(8):1458–1465.

56. Echevarria ME, Fangusaro J, Goldman S. Pediatric central nervous system germ cell tumors: a review. *Oncologist.* 2008;13(6):690–699.

57. Buckner JC, Peethambaram PP, Smithson WA, et al. Phase II trial of primary chemotherapy followed by reduced-dose radiation for CNS germ cell tumors. *J Clin Oncol.* 1999;17(3):933–940.

58. Shaikh F, Nathan PC, Hale J, Uleryk E, Frazier L. Is there a role for carboplatin in the treatment of malignant germ cell tumors? A systematic review of adult and pediatric trials. *Pediatr Blood Cancer.* 2013;60(4):587–592.

59. Feldman DR, Sheinfeld J, Bajorin DF, et al. TI-CE high-dose chemotherapy for patients with previously treated germ cell tumors: results and prognostic factor analysis. *J Clin Oncol.* 2010;28(10):1706–1713.

60. De Giorgi U, Rosti G, Slavin S, et al. Salvage high-dose chemotherapy for children with extragonadal germ-cell tumours. *Br J Cancer.* 2005;93(4):412–417.

61. Agarwal R, Dvorak CC, Stockerl-Goldstein KE, Johnston L, Srinivas S. High-dose chemotherapy followed by stem cell rescue for high-risk germ cell tumors: the Stanford experience. *Bone Marrow Transplant.* 2009;43(7):547–552.

62. HaDuong JH, Martin AA, Skapek SX, Mascarenhas L. Sarcomas *Pediatr Clin North Am.* 2015;62(1):179–200.

63. Meyers PA, Krailo MD, Ladanyi M, et al. High-dose melphalan, etoposide, total-body irradiation, and autologous stem-cell reconstitution as consolidation therapy for high-risk Ewing's sarcoma does not improve prognosis. *J Clin Oncol.* 2001;19(11):2812–2820.

64. Oberlin O, Rey A, Desfachelles AS, et al. Impact of high-dose busulfan plus melphalan as consolidation in metastatic Ewing tumors: a study by the Societe Francaise des Cancers de l'Enfant. *J Clin Oncol.* 2006;24(24):3997–4002.

65. Paulussen M, Ahrens S, Burdach S, et al. Primary metastatic (stage IV) Ewing tumor: survival analysis of 171 patients from the EICESS studies. European Intergroup Cooperative Ewing Sarcoma Studies. *Ann Oncol.* 1998;9(3):275–281.

66. Luksch R, Tienghi A, Hall KS, et al. Primary metastatic Ewing's family tumors: results of the Italian Sarcoma Group and Scandinavian Sarcoma Group ISG/SSG IV Study including myeloablative chemotherapy and total-lung irradiation. *Ann Oncol.* 2012;23(11):2970–2976.

67. Drabko K, Raciborska A, Bilska K, et al. Consolidation of first-line therapy with busulphan and melphalan, and autologous stem cell rescue in children with Ewing's sarcoma. *Bone Marrow Transplant.* 2012;47(12):1530–1534.

68. Dirksen U, Le Deley MC, Brennan B, et al. Efficacy of busulfan-melphalan high dose chemotherapy consolidation (BuMel) compared to conventional chemotherapy combined with lung irradiation in ewing sarcoma (ES) with primary lung metastases: results of EURO-EWING 99-R2pulm randomized trial (EE99R2pul). *J Clin Oncol.* 2016;34(15).

69. Whelan J, Le Deley MC, Dirksen U, et al. Efficacy of busulfan-melphalan high dose chemotherapy consolidation (BuMel) in localized high-risk Ewing sarcoma (ES): results of EURO-EWING 99-R2 randomized trial (EE99R2Loc). *J Clin Oncol.* 2016;34(15).

70. Rasper M, Jabar S, Ranft A, Jurgens H, Amler S, Dirksen U. The value of high-dose chemotherapy in patients with first relapsed Ewing sarcoma. *Pediatr Blood Cancer.* 2014;61(8):1382–1386.

71. Bacci G, Ferrari S, Mercuri M, et al. Multimodal therapy for the treatment of nonmetastatic Ewing sarcoma of pelvis. *J Pediatr Hematol Oncol.* 2003;25(2):118–124.

72. McTiernan AM, Cassoni AM, Driver D, Michelagnoli MP, Kilby AM, Whelan JS. Improving outcomes after relapse in Ewing's sarcoma: analysis of 114 patients from a single institution. *Sarcoma.* 2006;2006:83548.

73. Al-Faris N, Al Harbi T, Goia C, Pappo A, Doyle J, Gassas A. Does consolidation with autologous stem cell transplantation improve the outcome of children with metastatic or relapsed Ewing sarcoma? *Pediatr Blood Cancer.* 2007;49(2):190–195.

74. Whelan J, Seddon B, Perisoglou M. Management of osteosarcoma. *Curr Treat Options Oncol.* 2006;7(6):444–455.

75. Kager L, Zoubek A, Potschger U, et al. Primary metastatic osteosarcoma: presentation and outcome of patients treated on neoadjuvant Cooperative Osteosarcoma Study Group protocols. *J Clin Oncol.* 2003;21(10):2011–2018.

76. Kempf-Bielack B, Bielack SS, Jurgens H, et al. Osteosarcoma relapse after combined modality therapy: an analysis of unselected patients in the Cooperative Osteosarcoma Study Group (COSS). *J Clin Oncol.* 2005;23(3):559–568.

77. Rodriguez-Galindo C, Daw NC, Kaste SC, et al. Treatment of refractory osteosarcoma with fractionated cyclophosphamide and etoposide. *J Pediatr Hematol Oncol.* 2002;24(4):250–255.

78. Tabone MD, Kalifa C, Rodary C, Raquin M, Valteau-Couanet D, Lemerle J. Osteosarcoma recurrences in pediatric patients previously treated with intensive chemotherapy. *J Clin Oncol.* 1994;12(12):2614–2620.

79. Colombat P, Biron P, Coze C, et al. Failure of high-dose alkylating agents in osteosarcoma. Solid tumors working party. *Bone Marrow Transplant.* 1994;14(4):665–666.

80. Fagioli F, Aglietta M, Tienghi A, et al. High-dose chemotherapy in the treatment of relapsed osteosarcoma: an Italian sarcoma group study. *J Clin Oncol.* 2002;20(8):2150–2156.

81. Sauerbrey A, Bielack S, Kempf-Bielack B, Zoubek A, Paulussen M, Zintl F. High-dose chemotherapy (HDC) and autologous hematopoietic stem cell transplantation (ASCT) as salvage therapy for relapsed osteosarcoma. *Bone Marrow Transplant.* 2001;27(9):933–937.

82. Rosti G, Ferrante P, Ledermann J, et al. High-dose chemotherapy for solid tumors: results of the EBMT. *Crit Rev Oncol Hematol.* 2002;41(2):129–140.

83. Marec-Berard P, Segura-Ferlay C, Tabone MD, et al. High dose thiotepa in patients with relapsed or refractory osteosarcomas: experience of the SFCE group. *Sarcoma.* 2014;2014:475067.

84. Hong CR, Kang HJ, Kim MS, et al. High-dose chemotherapy and autologous stem cell transplantation with melphalan, etoposide and carboplatin for high-risk osteosarcoma. *Bone Marrow Transplant.* 2015;50(10):1375–1378.

85. Perez EA, Kassira N, Cheung MC, Koniaris LG, Neville HL, Sola JE. Rhabdomyosarcoma in children: a SEER population based study. *J Surg Res.* 2011;170(2):e243–e251.

86. Admiraal R, van der Paardt M, Kobes J, Kremer LC, Bisogno G, Merks JH. High-dose chemotherapy for children and young adults with stage IV rhabdomyosarcoma. *Cochrane Database Syst Rev.* 2010;(12):CD006669.

87. Peinemann F, Kroger N, Bartel C, et al. High-dose chemotherapy followed by autologous stem cell transplantation for metastatic rhabdomyosarcoma–a systematic review. *PLoS One.* 2011;6(2):e17127.

88. Peinemann F, Enk H, Smith LA. Autologous hematopoietic stem cell transplantation following high-dose chemotherapy for nonrhabdomyosarcoma soft tissue sarcomas. *Cochrane Database Syst Rev.* 2017;4:CD008216.

89. Bui-Nguyen B, Ray-Coquard I, Chevreau C, et al. High-dose chemotherapy consolidation for chemosensitive advanced soft tissue sarcoma patients: an open-label, randomized controlled trial. *Ann Oncol.* 2012;23(3):777–784.

90. Malogolowkin MH, Hemmer MT, Le-Rademacher J, et al. Outcomes following autologous hematopoietic stem cell transplant for patients with relapsed Wilms' tumor: a CIBMTR retrospective analysis. *Bone Marrow Transplant.* 2017.

91. Ha TC, Spreafico F, Graf N, et al. An international strategy to determine the role of high dose therapy in recurrent Wilms' tumour. *Eur J Cancer.* 2013;49(1):194–210.

FURTHER READING

1. Finkelstein-Shechter T, Gassas A, Mabbott D, et al. Atypical teratoid or rhabdoid tumors: improved outcome with high-dose chemotherapy. *J Pediatr Hematol Oncol.* 2010;32(5):e182–e186.

2. Gilman AL, Jacobsen C, Bunin N, et al. Phase I study of tandem high-dose chemotherapy with autologous peripheral blood stem cell rescue for children with recurrent brain tumors: a Pediatric Blood and Marrow Transplant Consortium study. *Pediatr Blood Cancer.* 2011;57(3):506–513.

CHAPTER 22

Pathophysiology and Management of Graft-Versus-Host Disease

RAGISHA GOPALAKRISHNAN, MD • MADAN JAGASIA, MBBS

ACUTE GVHD

Introduction

Acute graft-versus-host disease (aGVHD) is a complex, often multisystem disease that causes significant morbidity and mortality in hematopoietic transplant patients. Usually occurring within the first 100 days of transplant; aGVHD is a complex inflammatory disorder in which donor immune T cells attack native host tissue resulting in multisystem organ dysfunction. The increase in allogenic transplants has increased the incidence of acute GVHD over the past decade. In the 21st century, approximately 30%–50% of all hematopoietic stem cell transplant recipients will develop aGHVD. The hallmark of initial treatment is optimization of immunosuppression and initiation of steroids. Nevertheless, many patients will develop refractory acute GVHD and will require second-line therapy and beyond. This section of acute GHVD will examine the diagnostic criteria, pathophysiology, staging, and management of acute GVHD. We will also review new.

Definition

aGVHD generally occurs after allogenic hematopoietic stem cell transplant (HSCT) and is characterized as a reaction of donor immune cells against host tissues. It can involve single and/or multiorgan disease. Clinically, aGVHD is suspected when a patient of HSCT develops any of the following signs or symptoms which include dermatitis (skin rash), skin blisters, crampy abdominal pain, diarrhea, nausea, vomiting, and elevated liver enzymes (transaminitis). Usually symptoms of aGVHD start at the time of engraftment and present within the first 100 days after transplant. However, acute GVHD can be a difficult diagnosis as many infections or autoimmune

conditions can mimic the symptoms of aGVHD. Hence, histologic conformation is required to establish a diagnosis of aGVHD. The staging and further clinic symptom and diagnostic criteria are given in the following section.

Epidemiology

In the United States, more than 20,000 stem cell transplants are performed annually. The majority of these transplants are allogenic transplant (60%) and autologous (40%). As the number of allogenic transplants continues to rise, it is anticipated that as many as 35% of HSCT patients will develop acute GVHD. There are multiple risk factors that can increase the risk for acute GVHD, and it is anticipated that with the emergence of more allogenic transplant, more than 7000 patients annually may present with aGVHD. With the incorporation of posttransplantation chemotherapy after allogenic transplantation, it is projected that the incidence of aGVHD will decrease. Nevertheless, aGVHD will continue to remain a source of morbidity for HSCT if underdiagnosed or treated.

Risk Factors

There are a variety of risk factors that have been identified with the development of acute GVHD. One of the major risk factors is disparity between HLA antigens. Major histocompatibility antigens are located on the short arm of chromosome 6 in humans. It is associated with the major histocompatibility complex that triggers both cell-mediated and humoral immune responses. HLA matching and compatibility between donor and recipient is to reduce acute GVHD and improvement with engraftment. Numerous studies have demonstrated that matching transplant recipients with sibling donors who share identical HLA

Hematopoietic Cell Transplantation for Malignant Conditions. https://doi.org/10.1016/B978-0-323-56802-9.00022-5

antigens increases the rate of engraftment and reduced the incidence of GVHD compared to those have mismatched siblings. Nevertheless, aGVHD persists in patients with matched related donors and likely results from immune-related reactions to minor histocompatibility antigens. These antigens are peptides that result from degradation of intracellular proteins and are presented on MHC molecules on donor cells. aGVHD is triggered when alloreactivity occurs and minor histocompatibility antigens are presented by MHC class II receptors on the host and interact with donor T cells. Hence patients who have matched grafts have lower rates of GVHD than those receiving one, two, or three antigen mismatch grafts. However, for those patients who have unrelated donor transplants, the greater the degree of HLA mismatch, the higher the likelihood of developing acute GVHD and the worse the overall outcome.[9,10]

Other risk factors have been studied as well. There have been several studies that studied the risk factors for aGVHD. In particular, female sex, age above 35 years, TBI, and graft source were strongly associated with aGVHD but not always associated with chronic GVHD. Pretransplant comorbidities are associated with the incidence and severity of aGVHD. The incidence and severity of aGVHD also appear to increase with pretransplant comorbidities. In one study of 2985 patients who underwent myeloablative or reduced-intensity conditioning followed by AHCST for myeloid or lymphoid malignancies, the incidence and severity of aGVHD increased with increasing hematopoietic cell transplantation–specific comorbidity index.[20]

PATHOPHYSIOLOGY

In the past 2 decades the advances in clinical immunology have led to further understanding about the pathogenesis of GVHD. In essence, the development of acute GVHD can be summarized into 3 phases: an afferent phase, an efferent phase, and an effector phase.

The afferent phase begins before the allograft is infused during the condition regimens. From numerous studies, we know that the type of conditioning has a significant impact on the pathogenesis of acute GVHD. During the afferent phase, the type of conditioning that is used (ablative or nonmyeloablative) triggers an exaggerated inflammatory response leading to activation of dendritic antigen-presenting cells (APCs). This leads to cascade triggering tissue destruction which results in excess release of TNF alpha, IL6, and IL1. Subsequently this inflammatory cascade damages the intestinal epithelium, thereby triggering

release of bacteria and alteration of the gut microbiome triggering propagation of the immune response. This in turn triggers a cascade of inflammatory response which leads to further recruitment of APCs and further cross talk between APCs and donor T cells, thereby triggering the second phase of GVHD known as the efferent phase. Extensive strides in immunology have demonstrated that the activation and further recruitment of donor CD8 T cells are by host APCs. In contrast, donor CD4 T cells can also be activated by dendritic APCs within the GI tract.[6] Key to the recruitment is the IL2 and INF-γ. The role of INF-γ is found to be poorly defined and can have a paradoxical role. In the last phase, i.e., effector phase, the escalation of the inflammatory response triggers tissue damage which is mediated by donor effector T cells, NK T cells, and macrophages that cause end-organ damage and continual propagation of this pathway. A detailed discussion regarding the immunological mechanisms is too detailed for this chapter; but there are several excellent reviews that discussed the pathophysiology of aGVHD.

CLINICAL MANIFESTATIONS

The clinical manifestations of acute GVHD can be varied and represent the organ(s) involved. Many of the clinical symptoms represent the organs involved. aGVHD can affect the skin, gut, liver, and pulmonary. The earliest form and most common manifestation is skin manifestation of GVHD, and this usually occurs at the time of engraftment of donor cells. Patients can present with a maculopapular rash that starts anywhere in the body but usually involves the palms and soles. Pruritus and tenderness are often noted during the initial manifestations of the disease. While a detailed discussion of engraftment is too detailed for this context, there are several reviews that detail the signs of engraftment. The onset of skin GVHD and engraftment is largely dependent individually on the stem cell source and type of conditioning. With the advent of reduced-intensity regimens that do not cause marrow ablation, patients have a later onset of GVHD. Some have postulated that reduced induced intensity modulates the cytokine response which is responsible for initiating GVHD. Because acute GVHD can affect multiple organs, we have outlined the manifestations that can be seen in each organ.

Skin Manifestations

The most common early manifestations of skin GVHD is the development of a maculopapular rash that can

TABLE 22.1
Acute GVHD Staging (Organ System Based)

Organ	Grade 1	Grade 2	Grade 3	Grade 4
Skin	≤25% of body surface area (BSA) affected with rash	25%–50% of BSA affected with rash	≥50% BSA affected with rash; full-body erythroderma	Bullae formation
Liver	Conjugated bilirubin: 2–3 mg/dL	Conjugated bilirubin: 3.1–6 mg/dL	Conjugated bilirubin: 6–15 mg/dL	Conjugated bilirubin: >15 mg/dL
Gut	Diarrhea: ≥500 mL/day	Diarrhea: ≥1000 mL/day	Diarrhea: ≥1500 mL/day	Diarrhea: ≥2000 mL/day with abdominal pain ± ileus

start periengraftment. The usual distribution of this rash particularly in the early stages involve the nape of the neck, ears, shoulders, palms, and soles of the feet. Often these rashes are described as an early sunburn. Although most mild skin GVHD resolves spontaneously, some rashes may persist and develop into severe GVHD. With severe GVHD, skin lesions can often progress into widespread erythoderma and desquamation or may evolve into epidermal necrolysis. The progression of skin GVHD is summarized in Table 22.1. Diagnosis of acute skin GVHD is often complicated by presentation of viral and drug exanthems that can mimic the signs of skin GVHD. Hence expedited referral with histopathologic conformation is required to diagnose acute cutaneous GVHD. Unfortunately there are no pathognomic signs of acute GVHD that can present with langherans cell depletion, follicular involvement, intracellular edema, or basal cell necrosis. An area of investigation that has been promising is the development of skin biomarkers HLA-DR4 which can be used as the diagnostic aid for GVHD.

Hepatic Manifestations

Acute GVHD often affects the liver as well and can occur in the presence or absence of skin involvement from GVHD. Patients with liver aGVHD often present early with jaundice and immune-related cholestasis. Patients will often present with significant jaundice and elevations in conjugated bilirubin and alkaline phosphatase. It is suspected that CD8- T-cell–mediated damage to bile canaliculi leads to intrahepatic liver injury. Given the early manifestations of aGVHD, elevated transaminases are also seen in other causes including drug, sepsis, venoocclusive disease, and viral mediation which often happen during this period. A differentiator between these causes and liver aGVHD is that the aminotransferase level is normal. Similar

to other forms of GVHD, tissue diagnosis is key and should be ruled out if there is a high suspicion for the disease. Because establishing a histopathologic conformation is quite often difficult in these patients, transjugular approaches for liver biopsy are preferred over percutaneous liver biopsies as there is a lower risk for bleeding. During examination of histopathologic conformation, stains for hepatic damage including H&E and PAS with diastase (PASD), reticulin, iron, and CK7 should be used. Furthermore, liver GVHD is characterized by intrinsic damage to basement membrane of the biliary epithelium and bile duct loss. Often, patients with liver GVHD will have loss of nuclear polarity, overlap, and eosinophilia change of the cytoplasm with infiltration of lymphocytes into the biliary epithelium. For patients with cholestatic changes, tissue pathology will demonstrate accumulation of bile and plugs of the canalicular bile ducts. Bile duct proliferation is not seen which distinguishes these findings from other causes including drug and downstream obstruction. Staging of liver GVHD is summarized in Table 22.1.

Gastrointestinal Tract

Acute GVHD can effect multiple areas of the gut, and gut GVHD is the most severe and hardest to treat and diagnose. Patients can present with abdominal pain, nausea, vomiting, diarrhea, and a variety of gut dysmobilty syndromes. Because gut infections often occur within the first 100 days, cultures are often obtained to rule out infection; furthermore, prior risk factors such as the conditioning regimen may also trigger manifestations of diarrhea. Because the early presentation of GVHD can be nonspecific, endoscopic biopsy is often performed. There are no specific endoscopic findings of gut GVHD, and clinical endoscopic findings range from extreme edema, sloughing, bleeding, and normal gut GVHD. Gut GVHD can affect any organ along the

TABLE 22.2A
IBMTR Grading System

	DEGREE OF INVOLVEMENT BASED ON ORGAN			
Grade	Skin (Grade)	Liver (Grade)	Gut (Grade)	Performance Status
I	1–2	None	None	None
II	1–3	Stage I	Stage I	Mild decrease in PS
III	2–3	2–3	2–3	Marked decrease in PS
IV	2–4	2–4	2–3	Significant Decrease in PS

*Staging each organ system is described in Table 22.1.
IBMTR, International Bone Marrow Transplant Registry.

TABLE 22.2B
Glucksberg Grading System

	DEGREE OF INVOLVEMENT BASED ON ORGAN		
Grade	Skin (Grade)	Liver (Grade)	Gut (Grade)
I	1–2	None	None
II	1–3	Stage I	Stage I
III	2–3	2–3	2–3
IV	2–4	2–4	2–3

*Staging each organ system is described in Table 22.1.

GI tract but is most prominent in the ileum and ascending colon. On histologic tissue conformation, histology demonstrates crypt-cell necrosis and loss of adhesion molecules in Paneth cells. Upper GI GVHD is a rare variant that can be seen in the elderly patients during the early posttransplantation period. These patients present with food intolerance, nausea, vomiting, and dyspepsia which are recognized with biopsy of the upper GI tract and are treated with immunosuppressive treatment.

Endocrine and Hematologic Manifestations

GVHD can lead to lymphocyte proliferation and cause thymic atrophy, peripheral cytopenias (thrombocytopenia), and hypogammaglobulinemia (particularly IgA). The eyes are also affected with photophobia, hemorrhagic conjunctivitis, and lagophthalmos and kidneys with nephritis, nephrotic syndrome, e.g., membranous nephropathy.

GRADING OF ACUTE GVHD

At present, there is not a single universal grading system that exists for GVHD. Several systems for grading aGVHD have been developed, and the most commonly used are the International Bone Marrow Transplant Registry (IMBTR, shown in Table 22.2A) and the Glucksberg grade (I–IV). The severity of aGVHD is determined by a detailed examination of the degree of organ involvement including of the skin, liver, and gastrointestinal tract (Table 22.2B). Individual organ systems are graded based on involvement, combined with performance status (Glucksberg) or without the patient's performance status (IBMTR). The overall

composite grade then is evaluated, and the patient is given a grade as demonstrated in Tables 22.2A and B. Unfortunately, interpretation of the grading is clinician dependent and observer dependent and hence accounts for significant grading in the literature. However, despite significant interobserver variation, several studies have demonstrated that the overall grade has an impact on prognosis and survival particularly for those with grade III–IV aGVHD.

PREVENTION OF aGVHD

At present, there are no standardized preventive measures for aGVHD. The hallmark of prophylaxis approach is to modulate the T-cell response via pharmacologic measures such as medical immunosuppression and/or by T-cell depletion. Preventive measures are largely institutional based and vary based on the type of conditioning and desired GVL effect.

Pharmacologic Immunosuppression

Pharmacologic immunosuppression remains the primary strategy for prevention GVHD. The most widely adopted regimen for acute GVHD prevention in myeloablative allogenic hematopoietic transplant is a combination of methotrexate (given D + 1, D + 3, D + 6, D + 11 after HCT) in combination with a calcineurin inhibitor (cyclosporine or tacrolimus). This regimen was initially developed in early preclinical trials in the 1950s and widely adopted in the 1980s after multiple RCTs demonstrated superior outcomes in survival and response rates compared to single agent methotrexate or cyclosporine. The addition of a steroid to this prophylaxis regimen does not confer a benefit in prophylaxis and was often associated with higher infection rates, thereby negatively impacting survival.

Tacrolimus is now adopted in many centers over cyclosporine based on a 2000 trial suggesting greater efficacy in acute GVHD, but some studies have also shown an increased risk of relapsed risk with advanced disease.

For patients who receive nonmyeloablative conditioning before allogeneic HCT, a number of preventive regimens have been studied including a combination of calcineurin inhibitor in combination with mycophenolate mofetil (MMF).[11] Furthermore, given the high risk of genetic disparity between HLA-haploidentical transplant patients, the incorporation of posttransplant cyclophosphamide D + 3 and D + 4 allogenic transplant in combination with tacrolimus and MMF has reduced the rate of severe aGVHD to 5%–20%, but the continued occurrence of severe (and less severe but still clinically meaningful) aGVHD has stimulated a number of investigations into more effective prophylaxis against aGVHD.

T-Cell Depletion

The central role of donor T cells in initiating the cascade of acute GVHD has triggered interest into investigating T-cell depletion studies for GVHD. Although multiple studies have investigated ex vivo T-cell depletion, unfortunately these studies have been unsuccessful as they often demonstrated an increased risk of graft rejection, poor immune reconstitution, viral reactivation, and relapsed malignancy.[12] However, the incorporation of alemtuzumab and/or polyclonal antisera (e.g., antithymocyte globulin [ATG]) has revolutionized T-cell depletion. Soiffer et al.'s studies in 2011 which administered alemtuzumab or ATG resulted in a lower incidence of acute and chronic GVHD, with absolute risk reductions of 15%–20%. However, these had a negative impact of DFS, OS, and transplant-related mortality as both agents significantly increased the risk of relapse after T-cell depletion. There have now been studies demonstrating that ATG may prevent grade II, nonfatal aGVHD and does not increase secondary risk of malignancy. However, there was an increase of PTLD without a significant effect on OS or PFS at 2 years. Hence additional studies are required to be powered to assess the effect of ATG on survival outcomes long term.

Posttransplant cyclophosphamide has also been a promising method for T-cell depletion. Cyclophosphamide (Cytoxan) has been previously shown to be an immunosuppressant and lymphotoxin and preferentially inhibits expansion of activated lymphocytes. A study developed an approach in which patients receive bone marrow from an HLA-haploidentical donor, followed by cyclophosphamide at days +3 and +4 after HCT. This delay allowed T-cell interactions with antigen presentation and T-cell activation. Posttransplant day +3, cyclophosphamide semiselective ablates host-reactive donor T-cell clones which allows for host-specific donor tolerance while preserving donor-derived immunity against viruses and other pathogens.

Based on preclinical trials, a conditioning regimen of total-lymphoid irradiation (TLI) was combined with ATG. This regimen is thought to augment the host natural killer T (NKT) cells response, which are more radiation resistant than conventional T cells. These residual host NKT cells are then believed to interact with donor T cells to facilitate tolerance and prevent acute GVHD. Initially, clinical studies demonstrated low incidences of aGVHD but a high rate of relapse (60%). In addition, the high rate of relapse observed with this regimen is thought to be ablation of the impairment of the graft-versus-lymphoma effect from ATG. Given the high risk of relapse, TLI/ATG is only reserved for patients with low-risk disease but may require additional pharmacologic suppression as the Italian and Stanford group.[21]

B cells are often mediators in T-cell expansion and effector phase of aGVHD. Rituxan has shown to be effective in the treatment of refractory chronic GVHD with the anti-CD20 monoclonal antibody rituximab.[30,31] In preclinical models, depleting recipient B cells abrogates aGVHD.[33] A CIBMTR retrospective registry study demonstrated lower rates of GVHD who had received rituximab in the 6 months before allogeneic HCT.[34] However, prospective studies have not been as promising. Early prospective studies have demonstrated a persistent 11% chance of grade II–IV aGVHD in patients undergoing allogenic transplant for indolent non-Hodgkin lymphoma and observed an incidence of aGVHD grades II–IV of 11%. Hence additional studies, particularly prospective randomized controlled trials, would be required to clarify the role of rituximab in prevention of acute and chronic GVHD.

Sirolimus is a mammalian target of rapamycin (mTOR) pathway inhibitor that suppresses APC presentation and T-cell responses and regulates the regulatory T cell (Treg) expansion. It has been successful at preventing GVHD, but the results have been mixed. Some centers have demonstrated favorable responses; some have not. Sirolimus is better tolerated in patients with nonmyelobative conditioning but has higher rates of aGVHD and renal failure when combined with ablative regimens.[38,39]

Extracorporeal photopheresis (ECP) is a process in which leukocytes are harvested from the peripheral blood via apheresis, incubated ex vivo with 8-methoxypsoralen, treated with UV-A light, and then reinfused. The UV-A light exposure induces a conformational change in 8-methoxypsoralen, which then intercalates into DNA and interrupts transcription, inducing apoptosis in the treated leukocytes. ECP has an established role in the treatment of acute and chronic GVHD and has been explored in a limited fashion as a preventive agent. A 2010 pilot study tested prophylactic ECP in 62 patients undergoing myeloablative allogeneic HCT and reported rates of aGVHD grades II–IV of 30%–42%, a marginally statistically significant reduction compared to registry controls.[42] ECP is relatively logistically demanding but has few or no observed adverse effects and may prove amenable to larger controlled studies of aGVHD prevention.

Bortezomib is found to inhibit NK-kappa B and deplete alloreactive T cells and to decrease Th1 cytokine levels in murine models. It is well studied in multiple myeloma, and preclinical work suggests that this may be a potential efficacy against aGVHD. In a single-arm trial, bortezomib in combination with tacrolimus and methotrexate as GVHD prophylaxis was associated with a 13% incidence of aGVHD grades II–IV. This study has prompted further investigation into bortezomib as a future target for aGVHD.

Hypomethylating agents have been well studied in MDS and thought to expand regulatory T-cell populations both in vitro and in vivo. Because Tregs can suppress alloimmune reactions, these hypomethylating agents have generated interest as potential preventive approaches against GVHD, particularly in patients with myelodysplastic syndromes or acute myeloid leukemia, in whom these agents may also be effective against the underlying hematologic malignancy.

Novel Strategies for Prevention

Chemotaxis during T-cell migration to GVHD target organs is a new area of investigation for drug targets. Following is a table summarizing novel agents that are discussed in prevention of acute GVHD. Unfortunately, detailed discussions about these promising new targets are too detailed for this review (Table 22.3).

TREATMENT

First-Line Therapy for aGVHD

Frontline therapy for patients with aGVHD depends on the number of organs involved, extent of disease, and type of GVL effect. Most treatment options are based on the immunosuppression of donor T cells, which are responsible for the clinical manifestations of GVHD.

Stage I aGVHD

For patients with grade 1 GVHD, these patients usually present with single system (skin involvement, liver or

TABLE 22.3
Novel Targets in Prevention of Acute GVHD

Drug Target	Type of Study	Findings
CCR5 blockade and targeting agents	Phase II	CCR5 blockade prevented GVHD of the liver and the gut before day 100 particularly in myeloablative regimens
FTY720 (a sphingosine-1-phosphate receptor antagonist)	Preclinical studies	Reduced acute GVHD by trapping T cells in lymphoid organs and dendritic migration.
IL-22 inhibitors	Phase II (NCT02406651)	Lower GI and intestinal tract (grade 2 and grade 4),
α-GalCer, (glycolipid that expands and activates NKT cells)	Phase II	Ongoing study, results pending.
Janus kinase	Preclinical studies	Clinical studies currently being initiated and pending

GI, gastrointestinal; *GVHD,* graft-versus-host disease; *IL,* interleukin; *NKT,* natural killer T.

gut involvement only). For skin GVHD, the use of topical treatments such as topical steroids are often used. Antihistamines, nonirritating creams, and moisturizers are used to inhibit histamine-related pruritis which often accompanies the maculopapular rash. Topical immunosuppression has also been studied, and low-dose tacrolimus (0.1 mg) applied twice daily topically has shown promising results. For gastrointestinal GVHD, oral steroids such as budesonide are often used once aGVHD is diagnosed.

Stage II aGVHD

Steroids are the gold standard for treatment of grade II–IV aGVHD. The exact mechanism is not clear but involves a myriad of mechanisms including suppression of proinflammatory cytokines, as well as direct lymphotoxic effects. Patients are initially started on at least 1 mg/kg if not 2 mg/kg per day, and steroids are often escalated for persistent symptoms. Patients are subjected to chronic myopathy, hyperglycemia, insomnia, and many additional steroid-related side effects. Nevertheless, most patients will progress within 1–2 weeks of steroids, and additional lines of therapy are often required. There is not a clear second-line agent for steroid refractory GVHD.

Second-Line Therapy for aGVHD

Mycophenolate mofetil has many antimicrobial and antitumor properties. It has been evaluated for the treatment of glucocorticoid-resistant acute GVHD in small prospective trials. While MMF is often considered as part of second-line treatment, its true efficacy is limited, and more agents are needed. Phase III studies using MMF in conjunction with steroids were closed often early due to futility and leukopenia.

Etanercept, a recombinant human TNF-alpha receptor fusion protein, has been used alone or in combination to treat aGVHD. Patients treated with etanercept plus steroids were significantly more likely to attain complete remission (CR) after 28 days than those treated with steroids alone (69% vs. 33%). This difference was observed in HCT recipients of related donors (79% vs. 39%) as well as unrelated donors (53% vs. 26%). This translated to superior outcomes in patients at D100. However, etanercept also caused significant bacterial, viral, or invasive fungal infection with steroids.

Pentostatin, a purine analog, inhibits T-cell proliferation and function, has been used to prevent GVHD, and has had successful results. However, because many HSCT patients develop renal insufficiency, this medication should be used with caution in patients with renal insufficiency. Patients with renal insufficiency should often require a 50% dose reduction.

Alpha-one antitrypsin (AAT) has been shown to have activity in steroid-resistant acute GVHD. In phase II–III trials studies, 4 weeks of AAT showed improvement in survival and response. Sirolimus while studied in prevention has shown activity in treatment-related aGVHD. However, it is cautiously used as sirolimus is associated with sinusoidal obstruction syndrome (SOS) after myeloablative conditioning regimens and hence should be restricted to nonmyeloablative approaches.

Ruxolitinib (a Janus kinase (JAK) 1/2 inhibitor) is well known to be effective in primary myelofibrosis and polycythemia vera and shown activity in acute GVHD. JAK signaling is shown to help with chemotaxis and effector phase of acute GVHD development. Ruxolitinib has been shown to be effective at inhibiting JAK signaling and improve survival outcomes in patietns

with steroid refractory acute GVHD. However, this agent has shown to be effective more than placebo but has not been compared directly with other regimens. Most patients experience cytopenia and withdrawal syndrome.

ECP has shown to have poor and modest results for steroid refactory GVHD as well as often used for skin GVHD.

ATG is used in prevention and in refractory steroid acute GVHD for unrelated donor or haploidentical donor undergoing either myeloablative or reduced-intensity conditioning. For those who did not receive ATG as part of their prophylactic regimen, ATG can be considered for the management of patients with glucocorticoid-refractory acute GVHD. ATG has been used in patients with steroid and noted to have improved response rates and survival outcomes.

IL-2 monoclonal antibodies including daclizumab and basiliximab, inolimomab has shown to be effective in patients with steroid GVHD. However, they have not shown greater efficacy or safety than other treatments for glucocorticoid-resistant aGVHD. Further studies are needed to determine the efficacy of these monoclonal antibodies in this population. Owing to safety concerns, most of the agents have been removed from the market. Brentuximab vedotin (BV) is a monoclonal antibody-drug conjugate that is directed against CD30 which is expressed on T cells. In phase I trials, it has shown promise against GVHD. The humanized monoclonal anti-CD52 antibody alemtuzumab has shown retrospectively to improve outcomes in steroid acute GVHD. Cytomegalovirus reactivation, bacterial infection, and invasive aspergillosis were frequent complications, requiring careful monitoring and antiinfective supportive care.

Tocilizumab is an anti-interleukin-6 receptor antibody that is used in prophylaxis for chimeric antigen receptor T cell protocols is now been studied in the treatment of steroid refractory GVHD. While studies are often small prospective studies, additional studies need to be conducted to adequately its activity in steroid refractory GVHD.

FUTURE DIRECTIONS
Biomarkers in GVHD

The use of biomarkers for diagnosis and prognosis of aGVHD is an area of active research. An ideal biomarker would predict the diagnosis, appearance, and severity of acute GVHD and guide management. However, currently there is no individual biomarker ready for prime time. Summarized in Table 22.4 are biomarkers that are under investigation.

TABLE 22.4
Biomarkers for Acute GVHD

Biomarker	Mechanism	Study Findings:
ST2	a member of the interleukin-1 receptor family	study of 673 recipients of myeloablative conditioning found that ST2 (as early as 14 days after transplant) correlated with an increased risk of NRM and resistance to treatment of acute GVHD
REG3alpha	(regenerating islet-derived 3-alpha) is expressed by regenerating cells in the gastrointestinal epithelium (especially Paneth cells	Increased concentrations predict GVHD associated epithelial mucosal injury.
TNFR1	TNF receptor 1	Serum levels of TNFR1 correlate with onset of GVHD, mortality and overall survival.
Plasma and urine polypeptides for INF-a, IL-8, GF via proteomic analysis	Involved in cytokine and growth	Shown to predict onset of GVHD, prognostic information
Flow cytometry for CD30 and CD8	Mediated in effector response	Higher prediction of acute GVHD
TIM3, IL6, sTNFR1	Mediators in cytokine response	Predictor higher stage of GVHD and TRM from GVHD.

GF, growth factor; *GVHD*, graft-versus-host disease; *IL*, interleukin; *INF*, interferon; *TNF*, tumor necrosis factor.

Future Targets in aGVHD

A detailed analysis of all of the following therapies would be out of scope of this chapter. Hence future therapies are being summarized in Table 22.5.

aGVHD (CONCLUSION)

aGVHD continues to remain a major, life-threatening complication of hematopoietic transplantation that is associated with morbidity and mortality. Patients who are survive are immunodeficient for several years. Although we may have made significant strides in the biology and biomarkers for this disease, we have significant strides to be made in patients who develop steroid refractory disease. We have many promising targets that will hopefully improve the symptom burden and survival of patients with severe GVHD.

CHRONIC GVHD: INTRODUCTION

Chronic graft-versus-host disease (GVHD) is a frequent and potentially life-threatening complications of allogeneic hematopoietic stem cell transplantation. Till date, chronic GVHD remains the leading cause of long-term morbidity and mortality after allogenic hematopoietic stem cell transplantation. This is in part due to increased use of allogenic transplantation in elderly, and more

frequent use of unrelated donors has led to increased numbers of patients with this painful complication. With the implementation of reduced-intensity conditioning (RIC) regimens for allogenic transplantation, the overall mortality from allogenic transplant has decreased. However, these regimens have not be as effective at decreasing the late transplantation related mortality from chronic GVHD. There have been significant strides made in the advancement of the pathophysiology, prophylaxis, and treatment of GVHD. Nevertheless, we are still very early in our understanding for these diseases. With new pathophysiology targets emerging, we hope to have new and effective strategies in the future.

CHRONIC GVHD: RISK FACTORS AND EPIDEMIOLOGY

Although improvements in transplant practices have occurred, chronic GVHD continues to persist and be a source of major morbidity and mortality for those surviving after hematopoietic transplant. A 2015 study demonstrates an increase in the incidence of cGVHD, but significant strides have been made to reduce the nonrelapse mortality over time. Hence cGVHD continues to be a burden for many patients and is often fatal. There are a multitude of risk factors for GVHD, and these are similar to the risk factors in those patients who

TABLE 22.5
Current therapeutics that are actively being studied in clinical trials

Trial Number	Study Design	Diagnosis	Intervention	Status/Results
JAK KINASE INHIBITORS				
NCT02953678 **Ruxolitinib +**	Phase II SR-aGVHD	aGVHD	Ruxolitinib v. Best therapy +	Recruiting, results pending
Itacitinib – JAK1 inhibitor INCB039110	Phase II	aGVHD	Itactinib Itactinib + steroid in GRAVITAS trial	Day 28 ORR of 88.3% when used in the first-line setting as treatment for aGVHD, and 64.7% for SR disease
MONOCLONAL ANTIBODIES				
Natalizumab Ab α4-integrin NCT02176031	Phase II	aGVHD	Natalizumab in conjunction with steroids	Recruiting
Vedolizumab- Ab against for A4-integrin NCT02993783	Phase II	aGVHD	**Vedolizumab + steroids**	Recruiting
Brentuximab	Phase II	aGVHD	Brentixumab v. BSC	recruiting
Mesenchymal Stromal Cells	Meta-analysisn	Acute GVHD + chronic GVHD	Mesenchymal v. placebo	64% v. 49% placebo in 6 month.

aGVHD, acute graft-versus-host disease.

develop aGVHD. Risk factors include human leukocyte antigen (HLA) disparity, donor and recipient age, donor parity, donor and recipient gender, dose of total-body irradiation (TBI), conditioning regimen intensity, acute GVHD prophylaxis, splenectomy, immunoglobulin use, underlying disease, ABO compatibility, prior exposure to herpes viruses, donor transfusions, performance score, antibiotic gut decontamination, and posttransplant transfusions. However, much of these risk factors were derived from retrospective analyses before the NIH consensus criteria, and hence prospective studies have yet to be performed which validate these studies with the NIH consensus criteria.

CHRONIC GVHD: PATHOPHYSIOLOGY
Introduction
Chronic GVHD is a complex, poorly understood complex, immune syndrome. Although significant strides have been made, there are an underscored need for further research into understanding the biology of the disease further targets. Early models demonstrate that germinal center reactions donor and receipient CD4 T-cell and B-cell infiltration which was keep in the early development of lung fibrosis. This model postulates that patients with chronic GVHD frequently have

circulating auto and allo-antibodies that are reactive with recipient cells.[1-5] These alloreactive antibodies stimulate collagen production and subsequent dendritic recruitment which is often requirement for lung fibrosis. The hallmark of GVHD is that it is defined by loss of recognition of self and the development of autoimmune manifestations. Multiple murine models have proposed that donor CD4 Th1 T cells and irregularities in Treg cell reconstitution are instrumental in the development of GVHD pathophysiology. Donor T cells play an important role in the immune pathology of chronic GVHD by upregulating Th1 and Th17. This triggers a complex cascade which terminates in activation of IL-17 producing CD+8 T cells which mediate end-organ damage with fibrosis. The failure of Treg further propogates this damage, and the overall response is augmented and amplified by restricted deletion of MHC class II peptides of donor cells on the recipient.

Macrophages also play a key role in the GHVD pathogenesis by upregulating of macrophage function and stimulate macrophage accumulation.[8-10]

While extensive work has been done to understand the immunology behind GHVD, new preclinical data demonstrates that defects in Treg homeostasis are instrumental in GVHD. New strategies have been developed to enhance Treg numbers after SCT including

TABLE 22.6
Chronic GVHD Staging (Organ System Based)

Organ	Grade 1	Grade 2	Grade 3	Grade 4
Skin	≤25% of body surface area (BSA) affected with rash	25%–50% of BSA affected with rash	≥50% BSA affected with rash; full-body erythroderma	bullae formation
Liver	Conjugated Bilirubin: 2–3 mg/dL	Conjugated Bilirubin: 3.1–6 mg/dL	Conjugated Bilirubin: 6–15 mg/dL	Conjugated Bilirubin: >15 mg/dL
Gut	Diarrhea: ≥500 mL/day	Diarrhea: ≥1000 mL/day	Diarrhea: ≥1500 mL/day	Diarrhea: ≥2000 mL/day with abdominal pain± ileus

implementation of Treg adoptive therapy to reconstitute the Treg pool have been adopted from mice studies. Adoptive Treg transfer can be harnessed to help prevent and treat cGVHD and has been promising in preclinical models. IL-2 dysregulation is another area of focus as it is responsible for effector phase and chemotaxis of CD8 T cells. Finally, selective inhibition of CSF-1R in macrophages might prevent differentiation and survival and has shown to be a promising target in the setting of chronic GVHD.

CHRONIC GVHD: CLINICAL MANIFESTATIONS

Clinical manifestations of GVHD vary widely from manifestations of autoimmune collagen vascular diseases such as oral ulcerations (lichen planus), keratoconjunctivitis sicca, xerostomia polyserositis, esophagitis and stricture,[25] vaginal ulceration and stricture,[26] intrahepatic obstructive liver disease, obstructive pulmonary disease, scleroderma, morphea, fasciitis and myositis. The signs and symptoms of acute and chronic GVHD are summarized in Table 22.6.

Given the wide range and myriad of manifestations of GVHD, early recognition of GVHD and decision to initiate treatment remains a practical challenge. Tissue diagnosis is key to finalizing a diagnosis of chronic GVHD. The sections outlined below are the most common manifestation and do not represent an exhaustive list of clinical manifestations seen with GVHD.

Oral Mucosal Involvement

The oral mucosa is involved by chronic GVHD. Findings are nonspecific and range from erythema, leukoplakia, lichenoid lesions, ulcers, mucosal atrophy, and xerostomia. Symptoms can be masked by autoimmune phenomenon such as Sjögren's syndrome. GVHD involvement of salivary glands invariably leads to severe xerostomia and sialadenitis.

Skin and Soft Tissues

Cutaneous chronic GVHD is seen in two main forms: lichenoid and sclerodermatous types. The lichenoid form predominates and typically involves the periorbital regions, ears, palms, and soles and is seen in early GVHD. The sclerodermatous form which may present as inflammatory plaques over the extremities is seen later on in chronic GVHD and can be insidious. Unlike systemic sclerosis, patients with GVHD are less likely to develop Raynaud's phenomenon and are more likely to develop progressive restrictive lung disease due to diminished chest wall compliance from truncal involvement of GVHD. Subcutaneous involvement of nails including dystrophic changes of the nails, including vertical ridges, onycholysis, and telangiectasia of the nail fold are often seen. These nail changes occur frequently with fungal infection of the nail plate (onychomycosis) which can confound the clinical picture of chronic GVHD. Distinguishing between these active nail changes can be difficult, and biopsy and subungual accumulation of friable keratinous debris suggest the presence of onychomycosis.

Myofascitis, although a rare presentation, is not uncommon and often involves with proximal inflammatory aspects. Inflammatory changes of the overlying skin and subcutaneous tissue simulating cellulitis may be pronounced. As the inflammation subsides, the skin and subcutaneous tissue is replaced with fibrotic tissue leading to dimpling appearance of the skin and contracture.[22]

Ocular Involvement

Ocular involvement occurs in frequent symptom of patients with chronic GVHD with the most frequent ocular manifestations include keratoconjunctivitis sicca, and sterile conjunctivitis and uveitis. Xerophthalmia is often under recognized and can lead to serious complications such as corneal epithelial defects and ulceration. The Schirmer's test and urgent ophthalmology consult is required for suspicion of xeropthalmia and should be routinely performed in all patients early in the onset of chronic GVHD. If xerophthalmia is present, aggressive use of topical lubricants should be initiated. Patients should be advised to wear protective eyewear outdoors especially on windy days. For more severe cases, an ophthalmology consult and possible punctal occlusion or cauterization, bandage soft contact lenses, and/or tarsorrhaphy may be needed.[22,23]

Hepatic and Gastrointestinal Involvement

Chronic liver GVHD often presents with a mixed cholestasis clinical picture and can present with other signs of other organ involvement. The severity of chronic liver disease correlates with the histopathologic findings on biopsy; namely, the presence of bridging necrosis indicates extensive chronic GVHD. However, this cholestatic picture can concomitantly occur in patients with active hepatitis C; patients with chronic GVHD have shown to develop hepatic failure from hepatitis C or iatrogenic liver failure. However, in the absence of active hepatitis C or evidence of iatrogenic liver failure, progression of chronic GVHD to fulminant hepatic failure is rare is uncommon in long-term survivors. When hepatic failure occurs, the most frequent etiology is hepatitis C infection and iatrogenic liver failure.[15]

Esophageal involvement in chronic GVHD develops secondary from mucosal desquamation and development of fibrosis, esophageal webs, distal peptic esophagitis, and stricture. While acute GVHD has been associated with gastrointestinal dysmotility and pseudoobstruction, intestinal obstructions from chronic GVHD are less common. However, progression of intestinal forms of acute GVHD such as ileus or pseudoobstruction may lead to permanent damage, resulting in mechanical obstruction, diarrhea, stasis syndrome, and malabsorption which are often seen in long-term survivors from GVHD.

Pulmonary Complications

The most notorious side effect from pulmonary toxicity is interstitial lung disease which can develop from a range of etiologies which include regimen-related toxicity, infection, and immune-related fibrosis from acute GVHD. The most common restrictive interstitial lung disease is bronchiolitis in chronic GVHD. In these patients a mild cough may begin 3–20 months after transplantation and then progress to dyspnea, progressive airflow obstruction, and finally respiratory failure. A high-resolution CT scan may be normal or show hyperinflation, bronchial dilatation, consolidation, hypo-attenuated areas and vascular attenuation.[7] Patients with obstructive lung disease due to chronic GVHD infrequently respond to therapy, although some patients may survive long term.

Furthermore, additional restrictive physiologies from scleroderma skin changes or neuromuscular toxicity described below may lead to progressive restrictive physiologies that are often seen in long-term GVHD.[33–35]

Neuromuscular and CNS Involvement

While the incidence of neuromuscular involvement in chronic GVHD is rare, motor neuropathy, paraneoplastic, myositis, dermatomyositis, and mysthenia gravis have been reported and result from the toxicities of the preparative regimen. Neuropathy is frequently associated with treatment for GVHD, including thalidomid and occasionally tacrolimus or cyclosporine.[15–19]

Immunodeficiency

The most important complication associated with chronic GVHD is immunodeficiency, leading to susceptibility to wide ranges of opportunistic infections and frequently to death. Posttransplantation immune deficiency is multifactorial and can be secondary to either conditioning-induced thymic damage, age-associated thymic involution, thymic GVHD, or GVHD prophylaxis or treatment. It is a leading cause of morbidity and mortality from infections and relapse. In recent years, new strategies have been explored to enhance posttransplantation T-cell recovery and understand the process of immune reconstitution. In allogenic transplant patients, immune reconstitution can occur slowly than auto-transplanted patient and can take up to 18 months from day 0 of transplantation. Furthermore, this process is delayed in survivors with GVHD or those who have received prolonged immunosuppression. Chronic GVHD affects immune reconstitution of B cells and CD4– and CD8– T cells. Donor source and the degree of HLA compatibility between donor and recipient also affect the pace of immune reconstitution. Low B-cell count, inverted CD4:CD8 ratio, and a decreased IgA level are all risk factors associated with late infections. Hence, chronic

GVHD patients are susceptible to encapsulated bacteria. While fungal or cytomegalovirus infections are known to cause early mortality, reactivation of fungal and viral infections are notorious for causing morbidity and mortality in hospitalized patients with ongoing immune suppression for GVHD. Finally, late presentations of Pneumocystis jirovei infections are more common in patients receiving active treatment of chronic GVHD. Hence aggressive antimicrobial prophylaxis against Pneumocystis jirovei, cytomegalovirus (CMV) and pneumococcus is crucial in the prevention of potentially fatal infections. Long-term CMV prophylaxis may be needed in seropositive patients with chronic GVHD, especially those receiving immunosuppressive therapy. For additional details, please refer to the IDSA guidelines for infectious prophylaxis in stem cell transplant recipients, including patients with chronic GVHD.

Nonimmune, Late Effects after Transplantation and Chronic GVHD

While less common, nonmalignant complications involving ocular, bone, joint, and cardiovascular systems and impaired quality of life are very often directly or indirectly (through treatment) linked to chronic GVHD. Secondary malignancies are common, and squamous cell carcinomas (particularly of the head and neck) have been associated with chronic GVHD. It is not uncommon to have immune-suppressed patients, oncogenic viruses, such as human papillomavirus, may contribute to squamous cell cancers of the skin and buccal mucosa. Secondary increased risk for head and neck cancers including squamous cell cancers of the buccal cavity and skin are thought to develop from chronic lichen planus-like erosions, ionizing radiation, immunodeficiency and, conceivably, factors such as smoking or alcohol consumption.

DIAGNOSTIC CRITERIA FOR CHRONIC GVHD

Chronic GVHD is defined the arisement of symptoms outline above after D100 of transplant, and the NIH consensus criteria is used for the diagnosis of the disease.

There have been several retrospective and prospective studies that have validated the NIH Criteria Scale and now it has been widely adopted by several institutions worldwide. The NIH consensus criteria for GVHD is now used as a standard of care for the recognition and classification of acute and chronic forms of GVHD. While we have made significant strides in near universal adoption of the NIH Consensus Criteria for recognition of GVHD, their overall role in implementation of clinical practice is to be determined. At present, we cannot effectively use the NIH Criteria Scale to measure clinical response for GVHD as we lack effective biomarkers for measure clinical response for treatments targeted against GHVD.[13-15] We are in the present developing biomarkers to measure clinical response (Fig. 22.1).

CHRONIC GVHD PROPHYLAXIS AND TREATMENT

The hallmark of prevention therapy for chronic GVHD starts prior to engraftment and is summarized in the prevention section of acute GVHD. The main two agents that have been shown to improve prevention in chronic GVHD are ATG included within conditioning regimens has successfully lowered the incidence and severity of chronic GVHD. In addition to prevention, the progress in ancillary care has improved the treatment of chronic GVHD. While, detailed review of the ancillary therapy and supportive care is out of the scope of this book chapter, the most extensive review of ancillary therapy and supportive care was published by the NIH Consensus Conference in 2006. This review established extensive guidelines, including treatments for symptoms and recommendations for patient education, preventive measures, and appropriate follow-up. It provided guidelines for prevention and management of infections and other common complications of treatment of chronic GVHD. It highlighted that optimal care of patients with chronic GVHD often requires a multidisciplinary approach.

Current Treatment Strategies in Chronic GVHD

Front line systemic therapy for chronic GVHD

The choice of initial therapy for patients with chronic GVHD depends on the type and number of organs involved and the severity of their symptoms. The choice of primary treatment is also dictated by the prophylactic regimen that used previously, and based on the type of malignancy the graft-versus-tumor effect. The mainstay of treatment options is pharmacologic immunosuppression of donor T cells.

Steroids much like acute GVHD are also the first-line systemic therapy of choice for patients with moderate to severe chronic GVHD. Patients are usually started on 1 mg/kg/day of steroids. Some patients have an

	Score 0	Score 1	Score 2	Score 3
Performance score: KPS ECOG LPS	☐ Asymptomatic and fully active (ECOG 0; KPS or LPS 100%)	☐ Symptomatic, fully ambulatory, restricted only in physically strenuous activity (ECOG 1, KPS or LPS 80-90%)	☐ Symptomatic, ambulatory, capable of self-care, >50% of waking hours out of bed (ECOG 2, KPS or LPS 60-70%)	☐ Symptomatic, limited self-care, >50% of waking hours in bed (ECOG 3-4, KPS or LPS <60%)
Skin Clinical features: ☐ Maculopapular rash ☐ Lichen planus-like features ☐ Papulosquamous lesions or ichthyosis ☐ Hyperpigmentation ☐ Hypopigmentation ☐ Keratosis pilaris ☐ Erythema ☐ Erythroderma ☐ Poikiloderma ☐ Sclerotic features ☐ Pruritis ☐ Hair involvement ☐ Nail involvement % BSA involved	☐ No symptoms	☐ <18% BSA with disease signs but NO sclerotic features	☐ 19-50% BSA OR involvement with superficial sclerotic features "not hidebound" (able to pinch)	☐ >50% BSA OR deep sclerotic features "hidebound" (unable to pinch) OR impaired mobility, ulceration or severe pruritus
Mouth	☐ No symptoms	☐ Mild symptoms with disease signs but not limiting oral intake significantly	☐ Moderate symptoms with disease signs with partial limitation of oral intake	☐ Severe symptoms with disease signs on examination with major limitation of oral intake
Eyes Mean tear test(mm): ☐ >10 ☐ 6-10 ☐ ≤10 ☐ Not done	☐ No symptoms	☐ Mild dry eye symptoms not affecting ADL (requiring eyedrops ≤3 x per day) OR asymptomatic signs of keratoconjunctivitis sicca	☐ Moderate dry eye symptoms partially affecting ADL (requiring drops >3 x per day or punctal plugs), WITHOUT vision impairment	☐ Severe dry eye symptoms significantly affecting ADL (special eyeware to relieve pain) OR unable to work because of ocular symptoms OR loss of vision caused by keratoconjunctivitis sicca
GI tract	☐ No symptoms	☐ Symptoms such as dysphagia, nausea, vomiting, abdominal pain or diarrhoea without significant weight loss (<5%)	☐ Symptoms associated with mild to moderate weight loss (5-15%)	☐ Symptoms associated with significant weight loss >15%, requires nutritional supplement for most calorie needs OR oesophageal dilation
Liver	☐ Normal LFT	☐ Elevated Bilirubin, AP*, AST or ALT <2 x ULN	☐ Bilirubin >3 mg/dL or Bilirubin enzymes 2-5 x ULN	☐ Bilirubin or enzymes >5 x ULN

FIG. 22.1 NIH consensus criteria.

excellent responses and within 2 weeks to 1 month, steroids are often tapered by a steroid of 25%. Sometimes however, some patients may require extended courses of corticosteroids with treatment durations of two to 3 years. Given the risk of steroid induced myopathy, diabetes, other issues, steroids are modified in these situations to minimize the amount of corticosteroid necessary to control symptoms.

Steroids are often combined with site specific targeted therapy. For instance, for skin specific disease, creams and ointments are often used. Topical tacrolimus is also often combined with systemic steroids. In oral/mucosal involvement, topical fluoride and conjunction of dental hygiene is often emphasized.

Nevertheless, patients will still develop steroid refractory disease. . In general, per the NIH and CIBMTR guidelines, patients who have steroid responsive disease will remain stable and improve within 2 weeks of therapy. Patients who develop progression at 2 weeks or do not respond, need to be treatment with additional immunosuppression or sometimes switch therapy.

For patients who develop steroid refractory chronic GVHD, there is not a standard of care for second-line therapy. While combinations of immunosuppression have been tested with prednisone; the most promising has been the addition of calcineurin inhibitor (CsA cyclosporine and tacrolimus) to prednisone. Some studies have demonstrated improvement in overall survival; while others have not. The addition of a calcineurin inhibitor is institutional dependent, and patients are often enrolled in clinical trials. However, for those patients who are treated with either cyclosporine or tacrolimus, patients can expect to have electrolyte abnormalities, HTN and nephrotoxicity. Furthermore, transplant-associated thrombotic microangiopathy and neurotoxic effects that can lead to premature discontinuation.

In the setting of persistent disease or progressive disease despite adding a CsA (prednisone and a calcineurin inhibitor (cyclosporine or tacrolimus)), there is no standard third line agent and often clinical trials or novel therapeutic strategies are employed.

TABLE 22.7
Future Directions in Chronic GVHD Treatment

Drug	Mechanism	Results/Data
Ruxolitinib	JAK 2 Kinase inhibitor	The ORR was 85.4% with 32 (78%) patients achieving a PR and three patients achieving a CR. The median time to response was 3 (range 1–25) weeks
Baricitinib	JAK 2 Kinase inhibitor	Currently being investigated in trials
Ibrutinib	BTK inhibitor	ORR was 67% (28/42 patients; 21% CR; 45% PR). A total of 71% of responders had a sustained response of at least 20 weeks and improvement in QOL.
Fosmatinib	Spleen tyrosine kinase	Recruiting in phase I/II trial
ROCK Kinase inhibitors	ROCK kinase inhibiors	Recruiting in phase II trials
Abaterecept	CTLA-4	(44%) patients had a PR based On the NIH consensus criteria.
Bortezomib/Carfilzomib/Ixazomib	Proteasome Inhibitors:	ORR at week 15 of 80% with two (10%) complete responses and 14 (70%) PRs in 20 evaluable patients.
CD19, CD20 chimeric antigen receptor T (cART) cell therapy	CAR Therapy	Currently being studied in trials

ORR, overall response rate.

However, for the extremely elderly or patients who are ineligible for an RCT, non-pharmacologic approaches such as ECP or UVA can be used to treat chronic GVHD.

FUTURE DIRECTIONS AND NOVEL THERAPEUTICS

Chronic GVHD is a multisystem disease that causes significant immunodeficiency and can be challenging to treat given the increased risk of severe, life-threatening infections. As previously discussed while steroids are first-line, second-line treatment is often required. For those patients who fail the combination of calcineurin and prednisone, there is some promise that additional lines of pharmacologic immunosuppression may have a response rate of 25%–50%. However, no single medication has shown to be better than the other. The choice of third line therapy is general based on the individual patient, their comorbidities, organ involved and physician experience. Summarized below are new therapeutics that are being studied and are on the horizon; much of these therapeutics were previously mentioned with acute GVHD. However, there are a few therapeutics that are unique and specific to GVHD (Table 22.7).

BIOMARKERS

The use of biomarkers for diagnosis and prognosis of chronic GVHD is an area of active research. Much like for acute GVHD, an ideal biomarker would predict the diagnosis, appearance and severity of acute GVHD and guide management. However. There is not currently on an individual biomarker ready for prime time. Summarized in Table 22.8 below are biomarkers that are under investigation. Much of these biomarkers are being investigated in acute GVHD as well.

DISCUSSION

Acute and Chronic GVHD continue to remain a significant mortality and morbidity and burden in hematopoietic transplant patients. The treatment of acute chronic GVHD is determined in part by the severity of the disease. While most patients respond to steroids, patients still fail front line therapy and often require second-line therapy. There are promising new agents that are being developed and investigated. However, further understanding of the disease biology and immunological mechanisms are required to further enhance our treatment options for these challenging diseases.

TABLE 22.8
Current Biomarkers Currently Being Investigated in Clinical trials

Biomarker	Mechanism	Study Findings:
ST2	a member of the interleukin-1 receptor family	study of 673 recipients of myeloablative conditioning found that ST2 (as early as 14 days after transplant) correlated with an increased risk of NRM and resistance to treatment of acute GVHD
REG3alpha	(regenerating islet-derived 3-alpha) is expressed by regenerating cells in the gastrointestinal epithelium (especially Paneth cells	Increased concentrations predict GVHD associated epithelial mucosal injury.
TNFR1	TNF receptor 1	Serum levels of TNFR1 correlate with onset of GVHD, mortality and overall survival.
Plasma and urine polypeptides for INF-a, IL-8, GF via proteomic analysis	Involved in cytokine and growth	Shown to predict onset of GVHD, prognostic information
Flow cytometry for CD30 and CD8	Mediated in effector response	Higher prediction of acute GVHD
TIM3, IL6, sTNFR1	Mediators in cytokine response	Predictor higher stage of GVHD and TRM from GVHD.
CXCL9, matrix metalloproteinase-3,	Mediators in cytokine response	Currently under investigation
osteopontin, CXCL10, CXCL11, and CD163	Mediators in cytokine response	Currently under investigation

REFERENCES

1. Blazar BR, Murphy WJ, Abedi M. Advances in graft-versus-host disease biology and therapy. *Nat Rev Immunol.* 2012;12(6):443–458.
2. Chu YW, Gress RE. Murine models of chronic graft-versus-host disease: insights and unresolved issues. *Biol Blood Marrow Transpl.* 2008;14(4):365–378.
3. McDonald-Hyman C, Turka LA, Blazar BR. Advances and challenges in immunotherapy for solid organ and hematopoietic stem cell transplantation. *Sci Transl Med.* 2015;7(280):280rv2.
4. Schroeder MA, DiPersio JF. Mouse models of graft-versus-host disease: advances and limitations. *Dis Model Mech.* 2011;4(3):318–333.
5. Blazar, et al. Understanding chronic GVHD from different Angles. *Biol Blood Marrow Transpl.* 2012;18(suppl 1):S184–S188. https://doi.org/10.1016/j.bbmt. 2011.10.025.
6. Edinger M, Hoffmann P, Ermann J, et al. CD41 CD251 regulatory T cells preserve graft-versus tumor activity while inhibiting graft-versus-host disease after bone marrow transplantation. *Nat Med.* 2003;9(9):1144–1150.
7. Matsuoka K, Kim HT, McDonough S, et al. Altered regulatory T cell homeostasis in patients with CD41 lymphopenia following allogeneic hematopoietic stem cell transplantation. *J Clin Invest.* 2010;120(5):1479–1493.
8. Duffield JS, Forbes SJ, Constandinou CM, et al. Selective depletion of macrophages reveals distinct, opposing roles during liver injury and repair. *J Clin Invest.* 2005;115(1):56–65.
9. Gangadharan B, Hoeve MA, Allen JE, et al. Murine gammaherpesvirus-induced fibrosis is associated with the development of alternatively activated macrophages. *J Leukoc Biol.* 2008;84(1):50–58.
10. Alexander KA, Flynn R, Lineburg KE, et al. CSF-1-dependant donor-derived macrophages mediate chronic graft-versus-host disease. *J Clin Invest.* 2014;124(10):4266–4280.
11. Clancy RM, Buyon JP. Clearance of apoptotic cells: TGF-beta in the balance between inflammation and fibrosis. *J Leukoc Biol.* 2003;74(6):959–960. 115. Clancy J Jr, Tonder O, Boettcher CE. The effect of neonatal rat graft-vs-host disease (GVHD) on Fc receptor lymphocytes. *J Immunol.* 1976;116(1):210–217.
12. Sviland L. The pathology of bone marrow transplantation. *Curr Diag Pathol.* 2000;6:242–250.
13. Seber A, Khan SP, Kersey JH. Unexplained effusions: association with allogeneic bone marrow transplantation and acute or chronic graft-versus-host disease. *Bone Marrow Transpl.* 1996;17:207–211. MEDLINE.
14. McDonald GB, Shulman HM, Sullivan KM, et al. Intestinal and hepatic complications of human bone marrow transplantation. *Part II. Gastroenterol.* 1986;90:770–784.

15. DeLord C, Treleaven J, Shepherd J, et al. Vaginal stenosis following allogeneic bone marrow transplantation for acute myeloid leukaemia. *Bone Marrow Transpl.* 1999;23:523–525. MEDLINE.

16. Corson SL, Sullivan K, Batzer F, et al. Gynecologic manifestations of chronic graft-versus-host disease. *Obstet Gynecol.* 1982;60:488–492. MEDLINE.

17. Janin A, Socie G, Devergie A, et al. Fasciitis in chronic graft-versus-host disease. A clinicopathologic study of 14 cases. *Ann Int Med.* 1994;120:993–998.

18. Parker PM, Openshaw H, Forman SJ. Myositis associated with graft-versus-host disease. *Curr Opin Rheumatol.* 1997;9:513–519. MEDLINE.

19. Mackey JR, Desai S, Larratt L, et al. Myasthenia gravis in association with allogeneic bone marrow transplantation: clinical observations, therapeutic implications and review of literature. *Bone Marrow Transpl.* 1997;19:939–942. MEDLINE.

20. Redding SW, Callander NS, Haveman CW, et al. Treatment of oral chronic graft-versus-host disease with PUVA therapy: case report and literature review. *Oral Surg Oral Med Oral Pathol Oral Radiol Endo.* 1998;86:183–187.

21. Lindahl G, Lonnquist B, Hedfors E. Lymphocytic infiltrations of lip salivary glands in bone marrow recipients. A model for the development of the histopathological changes in Sjogren's syndrome? *J Autoimmun.* 1989;2:579–583.

22. Kami M, Kanda Y, Sasaki M, et al. Phimosis as a manifestation of chronic graft-versus-host disease after allogeneic bone marrow transplantation. *Bone Marrow Transpl.* 1998;21:721–723. MEDLINE.

23. Janin-Mercier A, Devergie A, Van Cauwenberge D, et al. Immunohistologic and ultrastructural study of the sclerotic skin in chronic graft-versus-host disease in man. *Am J Pathol.* 1984;115:296–306. MEDLINE.

24. Shulman HM, Sharma P, Amos D, et al. A coded histologic study of hepatic graft-versus-host disease after human bone marrow transplantation. *Hepatol.* 1988;8:463–470.

25. Strasser SI, Sullivan KM, Myerson D, et al. Cirrhosis of the liver in long-term marrow transplant survivors. *Blood.* 1999;93:3259–3266. MEDLINE.

26. McDonald GB, Sullivan KM, Schuffler MD, et al. Esophageal abnormalities in chronic graft-versus-host disease in humans. *Gastroenterol.* 1981;80:914–921.

27. Serota FT, Rosenberg HK, Rosen J, et al. Delayed onset of gastrointestinal disease in the recipients of bone marrow transplants. A variant graft-versus-host reaction. *Transplantation.* 1982;34:60–64. MEDLINE.

28. Carrigan DR, Drobyski WR, Russler SK, et al. Interstitial pneumonitis associated with human herpesvirus-6 infection after marrow transplantation. *Lancet.* 1991;338:147–149. MEDLINE.

29. Cone RW, Hackman RC, Huang ML, et al. Human herpesvirus 6 in lung tissue from patients with pneumonitis after bone marrow transplantation [see comments]. *New Engl J Med.* 1993;329:156–161. MEDLINE.

30. Cooke KR, Krenger W, Hill G, et al. Host reactive donor T cells are associated with lung injury after experimental allogeneic bone marrow transplantation. *Blood.* 1998;92:2571–2580. MEDLINE.

31. Epler GR. Bronchiolitis obliterans and airways obstruction associated with graft-versus-host disease. *Clin Chest Med.* 1988;9:551–556. MEDLINE.

32. Holland HK, Wingard JR, Beschorner WE, et al. Bronchiolitis obliterans in bone marrow transplantation and its relationship to chronic graft-v-host disease and low serum IgG. *Blood.* 1988;72:621–627. MEDLINE.

33. Ooi GC, Peh WC, Ip M. High-resolution computed tomography of bronchiolitis obliterans syndrome after bone marrow transplantation. *Respiration.* 1998;65:187–191. MEDLINE.

34. Clark JG, Crawford SW, Madtes DK, et al. Obstructive lung disease after allogeneic marrow transplantation. Clinical presentation and course. *Ann Int Med.* 1989;111:368–376.

35. Openshaw H. Peripheral neuropathy after bone marrow transplantation. *Biol Blood Marrow Transpl.* 1997;3:202–209. MEDLINE.

36. Castilla-Llorente C, Martin PJ, McDonald GB, et al. Prognostic factors and outcomes of severe gastrointestinal GVHD after allogeneic hematopoietic cell transplantation. *Bone Marrow Transpl.* 2014;49(7):966–971 (CrossRefPubMedGoogle Scholar).

37. Xhaard A, Rocha V, Bueno B, et al. Steroid-refractory acute GVHD: lack of long-term improved survival using new generation anticytokine treatment. *Biol Blood Marrow Transpl.* 2012;18(3):406–413 (CrossRefPubMedWeb of ScienceGoogle Scholar).

38. Paczesny S. Discovery and validation of graft-versus-host disease biomarkers. *Blood.* 2013;121(4):585–594 (Abstract/FREE Full TextGoogle Scholar).

39. Vander Lugt MT, Braun TM, Hanash S, et al. ST2 as a marker for risk of therapy-resistant graft-versus-host disease and death. *N Engl J Med.* 2013;369(6):529–539 (CrossRefPubMedWeb of ScienceGoogle Scholar).

40. Martin PJ, Furlong T, Rowley SD, et al. Evaluation of oral beclomethasone dipropionate for prevention of acute graft-versus-host disease. *Biol Blood Marrow Transpl.* 2012;18(6):922–929 (CrossRefPubMedGoogle Scholar).

41. Malone FR, Leisenring WM, Storer BE, et al. Prolonged anorexia and elevated plasma cytokine levels following myeloablative allogeneic hematopoietic cell transplant. *Bone Marrow Transpl.* 2007;40(8):765–772 (CrossRefPubMedGoogle Scholar).

42. Mielcarek M, Martin PJ, Leisenring W, et al. Graft-versus-host disease after nonmyeloablative versus conventional hematopoietic stem cell transplantation. *Blood.* 2003;102(2):756–762 (Abstract/FREE Full TextGoogle Scholar).

43. Levine JE, Huber E, Hammer ST, et al. Low Paneth cell numbers at onset of gastrointestinal graft-versus-host disease identify patients at high risk for nonrelapse mortality. *Blood.* 2013;122(8):1505–1509 (Abstract/FREE Full TextGoogle Scholar).

FURTHER READING

1. Socié G, Stone JV, Wingard JR, et al. Late effects working committee of the international bone marrow transplant registry. Long-term survival and late deaths after allogeneic bone marrow transplantation. *N Engl J Med.* 1999;341(1):14–21. PubMed: 10387937.

2. Wingard JR, Majhail NS, Brazauskas R, et al. Long-term survival and late deaths after allogeneic hematopoietic cell transplantation. *J Clin Oncol.* 2011;29(16):2230–2239. PMCID: PMC3107742. PubMed: 21464398.

3. Rezvani K, Mielke S, Ahmadzadeh M, et al. High donor FOXP3-positive regulatory T-cell (Treg) content is associated with a low risk of GVHD following HLA-matched allogeneic SCT. *Blood.* 2006;108(4):1291–1297.

4. Robb RJ, Lineburg KE, Kuns RD, et al. Identification and expansion of highly suppressive CD8(1) FoxP3(1) regulatory T cells after experimental allogeneic bone marrow transplantation. *Blood.* 2012;119(24):5898–5908.

5. Zhang P, Tey SK, Koyama M, et al. Induced regulatory T cells promote tolerance when stabilized by rapamycin and IL-2 in vivo. *J Immunol.* 2013;191(10):5291–5303.

6. Taylor PA, Lees CJ, Blazar BR. The infusion of ex vivo activated and expanded CD4(1)CD25(1) immune regulatory cells inhibits graft-versushost disease lethality. *Blood.* 2002;99(10):3493–3499.

7. Zorn E, Kim HT, Lee SJ, et al. Reduced frequency of FOXP31 CD41CD251 regulatory T cells in patients with chronic graft-versus-host disease. *Blood.* 2005;106(8):2903–2911.

8. Rieger K, Loddenkemper C, Maul J, et al. Mucosal FOXP31 regulatory T cells are numerically deficient in acute and chronic GvHD. *Blood.* 2006;107(4):1717–1723.

9. Erbel C, Akhavanpoor M, Okuyucu D, et al. IL-17A influences essential functions of the monocyte/macrophage lineage and is involved in advanced murine and human atherosclerosis. *J Immunol.* 2014;193(9):4344–4355.

10. Akpek G, Zahurak M, Piantadosi S, et al. Development of a prognostic model for grading chronic graft-versus-host disease. *Blood.* 2001;97:1219–1226. MEDLINE.

11. Artlett CM, Smith JB, Jimenez SA. New perspectives on the etiology of systemic sclerosis. *Mol Med Today.* 1999;5:74–78. MEDLINE.

12. Holmes JA, Livesey SJ, Bedwell AE, et al. Autoantibody analysis in chronic graft-versus-host disease. *Bone Marrow Transpl.* 1989;4:529–531. MEDLINE.

13. Woo SB, Lee SJ, Schubert MM. Graft-vs.-host disease. *Crit Rev Oral Biol Med.* 1997;8:201–216. MEDLINE.

14. Nakamura S, Hiroki A, Shinohara M, et al. Oral involvement in chronic graft-versus-host disease after allogeneic bone marrow transplantation. *Oral Surg Oral Med Oral Pathol Oral Radiol Endo.* 1996;82:556–563.

15. Manoussakis MN, Moutsopoulos HM. Sjogren's syndrome: autoimmune epithelitis. *Bailliere Clin Rheumatol.* 2000;14:73–95.

16. Nagler R, Marmary Y, Krausz Y, et al. Major salivary gland dysfunction in human acute and chronic graft-versus-host disease (GVHD). *Bone Marrow Transpl.* 1996;17:219–224. MEDLINE.

17. Singhal S, Mehta J, Rattenbury H, et al. Oral pilocarpine hydrochloride for the treatment of refractory xerostomia associated with chronic graft-versus-host disease. *Blood.* 1995;85:1147–1148. MEDLINE.

18. Vivino FB, Al Hashimi I, Khan Z, et al. Pilocarpine tablets for the treatment of dry mouth and dry eye symptoms in patients with Sjogren syndrome: a randomized, placebo-controlled, fixed-dose, multicenter trial. P92-01 Study Group. *Arc Int Med.* 1999;159:174–181.

19. Aractingi S, Chosidow O. Cutaneous graft-versus-host disease. *Arch Dermatol.* 1998;134:602–612. MEDLINE.

20. Ponec RJ, Saunders MD, Kimmey MB. Neostigmine for the treatment of acute colonic pseudo-obstruction. *New Engl J Med.* 1999;341:137–141. MEDLINE.

21. Fisk JD, Shulman HM, Greening RR, et al. Gastrointestinal radiographic features of human graft-vs.-host disease. *Am J Roentgenol.* 1981;136:329–336.

22. Pecego R, Hill R, Appelbaum FR, et al. Interstitial pneumonitis following autologous bone marrow transplantation. *Transplantation.* 1986;42:515–517. MEDLINE.

23. Weiner RS, Bortin MM, Gale RP, et al. Interstitial pneumonitis after bone marrow transplantation. Assessment of risk factors. *Ann Int Med.* 1986;104:168–175.

24. Wingard JR, Mellits ED, Sostrin MB, et al. Interstitial pneumonitis after allogeneic bone marrow transplantation. Nine-year experience at a single institution. *Medicine.* 1988;67:175–186. MEDLINE.

25. Ralph DD, Springmeyer SC, Sullivan KM, et al. Rapidly progressive air-flow obstruction in marrow transplant recipients. Possible association between obliterative bronchiolitis and chronic graft-versus-host disease. *Am Rev Resp Dis.* 1984;129:641–644. MEDLINE.

26. Greenspan A, Deeg HJ, Cottler-Fox M, et al. Incapacitating peripheral neuropathy as a manifestation of chronic graft-versus-host disease. *Bone Marrow Transpl.* 1990;5:349–352. MEDLINE.

27. Gabriel CM, Goldman JM, Lucas S, et al. Vasculitic neuropathy in association with chronic graft-versus-host disease. *J Neurol Sci.* 1999;168:68–70. MEDLINE.

28. Parker P, Chao NJ, Ben Ezra J, et al. Polymyositis as a manifestation of chronic graft-versus-host disease. *Medicine.* 1996;75:279–285. MEDLINE.

29. Leber B, Walker IR, Rodriguez A, et al. Reinduction of remission of chronic myeloid leukemia by donor leukocyte transfusion following relapse after bone marrow transplantation: recovery complicated by initial pancytopenia and late dermatomyositis. *Bone Marrow Transpl.* 1993;12:405–407. MEDLINE.

30. Tse S, Saunders EF, Silverman E, et al. Myasthenia gravis and polymyositis as manifestations of chronic graft-versus-host-disease. *Bone Marrow Transpl.* 1999;23:397–399. MEDLINE.

31. Bolger GB, Sullivan KM, Spence AM, et al. Myasthenia gravis after allogeneic bone marrow transplantation:

relationship to chronic graft-versus-host disease. *Neurology.* 1986;36:1087–1091. MEDLINE.

32. Smith CI, Aarli JA, Biberfeld P, et al. Myasthenia gravis after bone-marrow transplantation. Evidence for a donor origin. *N Engl J Med.* 1983;309:1565–1568. MEDLINE.

33. oley TA, Chien JW, Pergam SA, et al. Reduced mortality after allogeneic hematopoietic-cell transplantation. *N Engl J Med.* 2010;363(22):2091–2101 (CrossRefPubMedWeb of ScienceGoogle Scholar).

34. Levine JE, Braun TM, Harris AC, et al. For the Blood and Marrow Transplant Clinical Trials Network. A prognostic score for acute graft-versus-host disease based on biomarkers: a multicenter study. *Lancet Haematol.* 2015;2(1):e21–e29 (CrossRefGoogle Scholar).

35. Leisenring WM, Martin PJ, Petersdorf EW, et al. An acute graft-versus-host disease activity index to predict survival after hematopoietic cell transplantation with myeloablative conditioning regimens. *Blood.* 2006;108(2):749–755 (Abstract/FREE Full TextGoogle Scholar).

36. Van Lint MT, Milone G, Leotta S, et al. Treatment of acute graft-versus-host disease with prednisolone: significant survival advantage for day +5 responders and no advantage for nonresponders receiving anti-thymocyte globulin. *Blood.* 2006;107(10):4177–4181 (Abstract/FREE Full TextGoogle Scholar).

37. Ponce DM, Hilden P, Mumaw C, et al. High day 28 ST2 levels predict for acute graft-versus-host disease and transplant-related mortality after cord blood transplantation. *Blood.* 2015;125(1):199–205 (Abstract/FREE Full TextGoogle Scholar).

38. Rezvani AR, Storer BE, Storb RF, et al. Decreased serum albumin as a biomarker for severe acute graft-versus-host disease after reduced-intensity allogeneic hematopoietic cell transplantation. *Biol Blood Marrow Transpl.* 2011;17(11):1594–1601 (CrossRefPubMedWeb of ScienceGoogle Scholar).

39. Ferrara JL, Harris AC, Greenson JK, et al. Regenerating islet-derived 3-alpha is a biomarker of gastrointestinal graft-versus-host disease. *Blood.* 2011;118(25):6702–6708 (Abstract/FREE Full TextGoogle Scholar).

40. Hansen JA, Hanash SM, Tabellini L, et al. A novel soluble form of Tim-3 associated with severe graft-versus-host disease. *Biol Blood Marrow Transpl.* 2013;19(9):1323–1330 (CrossRefPubMedGoogle Scholar).

41. Holtan SG, Verneris MR, Schultz KR, et al. Circulating angiogenic factors associated with response and survival in patients with acute graft-versus-host disease: results from blood and marrow transplant clinical trials network 0302 and 0802. *Biol Blood Marrow Transpl.* 2015;21(6):1029–1036 (CrossRefPubMedGoogle Scholar).

42. Przepiorka D, Weisdorf D, Martin P, et al. 1994 consensus conference on acute GVHD grading. *Bone Marrow Transpl.* 1995;15(6):825–828 (PubMedWeb of Science-Google Scholar).

43. Mielcarek M, Storer BE, Boeckh M, et al. Initial therapy of acute graft-versus-host disease with low-dose prednisone does not compromise patient outcomes. *Blood.* 2009;113(13):2888–2894 (Abstract/FREE Full TextGoogle Scholar).

44. MacMillan ML, Robin M, Harris AC, et al. A refined risk score for acute graft-versus-host disease that predicts response to initial therapy, survival, and transplant-related mortality. *Biol Blood Marrow Transpl.* 2015;21(4):761–767 (CrossRefPubMedGoogle Scholar).

45. Rodriguez-Otero P, Porcher R, Peffault de Latour R, et al. Fecal calprotectin and alpha-1 antitrypsin predict severity and response to corticosteroids in gastrointestinal graft-versus-host disease. *Blood.* 2012;119(24):5909–5917 (Abstract/FREE Full TextGoogle Scholar).

46. Abraham J, Janin A, Gornet JM, et al. Clinical severity scores in gastrointestinal graft-versus-host disease. *Transplantation.* 2014;97(9):965–971 (PubMedGoogle Scholar).

47. Socié G, Mary J-Y, Lemann M, et al. Prognostic value of apoptotic cells and infiltrating neutrophils in graft-versus-host disease of the gastrointestinal tract in humans: TNF and Fas expression. *Blood.* 2004;103(1):50–57 (Abstract/FREE Full TextGoogle Scholar).

48. Epstein RJ, McDonald GB, Sale GE, Shulman HM, Thomas ED. The diagnostic accuracy of the rectal biopsy in acute graft-versus-host disease: a prospective study of thirteen patients. *Gastroenterology.* 1980;78(4):764–771 (PubMedWeb of ScienceGoogle Scholar).

49. DiCarlo J, Agarwal-Hashmi R, Shah A, et al. Cytokine and chemokine patterns across 100 days after hematopoietic stem cell transplantation in children. *Biol Blood Marrow Transpl.* 2014;20(3):361–369 (CrossRefPubMedGoogle Scholar).

50. Holtan SG, DeFor TE, Lazaryan A, et al. Composite end point of graft-versus-host disease-free, relapse-free survival after allogeneic hematopoietic cell transplantation. *Blood.* 2015;125(8):1333–1338 (Abstract/FREE Full TextGoogle Scholar).

51. Couriel DR, Hosing C, Saliba R, et al. Extracorporeal photochemotherapy for the treatment of steroid-resistant chronic GVHD. *Blood.* 2006;107:3074.

52. Marshall SR. Technology insight: ECP for the treatment of GvHD–can we offer selective immune control without generalized immunosuppression? *Nat Clin Pract Oncol.* 2006;3:302.

53. Knobler R, Barr ML, Couriel DR, et al. Extracorporeal photopheresis: past, present, and future. *J Am Acad Dermatol.* 2009;61:652.

54. Flowers ME, Apperley JF, van Besien K, et al. A multicenter prospective phase 2 randomized study of extracorporeal photopheresis for treatment of chronic graft-versus-host disease. *Blood.* 2008;112:2667.

55. Basara N, Blau WI, Römer E, et al. Mycophenolate mofetil for the treatment of acute and chronic GVHD in bone marrow transplant patients. *Bone Marrow Transpl.* 1998;22:61.

56. Couriel DR, Saliba R, Escalón MP, et al. Sirolimus in combination with tacrolimus and corticosteroids for the treatment of resistant chronic graft-versus-host disease. *Br J Haematol.* 2005;130:409.

57. Tefferi A, Pardanani A. Serious adverse events during ruxolitinib treatment discontinuation in patients with myelofibrosis. *Mayo Clin Proc.* 2011;86:1188.

58. Mori Y, Ikeda K, Inomata T, et al. Ruxolitinib treatment for GvHD in patients with myelofibrosis. *Bone Marrow Transpl.* 2016;51:1584.

59. Zeiser R, Burchert A, Lengerke C, et al. Ruxolitinib in corticosteroid-refractory graft-versus-host disease after allogeneic stem cell transplantation: a multicenter survey. *Leukemia.* 2015;2015:2062.

60. https://www.accessdata.fda.gov/drugsatfda_docs/label/2017/205552s017lbl.pdf.

61. Miklos D, Cutler CS, Arora M, et al. Multicenter open-label phase 2 study of ibrutinib in chronic graft versus host disease (cGVHD) after failure of corticosteroids (late breaking abstract-3). *Blood.* 2016.

62. Ratanatharathorn V, Carson E, Reynolds C, et al. Anti-CD20 chimeric monoclonal antibody treatment of refractory immune-mediated thrombocytopenia in a patient with chronic graft-versus-host disease. *Ann Intern Med.* 2000;133:275.

63. Canninga-van Dijk MR, van der Straaten HM, Fijnheer R, et al. Anti-CD20 monoclonal antibody treatment in 6 patients with therapy-refractory chronic graft-versus-host disease. *Blood.* 2004;104:2603.

64. Cutler C, Miklos D, Kim HT, et al. Rituximab for steroid-refractory chronic graft-versus-host disease. *Blood.* 2006;108:756.

65. Alousi AM, Uberti J, Ratanatharathorn V. The role of B cell depleting therapy in graft versus host disease after allogeneic hematopoietic cell transplant. *Leuk Lymphoma.* 2010;51:376.

66. Kim SJ, Lee JW, Jung CW, et al. Weekly rituximab followed by monthly rituximab treatment for steroid-refractory chronic graft-versus-host disease: results from a prospective, multicenter, phase II study. *Haematologica.* 1935;2010:95.

67. Clavert A, Chevallier P, Guillaume T, et al. Safety and efficacy of rituximab in steroid-refractory chronic GVHD. *Bone Marrow Transpl.* 2013;48:734.

68. Arai S, Pidala J, Pusic I, et al. A randomized phase II crossover study of imatinib or rituximab for cutaneous sclerosis after hematopoietic cell transplantation. *Clin Cancer Res.* 2016;22:319.

69. Magro L, Mohty M, Catteau B, et al. Imatinib mesylate as salvage therapy for refractory sclerotic chronic graft-versus-host disease. *Blood.* 2009;114:719.

70. Olivieri A, Locatelli F, Zecca M, et al. Imatinib for refractory chronic graft-versus-host disease with fibrotic features. *Blood.* 2009;114:709.

71. de Masson A, Bouaziz JD, Peffault de Latour R, et al. Limited efficacy and tolerance of imatinib mesylate in steroid-refractory sclerodermatous chronic GVHD. *Blood.* 2012;120:5089.

72. Olivieri A, Cimminiello M, Corradini P, et al. Long-term outcome and prospective validation of NIH response criteria in 39 patients receiving imatinib for steroid-refractory chronic GVHD. *Blood.* 2013;122:4111.

73. Stadler M, Ahlborn R, Kamal H, et al. Limited efficacy of imatinib in severe pulmonary chronic graft-versus-host disease. *Blood.* 2009;114:3718.

74. Fried RH, Murakami CS, Fisher LD, et al. Ursodeoxycholic acid treatment of refractory chronic graft-versus-host disease of the liver. *Ann Intern Med.* 1992;116:624.

75. Hillaire S, Boucher E, Calmus Y, et al. Effects of bile acids and cholestasis on major histocompatibility complex class I in human and rat hepatocytes. *Gastroenterology.* 1994;107:781.

76. Koreth J, Matsuoka K, Kim HT, et al. Interleukin-2 and regulatory T cells in graft-versus-host disease. *N Engl J Med.* 2011;2011:2055.

77. Koreth J, Kim HT, Jones KT, et al. Efficacy, durability, and response predictors of low-dose interleukin-2 therapy for chronic graft-versus-host disease. *Blood.* 2016;128:130.

78. Chiang KY, Abhyankar S, Bridges K, et al. Recombinant human tumor necrosis factor receptor fusion protein as complementary treatment for chronic graft-versus-host disease. *Transplantation.* 2002;73:665.

79. Vogelsang GB, Farmer ER, Hess AD, et al. Thalidomide for the treatment of chronic graft-versus-host disease. *N Engl J Med.* 1992;326:1055.

80. Parker PM, Chao N, Nademanee A, et al. Thalidomide as salvage therapy for chronic graft-versus-host disease. *Blood.* 1995;86:3604.

81. Jacobsohn DA, Chen AR, Zahurak M, et al. Phase II study of pentostatin in patients with corticosteroid-refractory chronic graft-versus-host disease. *J Clin Oncol.* 2007;25:4255.

82. Jacobsohn DA, Gilman AL, Rademaker A, et al. Evaluation of pentostatin in corticosteroid-refractory chronic graft-versus-host disease in children: a Pediatric Blood and Marrow Transplant Consortium study. *Blood.* 2009;114:4354.

CHAPTER 23

Graft Failure

RONI TAMARI, MD

Graft failure is a life-threatening complication after allogeneic hematopoietic stem cell transplantation (allo-HSCT). It was one of the major causes of treatment failure in the early era of allo-HSCT[1,2]; however, now a days, this complication is less prevalent, probably partly due to improved human leukocyte antigen (HLA) typing techniques, but when occurs, it remains a devastating complication after transplantation with very poor outcomes.[3,4]

DEFINITIONS

Graft failure (GF) after allo-HSCT is a complex syndrome characterized by pancytopenia and hypocellular or acellular bone marrow. Graft failure can be defined based on the mechanism leading to it or the timing of the event.

Graft rejection (GR): The best characterized form of graft failure is immune-medicated rejection. In this process, preexisting anti-HLA antibodies[5,6] or residual host T lymphocytes eliminate the donor stem cells, and typically these patients have only host cells.[7,8]

Poor graft function (PGF): This entity is characterized by the presence of full donor engraftment with hypocellular or acellular marrow and varies with the level of pancytopenia. This is due to qualitative or quantitative deficiencies or damage to the hematopoietic stem cells.

Primary graft failure: Characterized by the absence of initial donor cell engraftment; the patient never recovers from the neutropenia (absolute neutrophil count $< 0.5 \times 10^9$/L) induced by the conditioning regimen.

Secondary graft failure: Defined as loss of donor cells after initial engraftment occurred.

GRAFT REJECTION

Different immunological mechanism may result in GR. Most commonly it is due to immune recipient T cells, although natural killer (NK) cells-mediated rejection has also been demonstrated in animal models.[9–13] Whether antibodies can cause rejection is controversial,[14–18] although some data suggest that pretransplant donor-specific antiendothelial precursor cell antibodies augment the risk of GR in clinical allo-HSCT.[19] These studies indicate that cellular mechanisms are the major contributors to graft failure, but humoral mechanisms may also be important.

Olsson et al.[20] studied retrospectively 967 patients who underwent first allo-HSCT at a single center for various malignant and nonmalignant hematologic disease and reported the incidence of primary and secondary graft failure to be 5.6%, most of them being secondary GF, with primary GF reported only in six patients (0.6%). The following factors were found to be associated with increased risk for GF: (1) transplant after the year 2000 (6%–7%) compared with the ones performed previously (3%) $P = .05$, and (2) transplantation for nonmalignant disorders had a three times higher incidence of GF than those performed for malignant disease. In patients with malignant diseases, the incidence of GF was 20% for nonhematological malignancies, 10% in both chronic lymphocytic leukemia (CLL) and myeloproliferative disorders (MPDs)/myelofibrosis and 5% in myelodysplastic syndrome, whereas the incidence of GF was lower (2%–3%) in patients with acute leukemia. The intensity of the conditioning regimen was also an important factor in the risk for GF with 8% incidence of GF in patients who received a reduced intensity conditioning (RIC) and 19% in those who had a nonmyeloablative conditioning (NMA), in contrast to only 3% GF observed in patients who received a myeloablative conditioning (MAC). In multivariate analysis, patients conditioned with NMA (relative risk (RR), 4.5; $P < .01$) or RIC (RR, 2.58; $P < .01$) had a higher risk for GF than those treated with MAC. Stem cell source was also an important risk factor with higher incidence in recipients of cord blood transplants (CBTs) (18%) than peripheral blood stem cells (PBSCs) (5%) or bone marrow (BM) graft (6%), though this did not reach statistical significance ($P = .08$). In univariate analysis, both HLA and ABO mismatch between the patient and the donor were associated with increased incidence of GF. This was mostly pronounced for HLA-mismatched grafts, and in multivariate analysis, both transplant from a matched unrelated donor (MUD) and HLA-mismatched grafts had markedly increased

Hematopoietic Cell Transplantation for Malignant Conditions. https://doi.org/10.1016/B978-0-323-56802-9.00023-7

risk of GF. Moreover, GF rates were similar in 8 out of 8 or 6 out of 6 HLA-matched donor pairs ($P = .23$), and ABO incompatibility was almost a significant risk factor for GF in a multivariate analysis (RR, 1.36; $P = .06$). Cell dose was also a risk factor for GF, with risk of 10% in patients with a cell dose below 2.5×10^8 nucleated cells/kg compared with 5% in patients who received a higher cells dose. Patients with a CD34+ cell dose below 3×10^6/kg had an incidence of GF of 12%, which was significantly higher than the 1%–7% risk seen in patients who received a higher cell dose. Graft-versus-host disease (GVHD) prophylaxis with cyclosporine A (CsA) and methotrexate (MTX) were associated with a GF rate of 3%, which was lower than that of all other GVHD prophylaxis regimens ($P < .001$). In a multivariate analysis, there was a tendency for increased risk of GF using CsA and prednisolone (RR, 2.43; $P = .05$), and the risk was markedly increased using an ex vivo T-depleted graft (RR, 8.92; $P < .001$).

In a large and comprehensive retrospective analysis through the Center for Blood and Marrow Transplantation[21] in patients who received a MAC only including 23,272 allo-HSCTs between 1995 and 2008, GF was reported in 1278 patients (5.5%). This analysis looked into patient, disease, and transplant-related factors with relation to GF. Patient-related factors included younger age (<30 years) (odds ratio [OR] = 0.75; $P < .001$), female to male gender mismatch (OR = 1.28; $P = .001$), and Karnofsky/Lansky score < 90% (OR = 1.18; $P = .042$) as associated with increased risk. Disease-related factors included the diseases CLL (OR = 1.57; $P = .003$) and

chronic myeloid leukemia (CML) (OR = 1.88; $P < .001$) in comparison to acute myeloid leukemia (AML). In myelodysplastic syndrome (MDS) and myeloproliferative disorder (MPD) the risk for GF was dependent on the presence of absence of splenomegaly (MDS: OR = 2.34, $P = .002$; MPD: OR = 3.92, $P = .001$), whereas after splenectomy, patients with MDS and MPD did not have an increased risk for GF. In AML, acute lymphoblastic leukemia, and CML, the incidence of GF was higher in patients with advanced disease (OR = 1.54; $P < .001$). Transplant-related factors included busulfan/cyclophosphamide (Bu/Cy) as associated with increased risk for GF compared with total-body irradiation (TBI) and Cy (TBI/Cy) (OR = 1.35; $P = .002$). Well MUDs were associated with GF when compared with matched related donors (OR = 1.38; $P < .001$), and the highest risk for GF was seen in mismatched donors (OR = 1.79; $P < .001$). Major ABO mismatch was also associated with increased risk for GF (OR = 1.24; $P = .012$) as well as BM graft compared with PBSC (7.3% vs. 2.5%, $P < .001$). Total nucleated cell dose $\leq 2.4 \times 10^8$/kg was associated with GF (OR = 1.39; $P < .001$). Irrespective of graft source, cryopreservation was associated with GF (OR = 1.43; $P = .013$). GVHD prophylaxis with tacrolimus and MTX was associated with lower risk for GF (OR = 0.61; $P < .001$) in comparison to CsA/MTX. Interestingly ex vivo and in vivo T-cell depletion of the graft was not associated with increased risk of PGF, suggesting that the intensity of the conditioning regimen probably has a role in overcoming the immune-medicated GR. The findings of this large analysis are summarized in Table 23.1.

TABLE 23.1

Multivariate Risk Model for GF in a Cohort of Patients Who Underwent MAC Allo-HCT and Reported to the CIBMT Between 1995 and 2008[21]

Variable	N	OR	Lower	Upper	P Value
Recipient age (years)					<0.001
<30 years	9440	1			
≥30 years	13,815	0.75	0.65	0.86	<0.001
Donor/recipient gender match					<0.001
Other	18,166	1			
Female/male	4976	1.28	1.1	1.49	0.001
Unknown	113	1.39	0.64	2.99	0.406
Karnofsky/Lansky score (%)					0.005
≥90	16,431	1			
<90	5634	1.18	1.01	1.38	0.042
Unknown	1190	0.69	0.49	0.96	0.03

TABLE 23.1

Multivariate Risk Model for GF in a Cohort of Patients Who Underwent MAC Allo-HCT and Reported to the CIBMT Between 1995 and 2008[21] —cont'd

Variable		N	OR	Lower	Upper	P Value
Disease						<0.001
	AML	8296	1			
	ALL	5758	1.12	0.9	1.39	0.299
	CLL	843	1.57	1.17	2.1	0.003
	CML	5771	1.88	1.57	2.25	<0.001
	MDS	2126	1.38	1.07	1.79	0.013
	MPD	461	1.81	0.97	3.39	0.062
Disease status: AML/ALL/CML						<0.001
	Early	10,203	1			
	Intermediate	5534	0.98	0.84	1.15	0.816
	Advanced	3746	1.54	1.25	1.89	<0.001
	Unknown	342	0.85	0.52	1.4	0.533
Spleen status: MPD						<0.001
	Normal	181	1			
	Splenectomy	91	1.68	0.58	4.87	0.341
	Splenomegaly	161	3.92	1.79	8.55	0.001
	Unknown	28	0.82	0.1	6.76	0.854
Spleen status: MDS						0.007
	Normal	1671	1			
	Splenectomy	89	1.68	0.77	3.65	0.193
	Splenomegaly	174	2.34	1.36	4.03	0.002
	Unknown	192	1.5	0.84	2.66	0.167
Conditioning regimen						0.018
	TBI Cy and other	11,905	1			
	Bu Cy and other	7778	1.35	1.11	1.65	0.002
	Bu and other	1400	1.19	0.87	1.62	0.285
	Melphalan and other	166	1.27	0.6	2.66	0.533
	TBI and other	1418	1.3	0.98	1.73	0.069
	Unknown dosage	588	1.6	0.98	2.61	0.06
HLA match status						<0.001
	Related					
	• HLA identical sibling	10,059	1			
	Unrelated					
	• Well matched	7439	1.38	1.15	1.64	<0.001
	• Partially matched	3686	1.29	1.05	1.6	0.018
	• Mismatched	1829	1.79	1.41	2.27	<0.001
	• Unknown	242	1.79	1.09	2.94	0.021

Continued

TABLE 23.1
Multivariate Risk Model for GF in a Cohort of Patients Who Underwent MAC Allo-HCT and Reported to the CIBMT Between 1995 and 2008[21] — cont'd

Variable	N	OR	Lower	Upper	P Value
ABO incompatibilities					0.01
Matched	10,821	1			
Major	5584	1.24	1.05	1.46	0.012
Minor	4327	1.04	0.85	1.27	0.693
Unknown	2523	1.35	1.07	1.71	0.013
Graft type					<0.001
Splenomegaly	161	3.92	1.79	8.55	0.001
Unknown	28	0.82	0.1	6.76	0.854
Spleen status: MDS					0.007
Normal	1671	1			
Splenectomy	89	1.68	0.77	3.65	0.193
Splenomegaly	174	2.34	1.36	4.03	0.002
Unknown	192	1.5	0.84	2.66	0.167
Conditioning regimen					0.018
TBI Cy and other	11,905	1			
Bu Cy and other	7778	1.35	1.11	1.65	0.002
Bu and other	1400	1.19	0.87	1.62	0.285
Melphalan and other	166	1.27	0.6	2.66	0.533
TBI and other	1418	1.3	0.98	1.73	0.069
Unknown dosage	588	1.6	0.98	2.61	0.06
HLA match status					<0.001
Related					
• HLA identical sibling	10,059	1			
Unrelated					
• Well matched	7439	1.38	1.15	1.64	<0.001
• Partially matched	3686	1.29	1.05	1.6	0.018
• Mismatched	1829	1.79	1.41	2.27	<0.001
• Unknown	242	1.79	1.09	2.94	0.021
ABO incompatibilities					0.01
Matched	10,821	1			
Major	5584	1.24	1.05	1.46	0.012
Minor	4327	1.04	0.85	1.27	0.693
Unknown	2523	1.35	1.07	1.71	0.013
Graft type					<0.001

AML, acute myeloid leukemia; *Bu*, busulfan; *CML*, chronic myeloid leukemia; *CLL*, chronic lymphocytic leukemia; *Cy*, cyclophosphamide; *GF*, graft failure; *HLA*, human leukocyte antibody; *MPD*, myeloproliferative disorder; *OR*, odds ratio; *TBI*, total-body irradiation.

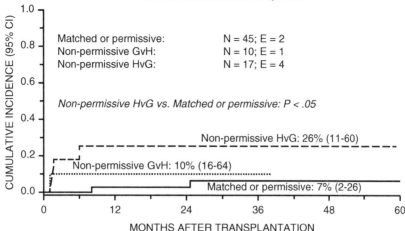

FIG. 23.1 The probability of graft rejection based on HLA-DPB1 match status.[25] Patients and donors were classified as follows: (1) matched for HLA-DPB1 or with a permissive mismatch (solid line; n=45); (2) matched for HLA-DPB1 with nonpermissive DPB1 mismatches in HvG direction (broken line; n=17); (3) matched for HLA-DPB1 with nonpermissive DPB1 mismatches in GvH direction (dotted line; n=10).*CI,* confidence interval; *HLA,* human leukocyte antibody; *HvG,* host-versus-graft.

This analysis highlights various factors associated with risk of GF, some modifiable and some not.

The diseases that were associated with higher risk for GF where diseases that usually require chemotherapy of low- or moderate-intensity pretransplant such as CLL and CML. The association between GF and MPD has been well recognized[22–24] and is probably multifactorial and includes a very distorted and fibrosed BM stroma, as well as splenomegaly and potentially allogenic immunization after multiple transfusions. The use of pretransplant treatment with JAK inhibitors may reduce the risk for GF due to its effects on splenomegaly and need for transfusions before allo-HSCT.

The conditioning regimen given before the infusion of the stem cells has to be tailored to the purpose of the BM transplantation. However, it always needs to be immunosuppressive and "space creating" to allow the donor cells to engraft. The numbers of functional T lymphocytes remaining in the host and present in the graft have reciprocal effects on GR (host-versus-graft) and GVHD. The higher incidence of GF in younger patients as reported by Olsson et al.[21] is likely reflecting a more robust immunity in children and young adult recipients than that in older patient population.

HLA compatibility between donor and recipient is of major importance of predicting GF. Olsson's

analysis highlights that having a transplant from an unrelated donor, even if well matched, was associated with increased risk for GF. When assessing for HLA-matched donor, match for HLA-A, HLA-B, HLA-C, and HLA-DRB1 (8/8 match) is mostly being done or at times also including HLA-DQ (10/10 HLA match). With that, more than 80% of well-matched donors are mismatched at DPB1. Fleischhauer et al.[25] reported on transplant outcomes in pediatric population who underwent allo-HSCT for thalassemia, where 10% (7 patients) of the study population had GF. None of the 7 patients were matched for both HLA-DPB1 alleles; 2 patients had permissive DPB1 mismatches, and 5 patients had nonpermissive HLA-DPB1 mismatched donors. The overall cumulative incidence of rejection in this group was 19% (95% confidence interval [CI], 9–43). Interestingly, in four of these cases, the mismatch was in host-versus-graft (HvG) direction, resulting in a significantly higher cumulative incidence of rejection in the HvG group (26%; 95% CI, 11–60) than that in the GvH group (10%; 95% CI, 2–64) (Fig. 23.1).

The impact of donor-specific antibodies (DSAs) on outcomes after transplantation has been extensively described in solid organ transplantation where HLA matching is not as important as that in allo-HSCT.[26] The presence of DSAs was described as a cause for GF

TABLE 23.2
Summary of Studies Reporting on the Incidence of DSA and Its Effect of GF Allo-HSCT

Reference	Patients (n)	Stem Cell Source	Conditioning	Anti-HLA %	DSA %	Graft Failure With/ Without DSA
Spellman et al.[5]	115	Mismatched unrelated	RIC	ND	9	24 versus 1%
Ciurea et al.[6]	592	10/10 and 9/10 unrelated	MAC or RIC	19.6	1.4	37.5 versus 2.7%
Yoshihara et al.[74]	79	Haploidentical	RIC	20.2	14	27 versus 3%
Ciurea et al.[6]	24	Haploidentical	RIC	ND	21	60 versus 5%
Chang et al.[75]	345	Haploidentical	MAC	25.2	11.3	61% (MFI > 10,000) versus 3.2%
Ciurea et al.[6]	122	Haploidentical	Nonspecified	ND	18	32 versus 4%
Takanashi et al.[28]	386	Single CBU	MAC	23.1	5	83 versus 32%
Cutler et al.[34]	73	Double CBU	MAC or RIC	ND	24	57 versus 5.5%
Ruggeri et al.[30]	294	Single and double CBU	RIC	23	5	81 versus 44%
Yamamoto et al.[76]	175	Single CBU	MAC or RIC	39.4	ND	50% if anti–HLA-C, DP, DQ, DRB1/2/3 versus 16%

Allo-HSCT, allogeneic hematopoietic stem cell transplantation; *DSA*, donor-specific antibody; *GF*, graft failure; *HLA*, human leukocyte antibody; *MAC*, myeloablative conditioning; *MFI*, median level of fluorescence intensity; *RIC*, reduced intensity conditioning; *ND*, not detected; *CBU*, cord blood unit.

in animal models of allo-HSCT. In a case control study, Spellman et al.[5] compared the presence of DSA among 37 patients who had primary GF to 78 controls, all received transplant from an unrelated donor. Among the patients with GF, 9 patients (24%) had DSA, of which 3 had it against class I HLA only, 4 against class II HLA only, and 2 against class I and II. In the control group, there was only 1 case of presence of DSA (against class I and II). This study found that the presence of DSA in the host against class I, II, or both before transplantation is significantly associated with GF. With the increased use of mismatched grafts, whether using a haploidentical donor, mis-MUD, or CBT, data are emerging on the importance of DSA as a risk factor for GF. Table 23.2 summarizes the incidence of presence of anti-HLA antibody and DSA and association with GF among several cohort of CBT and haploidentical transplants.[27]

In retrospective studies, the incidence of anti-HLA antibodies in CBT recipients varies from 15% to 41%,[28-32] and they are more commonly encountered in parous female patients. However, only a minority of patients with anti-HLA antibodies have DSAs with specificity against the CB graft(s). The incidence of preformed DSAs in single CBT is estimated as 5.2%–6.4%[28,30]

and 3.8%–24.7% in double CBT.[29,30,33] Ruggeri et al.[30] reported on the presence of DSA in 294 recipients of cord blood RIC transplant. Sixty-two patients (21%) had anti-HLA antibodies, and 14 were positive against the cord blood unit (DSA+). The cumulative incidence of engraftment was 77% in DSA-negative and 44% for DSA-positive patients (P = .003). The median level of fluorescence intensity (MFI) was 3900, and the intensity of the DSA measured by MFI was associated with graft failure. Of the 14 patients with DSA, 6 were engrafted and their median MFI was 2474 (1226–3650), whereas the median MFI among the 8 who were not engrafted was 7750 (2032–19,969). Cutler et al. reported similar findings in a cohort of 73 patients who underwent double CBT using an RIC or MAC conditioning regimen.[34] In contrast to what is mentioned previously, two other large centers have shown no discernible effect of anti-HLA antibodies or DSAs against one or both units on engraftment, unit dominance, or clinical outcomes after dCBT, with no MFI threshold effect.[29,32] These conflicting findings may be explained by differences in transplantation practices between centers including conditioning regimens and immunosuppression, including the use of in vivo T-cell depletion. In support of this hypothesis, a recent study suggested that the presence of DSAs correlates with the presence of cytotoxic T lymphocytes with specificity against the same HLA antigens as the DSAs that might mediate GR.[35] How to best incorporate the information about the presence and intensity of DSAs in the CB graft selection process requires further studies.

In haploidentical allo-HSCT with posttransplant cyclophosphamide (PTCy), Ciurea et al.[36] found that GF occurred in 75% of recipients with DSA compared with 5% of recipients without DSA and that antibodies to HLA-DRB1 were most frequent. Also in haplo-BMT with PTCy, Gladstone et al.[37] found that HLA-directed DSA occurred in 14.5% of all patients and 42% of women undergoing haplotransplant evaluation. DSA can be quantified by the solid phase immunoassay (SPI) using fluorescent beads coated with single phenotype and single-HLA antigens. SPI results can be correlated with cross-matching by flow cytometry or complement-dependent cytotoxicity assays and can be used as a "virtual crossmatch.[38] In subsequent analyses from Ciurea and colleagues[39] the overall incidence of DSA in haplo-BMT assessments was 18%; 32% of patients with DSA rejected their grafts. Median DSA MFI was 10,055 for patients who rejected versus 2065 for those who engrafted. In their study, graft failure was associated with a complement assay that detects C1q-binding DSA, with only one C1q-negative patient (who had an MFI of 6265) failing to engraft. Patients with C1q-binding DSA also had a higher median MFI of 15,279 versus 2471 for C1q-negative patients. All male patients were C1q-negative, and their median MFI levels were much lower. Pregnancy was associated with a much higher risk of developing DSA than transfusion of blood products. In an algorithm suggested by McCurdyn and Fuchs,[40] it is recommended to avoid donors to which the recipient has antidonor HLA antibodies, particularly for levels compatible with a positive complement-dependent cytotoxicity or flow cytometric crossmatch.

POOR GRAFT FUNCTION

PGF is a very different entity from GR, and it is characterized by evidence of donor engraftment, but with poor peripheral blood counts.[41] PGF occurs in 5%–27% of patients undergoing allo-HSCT,[42] and the severe form is associated with high morbidity and mortality due to infectious and hemorrhagic complications.[43] A number of factors are associated with PGF: (1) inadequate stem cell dose due to poor harvest/collection; (2) stem cell damage during ex vivo manipulation or storage; (3) mismatched donor; (4) GVHD[44]; (5) infections or medications used to treat an infection or noninfectious medications; and (6) use of a T-cell–depleted graft.[45]

PGF can be primary with suboptimal recovery of blood counts after the initial HSCT or secondary with decreasing blood counts after successful and prompt hematopoietic engraftment. PGF can be a transient event secondary to a reversible insult, such as an acute infection/sepsis or drugs, and blood counts can recover after removal of the insult. However, persistence of low blood counts requires further intervention, either in the form of a second transplant or infusion of more stem cells without further preinfusion conditioning therapy.

Tamari et al.[46] presented the outcomes of 182 patients who underwent ex vivo T-cell–depleted transplant (TCD) between 1997 and 2012 and reported a cumulative incidence of PGF of 18% at 1 year after transplantation (Fig. 23.2). Infections and antiviral therapies were the most common etiologies for PGF (87%), followed by GVHD, medications related, and unknown etiology in one case. It is important to note that although infections and antiviral therapies were the most common etiologies for PGF, treating the infection did not always result in improvement in graft function. At the time of analysis, 36% of patients who were diagnosed with PGF died from either infectious complications or GVHD, 33% patients had recovery of blood counts either after treatment of an identified offending agent (mostly viral infection) or discontinuation of medications, 15% had counts recovery after further cellular treatment (a TCD stem cell boost), 10% had persistent PGF, and in 6%, there was evidence of relapsed disease.

CLONAL HEMATOPIESIS AND GRAFT FAILURE

Clonal hematopoiesis (CH) resulting from an expansion of cells that harbor an initiating driver mutation has been recently shown to be an aspect of the aging hematopoietic system. There are limited data about CH among allo-HSCT donors and its impact on transplant outcomes. The risk of donor cell leukemia (DCL) has been reported in about 0.1% of allo-HSCT, and Gondek et al.[47] recently reported on two cases of DCL and demonstrated that it evolved from CH in the donor cells. Gibson et al.[48] studied a group of patients with unexplained cytopenia after allo-HSCT in the absence of evidence of disease relapse. They identified 89 patients (16%) of their transplant cohort, in whom a small group (6 patients, 7%) had "unexplained" cytopenia. Five of the six patients were found to have mutation in DNMT3A, which was confirmed to be of

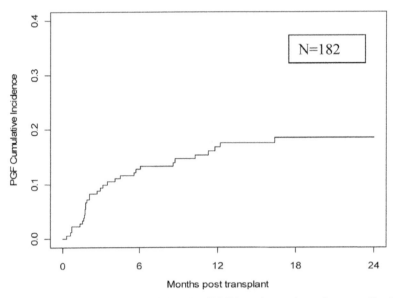

FIG. 23.2 Cumulative incidence of poor graft function (PGF) in patients who underwent a T-cell–depleted transplant.[46]

donor origin. In contrast, 24 of 84 patients (29%) with "explained" cytopenia after transplantation underwent next-generation sequencing as part of their evaluation, which was negative in all cases. It is important to note, however, that donor age was significantly higher in the group with "unexplained" cytopenia (median age 55 vs. 30 years, $P < .0001$). This observation requires validation in a larger cohort of patients-donor paired samples; however, this may suggest that donor screening for CH is important, particularly donors older than 50 years.

TREATMENT

Graft Rejection

After GR, a second stem cell transplant represents the best chance of long-term, disease-free survival for these patients. Achieving stable engraftment in patients who undergo a second transplant after GR is often difficult with engraftment rates as low as 33% reported in the literature.[49] Schreiber et al.[4] reported on a cohort of 122 patients who underwent a second allo-HSCT for GF and reported dismal outcomes with OS of only 11% at 1 year after second allo-HSCT. The engraftment rate at day 28 and 100 after second allo-HSCT was 66% and 74%, respectively. The most common causes of death were directly related to BM failure, such is infection and

bleeding. Interestingly, even among the patients who have engrafted, the OS was dismal, 19%, highlighting the general poor prognosis of this patient population. The key to success when planning a second transplant after GR is deep elimination of residual host immunity. Other considerations that need to be taken into account when planning a second transplant is the toxicity associated with the conditioning regimen because the second transplant is usually performed in proximity to the first transplant. Therefore, a strong immune ablative regimen which has a low-toxicity profile is needed. Chewning et al.[50] reported on 16 patients who underwent second allo-HSCT at a median of 45 days after GF secondary to GR. All patients, other than one (15 out of 16) had fludarabine-containing regimen: (1) fludarabine/anti thymocyte globulin (ATG) (N = 1), (2) fludarabine/Cy (N = 2), (3) fludarabine/Cy/ATG (N = 7), (4) fludarabine/thiotepa/ATG (N = 3), and (5) fludarabine/Thiotepa/CAMPATH (N = 2). One patient had a regimen of Cy/thiotepa/campath. The second transplant was unmodified in 8 patients, and a TCD graft was used in the rest of the patients. After the second transplant, all 16 patients engrafted in a median time of 12 days (range: 9–21 days). The OS at 3 years after second transplant was 35%. The median survival time was 44 days for the remaining patients (N = 10); 6 patients died within 100 days after second allo-HSCT, mostly from infectious causes. This small retrospective study demonstrated that all patients were able to achieve engraftment and that the cytoreduction was relatively well tolerated with no acute organ failure from toxicity, including no cases of veno-occlusive disease or grade III–IV mucositis. The authors concluded that fludarabine-based regimen including thiotepa or cyclophosphamide along with ATG, followed by a TCD PBSC transplant containing higher numbers of progenitor cells from a different donor, resulted in consistent engraftment.

Second allo-HSCT after GF is a medical emergency, and the goal is to proceed with identifying a graft source as early as possible to minimize the time of severe cytopenias. However, careful attention should be given to factors that can be modified to ensure engraftment of the second transplant. Ideally, a perfect HLA-matched donor to whom the patient does not have DSA should be picked for the second allo-HSCT, but if the patient has high DSA, intervention to reduce the DSA titer can be applied before second allo-HSCT. Gladstone et al.[37,51] found that plasmapheresis combined with anticytomegalovirus intravenous immunoglobulin, tacrolimus, and mycophenolate mofetil (MMF) starting 1–2 weeks before conditioning, depending on the level of DSA, was associated with a 64.4% mean reduction in DSA levels. Fifteen patients received this treatment, and the 14 patients who achieved DSA reduction to negative or weak levels underwent transplantation and were engrafted. Ciurea et al.[39] proposed an alternative desensitization method of plasma exchange, rituximab, and intravenous immunoglobulin, which they found to be only partially effective. However, combining the aforementioned regimen with the infusion of donor HLA antigens via a buffy coat 24 h before stem cell transplant was highly effective. They also reported that clearing of DSA may be unnecessary, with reduction to noncomplement binding levels sufficient to achieve engraftment.

POOR GRAFT FUNCTION
Stem Cell Boost From Original Donor
The best course of treatment for PGF is not well defined. Hematopoietic growth factors, namely granulocyte colony-stimulator factor, granulocyte-macrophage colony-stimulating factor, erythropoietin, or thrombopoietin receptor agonists have been used but often with less than optimal response.[52,53] The administration of additional hematopoietic stem cells after prior conditioning (second allo-HSCT) has had limited success secondary to toxicity of the conditioning regimen and high rates of grade III–IV GVHD.[54] An alternative approach is to administer additional donor-derived stem cells,

unmanipulated or TCD, without additional conditioning (stem cell boost). The use of unmanipulated donor stem cell boost, however, is associated with a high incidence of acute and chronic GVHD and poor survival rates.[55] A boost of TCD stem cells after conventional or TCD allo-HSCT has been more successful mainly related to the low incidence of GVHD.[56–58] An important study that demonstrated the benefit of a TCD boost for PGF compared patients treated with either a TCD boost, an unmanipulated stem cell boost, or supportive care alone. Trilineage recovery was more common, and nonrelapse mortality was lower in those receiving donor stem cells after TCD boost (CD34+ selection) compared with the other two groups. In addition, the incidence of GVHD was significantly lower in the TCD group than in the conventional boost arm[41,43] (Fig. 23.3).

Mesenchymal Stromal Cells
BM stromal cells such as mesenchymal stromal cells (MSCs) elaborate cytokines that nurture or stimulate the marrow microenvironment by several mechanisms.[59–61] MSCs can act as pericytes, wrapping around the endothelial cells of capillaries and venules, and secrete bioactive products that contribute to tissue regeneration.[62,63] MSCs could also be selectively immune-suppressive and could affect the production of inhibitory cytokines.[64,65] Hence it is possible that administration of MSCs in the setting of incomplete or delayed engraftment can modulate the milieu of the BM microenvironment, through both direct interaction with hematopoietic stem cells and through secretion of cytokines, to improve blood counts after transplantation.[66–68]

MSCs have inherently low immunogenicity, are poor targets for cytotoxic T cells and NK cells, do not activate allo-reactive T cells in vitro, and do not elicit allogeneic or xenogeneic immunologic response when transplanted. They have uniformly been determined to be safe and tolerable.[69] MSCs given at the time of HCT have been shown to improve engraftment, as well as have immunomodulatory effects in murine stem cell transplantation models.[70,71] MSCs can be found within multiple sites, including adipose tissue and BM.[72,73] The advantage of MSC over stem cell from original donor is that they can be used as "of-the-shelf" product without the need for a second mobilization process from a donor who may or may not be available for a second donation. Also, the lack of alloreactivity associated with MSC is another important advantage. However, further clinical studies are needed to assess the best source of MSC as well as doses and schedule of administration to ensure sustained engraftment.

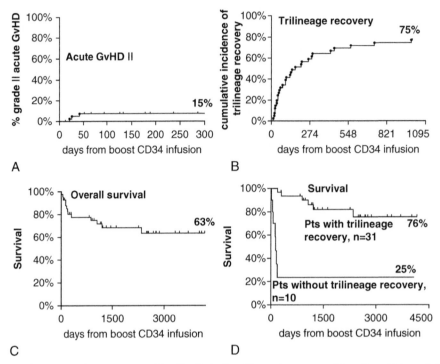

FIG. 23.3 Outcomes after treatment with a T-cell–depleted boost for poor graft function. (A) Cumulative incidence of acute GVHD. (B) Trilineage recovery. (C) Overall survival. (D) Comparison of survival based on counts recovery after TCD boost.[41] *GVHD*, Graft-versus-host disease; *TCD*, T-cell–depleted transplant.

APPROACH

In the case of lack of engraftment (primary graft failure) or loss of blood counts after initial engraftment occurred (secondary graft failure), the first and most important question to be addressed is the underlying mechanism, that is, whether there is rejection of the graft or PGF, as the nature of the required intervention is different between the two. When dealing with GR, a second transplant should be arranged as soon as possible particularly if MAC regimen was used for the initial transplant because the likelihood of autologous stem cell recovery is extremely low. If RIC or NMA conditioning regimens were used for the primary transplant, there is a chance of autologous stem cell recovery; however, that may give rise to the primary disease for which the transplant was done. When planning for a second transplant, attention needs to be given to further suppress the host immunity to prevent rejection of the second allo-graft. In the event that other factors have been identified as contributing to the GR, such as high DSA, host-donor mismatched, low cell dose, and so forth, they should be addressed if possible.

When dealing with PGF, attention should be given to all potential factors that may be affecting graft function including host nutritional status (i.e., B12/folic acid deficiencies), presence of enlarged spleen, medications that can be myelosuppressive (i.e., MMF, valacyclovir, and so forth), as well as infections that can be affecting stem cell recovery after allo-HSCT. If all identified reversible causes have been addressed without improvement in blood counts, a T-cell–depleted boost should be considered.

REFERENCES

1. Storb R, Thomas ED, Weiden PL, et al. A plastic anemia treated by allogeneic bone marrow transplantation: a report on 49 new cases from Seattle. *Blood.* 1976;48(6):817–841.
2. Johnson FL, Hartmann JR, Thomas ED, et al. Marrow transplantation in treatment of children with aplastic anaemia or acute leukaemia. *Arch Dis Child.* 1976;51(6): 403–410.
3. Remberger M, Mattsson J, Olsson R, Ringden O. Second allogeneic hematopoietic stem cell transplantation: a treatment for graft failure. *Clin Transplant.* 2011;25(1): E68–E76.
4. Schriber J, Agovi MA, Ho V, et al. Second unrelated donor hematopoietic cell transplantation for primary graft failure. *Biol Blood Marrow Transplant.* 2010;16(8): 1099–1106.

5. Spellman S, Bray R, Rosen-Bronson S, et al. The detection of donor-directed, HLA-specific alloantibodies in recipients of unrelated hematopoietic cell transplantation is predictive of graft failure. *Blood.* 2010;115(13):2704–2708.

6. Ciurea SO, Thall PF, Wang X, et al. Donor-specific anti-HLA Abs and graft failure in matched unrelated donor hematopoietic stem cell transplantation. *Blood.* 2011;118(22):5957–5964.

7. Donohue J, Homge M, Kernan NA. Characterization of cells emerging at the time of graft failure after bone marrow transplantation from an unrelated marrow donor. *Blood.* 1993;82(3):1023–1029.

8. Marijt WA, Kernan NA, Diaz-Barrientos T, et al. Multiple minor histocompatibility antigen-specific cytotoxic T lymphocyte clones can be generated during GR after HLA-identical bone marrow transplantation. *Bone Marrow Transplant.* 1995;16(1):125–132.

9. Cudkowicz G, Bennett M. Peculiar immunobiology of bone marrow allografts. II. Rejection of parental grafts by resistant F 1 hybrid mice. *J Exp Med.* 1971;134(6):1513–1528.

10. Murphy WJ, Kumar V, Bennett M. Acute rejection of murine bone marrow allografts by natural killer cells and T cells. Differences in kinetics and target antigens recognized. *J Exp Med.* 1987;166(5):1499–1509.

11. Kiessling R, Hochman PS, Haller O, Shearer GM, Wigzell H, Cudkowicz G. Evidence for a similar or common mechanism for natural killer cell activity and resistance to hemopoietic grafts. *Eur J Immunol.* 1977;7(9):655–663.

12. Raff RF, Deeg HJ, Loughran Jr TP, et al. Characterization of host cells involved in resistance to marrow grafts in dogs transplanted from unrelated DLA-nonidentical donors. *Blood.* 1986;68(4):861–868.

13. Raff RF, Sandmaier BM, Graham T, Loughran Jr TP, Pettinger M, Storb R. 'Resistance' to unrelated, DLA-nonidentical canine marrow grafts is unrestricted by the major histocompatibility complex. *Exp Hematol.* 1994;22(9):893–897.

14. Barge AJ, Johnson G, Witherspoon R, Torok-Storb B. Antibody-mediated marrow failure after allogeneic bone marrow transplantation. *Blood.* 1989;74(5):1477–1480.

15. Moeller E. Contact-induced cytotoxicity by lymphoid cells containing foreign isoantigens. *Science.* 1965;147(3660):873–879.

16. Storb R, Floersheim GL, Weiden PL, et al. Effect of prior blood transfusions on marrow grafts: abrogation of sensitization by procarbazine and antithymocyte serum. *J Immunol.* 1974;112(4):1508–1516.

17. Taylor PA, Ehrhardt MJ, Roforth MM, et al. Preformed antibody, not primed T cells, is the initial and major barrier to bone marrow engraftment in allosensitized recipients. *Blood.* 2007;109(3):1307–1315.

18. Warren RP, Storb R, Weiden PL, Su PJ, Thomas ED. Lymphocyte-mediated cytotoxicity and antibody-dependent cell-mediated cytotoxicity in patients with aplastic anemia: distinguishing transfusion-induced sensitization from possible immune-mediated aplastic anemia. *Transplant Proc.* 1981;13(1 Pt 1):245–247.

19. Nordlander A, Mattsson J, Sundberg B, Sumitran-Holgersson S. Novel antibodies to the donor stem cell population CD34+/VEGFR-2+ are associated with rejection after hematopoietic stem cell transplantation. *Transplantation.* 2008;86(5):686–696.

20. Olsson R, Remberger M, Schaffer M, et al. Graft failure in the modern era of allogeneic hematopoietic SCT. *Bone Marrow Transplant.* 2013;48(4):537–543.

21. Olsson RF, Logan BR, Chaudhury S, et al. Primary graft failure after myeloablative allogeneic hematopoietic cell transplantation for hematologic malignancies. *Leukemia.* 2015;29(8):1754–1762.

22. Abelsson J, Merup M, Birgegard G, et al. The outcome of allo-HSCT for 92 patients with myelofibrosis in the Nordic countries. *Bone Marrow Transplant.* 2012;47(3):380–386.

23. Ballen KK, Woolfrey AE, Zhu X, et al. Allogeneic hematopoietic cell transplantation for advanced polycythemia vera and essential thrombocythemia. *Biol Blood Marrow Transplant.* 2012;18(9):1446–1454.

24. Alchalby H, Yunus DR, Zabelina T, Ayuk F, Kroger N. Incidence and risk factors of poor graft function after allogeneic stem cell transplantation for myelofibrosis. *Bone Marrow Transplant.* 2016;51(9):1223–1227.

25. Fleischhauer K, Locatelli F, Zecca M, et al. GR after unrelated donor hematopoietic stem cell transplantation for thalassemia is associated with nonpermissive HLA-DPB1 disparity in host-versus-graft direction. *Blood.* 2006;107(7):2984–2992.

26. Patel AM, Pancoska C, Mulgaonkar S, Weng FL. Renal transplantation in patients with pre-transplant donor-specific antibodies and negative flow cytometry cross-matches. *Am J Transplant.* 2007;7(10):2371–2377.

27. Morin-Zorman S, Loiseau P, Taupin JL, Caillat-Zucman S. Donor-specific anti-HLA antibodies in allogeneic hematopoietic stem cell transplantation. *Front Immunol.* 2016;7:307.

28. Takanashi M, Atsuta Y, Fujiwara K, et al. The impact of anti-HLA antibodies on unrelated cord blood transplantations. *Blood.* 2010;116(15):2839–2846.

29. Brunstein CG, Noreen H, DeFor TE, Maurer D, Miller JS, Wagner JE. Anti-HLA antibodies in double umbilical cord blood transplantation. *Biol Blood Marrow Transplant.* 2011;17(11):1704–1708.

30. Ruggeri A, Rocha V, Masson E, et al. Impact of donor-specific anti-HLA antibodies on graft failure and survival after reduced intensity conditioning-unrelated cord blood transplantation: a Eurocord, Societe Francophone d'Histocompatibilite et d'Immunogenetique (SFHI) and Societe Francaise de Greffe de Moelle et de Therapie Cellulaire (SFGM-TC) analysis. *Haematologica.* 2013;98(7):1154–1160.

31. Takanashi M, Fujiwara K, Tanaka H, Satake M, Nakajima K. The impact of HLA antibodies on engraftment of unrelated cord blood transplants. *Transfusion.* 2008;48(4):791–793.

32. Dahi PB, Barone J, Devlin SM, et al. Sustained donor engraftment in recipients of double-unit cord blood transplantation is possible despite donor-specific human leukocyte antigen antibodies. *Biol Blood Marrow Transplant.* 2014;20(5):735–739.

33. Dahi PB, Ponce DM, Devlin S, et al. Donor-recipient allele-level HLA matching of unrelated cord blood units reveals high degrees of mismatch and alters graft selection. *Bone Marrow Transplant.* 2014;49(9):1184–1186.

34. Cutler C, Kim HT, Sun L, et al. Donor-specific anti-HLA antibodies predict outcome in double umbilical cord blood transplantation. *Blood.* 2011;118(25):6691–6697.

35. Hanajiri R, Murata M, Sugimoto K, et al. Integration of humoral and cellular HLA-specific immune responses in cord blood alloGR. *Bone Marrow Transplant.* 2015;50(9):1187–1194.

36. Ciurea SO, de Lima M, Cano P, et al. High risk of graft failure in patients with anti-HLA antibodies undergoing haploidentical stem-cell transplantation. *Transplantation.* 2009;88(8):1019–1024.

37. Gladstone DE, Zachary AA, Fuchs EJ, et al. Partially mismatched transplantation and human leukocyte antigen donor-specific antibodies. *Biol Blood Marrow Transplant.* 2013;19(4):647–652.

38. Zachary AA, Sholander JT, Houp JA, Leffell MS. Using real data for a virtual crossmatch. *Hum Immunol.* 2009;70(8):574–579.

39. Ciurea SO, Thall PF, Milton DR, et al. Complement-binding donor-specific anti-HLA antibodies and risk of primary graft failure in hematopoietic stem cell transplantation. *Biol Blood Marrow Transplant.* 2015;21(8):1392–1398.

40. McCurdy SR, Fuchs EJ. Selecting the best haploidentical donor. *Semin Hematol.* 2016;53(4):246–251.

41. Stasia A, Ghiso A, Galaverna F, et al. CD34 selected cells for the treatment of poor graft function after allogeneic stem cell transplantation. *Biol Blood Marrow Transplant.* 2014;20(9):1440–1443.

42. Dominietto A, Raiola AM, van Lint MT, et al. Factors influencing haematological recovery after allogeneic haemopoietic stem cell transplants: graft-versus-host disease, donor type, cytomegalovirus infections and cell dose. *Br J Haematol.* 2001;112(1):219–227.

43. Larocca A, Piaggio G, Podesta M, et al. Boost of CD34+-selected peripheral blood cells without further conditioning in patients with poor graft function following allogeneic stem cell transplantation. *Haematologica.* 2006;91(7):935–940.

44. Wolff SN. Second hematopoietic stem cell transplantation for the treatment of graft failure, GR or relapse after allogeneic transplantation. *Bone Marrow Transplant.* 2002;29(7):545–552.

45. Ash RC, Horowitz MM, Gale RP, et al. Bone marrow transplantation from related donors other than HLA-identical siblings: effect of T cell depletion. *Bone Marrow Transplant.* 1991;7(6):443–452.

46. Roni Tamari SR, Kuk D, Sauter CS, et al. *Poor Graft Function in Recipients of T Cell Depleted (TCD) Allogeneic Hematopoietic Stem Cell Transplants (HSCT) Is Mostly Related to Viral Infections and Anti-viral Therapy;* 2012.

47. Gondek LP, Zheng G, Ghiaur G, et al. Donor cell leukemia arising from clonal hematopoiesis after bone marrow transplantation. *Leukemia.* 2016;30(9):1916–1920.

48. Gibson CJ, Kennedy JA, Nikiforow S, et al. Donor-engrafted CHIP is common among stem cell transplant recipients with unexplained cytopenias. *Blood.* 2017;130(1):91–94.

49. Davies SM, Weisdorf DJ, Haake RJ, et al. Second infusion of bone marrow for treatment of graft failure after allogeneic bone marrow transplantation. *Bone Marrow Transplant.* 1994;14(1):73–77.

50. Chewning JH, Castro-Malaspina H, Jakubowski A, et al. Fludarabine-based conditioning secures engraftment of second hematopoietic stem cell allografts (HSCT) in the treatment of initial graft failure. *Biol Blood Marrow Transplant.* 2007;13(11):1313–1323.

51. Leffell MS, Jones RJ, Gladstone DE. Donor HLA-specific Abs: to BMT or not to BMT? *Bone Marrow Transplant.* 2015;50(6):751–758.

52. Vannucchi AM, Bosi A, Linari S, et al. High doses of recombinant human erythropoietin fail to accelerate platelet reconstitution in allogeneic bone marrow transplantation. Results of a pilot study. *Haematologica.* 1997;82(1):53–56.

53. Dyba J, Tinmouth A, Bredeson C, Matthews J, Allan DS. Eltrombopag after allogeneic haematopoietic cell transplantation in a case of poor graft function and systematic review of the literature. *Transfus Med.* 2016;26(3):202–207.

54. Guardiola P, Kuentz M, Garban F, et al. Second early allogeneic stem cell transplantations for graft failure in acute leukaemia, chronic myeloid leukaemia and aplastic anaemia. French Society of Bone Marrow Transplantation. *Br J Haematol.* 2000;111(1):292–302.

55. Remberger M, Ringden O, Ljungman P, et al. Booster marrow or blood cells for graft failure after allogeneic bone marrow transplantation. *Bone Marrow Transplant.* 1998;22(1):73–78.

56. Milone G, Tornello A, Leotta S, et al. CD34+ selected haematopoietic stem cell (HSC) not preceded by any immunosuppressive therapy as effective treatment for graft failure. *Bone Marrow Transplant.* 2005;35(5):521–522; author reply 522.

57. Mainardi C, Ebinger M, Enkel S, et al. CD34(+) selected stem cell boosts can improve poor graft function after paediatric allogeneic stem cell transplantation. *Br J Haematol.* 2018;180(1):90–99.

58. Klyuchnikov E, El-Cheikh J, Sputtek A, et al. CD34(+)-selected stem cell boost without further conditioning for poor graft function after allogeneic stem cell transplantation in patients with hematological malignancies. *Biol Blood Marrow Transplant.* 2014;20(3):382–386.

59. in 't Anker PS, Noort WA, Kruisselbrink AB, et al. Nonexpanded primary lung and bone marrow-derived mesenchymal cells promote the engraftment of umbilical cord blood-derived CD34(+) cells in NOD/SCID mice. *Exp Hematol.* 2003;31(10):881–889.

60. Noort WA, Kruisselbrink AB, in't Anker PS, et al. Mesenchymal stem cells promote engraftment of human umbilical cord blood-derived CD34(+) cells in NOD/SCID mice. *Exp Hematol.* 2002;30(8):870–878.

61. Metheny L, Eid SK, Lingas K, et al. Intra-osseous Cotransplantation of CD34-selected umbilical cord blood and mesenchymal stromal cells. *Hematol Med Oncol.* 2016;1(1):41–45.

62. da Silva Meirelles L, Caplan AI, Nardi NB. In search of the in vivo identity of mesenchymal stem cells. *Stem Cells.* 2008;26(9):2287–2299.

63. Crisan M, Yap S, Casteilla L, et al. A perivascular origin for mesenchymal stem cells in multiple human organs. *Cell Stem Cell.* 2008;3(3):301–313.

64. Caplan AI. Adult mesenchymal stem cells: when, where, and how. *Stem Cells Int.* 2015;2015:628767.

65. Ringden O. Mesenchymal stromal cells as first-line treatment of graft failure after hematopoietic stem cell transplantation. *Stem Cells Dev.* 2009;18(9):1243–1246.

66. Lazarus HM, Koc ON, Devine SM, et al. Cotransplantation of HLA-identical sibling culture-expanded mesenchymal stem cells and hematopoietic stem cells in hematologic malignancy patients. *Biol Blood Marrow Transplant.* 2005;11(5):389–398.

67. Koc ON, Gerson SL, Cooper BW, et al. Rapid hematopoietic recovery after coinfusion of autologous-blood stem cells and culture-expanded marrow mesenchymal stem cells in advanced breast cancer patients receiving high-dose chemotherapy. *J Clin Oncol.* 2000;18(2):307–316.

68. Fouillard L, Bensidhoum M, Bories D, et al. Engraftment of allogeneic mesenchymal stem cells in the bone marrow of a patient with severe idiopathic aplastic anemia improves stroma. *Leukemia.* 2003;17(2):474–476.

69. Chen X, Wang C, Yin J, Xu J, Wei J, Zhang Y. Efficacy of mesenchymal stem cell therapy for steroid-refractory acute graft-versus-host disease following allogeneic hematopoietic stem cell transplantation: a systematic review and meta-analysis. *PLoS One.* 2015;10(8):e0136991.

70. Carrancio S, Romo C, Ramos T, et al. Effects of MSC coadministration and route of delivery on cord blood hematopoietic stem cell engraftment. *Cell Transplant.* 2013;22(7):1171–1183.

71. Li ZY, Wang CQ, Lu G, Pan XY, Xu KL. Effects of bone marrow mesenchymal stem cells on hematopoietic recovery and acute graft-versus-host disease in murine allogeneic umbilical cord blood transplantation model. *Cell Biochem Biophys.* 2014;70(1):115–122.

72. Pontikoglou C, Deschaseaux F, Sensebe L, Papadaki HA. Bone marrow mesenchymal stem cells: biological properties and their role in hematopoiesis and hematopoietic stem cell transplantation. *Stem Cell Rev.* 2011;7(3):569–589.

73. Minteer D, Marra KG, Rubin JP. Adipose-derived mesenchymal stem cells: biology and potential applications. *Adv Biochem Eng Biotechnol.* 2013;129:59–71.

74. Yoshihara S, Maruya E, Taniguchi K, et al. Risk and prevention of graft failure in patients with preexisting donor-specific HLA antibodies undergoing unmanipulated haploidentical SCT. *Bone Marrow Transplant.* 2012;47(4):508–515.

75. Chang YJ, Zhao XY, Xu LP, et al. Donor-specific anti-human leukocyte antigen antibodies were associated with primary graft failure after unmanipulated haploidentical blood and marrow transplantation: a prospective study with randomly assigned training and validation sets. *J Hematol Oncol.* 2015;8:84.

76. Yamamoto H, Uchida N, Matsuno N, et al. Anti-HLA antibodies other than against HLA-A, -B, -DRB1 adversely affect engraftment and nonrelapse mortality in HLA-mismatched single cord blood transplantation: possible implications of unrecognized donor-specific antibodies. *Biol Blood Marrow Transplant.* 2014;20(10):1634–1640.

CHAPTER 24

Miscellaneous Complications Related to Hematopoietic Cell Transplantation

MUHAMMAD A. SAIF, MBBS, MRCP, FRCPATH, MD •
FIONA L. DIGNAN, MBCHB, FRCP, FRCPATH, MD

VENOOCCLUSIVE DISEASE (SINUSOIDAL OBSTRUCTION SYNDROME)

Hepatic venoocclusive disease (VOD) is caused by the conditioning administered before stem cell transplant and can be a serious and life-threatening complication. The condition is also known as sinusoidal obstruction syndrome (SOS), but in this chapter the initials VOD will be used. VOD is characterized by damage to the sinusoidal epithelial cells and hepatocytes in zone 3 of the hepatic acinus due to toxic metabolites from the conditioning regimen.[1] It typically presents in the first 3 weeks after stem cell infusion, but there are occasional reports of late-onset VOD. There are also reports of VOD occurring after chemotherapy alone or after monoclonal antibody therapy.[2] The incidence of VOD varies depending on the type of conditioning used and is estimated to be around 10%–15% after myeloablative conditioning and <5% after reduced-intensity allogeneic or autologous transplant in adults.[3–5] Severe VOD is associated with a high mortality rate of >80%.[6] The reported incidence is higher in children than in adults.[7]

A number of risk factors have been reported for VOD which have been reviewed previously.[8,9] These include transplant-related factors including myeloablative conditioning especially with high-dose TBI or oral or high-dose busulfan, unrelated donor transplants, and receipt of a second transplant. Patient factors are also important including preexisting hepatic disease, underlying diagnosis, age, and genetic factors. The concurrent use of hepatic toxic drugs or prior use of gemtuzumab ozogamicin or inotuzumab can also increase the risk of VOD occurring.

The diagnosis is primarily based on clinical grounds. Historically there have been two sets of diagnostic criteria that have tried to incorporate the classical clinical features of tender hepatomegaly, weight gain, and raised bilirubin. These include the Seattle criteria that were first reported in 1984 and include a triad of raised bilirubin, weight gain, and painful hepatomegaly within 20 days of transplant. Two out of three clinical features were required to make the diagnosis. There have been various minor modifications to these criteria over time.[10] The Baltimore criteria are similar requiring an elevated bilirubin >2 mg/dL within 21 days of transplant and two further criteria out of hepatomegaly and ascites.[11] More recently, the European society for Blood and Marrow transplantation has published revised diagnostic and severity criteria for VOD in adults and pediatrics. In adults, late-onset VOD is included occurring >21 days after transplant. Late-onset VOD includes patients with classical features or proven histology or two criteria out of bilirubin >2 mg/dL, painful hepatomegaly, weight gain or ascites on ultrasound, or measurement of hepatic venous pressure gradient.[8] In children the EBMT criteria include two or more clinical features of weight gain, hepatomegaly, ascites, refractory thrombocytopenia, or rapidly rising bilirubin at any time point after transplant.[12]

Although the key to diagnosis remains the presence of classical clinical features, additional diagnostic tests may be helpful in some patients. Ultrasound can be helpful to exclude other conditions and also to assess for the presence of hepatomegaly, ascites, and portal venous flow reversal. Liver biopsy can be difficult in patients with thrombocytopenia but may be helpful to exclude other causes.[9] Pathological features may include endothelial damage to small hepatic vein and sinusoidal endothelium, hepatocytic and sinusoidal fibrin, and small hepatic vein periadventitial factor VIII.[13]

The severity of VOD is also largely based on clinical features. Bearman originally associated a rapid gain in weight and rise in bilirubin with an increased likelihood of developing severe VOD.[14] The European society for Blood and Marrow transplantation has recently published revised severity criteria for adults which can be assigned prospectively and include bilirubin level, renal function, transaminases, weight increase, bilirubin level and kinetics, and time since symptom onset.[8] Similar criteria have also been developed for children.[12]

Prevention of VOD includes identification of preexisting risk factors and modification of these factors where possible. Various agents have been used in the prophylaxis of VOD, including antithrombin,[15] pentoxifylline,[16] heparin,[17] and prostaglandin E1,[14] but the evidence does not support their use. Ursodeoxycholic acid may be beneficial as a prophylactic agent although there are conflicting data from clinical studies. There are some data to suggest that defibrotide may have a role in prophylaxis in selected patients, but this agent is not currently approved for prophylactic use.[18]

Treatment of VOD includes careful fluid balance, use of diuretic therapy, and early involvement of critical care and hepatology. Defibrotide has antiischemic, antithrombotic, and antiinflammatory properties, and a number of recent clinical trials have shown efficacy of defibrotide in the management of VOD.[7,19] This agent is now approved for use in the United States and European Union.

Other agents have been investigated for use in VOD, including N-acetylcysteine[20] and tissue plasminogen activator,[21] but have not been found to be beneficial. There is limited evidence to suggest that methylprednisolone may occasionally be helpful.[22,23]

TRANSPLANT-ASSOCIATED THROMBOTIC MICROANGIOPATHY

Transplant-associated thrombotic microangiopathy (TA-TMA) is a distinct clinical entity, but it shares several features with other microangiopathies such as thrombotic thrombocytopenic purpura (TTP) and hemolytic uremic syndrome (HUS). Incidence of TA-TMA is variable and reported to be between 0.5% and 70% in different case series. This condition carries very high mortality (up to 75% in some studies).[24] A number of factors such as TBI, older age, graft-versus-host disease, unrelated donors, calcineurin inhibitors, sirolimus, haploidentical transplant, and use of busulfan are significant risk factors for development of TA-TMA. The pathophysiology of TA-TMA involves endothelial damage, activation of platelets and the complement system, and the release of proinflammatory cytokines. Dysfunctional activation of coagulation leads to fibrin stranding of microvasculature creating mechanical barriers to flow of cells. Other abnormalities include fibrinoid necrosis and inflammation of endothelial microvasculature.[25-28] These result in clinical manifestations such as nonimmune red cell hemolysis, thrombocytopenia, and organ dysfunction (renal failure, neurological involvement, etc.).[29] According to Blood and

Marrow Transplant Clinical Trials Network toxicity committee guidance,[30] TA-TMA is defined by following four features: (1) red blood cell fragmentation and ≥2 schistocytes per high-power field on peripheral smear, (2) concurrent increased serum Lactate dehydrogenase (LDH) above institutional baseline, (3) concurrent renal (doubling of serum creatinine from baseline or 50% decrease in creatinine clearance from baseline) and/or neurologic dysfunction without other explanations, and (4) negative direct and indirect Coombs test results.

Unlike TTP and HUS, thrombocytopenia is a less reliable diagnostic criteria in TA-TMA as many of these patients may have preexisting low platelet count. International working group criteria, however, include progressive thrombocytopenia (platelet count less than 5×10^9/L or a 50% or greater decrease in platelet number compared to baseline) within diagnostic criteria. It also incorporates serum haptoglobin concentration and defines hemolysis by 4 or more fragments per high-power field.[31] ADAMTS13 is not useful as its levels can be normal in TA-TMA.

Calcineurin inhibitors should be stopped if TA-TMA is suspected. Depending on the stage of transplantation, it may be necessary to substitute calcineurin inhibitor with an alternative agent such as corticosteroids or mycophenolate mofetil.

Plasma exchange has been used in treatment of TA-TMA. However, despite some patients experiencing initial improvement with plasma exchange, the outcome is very poor. Long-term mortality is reported to be around 70%–100%.[32-34] Complement-blocking therapy using eculizumab appears promising with reported survival of up to 60%.[35-39] However, one retrospective analysis involving 39 patients reported that despite good initial response, long-term survival was dismal, predominantly due to infection-related mortality (70%).[39a] Unlike HUS and Paroxysmal nocturnal hemoglobinurea (PNH), long-term treatment with eculizumab therapy may not be required as many patients achieve sustained response even after cessation of treatment. There is no consensus on optimum dose and duration of treatment, but monitoring of complement inhibition by CH50 assay may be helpful.[35] In our practice, when starting this therapy, we use initial treatment protocol similar to atypical HUS and reassess after 4 and 8 doses. We consider dose modification based on response.

RESPIRATORY COMPLICATIONS
Idiopathic Pneumonia Syndrome
Idiopathic pneumonia syndrome (IPS) usually occurs early after HSCT often within the first 3 months. The

condition is characterized by a restrictive pattern of pulmonary function tests, but clinical and chest radiograph features can be nonspecific and difficult to differentiate from pulmonary infection.[40] IPS rarely progresses to respiratory failure and has been associated with TBI, GVHD, older age, and pretransplant chemotherapy. Occasionally, patients develop late-onset restrictive defects of pulmonary function which may progress to respiratory failure. A small subset of patients develop diffuse alveolar hemorrhage which is a rare condition characterized by pulmonary infiltrates, hypoxia, and blood-stained broncho-alveolar lavage. It has been associated with older age, acute graft-versus-host disease, receipt of allogeneic transplant, and myeloablative conditioning. Treatment is with high-dose corticosteroids, but the condition is associated with a high mortality.[41] Periengraftment respiratory distress syndrome is sometimes included in IPS classification, but it has distinct manifestations characterized by progressive shortness of breath, hypoxia, cough, and signs of capillary leak including fluid retention and edema. Usually it presents within 5 days of neutrophil engraftment. This condition generally responds to diuresis and high-dose steroids. Reported mortality with this condition is up to 20%.

Cryptogenic Organizing Pneumonia

Cryptogenic organizing pneumonia (COP) was previously recognized as bronchiolitis obliterans organizing pneumonia and is a rare respiratory complication in allogeneic HSCT recipients. The condition tends to occur at a median of 100 days after HSCT with an incidence of 1%–10%.[42,43] It is characterized by fever, dyspnea, and dry cough. Pulmonary function tests typically show a restrictive pattern, and chest radiograph typically shows nodular opacities, patchy consolidation, and ground glass change.[40] The definitive diagnosis relies on a lung biopsy which shows granulation tissue within the lumen of alveolar ducts and alveoli. The condition is frequently associated with GVHD, and first-line treatment often includes corticosteroids.[40]

Bronchiolitis Obliterans

Bronchiolitis obliterans usually occurs in the setting of pulmonary GVHD, and the management of this condition is covered in Chapter 10.

Secondary Solid Cancers

Hematopoietic stem cell transplant recipients are at increased risk of secondary malignancies including posttransplant lymphoproliferative disorders, solid cancers, leukemia, and myelodysplasia. The increased risk of solid cancers appears to extend for many years after HSCT, and the incidence does not seem to reach a plateau even in studies with follow-up to 20 years. Compared to the general population, the risk of developing oral, skin, thyroid, esophagus, liver, nervous system, connective tissue, and bone cancers is all increased.[44,45]

Oral Cancer

Oropharyngeal cancer is the most common secondary solid cancer, with recipients of HSCT having a 7- to 16-fold higher risk than the general population.[44–47] Chronic GVHD requiring immunosuppression, male gender, and irradiation have been associated with an increased risk. Recommendations include education of patients about the increased risk of oral malignancy and the importance of regular review by a dentist or oral medicine specialist at least annually. Patients with chronic oral GVHD may benefit from more frequent review.[48]

Skin Cancer

Skin cancers can be divided into three types including squamous cell carcinoma, basal cell carcinoma, and malignant melanoma, and the incidence of all three subtypes is increased in recipients of HSCT.[41,49] Additional risk factors may include the use of voriconazole, chronic GVHD, younger age at the time of transplant, and total-body irradiation. Recommendations include patient education about early signs of skin cancer and risk of sun exposure and early investigation of suspicious skin lesions.[48]

Other Cancers

HSCT recipients are at higher risk of a number of other solid tumors than the general population, and patient awareness of the signs of secondary solid tumors may be beneficial. In cancers for which screening is available, e.g., cervical and breast cancer, patients should be encouraged to participate in national screening programmes. A full review of recommendations for clinical practice has recently been published by combined working party of the European Group for Blood and Marrow Transplantation and the Centre for International Blood and Marrow Transplant research.[48]

ENDOCRINE AND METABOLIC COMPLICATIONS

Thyroid Complications

Thyroid dysfunction is the most common endocrinopathy seen after HSCT. Thyroid dysfunction including subclinical or compensated hypothyroidism is seen in nearly half of the long-term survivors of allogeneic HSCT.[50-52] Thyroid complications can occur at any stage after transplantation. The incidence of thyroid abnormalities appears to be higher in recipients of allogeneic HSCT and those receiving total-body irradiation (TBI)–based conditioning regimens (particularly unfractionated TBI). Prior radiotherapy to neck as a part of treatment of lymphoma also increases the risk. Thyroid dysfunction mostly presents as hypothyroidism, hyperthyroidism, thyroiditis (including autoimmune thyroiditis), and thyroid neoplasia.[53,54]

It is important to distinguish functional thyroid abnormality from euthyroid sick syndrome (ESS) which is relatively common within the first 3 months of HSCT. ESS is characterized by transient low T3, with low or normal TSH (which may be elevated) and increased reverse T3 levels in the absence of prior hypothalamic-pituitary and thyroid gland dysfunction. T4 is usually normal but may be low in severe cases.[55,56] This condition reflects a higher conversion of T3 and T4 into metabolically inactive reverse T3 and does not point toward dysregulation of thyroid pituitary axis. This condition can be confused with primary hypothyroidism in which there is persistent low free T3 and T4 associated with high TSH and normal reverse T3. Suppression of free T3/T4 and TSH indicates secondary hypothyroidism due to underactive pituitary gland. Hyperthyroidism is diagnosed when there is a high level of T3/T4 with suppressed TSH. ESS is associated with poor transplant outcome.[57] It has been hypothesized that ESS is a surrogate marker for general endocrine dysfunction and poor health. While ESS does not require treatment, functional hypothyroidism is treated with thyroid replacement therapy. The recommended starting dose of Levothyroxine ranges from 50 to 200 mcg per day (consider dose escalation while monitoring thyroid function every 4–6 weeks). Older patients require lower doses, and consultation with an endocrinologist is advised. Hyperthyroidism could be treated with antithyroid drugs (e.g., propylthiouracil or carbimazole), surgery (sub-total thyroidectomy), or radioactive iodine. Antithyroid medication can result in agranulocytosis, and hence monitoring of blood counts is required.

Diabetes Mellitus

Posttransplant diabetes mellitus (PTDM) and impaired glucose tolerance are relatively common complications after HSCT, with an incidence of up to 30%.[58] They can occur immediately after HSCT, mostly due to the use of immunosuppressive therapy such as corticosteroid and sirolimus or late after HSCT due to altered body homeostasis and persistence of inflammation.[59] Recipients of TBI are at a high risk of developing PTDM. Regular glucose monitoring is mandatory in patients receiving high dose of steroids. In patients with hyperglycemia, sliding scale insulin can be used to control very high levels of glucose. However, basal bolus insulin may be more effective. Patients with persistently high blood glucose need referral to an endocrinologist to commence regular hypoglycemics or a regular insulin regimen. This may require close monitoring as the requirement for therapy may alter particularly if the patient is on variable dose corticosteroid therapy.[60,61]

Long-term survivors of HSCT require life-long monitoring for early detection of PTDM. The diagnostic criteria for PTDM is same as those for type 2 diabetes mellitus; a fasting plasma glucose of 126 mg/dL (7 mmol/L), random plasma glucose 200 mg/dL (11.1 mmol/L), 2-hour plasma glucose after oral glucose tolerance test of 200 mg/dL (11.1 mmol/L), or HbA1c 6.5% or more would indicate PTDM.[62] Life style advice, risk factor modification, and dietary advice should be a part of comprehensive management plan for these patients.[63]

ADRENAL COMPLICATIONS

Primary hypoadrenalism is rare after allogeneic HSCT, whereas secondary hypoadrenalism caused by exogenous steroid therapy is relatively common. Duration and length of treatment predict suppression of adrenal gland secretion. While 2- to 3-week treatment with lower doses of steroid may result in clinically significant adrenal suppression, a very high dose of steroid could result in hypoadrenalism within 3 days of treatment. Baseline serum cortisol is not always helpful, and all patients suspected of hypoadrenalism should have ACTH stimulation test (short synacthen test). This test involves administration of synacthen and measurement of cortisol levels at base line and 30 min after administration of synacthen. Ongoing steroid therapy can interfere with these results, and hence discussion with an endocrinologist is recommended while interpreting results in patients on steroids. A tapering regimen of systemic steroids in patients who had prolonged course of steroids is recommended to avoid Addisonian crisis or clinically significant hypoadrenalism.

Osteoporosis and Bone Complications

Dysregulation of bone metabolism is a common complication of HSCT. Osteopenia is seen in about half of the patients after HSCT while the incidence of osteoporosis is nearly 20%. Time to development of osteopenia and osteoporosis is variable, ranging from a few weeks to over a decade. Most patients present at around 1 year after HSCT.[64-66] High age at HSCT, female gender, and use of steroids are risk factors for developing metabolic bone disorder. After HSCT, dysregulation of hormones such as estrogen and testosterone, altered calcium levels, and secondary hyperparathyroidism lead to development of osteoporosis.[67,68] Loss of bone mineral density (BMD) is known to increase the risk of bone fracture. This risk doubles with a decline in BMD of 10%–15% leading to a significant compromise in the quality of life.[69] While dual-energy X-ray absorptiometry (DEXA) scan remains one of the most widely used tools for evaluation of metabolic bone disease in many centers, other modalities such as dual photon absorptiometry (DPA), quantitative computed tomography, and magnetic resonance imaging could also be used to assess BMD.

It is recommended that all patients should have a regular DEXA scan starting at around 1 year after allogeneic HSCT (or earlier if prior bone disease or high risk of developing osteoporosis). Depending on DEXA scan, patients' results are compared to either young healthy adults (T-score) or age- and sex-matched population (Z-score). According to WHO criteria, a T-score within one standard deviation (SD) is considered normal, result between 1 and 2.5 SD indicates osteopenia, and any result above 2.5 SD is considered as established oeteoporosis.[70] All patients on long-term steroids should receive calcium, vitamin D supplements, and bisphosphonate therapy (e.g., alendronic acid).

Patients with osteopenia could be managed with calcium and vitamin D supplements alone. Established osteoporosis requires bisphosphonate therapy in addition to calcium and vitamin D supplements. While on bisphosphonate, patients should be monitored for signs of osteonecrosis even though the incidence of osteonecrosis in this context seems to be very low. If hypogonadism is found to be the cause of osteoporosis, hormone replacement therapy should be considered. Other treatment options include denosumab (monoclonal antibody against nuclear kappa B ligand), raloxifene (second-generation selective estrogen receptor modulator), and teriparatide (Recombinant human parathyroid hormone).[71,72]

Gonadal Dysfunction

Hypogonadism can have significant impact on the quality of life of patients after allogeneic HSCT. Common symptoms of hypogonadism in men include tiredness, reduced or loss of libido, erectile dysfunction, gynecomastia, and infertility/subfertility. This can be caused by either primary testicular failure or dysfunction of hypothalamic-pituitary axis. Evaluation of gonadal dysfunction in men includes testing of testosterone, luteinizing hormone (LH), and follicle-stimulating hormone (FSH) levels. A suppression of all three hormones points toward a disorder of hypothalamic-pituitary axis, whereas low testosterone in the presence of raised LH and FSH indicates primary testicular failure. Androgen replacement may improve symptoms, but careful assessment of the risks should be undertaken before commencing this treatment. Androgen therapy in men can lead to prostate hypertrophy, prostate carcinoma, liver dysfunction, and fluid retention. Monitoring of prostate-specific antigen, regular liver function test, and lipid profile is recommended in patients on androgen therapy. For patients with erectile dysfunction, careful assessment should be made of psychosocial issues.[73]

In women, common presentation of hypogonadism is infertility and symptoms similar to menopausal state.[54] LH, FSH, estrogen, and prolactin are needed for evaluation. In case of loss of libido, testosterone should also be tested. Depression of all hormones indicates hypothalamic/pituitary axis dysfunction. Primary ovarian failure will cause a rise in FSH levels and low estrogen. Raised prolactin with suppression of FSH and estrogen may indicate prolactin-secreting tumor. Indications for hormone replacement therapy (after careful consideration and discussion on risks of treatment) include symptoms of hypogonadism and prevention of metabolic bone disease leading to loss of BMD.

Fertility

Discussion on loss of fertility, an issue in young patients, is an important issue in pretransplant clinic. Although some conditioning regimens may not render a patient infertile, the use of TBI (especially myeloablative dose) and chemotherapeutic agents such as cyclophosphamide, ifosfamide, melphalan, and busufan are likely to lead to infertility. Dose of chemotherapeutic agents, age, prior treatment, and pretransplant subfertility are important predictors for posttransplant infertility.

Many patients with malignant disorders would have received prior chemotherapy and should have fertility preservation options discussed before their initial treatment. The options for fertility preservation include sperm cryopreservation in men (naturally or by sperm extraction) and embryo cryopreservation (if a partner is available), oocyte cryopreservation after ovarian stimulation, and ovarian tissue cryopreservation in females.

RENAL COMPLICATIONS

Acute kidney injury (AKI) is a common complication after HSCT. There is no clear consensus on the definition of AKI, and several definitions and classifications of AKI are currently in use. Commonly used criteria include those proposed by acute kidney injury network, Kidney Disease Improving Global Outcomes (KDIGO), and RIFLE (Risk, Injury, Failure, Loss of kidney function, and End-stage kidney disease) criteria.[74–77] After HSCT, AKI can be caused by direct conditioning toxicity (including radiation nephritis), nephrotoxic medication, sepsis, tumor lysis syndrome, ABO incompatibility, and dehydration (due to excessive fluid loss).[78–80] Renal failure in association with TMA and SOS is covered in separate sections. National kidney foundation defines chronic kidney disease (CKD) as persistent renal impairment for 3 or more months. Five stages of CKD are described based on Estimated glomerular filtration rate (eGFR). Stage 1 involves kidney damage with eGFR above 90 mL/min per 1.73 m^2, and stage 2, 3, 4, and 5 are defined by declining eGFR with 60–89, 30–59, 15–29, and less than 15 mL/min per 1.73 m^2, respectively.[81] Cumulative incidence of CKD is reported to be up to 60% in adult population. Preexisting AKI, TMA, long-term immunosuppression with calcineurin inhibitor (CNI), and GVHD increase the risk of CKD. In some cases, chronic renal failure can present with nephrotic syndrome. The majority of cases of nephrotic syndrome in the context of HSCT are either membranous nephropathy or minimal change disease.[82,83] There is association of this presentation with GVHD. Systemic steroids and CNI may be helpful in these cases.

HEMORRHAGIC CYSTITIS

Hemorrhagic cystitis (HC) is a common complication of HSCT described in up to 40%–50% of patients within first year of allogeneic HSCT.[84] HC after HSCT may be due to a number of different etiologies. Irrespective of the cause of HC, its grading is based on clinical features. Commonly used grading criteria are described by the National Cancer Institute. According to toxicity criteria, grade 1 toxicity is defined as microscopic hematuria with minimal symptoms of cystitis (urgency, frequency, and nocturia). Grade 2 toxicity involves macroscopic hematuria with moderate symptoms, often requiring urinary catheterization or bladder irrigation. This has impact on activities of daily living. Grade 3 is a more severe form with gross hematuria with clots in which case transfusion may be required. Radiological and endoscopic interventions are usually needed to control this grade of HC. Grade 4 hematuria is life-threatening bleed with hemodynamic compromise, requiring urgent surgical or radiological intervention.

Timing of HC after HSCT may depend on the etiology. Usually, early-onset HC (occurring within 48 hours of HSCT) is caused by direct toxicity of conditioning. The most common cause for HC is cyclophosphamide. Inflammation of bladder mucosa after cyclophosphamide infusion is due to acrolein which is a breakdown product of cyclophosphamide. Severity of HC is dependent on the dose of cyclophosphamide. Several factors increase the risk of HC including pelvic radiotherapy, type of conditioning (increased incidence in haploidentical transplant), ifosfamide use, etc. Late-onset HC can occur any time after 48 hours and is usually caused by viruses such as polyoma viruses (JC and BK virus) and adenovirus. A proportion of 90% of adult population is exposed to Polyoma virus during early life and hence in a vast majority of patients HC is caused by reactivation of this virus. Disabling hematuria could be delayed by several months after HSCT. High level of polyoma virus in blood is associated with increased incidence of viral HC.[85,86] Risk factors for developing late HC include male gender, older age, use of busulfan, myeloablative conditioning, GVHD, haploidentical transplantation, and unrelated donor.[87–89]

A detailed clinical assessment and relevant microbiological tests are needed to establish the cause of HC. This assessment should include mid-stream specimen of urine to rule out bacterial, fungal, and parasitic infection and relevant virology tests including PCR for BK and JC virus. Imaging may be needed if there is suspicion of hydronephrosis or other structural lesions.

Treatment depends on the severity and etiology of HC. Early-onset HC caused by cyclophosphamide may require additional doses of Mercaptoethane sulfonate (MESNA) and hydration. Late HC caused by polyoma viruses could be treated with simple hyperhydration and urinary alkalinization. Smooth muscle relaxants (oxybutynin/buscopan) can be used for symptom control. Diuretics could be used to avoid fluid overload and maintain good urine output during hyperhydration. Significant hematuria may require reduction of platelet transfusion threshold and correction of coagulopathy. Recombinant factor VIIa should be considered in serious life-threatening bleed, but the risk of thrombosis needs to be evaluated before its use. Tranexamic acid should be avoided due to risk of clot colic and hydronephrosis. Review from urology and bladder irrigation should be sought early if dealing with significant hematuria. There are reports of improvement in conditioning with the use of antibiotics such as quinolones.

Cidofovir (intravenous and intravesicular) for polyoma virus and intravenous ribavirin for adenovirus-related HC may be effective. Leflunomide, prostaglandins, sodium hyalorunate, and silver nitrate have all been used to treat HC with variable success.[90–94] Cellular therapy against polyoma virus is an effective treatment strategy,[95] but access to this treatment and cost may be prohibitive for many transplant centers.

CARDIAC COMPLICATIONS

Compared to the general population, the life time risk of developing cardiac complications is 2–4 times higher in recipients of stem cell transplantation.[96] Cumulative incidence of cardiovascular event in recipients of HSCT is reported to be around 7.5% at 15 years, increasing to 22% at 25 years. This number is lower for autologous HSCT (2.5% at 15 years).[97] This translates into increased risk of death in this patient population mainly due to acute cardiovascular events when compared to the general population.[98] Median time to development of coronary artery disease is 4–9 years. Use of anthracycline, preexisting cardiac disease risk factors, radiotherapy, and graft-versus-host disease increase the risks of coronary artery disease after HSCT.[99] Early recognition and management of cardiac risk factors in late effect survivorship clinics is recommended.

Fluid overload and congestive cardiac failure (CCF) can occur early after transplantation due to the toxicity of conditioning regimen as well as the high fluid load in the early phase of transplantation. This can be aggravated by preexisting cardiac systolic or diastolic dysfunction. Incidence of late CCF appears especially high in recipients of autologous and allogeneic HSCT.[99,100]

The risk of pericarditis after HSCT is mostly related to prior radiotherapy particularly in patients with lymphoma who had radiotherapy during the course of treatment. Pericarditis tends to manifest in constrictive form mostly associated with heart failure. Valvular abnormalities could be secondary to infective endocarditis, acute coronary event, and chronic heart disease. Cardiac arrhythmia is another serious complication of HSCT which can present early (due to toxicity of conditioning) or late due to coronary artery disease, conduction defects, cardiomyopathy, etc. Anthracycline- and etoposide-based conditioning can rarely trigger serious cardiac arrhythmias particularly if there is prior cardiovascular risk. Survivorship guidelines focusing on mitigating cardiovascular risks recommend monitoring patients to identify and address the risks of cardiovascular disease, life style modification, and early treatment and referral to cardiology if indicated.

NEUROLOGICAL COMPLICATIONS

Posterior Reversible Encephalopathy Syndrome

Posterior reversible encephalopathy syndrome (PRES) is a rare complication of HSCT mostly described in association with the use of CNIs. Clinical symptoms of this condition include headache, confusion, cognitive impairment, neurological deficit, visual disturbance, and delirium. MRI may show signal changes in frontal, temporal, and parietal lobes in addition to occipital cortex or subcortical regions. PRES is often associated with high blood pressure. Pathophysiology of this condition remains unknown. Incidence of PRES appears to be higher in patients with GVHD.[101] The overall incidence of PRES was reported to be around 1.6% in recipients of HSCT. It seems to be slightly higher in recipients of cord blood transplantation (7.1%) than in those of unrelated donor transplantation (3%–5%).[102] Optimizing blood pressure control, consideration of alternative CNI, or temporary discontinuation of CNI may lead to complete resolution of symptoms. In some patients, no recurrence of symptoms was observed despite restarting the CNI.

Progressive Multifocal Leukoencephalopathy

In the context of HSCT, progressive multifocal leukoencephalopathy (PML) is mostly associated with polyoma virus. PML is well known to be associated with the use of treatments such as fludarabine, anti-CD 20 immunotherapy (rituximab), and natalizumab.[103,104] Usual onset of PML is around 1 month or longer after allogeneic HSCT.[105] Clinical manifestations of this conditions after transplant are variable and include confusion, neurological deficit (motor and sensory), or cognitive dysfunction and encephalopathy.[106] Diagnosis requires magnetic resonance imaging (MRI) of brain and analysis of CSF. Depending on the severity of illness, the radiological finding may vary from subtle white matter changes to discrete lesions with gadolinium enhancement on MRI. Analysis of CSF (PCR for polyoma virus and neuropathic viruses) is mandatory and has high sensitivity and specificity.[107] PML has extremely poor prognosis and no effective treatment. Quick taper of immune suppression to facilitate immune reconstitution may help. Other treatments which have been used include Interleukin 2 (IL2), mefloquin, and cidofovir[104,106,108–110].

Immune-Mediated Complications of Central and Peripheral Nervous System

Polymyositis (2%–3%), acute inflammatory demyelination mimicking Guillain Barre syndrome, chronic inflammatory demyelinating polyneuropathy (1%–2%), myasthenia gravis (<1%), extrapyramidal syndrome, and peripheral neuropathy are reported in association with HSCT and seem to have a higher incidence in patients with GVHD.[111-113] Polymyositis, particularly in isolation, should be treated as GVHD with immunosuppression. Inflammatory demyelinating neuropathy requires treatment with intravenous immunoglobulins, plasma exchange, and immunosuppressive therapy such as steroids, CNI, and metabolite mycophenolate mofetil. A multidisciplinary approach involving neurologist and neurorehabilitation services is advised. Diagnosis of MG may often be difficult and requires assessment by neurologists. Antiacetylcholine receptor antibody may help in diagnosis, but it can be false positive in some HSCT recipients without a clinical diagnosis of MG. Oral cholinesterase inhibitor, immunosuppression, intravenous immunoglobulins, and plasma exchange are used for treatment of MG.[114-116]

Complications Due to CNIs

Use of CNI can lead to common neurotoxicities such as tremors (15%–20%), headache (20%), and neuropathy (about 10%). Less common complications of this treatment include altered conscious level, psychiatric disorders (e.g., mania), seizures, ataxia, PRES, TMA, psudobulbar palsy, and extrapyramidal syndrome. While dealing with these complications, based on severity of clinical presentation, alternative immunosuppression should be considered.

GASTROINTESTINAL COMPLICATIONS

Gastrointestinal complications are discussed in detail in chapter number 27.

PSYCHOLOGICAL COMPLICATIONS

Psychological complications are common after stem cell transplantation. History of psychiatric disturbance is recognized as an independent risk factor for poor outcome after SCT.[117] These disorders can manifest in several forms including depression, anxiety, psychotic illness, and features suggestive of posttraumatic stress disorder (PTSD). Younger age, female gender, presence of chronic pain, chronic GVHD, prolonged hospital/intensive care admission, and pharmacological treatment, e.g., steroids, are known to increase the risk of psychological complications.[118] In one prospective study 15% patients after SCT showed features of PTSD at least once during posttransplant recovery.[119] Depression is seen in up to 45% of patients, whereas anxiety

is seen in up to 20% patients undergoing HSCT. Coping strategies and psychotherapy could be beneficial.[120] Several classes of antidepressants are available for pharmacological treatment which have a different therapeutic and side effect profile. Choice of antidepressants in patients suffering from clinical depression should be based on "predominant symptoms of depression" such as insomnia, anorexia, etc. and any "associated symptoms or comorbidities" such as pain, obesity, etc. A careful assessment of potential side effects of treatment and drug interactions should be done before commencing new antidepressant treatment. Refractory depression will need careful clinical evaluation of patients to exclude other medical illnesses mimicking depression such as hypothyroidism and vitamin D deficiency. A combination of antidepressants can be used in difficult cases, but consultation and discussion with a psychiatrist is recommended before these strategies.

REFERENCES

1. Shulman HM, Fisher LB, Schoch HG, Henne KW, McDonald GB. Veno-occlusive disease of the liver after marrow transplantation: histological correlates of clinical signs and symptoms. *Hepatology.* 1994;19(5):1171–1181. http://www.ncbi.nlm.nih.gov/pubmed/8175139.
2. Wadleigh M, Richardson PG, Zahrieh D, et al. Prior gemtuzumab ozogamicin exposure significantly increases the risk of veno-occlusive disease in patients who undergo myeloablative allogeneic stem cell transplantation. *Blood.* 2003;102(5):1578–1582. https://doi.org/10.1182/blood-2003-01-0255.
3. Carreras E, Bertz H, Arcese W, et al. Incidence and outcome of hepatic veno-occlusive disease after blood or marrow transplantation: a prospective cohort study of the European group for blood and marrow transplantation. *Blood.* 1998;92(10):3599–3604. http://bloodjournal.hematologylibrary.org/content/92/10/3599.abstract.
4. Carreras E, Díaz-Beyá M, Rosiñol L, Martínez C, Fernández-Avilés F, Rovira M. The incidence of veno-occlusive disease following allogeneic hematopoietic stem cell transplantation has diminished and the outcome improved over the last decade. *Biol Blood Marrow Transplant.* 2011;17(11):1713–1720. https://doi.org/10.1016/j.bbmt.2011.06.006.
5. Yakushijin K, Atsuta Y, Doki N, et al. Sinusoidal obstruction syndrome after allogeneic hematopoietic stem cell transplantation: incidence, risk factors and outcomes. *Bone Marrow Transplant.* 2016;51(3):403–409. https://doi.org/10.1038/bmt.2015.283.
6. Richardson PG, Elias a D, Krishnan a, et al. Treatment of severe veno-occlusive disease with defibrotide: compassionate use results in response without significant toxicity in a high-risk population. *Blood.* 1998;92(3):737–744. doi:9680339.

7. Corbacioglu S, Carreras E, Mohty M, et al. Defibrotide for the treatment of hepatic veno-occlusive disease: final results from the international compassionate-use program. *Biol Blood Marrow Transplant.* 2016;22(10):1874–1882. https://doi.org/10.1016/j.bbmt.2016.07.001. .

8. Mohty M, Malard F, Abecassis M, et al. Revised diagnosis and severity criteria for sinusoidal obstruction syndrome/veno-occlusive disease in adult patients: a new classification from the European Society for Blood and Marrow Transplantation. *Bone Marrow Transplant.* 2016;51(7):906–912. https://doi.org/10.1038/bmt.2016.130.

9. Dignan FL, Wynn RF, Hadzic N, et al. BCSH/BSBMT guideline: diagnosis and management of veno-occlusive disease (sinusoidal obstruction syndrome) following haematopoietic stem cell transplantation. *Br J Haematol.* 2013;163(4):444–457. https://doi.org/10.1111/bjh.12558.

10. Mcdonald GB, Sharma P, Matthews DE, Shulman HM, Thomas ED. Venocclusive disease of the liver after bone marrow transplantation: diagnosis, incidence, and predisposing factors. *Hepatology.* 1984;4(1):116–122. https://doi.org/10.1002/hep.1840040121.

11. Jones RJ, Lee KS, Beschorner WE, et al. Venoocclusive disease of the liver following bone marrow transplantation. *Transplantation.* 1987;44(6):778–783.

12. Corbacioglu S, Carreras E, Ansari M, et al. Diagnosis and severity criteria for sinusoidal obstruction syndrome/veno-occlusive disease in pediatric patients: a new classification from the European society for blood and marrow transplantation. *Bone Marrow Transplant.* 2017;51(7):906–912. https://doi.org/10.1038/bmt.2017.161.

13. Shulman HM, Gown AM, Nugent DJ. Hepatic veno-occlusive disease after bone marrow transplantation. Immunohistochemical identification of the material within occluded central venules. *Am J Pathol.* 1987;127(3):549–558.

14. Bearman SI, Shen DD, Hinds MS, Hill HA, Mcdonald GB. A phase-I phase-II study of prostaglandin-E1 for the prevention of hepatic venocclusive disease after bone-marrow transplantation. *Br J Haematol.* 1993;84(4):724–730. https://doi.org/10.1111/j.1365-2141.1993.tb03152.x.

15. Haussmann U, Fischer J, Eber S, Scherer F, Seger R, Gungor T. Hepatic veno-occlusive disease in pediatric stem cell transplantation: impact of pre-emptive antithrombin III replacement and combined antithrombin III/defibrotide therapy. *Haematologica.* 2006;91(6):795–800. https://doi.org/10.3324/haematol.13619.

16. Attal M, Huguet F, Rubie H, et al. Prevention of regimen-related toxicities after bone marrow transplantation by pentoxifylline: a prospective, randomized trial. *Blood.* 1993;82(3):732–736. http://www.ncbi.nlm.nih.gov/entrez/query.fcgi?cmd=Retrieve&db=PubMed&dopt=Citation&list_uids=8338943.

17. Imran H, Tleyjeh IM, Zirakzadeh A, Rodriguez V, Khan SP. Use of prophylactic anticoagulation and the risk of hepatic veno-occlusive disease in patients undergoing hematopoietic stem cell transplantation: a systematic review and meta-analysis. *Bone Marrow Transplant.* 2005;2006(37):677–686. https://doi.org/10.1038/sj.bmt.1705297.

18. Corbacioglu S, Cesaro S, Faraci M, et al. Defibrotide for prophylaxis of hepatic veno-occlusive disease in paediatric haemopoietic stem-cell transplantation: an open-label, phase 3, randomised controlled trial. *Lancet.* 2012;379(9823):1301–1309. https://doi.org/10.1016/S0140-6736(11)61938-7.

19. Richardson PG, Riches ML, Kernan NA, et al. Phase 3 trial of defibrotide for the treatment of severe veno-occlusive disease and multi-organ failure. *Blood.* 2016;127(13):1656–1665. https://doi.org/10.1182/blood-2015-10-676924.

20. Barkholt L, Remberger M, Hassan Z, et al. A prospective randomized study using N-acetyl-L-cysteine for early liver toxicity after allogeneic hematopoietic stem cell transplantation. *Bone Marrow Transplant.* 2008;41(9):785–790. https://doi.org/10.1038/sj.bmt.1705969.

21. Bearman SI, Lee JL, Baron AE, McDonald GB. Treatment of hepatic venocclusive disease with recombinant human tissue plasminogen activator and heparin in 42 marrow transplant patients. *Blood.* 1997;89(5):1501–1506. http://www.ncbi.nlm.nih.gov/pubmed/9057629.

22. Myers KC, Lawrence J, Marsh RA, Davies SM, Jodele S. High-dose methylprednisolone for veno-occlusive disease of the liver in pediatric hematopoietic stem cell transplantation recipients. *Biol Blood Marrow Transplant.* 2013;19(3):500–503. https://doi.org/10.1016/j.bbmt.2012.11.011.

23. Al Beihany A, Al Omar H, Sahovic E, et al. Successful treatment of hepatic veno-occlusive disease after myeloablative allogeneic hematopoietic stem cell transplantation by early administration of a short course of methylprednisolone. *Bone Marrow Transplant.* 2008;41(3):287–291. https://doi.org/10.1038/sj.bmt.1705896.

24. George JN, Li X, McMinn JR, Terrell DR, Vesely SK, Selby GB. Thrombotic thrombocytopenic purpura-hemolytic uremic syndrome following allogeneic HPC transplantation: a diagnostic dilemma. *Transfusion.* 2004;44(2):294–304. https://doi.org/10.1111/j.1537-2995.2004.00700.x.

25. Rosenthal J. Hematopoietic cell transplantation-associated thrombotic microangiopathy: a review of pathophysiology, diagnosis, and treatment. *J Blood Med.* 2016;7:181–186. https://doi.org/10.2147/jbm.s102235.

26. Zeigler ZR, Shadduck RK, Nemunaitis J, Andrews DF, Rosenfeld CS. Bone marrow transplant-associated thrombotic microangiopathy: a case series. *Bone Marrow Transplant.* 1995;15(2):247–253. http://www.ncbi.nlm.nih.gov/pubmed/7773214.

27. Iacopino P, Pucci G, Arcese W, et al. Severe thrombotic microangiopathy: an infrequent complication of bone marrow transplantation. *Bone Marrow Transplant.* 1999;24(1):47–51. https://doi.org/10.1038/sj.bmt.1701830.

28. Ruutu T, Hermans J, Niederwieser D, et al. Thrombotic thrombocytopenic purpura after allogeneic stem cell transplantation: a survey of the European Group for Blood and Marrow Transplantation (EBMT). *Br J Haematol.* 2002;118(4):1112–1119. doi:3721 [pii].

29. Fuge R, Bird JM, Fraser A, et al. The clinical features, risk factors and outcome of thrombotic thrombocytopenic purpura occurring after bone marrow transplantation. *Br J Haematol.* 2001;113(1):58–64. doi:bjh2799 [pii].

30. Ho VT, Cutler C, Carter S, et al. Blood and marrow transplant clinical trials network toxicity committee consensus summary: thrombotic microangiopathy after hematopoietic stem cell transplantation. *Biol Blood Marrow Transplant.* 2005;11(8):571–575. https://doi.org/10.1016/j.bbmt.2005.06.001.

31. Ruutu T, Barosi G, Benjamin RJ, et al. Diagnostic criteria for hematopoietic stem cell transplant-associated microangiopathy: results of a consensus process by an International Working Group. *Haematologica.* 2007;92(1):95–100. https://doi.org/10.3324/haematol.10699.

32. Silva VA, Frei-Lahr D, Brown RA, Herzig GP. Plasma exchange and vincristine in the treatment of hemolytic uremic syndrome/thrombotic thrombocytopenic purpura associated with bone marrow transplantation. *J Clin Apher.* 1991;6(1):16–20. http://www.ncbi.nlm.nih.gov/pubmed/2045377.

33. Roy V, Rizvi MA, Vesely SK, George JN. Thrombotic thrombocytopenic purpura-like syndromes following bone marrow transplantation: an analysis of associated conditions and clinical outcomes. *Bone Marrow Transplant.* 2001;27(6):641–646. https://doi.org/10.1038/sj.bmt.1702849.

34. Dua A, Zeigler ZR, Shadduck RK, Nath R, Andrews DF, Agha M. Apheresis in grade 4 bone marrow transplant associated thrombotic microangiopathy: a case series. *J Clin Apher.* 1996;11(4):176–184. doi:10.1002/(SICI)1098-1101(1996)11:4<176::AID-JCA2>3.0.CO;2-8.

35. Jodele S, Fukuda T, Vinks A, et al. Eculizumab therapy in children with severe hematopoietic stem cell transplantation-associated thrombotic microangiopathy. *Biol Blood Marrow Transplant.* 2014;20(4):518–525. https://doi.org/10.1016/j.bbmt.2013.12.565.

36. Fernandez C, Lario A, Fores R, Cabrera R. Eculizumab treatment in a patient with hematopoietic stem cell transplantation-associated thrombotic microangiopathy and steroid-refractory acute graft versus host disease. *Hematol Rep.* 2015;7(4):6107. https://doi.org/10.4081/hr.2015.6107.

37. Jodele S, Dandoy CE, Myers KC, et al. New approaches in the diagnosis, pathophysiology, and treatment of pediatric hematopoietic stem cell transplantation-associated thrombotic microangiopathy. *Transfus Apher Sci.* 2016;54(2):181–190. https://doi.org/10.1016/j.transci.2016.04.007.

38. de Fontbrune FS, Galambrun C, Sirvent A, et al. Use of eculizumab in patients with allogeneic stem cell transplant-associated thrombotic microangiopathy. *Transplantation.* 2015;99(9):1953–1959. https://doi.org/10.1097/TP.0000000000000601.

39. De Latour RP, Xhaard A, Fremeaux-Bacchi V, et al. Successful use of eculizumab in a patient with post-transplant thrombotic microangiopathy. *Br J Haematol.* 2013;161(2):279–280. https://doi.org/10.1111/bjh.12202.

39a. Bohl SR, Kuchenbauer F, von Harsdorf S, et al. Thrombotic microangiopathy after allogeneic stem cell transplantation: a comparison of eculizumab therapy and conventional therapy. *Biol Blood Marrow Transplant.* 2017;23(12):2172–2177.

40. Tichelli A, Rovó A, Gratwohl A. Late pulmonary, cardiovascular, and renal complications after hematopoietic stem cell transplantation and recommended screening practices. *Hematol Am Soc Hematol Educ Program.* 2008:125–133. https://doi.org/10.1182/asheducation-2008.1.125.

41. Majhail NS, Parks K, Defor TE, Weisdorf DJ. Diffuse alveolar hemorrhage and infection-associated alveolar hemorrhage following hematopoietic stem cell transplantation: related and high-risk clinical syndromes. *Biol Blood Marrow Transplant.* 2006;12(10):1038–1046. https://doi.org/10.1016/j.bbmt.2006.06.002.

42. Yoshihara S, Yanik G, Cooke KR, Mineishi S. Bronchiolitis obliterans syndrome (BOS), bronchiolitis obliterans organizing pneumonia (BOOP), and other late-onset noninfectious pulmonary complications following allogeneic hematopoietic stem cell transplantation. *Biol Blood Marrow Transplant.* 2007;13(7):749–759. https://doi.org/10.1016/j.bbmt.2007.05.001.

43. Afessa B, Litzow MR, Tefferi A. Bronchiolitis obliterans and other late onset non-infectious pulmonary complications in hematopoietic stem cell transplantation. *Bone Marrow Transplant.* 2001;28(5):425–434. https://doi.org/10.1038/sj.bmt.1703142.

44. Majhail NS, Brazauskas R, Douglas Rizzo J, et al. Secondary solid cancers after allogeneic hematopoietic cell transplantation using busulfan-cyclophosphamide conditioning. *Blood.* 2011;117(1):316–322. https://doi.org/10.1182/blood-2010-07-294629.

45. Rizzo JD, Curtis RE, Socié G, et al. Solid cancers after allogeneic hematopoietic cell transplantation. *Blood.* 2009;113(5):1175–1183. https://doi.org/10.1182/blood-2008-05-158782.

46. Curtis RE, Rowlings PA, Deeg HJ, et al. Solid cancers after bone marrow transplantation. *N Engl J Med.* 1997;336(13):897–904. https://doi.org/10.1056/NEJM199703273361301.

47. Atsuta Y, Suzuki R, Yamashita T, et al. Continuing increased risk of oral/esophageal cancer after allogeneic hematopoietic stem cell transplantation in adults in association with chronic graft-versus-host disease. *Ann Oncol.* 2014;25(2):435–441. https://doi.org/10.1093/annonc/mdt559.

48. Inamoto Y, Shah NN, Savani BN, et al. Secondary solid cancer screening following hematopoietic cell transplantation. *Bone Marrow Transplant.* 2015;50(8):1013–1023. https://doi.org/10.1038/bmt.2015.63.

49. Baker KS, DeFor TE, Burns LJ, Ramsay NKC, Neglia JP, Robison LL. New malignancies after blood or marrow stem-cell transplantation in children and adults: incidence and risk factors. *J Clin Oncol.* 2003;21(7):1352–1358. https://doi.org/10.1200/JCO.2003.05.108.

50. Berger C, Le-Gallo B, Donadieu J, et al. Late thyroid toxicity in 153 long-term survivors of allogeneic bone marrow transplantation for acute lymphoblastic leukaemia. *Bone Marrow Transplant.* 2005;35(10):991–995. https://doi.org/10.1038/sj.bmt.1704945.

51. Al-Fiar FZ, Colwill R, Lipton JH, Fyles G, Spaner D, Messner H. Abnormal thyroid stimulating hormone (TSH) levels in adults following allogeneic bone marrow transplants. *Bone Marrow Transplant.* 1997;19(10):1019–1022. https://doi.org/10.1038/sj.bmt.1700771.

52. Borgstrom B, Bolme P. Thyroid function in children after allogeneic bone marrow transplantation. *Bone Marrow Transplant.* 1994;13(1):59–64.

53. Ishiguro H, Yasuda Y, Tomita Y, et al. Long-term follow-up of thyroid function in patients who received bone marrow transplantation during childhood and adolescence. *J Clin Endocrinol Metab.* 2004;89(February):5981–5986. https://doi.org/10.1210/jc.2004-0836.

54. Orio F, Muscogiuri G, Palomba S, et al. Endocrinopathies after allogeneic and autologous transplantation of hematopoietic stem cells. *Sci World J.* 2014;2014. https://doi.org/10.1155/2014/282147.

55. Fliers E, Bianco AC, Langouche L, Boelen A. Thyroid function in critically ill patients. *Lancet Diab Endocrinol.* 2015;3(10):816–825. https://doi.org/10.1016/S2213-8587(15)00225-9.

56. Lee S, Farwell AP. Euthyroid sick syndrome. *Compr Physiol.* 2016;6(2):1071–1080. https://doi.org/10.1002/cphy.c150017.

57. Jung YJ, Jeon YJ, Cho WK, et al. Risk factors for short term thyroid dysfunction after hematopoietic stem cell transplantation in children. *Korean J Pediatr.* 2013;56(7):301–306. https://doi.org/10.3345/kjp.2013.56.7.301.

58. Majhail NS, Challa TR, Mulrooney DA, Baker KS, Burns LJ. Hypertension and diabetes mellitus in adult and pediatric survivors of allogeneic hematopoietic cell transplantation. *Biol Blood Marrow Transplant.* 2009;15(9):1100–1107. https://doi.org/10.1016/j.bbmt.2009.05.010.

59. F S, R A, O K, et al. How do I manage hyperglycemia/post-transplant diabetes mellitus after allogeneic HSCT. *Bone Marrow Transplant.* 2016;51(8):1041–1049. https://doi.org/10.1038/bmt.2016.81.

60. Michota F. What are the disadvantages of sliding-scale insulin? *J Hosp Med.* 2007;2(suppl 1):20–22. https://doi.org/10.1002/jhm.183.

61. Umpierrez GE, Smiley D, Jacobs S, et al. Randomized study of basal-bolus insulin therapy in the inpatient management of patients with type 2 diabetes undergoing general surgery (RABBIT 2 surgery). *Diabetes Care.* 2011;34(2):256–261. https://doi.org/10.2337/dc10-1407.

62. Sharif A, Hecking M, De Vries APJ, et al. Proceedings from an international consensus meeting on posttransplantation diabetes mellitus: recommendations and future directions. *Am J Transplant.* 2014;14(9):1992–2000. https://doi.org/10.1111/ajt.12850.

63. Handelsman Y, Bloomgarden ZT, Grunberger G, et al. American association of clinical endocrinologists and american college of endocrinology - clinical practice guidelines for developing a diabetes mellitus comprehensive care plan - 2015. *Endocr Pract.* 2015;21(4):1–87. https://doi.org/10.4158/EP15672.GL.

64. Schulte C, Beelen DW, Schaefer UW, Mann K. Bone loss in long-term survivors after transplantation of hematopoietic stem cells: a prospective study. *Osteoporos Int.* 2000;11(4):344–353. https://doi.org/10.1007/s001980070124.

65. Schulte CMS, Beelen DW. Bone loss following hematopoietic stem cell transplantation: a long-term follow-up. *Blood.* 2004;103(10):3635–3643. https://doi.org/10.1182/blood-2003-09-3081.

66. Kaste SC, Shidler TJ, Tong X, et al. Bone mineral density and osteonecrosis in survivors of childhood allogeneic bone marrow transplantation. *Bone Marrow Transplant.* 2004;33(4):435–441. https://doi.org/10.1038/sj.bmt.1704360.

67. Stern JM, Chesnut 3rd CH, Bruemmer B, et al. Bone density loss during treatment of chronic GVHD. *Bone Marrow Transplant.* 1996;17(3):395–400. http://www.embase.com/search/results?subaction=viewrecord&from=export&id=L26114498%5Cnhttp://elvis.ubvu.vu.nl:9003/vulink?sid=EMBASE&issn=02683369&id=doi:&atitle=Bone+density+loss+during+treatment+of+chronic+GVHD&stitle=BONE+MARROW+TRANSPLANT.&title=Bone+.

68. Weilbaecher KN. Mechanisms of osteoporosis after hematopoietic cell transplantation. *Biol Blood Marrow Transplant.* 2000;6(2A):165–174. https://doi.org/10.1016/S1083-8791(00)70039-5.

69. Yao S, McCarthy PL, Dunford LM, et al. High prevalence of early-onset osteopenia/osteoporosis after allogeneic stem cell transplantation and improvement after bisphosphonate therapy. *Bone Marrow Transplant.* 2008;41(4):393–398. https://doi.org/10.1038/sj.bmt.1705918.

70. Kanis JA, Kanis JA. Assessment of fracture risk and its application to screening for postmenopausal osteoporosis: synopsis of a WHO report. *Osteoporos Int.* 1994;4(6):368–381. https://doi.org/10.1007/BF01622200.

71. Cranney A, Adachi JD. Benefit-risk assessment of raloxifene in postmenopausal osteoporosis. *Drug Saf.* 2005;28(8):721–730. https://doi.org/10.2165/00002018-200528080-00006.

72. Bodenner D, Redman C, Riggs A. Teriparatide in the management of osteoporosis. *Clin Interv Aging.* 2007;2(4):499–507.

73. Roziakova L, Mladosievicova B. Endocrine late effects after hematopoietic stem cell transplantation. *Oncol Res.* 2010;18(11–12):607–615. http://gateway.ovid.com/ovidweb.cgi?T=JS&CSC=Y&NEWS=N&PAGE=fulltext&D=medl&AN=20939437%5Cnhttp://sfx.nottingham.ac.uk:80/sfx_local?genre=article&atitle=Endocrine+late+effects+after+hematopoietic+stem+cell+transplantation.&title=Oncology+Research&issn=0965.

74. Englberger L, Suri RM, Li Z, et al. Clinical accuracy of RIFLE and Acute Kidney Injury Network (AKIN) criteria for acute kidney injury in patients undergoing cardiac surgery. *Crit Care.* 2011;15(1):R16. https://doi.org/10.1186/cc9960.

75. Lopes JA, Jorge S. The RIFLE and AKIN classifications for acute kidney injury: a critical and comprehensive review. *Clin Kidney J.* 2013;6(1):8–14. https://doi.org/10.1093/ckj/sfs160.

76. Kellum J a, Lameire N, Aspelin P, et al. KDIGO clinical practice guideline for acute kidney injury. *Kidney Int Suppl.* 2012;2(1):1–138. https://doi.org/10.1038/kisup.2012.7.

77. Mehta RL, Kellum JA, Shah SV, et al. Acute Kidney Injury Network: report of an initiative to improve outcomes in acute kidney injury. *Crit Care.* 2007;11(2):R31. https://doi.org/10.1186/cc5713.

78. McDonald GB, Hinds MS, Fisher LD, et al. Veno-occlusive disease of the liver and multiorgan failure after bone marrow transplantation: a cohort study of 355 patients. *Ann Intern Med.* 1993;118(4):255–267. https://doi.org/10.7326/0003-4819-118-4-199302150-00003.

79. Parikh CR, Coca SG. Acute renal failure in hematopoietic cell transplantation. *Kidney Int.* 2006;69(3):430–435. https://doi.org/10.1038/sj.ki.5000055.

80. G E, B C, T JF, et al. Acute renal failure in patients following bone marrow transplantation: prevalence, risk factors and outcome. *Am J Nephrol.* 1995;15(6):473–479. http://ovidsp.ovid.com/ovidweb.cgi?T=JS&PAGE=reference&D=emed3&NEWS=N&AN=1995315978.

81. Levey AS, Coresh J, Balk E, et al. National kidney foundation practice guidelines for chronic kidney disease: evaluation, classification, and stratification. *Ann Intern Med.* 2003;139(2). 137–147+I36. doi:200307150-00013 [pii].

82. Colombo AA, Rusconi C, Esposito C, et al. Nephrotic syndrome after allogeneic hematopoietic stem cell transplantation as a late complication of chronic graft-versus-host disease. *Transplantation.* 2006;81(8):1087–1092. https://doi.org/10.1097/01.tp.0000209496.26639.cb.

83. Reddy P, Johnson K, Uberti JP, et al. Nephrotic syndrome associated with chronic graft-versus-host disease after allogeneic hematopoietic stem cell transplantation. *Bone Marrow Transplant.* 2006;38(5):351–357. https://doi.org/10.1038/sj.bmt.1705446.

84. Tomonari A, Takahashi S, Ooi J, et al. Hemorrhagic cystitis in adults after unrelated cord blood transplantation: a single-institution experience in Japan. *Int J Hematol.* 2006;84(3):268–271. https://doi.org/10.1532/IJH97.05169.

85. Megged O, Stein J, Ben-Meir D, et al. BK-virus-associated hemorrhagic cystitis in children after hematopoietic stem cell transplantation. *J Pediatr Hematol Off J Am Soc Pediatr Hematol.* 2011;33(3):190–193. https://doi.org/10.1097/MPH.0b013e3181fce388.

86. Leung AYH, Suen CKM, Lie AKW, Liang RHS, Yuen KY, Kwong YL. Quantification of polyoma BK viruria in hemorrhagic cystitis complicating bone marrow transplantation. *Blood.* 2001;98(6):1971–1978. https://doi.org/10.1182/blood.V98.6.1971.

87. Ruggeri A, Roth-Guepin G, Battipaglia G, et al. Incidence and risk factors for hemorrhagic cystitis in unmanipulated haploidentical transplant recipients. *Transpl Infect Dis.* 2015;17(6):822–830. https://doi.org/10.1111/tid.12455.

88. Silva L de P, Patah PA, Saliba RM, et al. Hemorrhagic cystitis after allogeneic hematopoietic stem cell transplants is the complex result of BK virus infection, preparative regimen intensity and donor type. *Haematologica.* 2010;95(7):1183–1190. https://doi.org/10.3324/haematol.2009.016758.

89. Lunde LE, Dasaraju S, Cao Q, et al. Hemorrhagic cystitis after allogeneic hematopoietic cell transplantation : risk factors, graft source and survival. *Bone Marrow Transplant.* 2015;50(11):1432–1437. https://doi.org/10.1038/bmt.2015.162.

90. Mackey MC. Intravesicular cidofovir for the treatment of polyomavirus-associated hemorrhagic cystitis. *Ann Pharmacother.* 2012;46:442–446. https://doi.org/10.1345/aph.1Q430.

91. Savona MR, Newton D, Frame D, Levine JE, Mineishi S, Kaul DR. Low-dose cidofovir treatment of BK virus-associated hemorrhagic cystitis in recipients of hematopoietic stem cell transplant. *Bone Marrow Transplant.* 2007;39(12):783–787. https://doi.org/10.1038/sj.bmt.1705678.

92. C CL. Use of prostaglandin F2 alpha for cyclophosphamide-induced hemorrhagic cystitis. *J Pharm Technol.* 1994;10(5):204–206. http://www.embase.com/search/results?subaction=viewrecord&from=export&id=L24301107.

93. Iavazzo C, Athanasiou S, Pitsouni E, Falagas ME. Hyaluronic acid: an effective alternative treatment of interstitial cystitis, recurrent urinary tract infections, and hemorrhagic cystitis? *Eur Urol.* 2007;51(6):1534–1541. https://doi.org/10.1016/j.eururo.2007.03.020.

94. Montgomery BD, Boorjian SA, Ziegelmann MJ, Joyce DD, Linder BJ. Intravesical silver nitrate for refractory hemorrhagic cystitis. *Turk Urol Derg.* 2016;42(3):197–201. https://doi.org/10.5152/tud.2016.38445.

95. Mani J, Jin N, Schmitt M. Cellular immunotherapy for patients with reactivation of JC and BK polyomaviruses after transplantation. *Cytotherapy.* 2014;16(10):1325–1335. https://doi.org/10.1016/j.jcyt.2014.04.003.

96. Bhatia S, Francisco L, Carter A, et al. Late mortality after allogeneic hematopoietic cell transplantation and functional status of long-term survivors: report from the Bone Marrow Transplant Survivor study. *Blood.* 2007;110(10):3784–3792. https://doi.org/10.1182/blood-2007-03-082933.

97. Tichelli A, Bucher C, Rovó A, et al. Premature cardiovascular disease after allogeneic hematopoietic stem-cell transplantation. *Blood*. 2007;110(9):3463–3471. https://doi.org/10.1182/blood-2006-10-054080.

98. Chow EJ, Mueller BA, Baker KS, et al. Cardiovascular hospitalizations and mortality among recipients of hematopoietic stem cell transplantation. *Ann Intern Med*. 2011;155(1):21–37. https://doi.org/10.1378/chest.06-3048.

99. Armenian SH, Chow EJ. Cardiovascular disease in survivors of hematopoietic cell transplantation. *Cancer*. 2014;120(4):469–479. https://doi.org/10.1002/cncr.28444.

100. Armenian SH, Sun C-L, Shannon T, et al. Incidence and predictors of congestive heart failure after autologous hematopoietic cell transplantation. *Blood*. 2011;118(23):6023–6029.https://doi.org/10.1182/blood-2011-06-358226.

101. Aisa Y, Mori T, Shimizu T, et al. Retrospective analysis of posterior reversible encephalopathy syndrome after allogeneic stem cell transplantation. [Japanese] *Rinsho Ketsueki*. 2009;50(1):9–15. http://ovidsp.ovid.com/ovidweb.cgi?T=JS&CSC=Y&NEWS=N&PAGE=fulltext&D=emed12&AN=354481451%5Cnhttp://www.tdnet.com/AalSy/resolver?sid=OVID:embase&id=pmid:19225223&id=doi:&issn=0485-1439&isbn=&volume=50&issue=1&spage=9&pages=9-15&date=2009&title=%5BRinsho+ke.

102. WongGZ,DeLimaM,GiraltSA,etal.Tacrolimus-associated posterior reversible encephalopathy syndrome after allogeneic haematopoietic stem cell transplantation. *Br J Haematol*. 2003;122(1):128–134. https://doi.org/10.1046/j.1365-2141.2003.04447.x.

103. Saumoy M, Castells G, Escoda L, Marés R, Richart C, Ugarriza A. Progressive multifocal leukoencephalopathy in chronic lymphocytic leukemia after treatment with fludarabine. *Leuk Lymphoma*. 2002;43(2):433–436. https://doi.org/10.1080/10428190290006297.

104. Kiewe P, Seyfert S, Körper S, Rieger K, Thiel E, Knauf W. Progressive multifocal leukoencephalopathy with detection of JC virus in a patient with chronic lymphocytic leukemia parallel to onset of fludarabine therapy. *Leuk Lymphoma*. 2003;44(10):1815–1818. https://doi.org/10.1080/1042819031000116625.

105. Kharfan-Dabaja MA, Ayala E, Greene J, Rojiani A, Murtagh FR, Anasetti C. Two cases of progressive multifocal leukoencephalopathy after allogeneic hematopoietic cell transplantation and a review of the literature. *Bone Marrow Transplant*. 2007;39(2):101–107. https://doi.org/10.1038/sj.bmt.1705548.

106. Buckanovich RJ, Liu G, Stricker C, et al. Nonmyeloablative allogeneic stem cell transplantation for refractory Hodgkin's lymphoma complicated by interleukin-2 responsive progressive multifocal leukoencephalopathy. *Ann Hematol*. 2002;81(7):410–413. https://doi.org/10.1007/s00277-002-0481-4.

107. Pruitt AA, Graus F, Rosenfeld MR. Neurological complications of transplantation. *Neurohospital*. 2013;3(1):24–38. https://doi.org/10.1177/1941874412455338.

108. Gofton TE, Al-Khotani a, O'Farrell B, Ang LC, McLachlan RS. Mefloquine in the treatment of progressive multifocal leukoencephalopathy. *J Neurol Neurosurg Psychiat*. 2011;82(4):452–455. https://doi.org/10.1136/jnnp.2009.190652.

109. Kishida S, Tanaka K. Mefloquine treatment in a patient suffering from progressive multifocal leukoencephalopathy after umbilical cord blood transplant. *Intern Med*. 2010;49(22):2509–2513. https://doi.org/10.2169/internalmedicine.49.3227.

110. Brickelmaier M, Lugovskoy A, Kartikeyan R, et al. Identification and characterization of mefloquine efficacy against JC virus in vitro. *Antimicrob Agents Chemother*. 2009;53(5):1840–1849. https://doi.org/10.1128/AAC.01614-08.

111. Michelis FV, Bril V, Lipton JH. A case report and literature review of chronic graft-versus-host disease manifesting as polymyositis. *Int J Hematol*. 2015;102(1):144–146. https://doi.org/10.1007/s12185-015-1768-2.

112. Cocito D, Romagnolo A, Rosso M, Peci E, Lopiano L, Merola A. CIDP-like neuropathies in graft versus host disease. *J Peripher Nerv Syst*. 2015;20(1):1–6. https://doi.org/10.1111/jns.12108.

113. Rodriguez V, Kuehnle I, Heslop HE, Khan S, Krance RA. Guillain-Barre syndrome after allogeneic hematopoietic stem cell transplantation. *Bone Marrow Transplant*. 2002;29(6):515–517. https://doi.org/10.1038/sj.bmt.1703412.

114. Burns TM. Guillian Barre syndrome. *Semin Neurol*. 2008;1(212):152–167. https://doi.org/10.1055/s-2008-1062261.

115. D KJ, S VK, S RB. Guillian-Barre syndrome: a comparative study of treatment modality-intravenous immunoglobulin versus plasmapheresis and outcome in our intensive care unit. *Indian J Crit Care Med*. 2014;18:S31. http://www.embase.com/search/results?subaction=viewrecord&from=export&id=L71398652%5Cnhttp://linksource.ebsco.com/linking.aspx?sid=EMBASE&issn=09725229&id=doi:&atitle=Guillian-Barre+syndrome:+A+comparative+study+of+treatment+modality-intravenous+immunoglo.

116. Xu X, Jia L, Chen L, Zhang W, Wang J. Guillain-Barre syndrome after allogeneic hematopoietic stem cell transplantation: two cases report and literature review. *Zhonghua Xue Ye Xue Za Zhi*. 2014;35(8):694–697. https://doi.org/10.3760/cma.j.issn.0253-2727.2014.08.005.

117. Sorror ML, Maris MB, Storb R, et al. Hematopoietic cell transplantation (HCT)-specific comorbidity index: a new tool for risk assessment before allogeneic HCT. *Blood*. 2005;106(8):2912–2919. https://doi.org/10.1182/blood-2005-05-2004.

118. Jim HSL, Sutton SK, Jacobsen PB, Martin PJ, Flowers ME, Lee SJ. Risk factors for depression and fatigue among survivors of hematopoietic cell transplantation. *Cancer*. 2016;122(8):1290–1297. https://doi.org/10.1002/cncr.29877.

119. Kuba K, Esser P, Scherwath A, et al. Cancer-and-treatment-specific distress and its impact on posttraumatic stress in patients undergoing allogeneic hematopoietic stem cell transplantation (HSCT). *Psycho Oncol.* 2016. https://doi.org/10.1002/pon.4295.

120. Barata A, Gonzalez BD, Sutton SK, et al. Coping strategies modify risk of depression associated with hematopoietic cell transplant symptomatology. *J Health Psychol.* 2016:1359105316642004. https://doi.org/10.1177/1359105316642004.

CHAPTER 25

Prophylaxis and Management of Infectious Complications After Hematopoietic Cell Transplantation

MUFTI NAEEM AHMAD, MD, KELLY E. PILLINGER, PharmD,
ZAINAB SHAHID, MD, FACP

BACKGROUND

Infections are common and serious complications after hematopoietic cell transplantation (HCT). Management of infectious complications requires an understanding of host risk factors at different points after transplant, epidemiology of most common infections at those time points, different clinical syndromes, type of conditioning regimens, and transplantation techniques and immune reconstitution.[1] Overall risk of infections is higher in allogeneic HCT than in autologous HCT. Classically, posttransplant complications have been divided into early (until day +100) and late (after day 100) period due to expected period of immunosuppression. Early period is also divided into preengraftment and postengraftment period based on risk of infection before neutrophil recovery (Fig. 25.1).

PREENGRAFTMENT RISK PERIOD

Preengraftment risk period starts with the onset of conditioning regimen and continues approximately until day 30. Days to engraftment can vary based on the type of conditioning regimen, type of transplant, and HCT source. Risk of infection is driven by lack of neutrophils and lymphocyte during this phase.

Bacterial infections are common during this phase, including bacteremia, sepsis syndrome, pneumonia, oropharyngitis, sinusitis, proctitis, and cellulitis. Oral prophylaxis with oral quinolone reduces the frequency of febrile neutropenic episodes and mortality among neutropenic patients.[2] Risk factors for infections include mucositis, duration of neutropenia, and sinusoidal occlusive syndrome (SOS). The use of acyclovir prophylaxis risk of herpes simplex virus (HSV) reactivation from 70% to 1%. Candidemia and early invasive aspergillosis (IA) can be seen in this phase. Either fluconazole or an echinocandin prophylaxis is used to avoid these infections.

POSTENGRAFTMENT RISK PERIOD

Early Risk Period

There is resurgence of innate cellular immunity and recovery from mucosal injury, but risk of infection remains due to B- and T-cell quantitative and qualitative deficiency. Autologous HCT recipients start to recover T lymphocytes. There is continued risk of respiratory tract infections including viral, bacterial, and pneumocystis jirovecii pneumonia. PJP prophylaxis is used in recipients with continued low CD4 counts. Acyclovir is continued during this phase to prevent herpes zoster (VZV) and simplex (HSV) reactivation. Cytomegalovirus (CMV) reactivation can be seen in up to 40% of autologous HCT recipients, but routine CMV surveillance is not recommended due to low likelihood of progression from reactivation to disease.[3] Exceptions include tandem transplantations, CD 34–depleted grafts, history of CMV infection, and treatment with fludarabine, cladribine, or alemtuzumab.[4,5]

Allogeneic HCT recipients are on immunosuppression for graft-versus-host disease (GVHD) prophylaxis during this period which interferes with immune reconstitution. Owing to increased risk of encapsulated organisms, prophylaxis is given with PCN, azithromycin, or a quinolone with GVHD requiring systemic steroids. Invasive fungal infection (IFI) prophylaxis with voriconazole or posaconazole is used in high-risk patients, although practices vary among transplant centers. Antifungal prophylaxis is used till GVHD immunoprophylaxis is continued (usually day +100) or longer in the presence of GVHD. PJP risk remains during this period, and prophylaxis can be given with trimethoprim-sulfamethoxazole or dapsone, inhaled or IV pentamidine or atovaquone. Acyclovir is continued for HSV and VZV prophylaxis. CMV reactivation/infection can occur in up to 70% of allogeneic HCT recipients at risk of CMV. CMV virus surveillance is performed, and mainly preemptive strategy is used to manage CMV reactivation (Table 25.1).

Hematopoietic Cell Transplantation for Malignant Conditions. https://doi.org/10.1016/B978-0-323-56802-9.00025-0

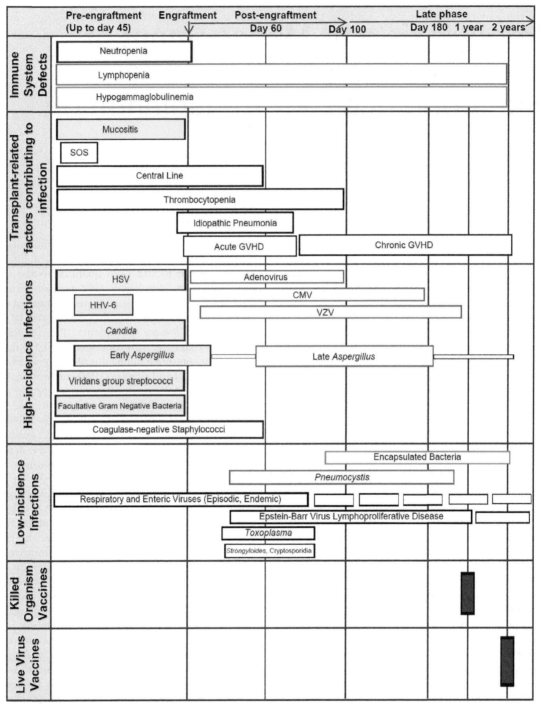

FIG. 25.1 Expected opportunistic infections at different phases of immunosuppression after Hematopoietic Cell Transplantation. *CMV*, cytomegalovirus; *GVHD*, graft-versus-host disease; *HHV*, human herpesvirus; *HSV*, herpes simplex virus; *SOS*, sinusoidal occlusive syndrome; *VZV*, varicella zoster virus. (Adapted and modified from Van Burik J-AH, Freifeld AG. Infection in severely immunocompromised host. In: Abeloff MD, Armitage JO, Niederhuber JE, et al., eds. *Clinical Oncology* third ed. Philadelphia: Churchill Livingstone; 2004:942.)

TABLE 25.1
Antimicrobial Prophylaxis Recommendations in Allogeneic Hematopoietic Cellular Recipients

Risk Period	Bacterial	Fungal	VIRAL		
			HSV (+) or VZV (+)	CMV	PJP
Early posttransplant (within day +100)	Levofloxacin 500mg PO daily[a] If quinolone allergy or intolerance, use cefepime 2 gm IV q8h, starting on day −1 until hematopoietic recovery[b] and resolution of mucositis	Micafungin 50mg IV daily starting day +1 until tolerating oral therapy, when patient can be transitioned to oral voriconazole if high risk for IFI[c]	Acyclovir 400mg PO BID, starting on admission (if not on previously) and continue for at least 2 years or longer (or until 6 months after immunosuppression is discontinued, whichever is later)	Preemptive approach[e]: If high-risk CMV (i.e., D+/R−, D+/R+, D−/R+), use preemptive approach and check CMV PCR twice weekly and initiate therapy (foscarnet, ganciclovir, valganciclovir) upon CMV reactivation Prophylaxis approach: For CMV R (+), prophylactic letermovir from thru week 14 with CMV monitoring OR IV ganciclovir or PO valganciclovir with CMV monitoring	SMX/TMP SS 1-tab PO daily preferred after hematopoietic recovery[i] If SMX/TMP allergy or intolerance, use dapsone PO or pentamidine inhaled or IV Continue for at least 6 months until CD4>200 or longer if still on immunosuppression
Late posttransplant (after day +100)	N/A	Risk assessment for antifungal therapy[f]			See above
GVHD (if receiving systemic corticosteroids)	Levofloxacin 500mg PO daily If quinolone allergy or intolerance, use Penicillin VK 500mg PO daily or Azithromycin 500mg PO daily[d]	Voriconazole or posaconazole[g]	Acyclovir 400mg PO BID[h] until off immunosuppression VZV (IgG+) acyclovir 800mg PO BID until on immunosuppression	CMV monitoring is continued in high-risk patient e.g., history of CMV reactivation or disease	

(−), seronegative; (+), seropositive; CMV, cytomegalovirus; D, donor; GVHD, graft-versus-host disease; HSV, herpes simplex virus; PJP, Pneumocystis jirovecii pneumonia; R, recipient; SMX/TMP, sulfamethoxazole/trimethoprim; SS, single strength; VZV, varicella zoster virus.

[a]Primarily for gram-negative rods, including Pseudomonas.
[b]Defined as ANC >500×3days or >5000×1day, whichever comes first.
[c]High-risk factors for IFI include prolonged neutropenia, myeloablative regimens and presence of GvHD.
[d]Primarily for streptococcus pneumoniae coverage, agent of choice can vary by institutions.
[e]Cytomegalovirus is managed using preemptive approach, historically prophylactic approach has not shown survival benefit, more data to come with newer agents.
[f]Allogeneic HCT recipients receiving myeloablative conditioning regimens are considered high risk for fungal infections.
[g]Continued based on the net state of immunosuppression including dose and duration of steroids, agents of choice vary by institutions.
[h]Some institutions use acyclovir 800mg PO BID.
[i]In cases of delayed engraftment as defined by lack of hematopoietic recovery by D + 30, consider starting alternative PJP prophylaxis.

TABLE 25.2
Management of Neutropenic Fever in High-Risk Patients[10]

Initial Empiric Therapy	If Concern for Methicillin Resistant Staphylococcus Aureus (MRSA)[a]	If Risk for MDR Organisms
Antipseudomonal beta-lactam (i.e., cefepime, piperacillin/ tazobactam, imipenem, meropenem)[a]	Addition of vancomycin (alternatives: linezolid, daptomycin)	**Extended spectrum beta-lactamase (ESBL)**: carbapenem
		Carbapenem Resistant Enterobacteriaceae (CRE): combination therapy based on susceptibilities (i.e., ceftazidime/avibactam, polymyxin B, colistin, tigecycline)
		VRE: daptomycin or linezolid

[a]Indications for empiric MRSA coverage include suspicions of catheter-related bloodstream infection, skin and soft tissue infection, pneumonia, hemodynamic instability, or history of MRSA infection/colonization.
MDR, multidrug resistant; *VRE*, vancomycin-resistant Enterococcus.

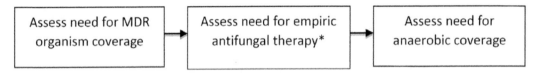

*Recommended if persistent fever after 4 – 7 days on antibiotics

FIG. 25.2 Antimicrobial therapy for persistent neutropenic fever.[2] *MDR*, multidrug-resistant.

Late Risk Period

Late risk period begins after day +100, and risk of infection is variable based on the host factors. Among autologous HCT recipients, recovery of cellular and humoral immunity can be observed within 6–12 months, whereas for allogeneic HCT recipients, it may take more than 2 years.[6] Immune reconstitution can be monitored during this period with quantitative and qualitative assay for T and B cells to help determine the risk of infection. Bacterial infections are common in the setting of GVHD and ongoing immune suppression.[7] Late CMV infection is also observed with ongoing immunosuppression. CMV surveillance should be continued during this period to avoid CMV disease. GVHD patients remain at risk of VZV reactivation, infections with encapsulated bacteria (*Streptococcal pneumonia* and *Hemophilus influenza*), and invasive aspergillosis, and prophylaxis is continued against these infections among such patients. Posttransplant vaccinations are also initiated to reduce infectious risk.[8]

MANAGEMENT OF DIFFERENT INFECTIONS
Neutropenic Fever Syndromes

Neutropenic fever is the most common syndrome seen in the preengraftment period and is associated with an in-hospital mortality rate of about 10%.[9] The most common cause of neutropenic fever is bloodstream infections, mostly caused by gram-positive organisms followed by gram-negative organisms.[10,11] However, the incidence of positive blood cultures is impacted by antimicrobial prophylaxis, and only 10%–25% of all patients with neutropenic fevers will be found bacteremic.[10,12] Mucosal barrier injury predisposes these patients to bloodstream infections. HCT recipients with neutropenic fevers can develop bacterial pneumonia, with a reported incidence of 20%–50% in the preengraftment phase.[13] Neutropenic typhlitis is also observed during this period. In recent years, HCT recipients have become increasingly at risk for infections due to multidrug-resistant (MDR) organisms, including vancomycin-resistant Enterococcus (VRE) and carbapenem-resistant Enterobacteriaceae (CRE).[14]

Empiric antibiotic selection should be guided by patient-specific factors and the institutional antibiogram. Table 25.2 describes the algorithmic approach to the treatment of neutropenic fevers in high-risk patients. If neutropenic fever does not respond to initial therapy, antimicrobial coverage may need to be broadened to cover for possible MDR organisms and/ or broader spectrum antifungal therapy.[10] Fig. 25.2 describes considerations for antimicrobial coverage with persistent neutropenic fever. Serum surveillance with galactomannan and beta D-glucan is helpful in early diagnosis of invasive fungal infections.[10] Historically, amphotericin B was used as first-line antifungal therapy, but recent studies have shown that voriconazole or an echinocandin is as effective and better tolerated as empiric therapy for fungal infection.[15–18] Patients already receiving antifungal prophylaxis should be changed to a different class of antimold coverage.[10]

It remains controversial if broad-spectrum antibiotics can be deescalated before marrow recovery after an appropriate treatment course.[10] Several studies suggest that the latter strategy may be safe and effective and result in less overall antimicrobial exposure.[19,20]

Growth Factors

Hematopoietic stimulating factors are used to shorten the duration of neutropenia and hasten marrow recovery.[21,22] They include granulocyte colony-stimulating factor (G-CSF) and granulocyte macrophage colony-stimulating factor(GM-CSF). In a metaanalysis of clinical trials that compared G-CSF primary prophylaxis (PP) versus no G-CSF PP or placebo, G-CSF PP reduced the risk of FN among chemotherapy recipients along with reduction in infection-related and all-cause mortality.[22]

Granulocyte Transfusions

Pioneering studies indicated that repeated granulocyte transfusions (GTs) to neutropenic patients were effective in clinical management of neutropenic patients with gram-negative septicemia.[23] Disappointedly no metaanalysis of randomized control trials or any phase III trials has shown any benefit of GTs in terms of mortality or reversal of clinical infection.[21] Despite that, GTs are still perceived as a tool to support neutropenic patients with life-threatening infections.

MANAGEMENT OF FUNGAL INFECTIONS

IFIs remain an important cause of morbidity and mortality among allogeneic and autologous HCT recipients.[24] IFIs are defined by European Organizarion for Research & Treatment of Cancer (EROCT) criteria.[25]

Invasive Candidiasis

Candida blood stream infection is the most common form if invasive candidiasis (IC).[24] Other manifestations of IC include hepatosplenic candidiasis and candida endophthalmistis among HCT recipients. IC is associated with high morbidity and mortality.[24] Blood cultures remain the most common diagnostic modality but have low diagnostic yield.[26] Noncultures diagnostics includes candida antigen and antibody detection, serum

TABLE 25.3
First-Line Therapy for Different Candida Species Among HCT Recipients

Candida Species	First-Line Therapy	Alternative Agent
C. glabrata C. Krusii	Echinocandins	Liposomal amphotericin B
C. Albicans	Echinocandins	Fluconazole
C. parasilosis	Flucoanzole	Echinocandins
C. tropicalis	Fluconazole	Enchinocandins

HCT, hematopoietic cell transplantation

beta-D-glucan measurement, and polymerase chain reaction (PCR). Metaanalysis of 14 studies showed that the sensitivity/specificity for the diagnosis of IC of mannan and antimannan IgG individually were 58%/93% and 59%/83%, respectively.[27] In a single-center study of prospectively enrolled patients, the sensitivities/specificities of the β-D-glucan (BDG) assay and a real-time quantitative PCR assay (ViraCor-IBT, Lee's Summit, Missouri) for invasive candidiasis were 56%/73% and 80%/70%, respectively.[28] Commercially available multiplex PCR now can readily identify most common species of candida in blood.[29] Management of candidiasis also includes source when possible e.g., removal central venous catheters along with early directed therapy. Table 25.3 describes the common antifungal used for the treatment of candidemia.[30,31] Duration of treatment depends on the clinical entity of IC. For example, hepatosplenic candidiasis requires longer duration of therapy.

Invasive Aspergillosis

Invasive aspergillosis (IA) is the most common IFI among allogeneic HCT recipients and is associated with significant mortality.[32,33] Allogeneic HCT recipients are more likely than autologous HCT recipients to develop IA, and common risk factors for IA include prolonged neutropenia (disease and treatment related) and immunosuppression during the treatment of both acute and chronic GVHD.[7,34]

Despite antifungal prophylaxis, studies suggest that between 5% and 10% of HCT recipients will develop IA infection.[32,35,36] Molecular methods for diagnosis of IA include the use of serum, bronchoalveolar lavage (BAL), CSF galactomannan, and serum BDG, although the latter is nonspecific for IA. Aspergillus PCR should only be used in conjunction with other diagnostic tests due to lack of validated tests.[34] Chest CT and BAL testing are important tools for diagnosis as the most common site of IA infection is pulmonary.[34,37]

TABLE 25.4
Antifungal Therapy Recommendations for the Treatment of Invasive Aspergillosis

Place in Therapy	Antifungal Therapy
First Line	Voriconazole[a]
Alternatives	Isavuconazole or liposomal amphotericin B
High-Risk Patients or Salvage Therapy	Combination therapy (voriconazole plus echniocandin)

[a]Therapeutic drug monitoring recommended.

Voriconazole is first-line, primary treatment for IA,[34] based on a landmark trial by Herbrecht et al. in which voriconazole was compared to amphotericin B deoxycholate and was shown to have a significantly higher rate of successful outcomes, lower mortality, and fewer adverse effects.[38] Further cohort studies have supported this finding of improved survival in patients treated with voriconazole.[34] Alternative antifungal therapy for IA includes isavuconazole and liposomal amphotericin B. A randomized controlled trial by Maertens et al. found isavuconazole to be noninferior to voriconazole in terms of all-cause mortality in the treatment of IA. Isavuconazole was associated with fewer adverse effects than voriconazole, including hepatobiliary disorders (9% vs. 16%, $P = .016$), eye disorders (15% vs. 27%, $P = .002$), and skin and subcutaneous tissue disorders (33% vs. 42%, $P = .037$).[39] Treatment options for IA are listed in Table 25.4.

Combination therapy with voriconazole plus an echinocandin can be considered for certain patients such as those with severe disease and profound, persistent neutropenia or as salvage therapy.[34]

Echinocandin monotherapy is not recommended unless there is a contraindication to the extended spectrum azoles and polyenes. Duration of therapy is not well defined but generally should be at least 6–12 weeks, depending on duration of neutropenia and immunosuppression.[34]

Mucormycosis

Mucormycosis refers to infections due to fungi in Mucorales order. It is difficult to understand its epidemiology, but incidence is about 8% in HSCT recipients with 1-year cumulative incidence of 0.29%.[40] Risk factors include diagnosis of myelodysplastic syndrome, male sex, and presence of severe GVHD.[41] Previous exposure to voriconazole also has been reported as a risk factor.[42] Most common site of involvement includes sinuses, lungs, skin, and gastrointestinal (GI) tract. Diagnosis is challenging and primarily depends on histopathology and cultures. Serum galactomannan in serum is usually negative. New molecular PCR assay is now available to test tissue specimens, BAL, and serum, although these are not readily available.[43,44] Treatment includes surgical debridement when possible along with antifungal therapy. First-line antifungal agent is amphotericin B. Posaconazole and isavuconazole can be used as salvage therapy. Echinocandin has no activity against mucormycosis. Echinocandins have shown in vitro synergy with AMB against *Rhizopus oryzae*.[45] There are no enough data to recommend combination therapy although frequently used in clinical practice. Other non-aspergillus molds include fusarium, scedosporium, and dematiaceous molds.

Pneumocystis Jiroveci Pneumonia

Pneumocystis jiroveci pneumonia (PJP) in an important fungal infection after HSCT which has been associated with high mortality rates (34%–53%).[46] Preprophylaxis literature states incidence as high as 37% of HCT patients.[47–49] More recent reports from the Center of International Board and Marrow Transplant Research show incidence of 0.63% after allogeneic HCT and 0.28% after autologous HCT with 50% of cases occurring between 60 and 270 days. PJP diagnosis was associated with poor overall survival. Risk factors associated for PJP included GVHD and poor immune reconstitution. Clinical presentation may be associated with fevers, dyspnea, and nonproductive cough.[50] LDH may be elevated. Serum BDG has sensitivity of 90%–100% and specificity of 88%–96% for PJP diagnosis. CT imaging is nonspecific. BAL fluid testing remains the gold standard for PCP diagnosis.[48] Immunofluorescence testing has lower yield. Quantitative PCR on BAL has improved sensitivity and specificity.[51] First-line treatment includes trimethprim/sulfamethaxazole. Other agents include IV pentamidine, primaquine/clindamycin, and atovaquone. Routine adjunctive therapy with steroids is not recommended in non-HIV patients and is decided on an individual basis.[50] Usually, duration of treatment is 3 weeks. Secondary prophylaxis should be considered after treatment till immune system is recovered.

MANAGEMENT OF VIRAL INFECTIONS
Cytomegalovirus Infection

CMV infection is an important cause of morbidity and mortality after HCT both in autologous and allogeneic setting. CMV infection has classically been associated with allogeneic setting with mortality up 25% in early transplantation periods.[53] Risk factors for CMV infection after allogeneic HCT include recipients with CMV-seropositive status before HCT, in vivo T-cell depletion e.g., alemtuzumab, in vitro T-cell depletion, HLA mismatch, source of stem cell (e.g., umbilical cord), and GVHD.[52,53] Among autologous HCT recipient, tandem transplantation with CD34 selection increases the risk of CMV infection.[4,5]

CMV Infection and Disease

CMV viremia or CMV reactivation is the most common CMV infection (50%–70%). CMV viremia is frequently asymptomatic but can be associated with fevers. CMV disease is defined as isolation of CMV from an appropriate tissue specimen along with compatible signs and symptoms. Common sites include gastrointestinal (GI) tract, liver, and lung. CMV involving the GI tract presents similarly to GI GVHD and may require biopsy of the GI tract to differentiate the two. CMV pneumonitis was the most common presentation before the preemptive therapy era. It is diagnosed by isolation of CMV either in lung tissue or BAL with respiratory tract symptoms. More recently, quantitative polymerase chain reaction (qPCR) in BAL may be helpful in diagnosis of CMV pneumonitis.[54] Less commonly, CMV can involve the central nervous system including the eye. CMV retinitis is diagnosed by retinal necrosis, ± retinal hemorrhage in the presence of CMV viremia. CMV viremia may not precede or accompany CMV disease, especially in GI and CNS involvement.[55] CMV can rarely involve kidneys, bladder, gall bladder, heart, and pancreas.

At the time of donor selection, CMV status of the donor and recipient should be taken into consideration. The use of CMV-specific immunoglobulins has not shown any difference in disease incidence when used in seronegative recipients who received HCT from seropositive donors.[56] Studies have failed to show consistent results regarding CMV-related complications or survival benefits of CMV-specific immunoglobulin.[57,58]

Routine surveillance for CMV reactivation is not usually performed in autologous HCT setting unless it is a high-risk setting for CMV reactivation. During early transplantation era, both acyclovir and ganciclovir were explored for the prevention of CMV therapy. High-dose acyclovir when compared to low-dose acyclovir did not affect the incidence of CMV disease.[59]

Prophylaxis of ganciclovir in RCTs has shown reduction in CMV infection but did not show any survival advantage, and severe neutropenia was observed. Most recently, oral valganciclovir prophylaxis when compared to preemptive approach did not show any

difference in CMV disease, invasive bacterial, or fungal infections, and more patients received growth factors in the valganciclovir group.[60–63]

Preemptive approach in CMV infection refers to timely detection of virus in whole blood and serum by PCR technique or quantitative pp65 antigen test. Antiviral treatment is implemented immediately on viral detection to prevent CMV disease as viral replication is predictive of disease. This requires availability of frequent (at least weekly) and standardized testing with reliable sample collection.[64]

Viral thresholds may be different among institution to start empiric therapy. Owing to low sensitivity of pp65 antigenemia, any level of antigen detection therapy is recommended. For CMV-quantitative PCR, preemptive therapy threshold is between 500 copies/mL and 10,000 copies/ml in standard recipients, whereas for high-risk patients, e.g., T-cell depleted, steroids therapy or umbilical cord transplants, any detectable level should prompt therapy.

Table 25.5 describes the treatment strategy for CMV reactivation and disease. IV ganciclovir is the first-line treatment for preemptive therapy, but IV foscarnet is also used with similar results in reports. IV ganciclovir is associated with neutropenia, whereas foscarnet causes nephrotoxicity and electrolyte abnormalities.[65] Oral valganciclovir has been used in the preemptive approach, but there are limited data in this setting.[66] Pooled immunoglobulins or CMV hyperimmunoglobulins have not shown to be effective in preventing CMV reactivation and are not routinely recommended.[67] Cidofovir is used as a third-line agent in allogeneic HCT setting for CMV disease but has significant renal and marrow toxicities.[68,69] It is also observed that initiation of therapy at low CMV levels is associated with shorter duration of viremia and treatment.[70]

For autologous and low-risk setting, it may be reasonable to observe till a certain threshold as the viremia may resolve spontaneously. CMV surveillance is continued till day +100 and after day +100 continued in high-risk patients.

Ganciclovir resistance is rare, and the previous exposure is mostly associated to ganciclovir with prolonged subclinical reactivation. Ganciclovir resistance results from viral phosphotransferase gene (UL97) causing low-level resistance followed by DNA polymerase (UL 54) causing more severe resistance and is commercially available. Drug resistance is suspected when the viral load continues to rise for >2 weeks on induction doses of the drug.

Novel agents include Marabivir, which is a UL 97 polymerase inhibitor being evaluated for resistant or

TABLE 25.5
Duration of Therapy for CMV Infection and Disease

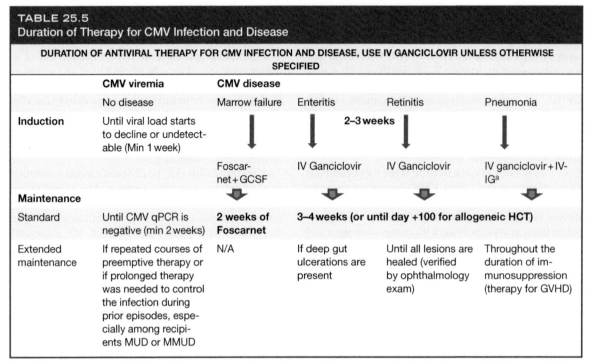

DURATION OF ANTIVIRAL THERAPY FOR CMV INFECTION AND DISEASE, USE IV GANCICLOVIR UNLESS OTHERWISE SPECIFIED					
	CMV viremia	**CMV disease**			
	No disease	Marrow failure	Enteritis	Retinitis	Pneumonia
Induction	Until viral load starts to decline or undetectable (Min 1 week)	↓	↓ 2–3 weeks ↓		↓
		Foscarnet + GCSF	IV Ganciclovir	IV Ganciclovir	IV ganciclovir + IV-IG[a]
Maintenance					
Standard	Until CMV qPCR is negative (min 2 weeks)	**2 weeks of Foscarnet**	**3–4 weeks (or until day +100 for allogeneic HCT)**		
Extended maintenance	If repeated courses of preemptive therapy or if prolonged therapy was needed to control the infection during prior episodes, especially among recipients MUD or MMUD	N/A	If deep gut ulcerations are present	Until all lesions are healed (verified by ophthalmology exam)	Throughout the duration of immunosuppression (therapy for GVHD)

[a]For CMV pneumonia, give IVIG 500 mg/KG every other day for 2 weeks, then IVIG once a week for the duration of anti-CMV therapy. IVIG 500 mg/kg is equivalent to CMV-IGIV 150 mg/kg (same schedule for therapy). Use CMV-IGIV if volume consideration prohibits the use of IVIG or if IVIG is not available. GvHD; graft-versus-host disease.[133,134]

refractory CMV disease. Levemir is a terminase inhibitor; early studies are promising. More studies are underway in prophylaxis settings. Brincidofovir is an oral UL54 DNA polymerase inhibitor being evaluated for CMV prophylaxis in HCT setting. CMV vaccines are still in early phases of development. ASP0113 and CMVPepVax have both shown to decrease the incidence of viremia. Tetanus-CMV fusion peptide vaccine with PF-03512676 adjuvant and multi-antigen CMV-MVA triplex vaccine are still in phase I and phase II clinical trial. CMV-specific T cells are also used for adaptive cell-mediated immunity against CMV. Early reports have shown to decrease disease recurrence and/or late CMV infection and decrease antiviral immunity after allogeneic stem cell transplantation.[71] More trials are underway to study third party cytotoxic T-cell lymphocytes in prophylaxis and treatment settings.

Hemorrhagic Cystitis

Hemorrhagic cystitis (HC) is an inflammatory condition of urinary bladder resulting in bladder wall bleeding. Incidence of HC is reported between 10% and 70% with known morbidity and mortality.[72]

Early HC is thought to be related to chemotherapeutic agents such as cyclophosphamide, ifosfamide, busalphan, and thiotepa. Delayed HC (after 72 h insulting agent) is likely related to viral infections of polyoma BK virus, CMV, and adenovirus.[73] It is typically seen after 30 days of transplantation, but urinary shedding can be seen in the first 2–3 weeks.[74-77]

Patients may present with increased urinary frequency, urgency, lower abdominal pain, change in the color of urine, presence of blood clots, and urinary retention. Diagnosis is made by evaluating urinalysis and testing urine for the presence of viruses by commercially available quantitative PCR testing.

Risk factors identified for development of HC include age, donor-recipient gender mismatch, stem cell sources, conditioning regimen, and use of immunosuppressive agents.[74,78,79]

Prophylactic strategies in high-risk patients include hyperhydration, and use of mercaptoethane-sodium sulfonate therapy with cyclophosphamide oral ciprofloxacin has also shown to prevent severe BK HC (due to inhibitory activity against prokaryotic DNA gyrase subunit A) and viral replication.[80]

Treatment includes hyperhydration and management of symptoms with phenazopyridine and systemic opioids. Continued bladder irrigation may be required in case of urinary retention or excessive clots. Pooled immunoglobulins are used due the presence of potential anti-BK virus activity.[81] For BK-associated HC, IV cidofovir is shown to be an effective treatment with associated nephrotoxicity.[82] Low-dose cidofovir (1 mg/kg) may be an alternative option to avoid nephrotoxicity.[83] Intravesicular cidofovir has been used but requires continued bladder irrigation.[84] Leflunomide is also an alternative option for BK-HC.[85] Early reports show successful treatment of BK-HC with BK-specific cytotoxic T-cell lymphocytes.[86]

Human Herpesvirus 6

Human herpesvirus 6 (HHV-6) usually infects during childhood and rarely causes disease in immunocompetent individuals. HHV-6 A and HHV-6B are distinct species. HHV-6B causes Roseola among children and infects most kids. HHV-6A significance is not very well understood.[87,88]

HHV-6A and HHV-6b have the unique ability to integrate into human chromosome. If viral integration occurs in germline cell, vertical transmission of chromosomally integrated HHV-6 (ciHHV-6) results in offspring with a copy of HHV-6 genome in all nucleated cells. Population-based studies show that almost 1% of the world's population has ciHHV-6.[89] HHV-6 reactivation can be differentiated from ciHHV-6 by newer droplet digital PCR.[90] HHV-6B reactivation is experienced among 33%–48% allogeneic HCT recipients.[91] Most recently it is also recognized to cause febrile illness and disease among autologous HCT recipients.[91] Among allogeneic HCT recipients, HHV-6 reactivation is usually detected in 2–4 weeks by PCR. HHV-6 reactivation is associated with febrile rash, hepatitis, pneumonitis, enteritis, myelosuppression, and encephalitis. Risk factors include HHV-6, cord blood transplantation, engraftment syndrome, and history of allogeneic HCT. HHV-6 encephalitis is associated with poorer outcomes and neurological sequalae. HHV-6 can be isolated by molecular PCR testing from different body fluids such as CSF and BAL to help in diagnosis, but there are no standard syndrome definitions. Role of HHV-6 in posttransplant setting is still being evaluated.

HHV-6 reactivation was associated with CMV reactivation and GVHD and increased overall mortality. Antiviral agents such as ganciclovir, foscarnet, and cidofovir inhibit viral replication and are commonly used for treatment. IVIG does not have a defined role. There are no preemptive or prophylactic strategies available. HHV-6–specific T-cell lymphocyte has also been used for the treatment of HHV-6 infection, but this treatment modality is not readily available.[86]

Varicella Zoster Virus Infection

VZV infection can occur as a primary infection or as reactivation in about 17%–50% allogeneic HCT recipients and 14%–28% autologous HCT recipients observed during the first year of transplant.[92,93]

Clinical presentation may be localized lesions or disseminated disease. Localized lesions may have atypical presentation, so laboratory diagnosis is recommended. Diagnosis can be made by performing a DFA of cell on skin scrapping with VZV-specific monoclonal antibodies. Viral cultures have low yield. Quantitative PCR testing is also available on blood, BAL, CSF, and tissue specimen including bone marrow.

VZV disease can present with pulmonary hemorrhage, hepatitis, encephalitis, abdominal pain, thrombocytopenia, and retinal necrosis. Syndrome of inappropriate antidiuretic hormone secretion has been associated with disseminated disease and can precede skin manifestations. Postherpetic neuralgia can occur in up to 35% of HCT recipients with skin manifestations. GVHD is a strong predictor of disseminated disease.[94]

Prolonged antiviral prophylaxis for at least 1 year significantly reduces VZV in HCT recipients irrespective of the type of transplant.[95] Net immunosuppression should help determine optimal duration of prophylaxis. High-dose IV acyclovir at 10 mg/kg every 8 hours is the initial treatment for disseminated disease. Oral therapy with acyclovir or valacyclovir can be used as an initial therapy for localized infection.

When a seronegative HCT recipient is exposed to active or incubating varicella infection, varicella zoster immunoglobulins (VZIGs) should be given to prevent primary VZV infection.[96]

Herpes Simplex Virus

Herpes simplex virus (HSV) reactivation usually causes mucocutaneous lesions but can also cause visceral disease including esophagitis, tracheobronchitis, and pneumonitis. Rarely it can also cause Bell's palsy, hepatitis, and encephalitis in patients undergoing HCT. Up to 80% of seropositive patients undergoing autologous or allogeneic HCT can experience reactivation usually in early risk period. HSV reactivation rate has been decreased to less than 5% with acyclovir prophylaxis.[97,98] Oral acyclovir, IV acyclovir, or oral valacyclovir has been used in these settings.[99]

Acyclovir-resistant HSV can develop with prolonged and repeated courses of acyclovir. In allogeneic HCT grade II GVHD and lack of ganciclovir, prophylaxis was shown to be associated with acyclovir-resistant HSV. The prevalence of antiviral resistant can be as high as 27%. Foscarnet, cidofovir, famciclovir, and brincidofovir can be helpful in such clinical settings.[100] Topical forms of foscarnet and cidofovir have also been used.[101]

Ebstein-Barr Virus

Ebstein-Barr virus (EBV) infects about 90% of the adults.[102] EBV usually infects human B cells and has been associated with EBV-driven B-cell proliferation leading to posttransplant lymphoproliferation disorder (PTLD) after allogeneic HCT. EBV reactivation is observed in allogenic HCT both in unmanipulated and T-cell deplete HCT mostly during in the early risk period.[102] PTLD also has been described in autologous setting.[103] EBV reactivation also been described with hemophagocytic syndrome. Although IV ganciclovir inhibits linear EBV DNA, it is not effective against episomal DNA and does not prevent B-cell proliferation. EBV reactivation predict EBV-associated PTLD on high-risk setting (T-cell depletion, age >50, second allogeneic HCT, acute and chronic GVHD, cord blood transplant, and haploidentical transplant).[104] Rituximab has been used for preemptive therapy to control EBV reactivation in such settings[105] EBV-specific cytotoxic T-cell lymphocytes have been used both in prophylactic and preemptive setting with promising results.[106]

Respiratory Viral Infection

Respiratory viruses include respiratory syncytial virus (RSV), parainfluenza virus (PIV), human metapneumovirus (hMPV), rhinovirus, adenovirus (ADV), and influenza virus.[107–109] Respiratory viral infections in HCT recipients can quickly progress from upper respiratory tract (URT) to lower respiratory tract (LRT) and result in death, with a reported mortality rate of 10%–50%.[107–109] Risk factors for progression include neutropenia, preengraftment, lymphopenia, elderly, GVHD, mismatched or unrelated donor, and corticosteroid use.[109] Viral multiplex PCR panels, which are highly sensitive and specific, are the preferred method for diagnosis as viral culture can take up to a week to become positive.[109] Treatment options for respiratory viruses are limited, and infections are often primarily managed with supportive care.[107–109] See Table 25.6 for antiviral therapies.

Treatment of RSV in HCT recipients includes supportive care and ribavirin. Although there is a lack of high-quality, randomized control trials, studies suggest

TABLE 25.6
Antiviral Therapies for Respiratory Viral Infections[11,108,112]

Respiratory Virus	Treatment Modalities
Respiratory syncytial virus	Ribavirin (oral, aerosolized, intravenous) ± immune globulin (IVIG)
Parainfluenza virus	Currently available antivirals do not show benefit
Human metapneumovirus	Currently available antivirals do not show benefit
Rhinovirus	Currently available antivirals do not show benefit
Adenovirus	Brincidofovir[a], Cidofovir
Influenza	Oseltamivir, Zanamivir, Peramivir

[a]Brincidofovir is currently under development and not FDA-approved.

that aerosolized ribavirin may help prevent progression of RSV from URT to LRT infection and death.[110,111]

Brincidofovir is currently being studied in the setting of treatment for adenovirus. A recent open-label study in pediatric and adult HCT recipients showed reductions in ADV viral loads. The effects of therapy were more pronounced in pediatric HCT recipients who had lower all-cause mortality rates than adults.[112]

Treatment with antiviral therapy for influenza should occur promptly within 48 hours of onset of symptoms if possible.[113] Prompt treatment may reduce mortality to less than 10%.[108]

PARASITIC INFECTIONS

Parasitic infections are uncommon and affect <1% of the HSCT patients. Toxoplasma is the most common infection and usually affects within first 100 days of transplant. It is typically seen in allo-HCT patients as a reactivation of their own latent infection.[114] Prophylaxis with Pyrimethamine-sulphadoxine is considered efficient but is mostly recommended in high prevalence areas of the world in seropositive recipients.[115] Cryptosporidium, microsporadium, and Giardia infection have also been reported.[116]

DIFFERENT SYNDROMES

Pulmonary Complications

Lung injury is common in HSCT patients and is associated with high morbidity and mortality. Lungs generally respond to injury with overlapping clinical and

<table>
<tr><td colspan="2">**TABLE 25.7**
Diagnostic Yield of Non-invasive diagnostic Techniques</td></tr>
<tr><td>Blood Cultures</td><td>18%[117]</td></tr>
<tr><td>Nasopharyngeal swab (PCR)</td><td>75%[117]</td></tr>
<tr><td>Computed tomography (CT scan)</td><td>31%[117]</td></tr>
<tr><td>Bronchi-alveolar lavage (BAL)</td><td>29.4%–73%</td></tr>
</table>

PCR, polymerase chain reaction.

radiographic features. Diagnostic algorithms including flexible bronchoscopy with BAL and noninvasive workup (see Table 25.7) have been validated in prospective studies.[117] PCR-based analysis of the BAL, nasopharyngeal swab, and blood has increased diagnostic yield and shortens the turnaround time for tests. Idiopathic pneumonia syndrome (IPS) is defined as an idiopathic syndrome of pneumopathy after HSCT, with evidence of widespread alveolar injury and in which infectious etiologies and cardiac dysfunction, acute renal failure, or iatrogenic fluid overload have been excluded.[118] Important differential on the IPS spectrum includes diffuse alveolar hemorrhage (DAH), engraftment syndrome, and bronchiolitis obliterans with organizing pneumonia.

DAH generally develops in the immediate post-HSCT period and is characterized by progressive shortness of breath, cough, and hypoxemia with or without fever. Mortality from DAH ranges from 60% to 100% despite treatment with high-dose corticosteroids. Engraftment syndrome represents another clinical subset of IPS. It occurs within 5 days of engraftment and can account for 33% of IPS cases after allogeneic HSCT. Corticosteroids are an important part of the treatment.[118]

Hepatitis

Hepatic injury could range from mild asymptomatic liver dysfunction to fulminant hepatic failure (see Table 25.8). Preexisting hepatic fibrosis, cholestasis, chronic HCV, or HBV infections are associated with increased risk of mortality.[119] Cholestasis may be reversible. Prophylactic ursodiol reduces the frequency of cholestasis in general and GVHD-related cholestasis in specific and improves outcomes when compared to placebo.[120] HCT recipients with preexisting cirrhosis should not receive high-dose conditioning regimens and may not be considered suitable candidates for HCT.[121]

HCV-infected patients have an overall poor survival related to infection. Hepatitis B–infected HCT recipients are at an additional risk for fulminant liver failure. This risk can be reduced by administration of antiviral

TABLE 25.8
Acute Liver Injury Can Occur Due to Multiple Reasons as Summarized in the Table Below[116]

First 3-week posttransplant
Drug toxicity
Conditioning regimens (cyclophosphamide, total body irradiation, bis-chloroethylnitrosourea, busulfan)
Calcineurin inhibitors
Azole antifungals
SOS
Sepsis, candidiasis
Ischemic liver disease

From 3 weeks to 3-month posttransplant
Acute GVHD
Drug toxicity
SOS
Hepatitis (fulminant, acute or chronic):
Viral (HBV, HCV, HSV, VZV, adenovirus) reactivation
Bacterial or fungal Infection
Fungal abscess
Gall bladder disease/cholecystitis
Hyperalimentation
Posttransplant lymphoproliferative disorder (EBV-related)

After 3-month posttransplant
Chronic GVHD
Iron overload
Chronic viral hepatitis
Drug toxicity
Liver fibrosis or cirrhosis: SOS Viral infections Hemosiderosis
Disease recurrence or new malignancy including hepatocellular carcinoma, lymphoproliferative disorder
Nodular regenerative hyperplasia
Gallbladder disease

CMV, cytomegalovirus; *EBV*, Ebstein-Barr virus; *GVHD*, graft-versus-host disease; *HCT*, hematopoietic cell transplantation; *HSV*, herpes simplex virus.
Adapted from Tuncer HH, Rana N, Milani C, et al. Gastrointestinal and hepatic complications of stem cell transplantation. *World J Gastroenterol.* 2012;18:1851–1860.

drugs throughout the transplant process.[122] Patients with symptomatic gallbladder or common duct stones should be considered for cholecystectomy or endoscopic intervention before HCT.

Sinusoidal occlusive syndrome (SOS) affects 13.7% of HCT recipients, and in severe cases it is associated with a mortality rate of 84.3%. Clinically, SOS presents with tender hepatomegaly, rapid weight gain, ascites, and jaundice. Management should focus on supportive care with intravenous fluids to maintain intravascular volume, electrolyte management, and dopamine in patients with renal failure dopamine hepatorenal syndrome.[116]

Diarrhea

Diarrhea affects 43%–91% of transplant recipients and is a major cause of morbidity and discomfort. Diarrhea in transplant recipients is mostly caused by noninfectious factors including toxic conditioning regimens leading intestinal mucosal inflammation, neutropenic enterocolitis, and prophylactic antibiotic use leading to irritable bowel syndrome, use of motility agents as antiemetic, immune-related colitis, and development of acute GVHD.[123]

Clostridium difficile (C-diff) accounts for 13%–30% of the intestinal infections.[123] Clinical sign and symptoms of infectious and acute GVHD can be similar; therefore clinical vigilance and stool assessment for C-diff toxin are strongly recommended. Recently gastrointestinal pathogen panels have been developed which can perform multiple molecular assay for simultaneous detection of bacteria, viral, and parasitic causes of infectious diarrhea.[124] Management of diarrhea includes supportive care in general and may require specific treatment of the underlying etiology. Various causes of diarrhea are summarized in Table 25.9.

Rash

Skin manifestations of acute and chronic GVHD are the most common cutaneous manifestations after HSCT. GVHD should be diagnosed in the context of concomitant liver and GI signs and symptoms. Other important differentials include drug eruptions (e.g., antibiotics), viral exanthems (e.g., Shingles), conditioning chemotherapy or radiation therapy, and skin involvement in IA or toxoplasmosis.

DONOR-DRIVEN INFECTIONS

Donor-derived infectious (DDI) diseases are infections that are present in a donor and have the potential to be transmitted to the transplant recipient. Unfortunately, diseases that are not expected or are not identified in the donor can also be transmitted to the recipient related to latent pathogens and/or unavoidable timing[125] (also see Table 25.10).

Exact incidence of DDIs in bone marrow transplant recipients is unknown, but they appear to affect 0.13% of all transplant procedures.[126] Bacteria remain the most common donor-derived infectious pathogen.[126] Other common infections include human immunodeficiency virus (HIV), hepatitis B virus (HBV), human T-cell leukemia virus (HTLV) - I/- II, hepatitis C virus (HCV), toxoplasmosis, and West Nile Virus. Some infections such as strongyloides stercoralis or coccidioidomycosis may emerge decades after initial exposure.[127] Donors should be tested as close as possible

TABLE 25.9
Differential Diagnosis of Post HCT Diarrhea
Conditioning regimen toxicity
Acute GVHD
Drug toxicity
Antibiotic-related
Opioid withdrawal
Mycophenolate mofetil toxicity
Tacrolimus (thrombotic microangiopathy)
Proton pump inhibitors
Promotility agents
Magnesium salts
Metoclopramide
Infectious
Clostridium difficile
CMV
Rotavirus
Adenovirus
EBV
HSV
Astrovirus
Norovirus
Bacterial infections including ESBL
Fungal infections
Parasitic infections (*Cryptosporidium, Microsporidia, Giardia*)
Mycobacterial infections
Others
Lactose intolerance
Malabsorption
Pancreatic insufficiency

CMV, cytomegalovirus; *EBV*, Ebstein-Barr virus; *GVHD*, graft-versus-host disease; *HCT*, hematopoietic cell transplantation; *HSV*, herpes simplex virus.
Adapted from Tuncer HH, Rana N, Milani C, et al. Gastrointestinal and hepatic complications of stem cell transplantation. *World J Gastroenterol*. 2012;18:1851–1860.

to the time of donation but at least within 28-day time period before transplant.[128]

LONG-TERM FOLLOW-UP—VACCINATION

Vaccines are proven interventions to reduce preventable disease. Vaccines are particularly important in HCT recipients who may lose acquired immunity to previously encountered pathogens. The severity of loss of this immunity can vary depending on the type of transplant (Allo vs. Auto HCT), recipients underlying malignancy, presence of GvHD, and chemotherapeutic and immunosuppressive regimens. Immunosuppression is also linked with higher virulence and chronic complications from the pathogens. This leads to HCT recipients more susceptible to infections from vaccine-preventable diseases than the general population.[129–131]

Vaccines are recommended for all HCT recipients (see Tables 25.11 and 25.12). In some cases, vaccines are also recommended for the family members, household contacts, and healthcare workers to lessen the exposure of vaccine-preventable diseases to HCT recipients. Vaccines are usually not recommended for donors due to practical and ethical difficulties with it.[132]

TABLE 25.10

Estimated Probability of Viremia Undetected by Testing Methods at the Time of Tissue Donation, According to the Blood-Donor Approach and the General-Population Approach

Pathogen	Window Period (days) for Positive Serology	Window Period (days) for Positive for Nucleic Acid Amplification
HCV	70	7
HBsAg[a]	59	20
HTLV −I/−II[b]	51	
HIV	22	7

HCT, hematopoietic cell transplantation.
[a]Testing for Hepatitis core antibody (IgM type) significantly reduces HBV transmission.[135]
[b]Serologic and molecular assays difficult to interpret.[136]
Adapted from Probability of viremia with HBV, HCV, HIV, and HTLV among tissue donors in the United States. *N Engl J Med*. 2004;351:751–759.

TABLE 25.11

Vaccination Recommendations for Both Autologous and Allogeneic HCT Recipients

Vaccine	Recommended for Use After HCT	Time Post-HCT to Initiate Vaccine	No of Doses
Pneumococcal conjugate (PCV)[a]	Yes	3–6 months	3–4
Tetanus, diphtheria, acellular pertussis[b]	Yes	6–12 months	3
Haemophilus influenazae conjugate	Yes	6–12 months	3
Meningococcal conjugate	Varies per each country recommendations	6–12 months	1
Inactivated Polio	Yes	6–12 months	3
Recombinant hepatitis B	Varies per each country recommendations	6–12	3
Inactivated influenza (yearly)[c]	Yes	4–6	1–2
Measles-Mumps-Rubella[d]	Yes	24	1–2

HCT, hematopoietic cell transplantation
[a]Conjugated 13 valent vaccine, upon completion of PCV-13 series then PPSV23. For patients with chronic GVHD who are likely to respond poorly to PPSV23, a fourth dose of the PCV should be considered instead of PPSV23.
[b]DTaP (diphtheria tetanus pertussis vaccine) is preferred, however, if only Tdap (tetanus toxoid–reduced diphtheria–toxoid reduced acellular pertussis vaccine) is available (for example, because DTaP is not licensed for adults), administer Tdap. Acellular pertussis vaccine is preferred, but the whole-cell pertussis vaccine should be used if it is the only pertussis vaccine available.
[c]Children <9 years of age, two doses are recommended yearly between transplant and 9 year of age.
[d]Measles, mumps and rubella vaccines are usually given together as combination vaccine. In females with pregnancy potential vaccination with rubella vaccine ether as a single or a combination vaccine is indicated.
Adapted from Ljungman P, Cordonnier C, Einsele H, et al. Vaccination of hematopoietic cell transplant recipients. *Bone Marrow Transplant*. 2009;44(8):521–526. Tomblyn M, Chiller T, Einsele H, et al. Guidelines for preventing infectious complications among hematopoietic cell transplantation recipients: a global perspective. *Biol Blood Marrow Transplant*. 2009;15(10):1143–1238. Tomblyn M, Chiller T, Einsele H, et al. Guidelines for preventing infectious complications among hematopoietic cell transplant recipients: a global perspective. *Pref Bone Marrow Transplant*. 2009;44(8):453–455, Copyright 2009, with permission from Macmillan Publishers Ltd.

TABLE 25.12
Optional Vaccines for Both Autologous and Allogeneic HCT Recipients

Vaccine	Recommended for Use After HCT	Time Post-HCT to Initiate Vaccine	No of Doses
Hepatitis A	Optional but strongly consider	6–12	2
Varicella (Live)	Optional	>24 months post-HCT, active GVHD or on immunosuppression	1

GVHD, graft-versus-host disease; *HCT*, hematopoietic cell transplantation.
Adapted from Ljungman P, Cordonnier C, Einsele H, et al. Vaccination of hematopoietic cell transplant recipients. *Bone Marrow Transplant.* 2009;44(8):521–526, Copyright 2009, with permission from Macmillan Publishers Ltd.

REFERENCES

1. Sahin U, Toprak SK, Atilla PA, Atilla E, Demirer T. An overview of infectious complications after allogeneic hematopoietic stem cell transplantation. *J Infect Chemother.* 2016;22(8):505–514.
2. Imran H, Tleyjeh IM, Arndt CA, et al. Fluoroquinolone prophylaxis in patients with neutropenia: a meta-analysis of randomized placebo-controlled trials. *Eur J Clin Microbiol Infect Dis.* 2008;27(1):53–63.
3. Mengarelli A, Annibali O, Pimpinelli F, et al. Prospective surveillance vs clinically driven approach for CMV reactivation after autologous stem cell transplant. *J Infect.* 2016;72(2):265–268.
4. Kim JH, Goulston C, Sanders S, et al. Cytomegalovirus reactivation following autologous peripheral blood stem cell transplantation for multiple myeloma in the era of novel chemotherapeutics and tandem transplantation. *Biol Blood Marrow Transplant.* 2012;18(11):1753–1758.
5. Ljungman P, de la Camara R, Cordonnier C, et al. Management of CMV, HHV-6, HHV-7 and Kaposi-sarcoma herpesvirus (HHV-8) infections in patients with hematological malignancies and after SCT.. *Bone Marrow Transplant.* 2008;42(4):227–240.
6. Bosch M, Dhadda M, Hoegh-Petersen M, et al. Immune reconstitution after antithymocyte globulin-conditioned hematopoietic cell transplantation. *Cytotherapy.* 2012;14(10):1258–1275.
7. Miller HK, Braun TM, Stillwell T, et al. Infectious risk after allogeneic hematopoietic cell transplantation complicated by acute graft-versus-host disease. *Biol Blood Marrow Transplant.* 2017;23(3):522–528.
8. Small TN, Cowan MJ. Immunization of hematopoietic stem cell transplant recipients against vaccine-preventable diseases. *Expert Rev Clin Immunol.* 2011;7(2):193–203.
9. Klastersky J, de Naurois J, Rolston K, et al. Management of febrile neutropaenia: ESMO clinical practice guidelines. *Ann Oncol.* 2016;27(suppl 5):v111–v118.
10. Freifeld AG, Bow EJ, Sepkowitz KA, et al. Clinical practice guideline for the use of antimicrobial agents in neutropenic patients with cancer: 2010 Update by the Infectious Diseases Society of America. *Clin Infect Dis.* 2011;52(4):427–431.
11. Celebi H, Akan H, Akcaglayan E, Ustun C, Arat M. Febrile neutropenia in allogeneic and autologous peripheral blood stem cell transplantation and conventional chemotherapy for malignancies. *Bone Marrow Transplant.* 2000;26(2):211–214.
12. de Naurois J, Novitzky-Basso I, Gill MJ, Marti FM, Cullen MH, Roila F. Management of febrile neutropenia: ESMO clinical practice guidelines. *Ann Oncol.* 2010;21(suppl 5):v252–256.
13. Chi AK, Soubani AO, White AC, Miller KB. An update on pulmonary complications of hematopoietic stem cell transplantation. *Chest.* 2013;144(6):1913–1922.
14. Aitken SL, Tarrand JJ, Deshpande LM, et al. High rates of nonsusceptibility to ceftazidime-avibactam and identification of New Delhi metallo-beta-lactamase production in Enterobacteriaceae bloodstream infections at a major cancer center. *Clin Infect Dis.* 2016;63(7):954–958.
15. Chen K, Wang Q, Pleasants RA, et al. Empiric treatment against invasive fungal diseases in febrile neutropenic patients: a systematic review and network meta-analysis. *BMC Infect Dis.* 2017;17(1):159.
16. Kubiak DW, Bryar JM, McDonnell AM, et al. Evaluation of caspofungin or micafungin as empiric antifungal therapy in adult patients with persistent febrile neutropenia: a retrospective, observational, sequential cohort analysis. *Clin Ther.* 2010;32(4):637–648.
17. Walsh TJ, Teppler H, Donowitz GR, et al. Caspofungin versus liposomal amphotericin B for empirical antifungal therapy in patients with persistent fever and neutropenia. *N Engl J Med.* 2004;351(14):1391–1402.
18. Walsh TJ, Pappas P, Winston DJ, et al. Voriconazole compared with liposomal amphotericin B for empirical antifungal therapy in patients with neutropenia and persistent fever. *N Engl J Med.* 2002;346(4):225–234.
19. Mokart D, Slehofer G, Lambert J, et al. De-escalation of antimicrobial treatment in neutropenic patients with severe sepsis: results from an observational study. *Intensive Care Med.* 2014;40(1):41–49.
20. Kaya AH, Tekgündüz E, Duygu F, et al. Risk adapted management of febrile neutrepenia and early cessation of empirical antibiotherapy in hematopoietic stem cell transplantation setting. *Balkan Med J.* 2017;34(2):132–139.

21. Valentini CG, Farina F, Pagano L, Teofili L. Granulocyte transfusions: a critical reappraisal. *Biol Blood Marrow Transplant*. 2017.

22. Wang L, Baser O, Kutikova L, Page JH, Barron R. The impact of primary prophylaxis with granulocyte colony-stimulating factors on febrile neutropenia during chemotherapy: a systematic review and meta-analysis of randomized controlled trials. *Support Care Cancer*. 2015;23(11):3131–3140.

23. Graw Jr RG, Herzig G, Perry S, Henderson ES. Normal granulocyte transfusion therapy: treatment of septicemia due to gram-negative bacteria. *N Engl J Med*. 1972;287(8):367–371.

24. Neofytos D, Horn D, Anaissie E, Steinbach W, Olyaei A, Fishman J. Epidemiology and outcome of invasive fungal infection in adult hematopoietic stem cell transplant recipients: analysis of Multicenter Prospective Antifungal Therapy (PATH) Alliance registry. *Clin Infect Dis*. 2009;48.

25. De Pauw B, Walsh TJ, Donnelly JP, et al. Revised definitions of invasive fungal disease from the European Organization for research and treatment of cancer/invasive fungal infections cooperative group and the National Institute of Allergy and Infectious Diseases Mycoses Study Group (EORTC/MSG) Consensus group. *Clin Infect Dis*. 2008;46(12):1813–1821.

26. Thaler M, Pastakia B, Shawker TH, O'Leary T, Pizzo PA. Hepatic candidiasis in cancer patients: the evolving picture of the syndrome. *Ann Intern Med*. 1988;108(1):88–100.

27. Mikulska M, Calandra T, Sanguinetti M, Poulain D, Viscoli C. The use of mannan antigen and anti-mannan antibodies in the diagnosis of invasive candidiasis: recommendations from the Third European Conference on Infections in Leukemia. *Crit Care*. 2010;14(6):R222.

28. Nguyen MH, Wissel MC, Shields RK, et al. Performance of Candida real-time polymerase chain reaction, beta-D-glucan assay, and blood cultures in the diagnosis of invasive candidiasis. *Clin Infect Dis*. 2012;54(9):1240–1248.

29. Lau A, Halliday C, Chen SC, Playford EG, Stanley K, Sorrell TC. Comparison of whole blood, serum, and plasma for early detection of candidemia by multiplex-tandem PCR. *J Clin Microbiol*. 2010;48(3):811–816.

30. Tissot F, Agrawal S, Pagano L, et al. ECIL-6 guidelines for the treatment of invasive candidiasis, aspergillosis and mucormycosis in leukemia and hematopoietic stem cell transplant patients. *Haematologica*. 2017;102(3):433–444.

31. Pappas PG, Kauffman CA, Andes DR, et al. Clinical practice guideline for the management of candidiasis: 2016 update by the Infectious Diseases Society of America. *Clin Infect Dis*. 2016;62(4):e1–e50.

32. Harrison N, Mitterbauer M, Tobudic S, et al. Incidence and characteristics of invasive fungal diseases in allogeneic hematopoietic stem cell transplant recipients: a retrospective cohort study. *BMC Infect Dis*. 2015;15(1):584.

33. Corzo-Leon DE, Satlin MJ, Soave R, et al. Epidemiology and outcomes of invasive fungal infections in allogeneic haematopoietic stem cell transplant recipients in the era of antifungal prophylaxis: a single-centre study with focus on emerging pathogens. *Mycoses*. 2015;58(6):325–336.

34. Patterson TF, Thompson III GR, Denning DW, et al. Practice guidelines for the diagnosis and management of aspergillosis: 2016 update by the Infectious Diseases Society of America. *Clin Infect Dis*. 2016;63(4):e1–e60.

35. Labbe AC, Su SH, Laverdiere M, et al. High incidence of invasive aspergillosis associated with intestinal graft-versus-host disease following nonmyeloablative transplantation. *Biol Blood Marrow Transplant*. 2007;13(10):1192–1200.

36. Miyakoshi S, Kusumi E, Matsumura T, et al. Invasive fungal infection following reduced-intensity cord blood transplantation for adult patients with hematologic diseases. *Biol Blood Marrow Transplant*. 2007;13(7):771–777.

37. Chellapandian D, Lehrnbecher T, Phillips B, et al. Bronchoalveolar lavage and lung biopsy in patients with cancer and hematopoietic stem-cell transplantation recipients: a systematic review and meta-analysis. *J Clin Oncol*. 2015;33(5):501–509.

38. Herbrecht R, Denning DW, Patterson TF, et al. Voriconazole versus amphotericin B for primary therapy of invasive aspergillosis. *N Engl J Med*. 2002;347(6):408–415.

39. Maertens JA, Raad II, Marr KA, et al. Isavuconazole versus voriconazole for primary treatment of invasive mould disease caused by Aspergillus and other filamentous fungi (SECURE): a phase 3, randomised-controlled, non-inferiority trial. *Lancet*. 2016;387(10020):760–769.

40. Park BJ, Pappas PG, Wannemuehler KA, et al. Invasive non-Aspergillus mold infections in transplant recipients, United States, 2001–2006. *Emerg Infect Dis*. 2011;17(10):1855–1864.

41. Marr KA, Carter RA, Crippa F, Wald A, Corey L. Epidemiology and outcome of mould infections in hematopoietic stem cell transplant recipients. *Clin Infect Dis*. 2002;34(7):909–917.

42. Kontoyiannis DP, Lionakis MS, Lewis RE, et al. Zygomycosis in a tertiary-care cancer center in the era of Aspergillus-active antifungal therapy: a case-control observational study of 27 recent cases. *J Infect Dis*. 2005;191(8):1350–1360.

43. Millon L, Herbrecht R, Grenouillet F, et al. Early diagnosis and monitoring of mucormycosis by detection of circulating DNA in serum: retrospective analysis of 44 cases collected through the French Surveillance Network of Invasive Fungal Infections (RESSIF). *Clin Microbiol Infect*. 2016;22(9):810.e811–810.e818.

44. Walsh TJ, Gamaletsou MN, McGinnis MR, Hayden RT, Kontoyiannis DP. Early clinical and laboratory diagnosis of invasive pulmonary, extrapulmonary, and disseminated mucormycosis (zygomycosis). *Clin Infect Dis*. 2012;54(suppl 1):S55–S60.

45. Ibrahim AS, Gebremariam T, Fu Y, Edwards Jr JE, Spellberg B. Combination echinocandin-polyene treatment of murine mucormycosis. *Antimicrob Agents Chemother.* 2008;52(4):1556–1558.

46. Sepkowitz KA, Brown AE, Telzak EE, Gottlieb S, Armstrong D. Pneumocystis carinii pneumonia among patients without AIDS at a cancer hospital. *Jama.* 1992;267(6):832–837.

47. Rodriguez M, Fishman JA. Prevention of infection due to Pneumocystis spp. in human immunodeficiency virus-negative immunocompromised patients. *Clin Microbiol Rev.* 2004;17(4):770–782.

48. Williams KM, Ahn KW, Chen M, et al. The incidence, mortality and timing of Pneumocystis jiroveci pneumonia after hematopoietic cell transplantation: a CIBMTR(®) analysis. *Bone Marrow Transplant.* 2016;51(4):573–580.

49. Cordonnier C, Cesaro S, Maschmeyer G, et al. Pneumocystis jirovecii pneumonia: still a concern in patients with haematological malignancies and stem cell transplant recipients. *J Antimicrob Chemother.* 2016;71(9):2379–2385.

50. Maschmeyer G, Helweg-Larsen J, Pagano L, Robin C, Cordonnier C, Schellongowski P. ECIL guidelines for treatment of Pneumocystis jirovecii pneumonia in non-HIV-infected haematology patients. *J Antimicrob Chemother.* 2016;71(9):2405–2413.

51. Song Y, Ren Y, Wang X, Li R. Recent advances in the diagnosis of Pneumocystis pneumonia. *Med Mycol J.* 2016;57(4):E111–e116.

52. Boeckh M, Nichols WG, Papanicolaou G, Rubin R, Wingard JR, Zaia J. Cytomegalovirus in hematopoietic stem cell transplant recipients: current status, known challenges, and future strategies. *Biol Blood Marrow Transplant.* 2003;9(9):543–558.

53. Rowe RG, Guo D, Lee M, Margossian S, London WB, Lehmann L. Cytomegalovirus infection in pediatric hematopoietic stem cell transplantation: risk factors for primary infection and cases of recurrent and late infection at a single center. *Biol Blood Marrow Transplant.* 2016;22(7):1275–1283.

54. Tan SK, Burgener EB, Waggoner JJ, et al. Molecular and culture-based bronchoalveolar lavage fluid testing for the diagnosis of cytomegalovirus pneumonitis. *Open Forum Infect Dis.* 2016;3(1):ofv212.

55. Machado CM, Dulley FL, Boas LS, et al. CMV pneumonia in allogeneic BMT recipients undergoing early treatment of pre-emptive ganciclovir therapy. *Bone Marrow Transplant.* 2000;26(4):413–417.

56. Ruutu T, Ljungman P, Brinch L, et al. No prevention of cytomegalovirus infection by anti-cytomegalovirus hyperimmune globulin in seronegative bone marrow transplant recipients. The Nordic BMT Group. *Bone Marrow Transplant.* 1997;19(3):233–236.

57. Messori A, Rampazzo R, Scroccaro G, Martini N. Efficacy of hyperimmune anti-cytomegalovirus immunoglobulins for the prevention of cytomegalovirus infection in recipients of allogeneic bone marrow transplantation: a meta-analysis. *Bone Marrow Transplant.* 1994;13(2):163–167.

58. Zikos P, Van Lint M, Lamparelli T, et al. A randomized trial of high dose polyvalent intravenous immunoglobulin (HDIgG) vs. Cytomegalovirus (CMV) hyperimmune IgG in allogeneic hemopoietic stem cell transplants (HSCT). *Haematologica.* 1998;83(2):132–137.

59. Prentice HG, Gluckman E, Powles RL, et al. Impact of long-term acyclovir on cytomegalovirus infection and survival after allogeneic bone marrow transplantation. European Acyclovir for CMV Prophylaxis Study Group. *Lancet.* 1994;343(8900):749–753.

60. Boeckh M, Nichols W, Chemaly RF, et al. Valganciclovir for the prevention of complications of late cytomegalovirus infection after allogeneic hematopoietic cell transplantation: a randomized trial. *Ann Intern Med.* 2015;162(1):1–10.

61. Boeckh M, Gooley T, Myerson D, Cunningham T, Schoch G, Bowden R. Cytomegalovirus pp65 antigenemia-guided early treatment with ganciclovir versus ganciclovir at engraftment after allogeneic marrow transplantation: a randomized double-blind study. *Blood.* 1996;88(10):4063–4071.

62. Goodrich JM, Bowden RA, Fisher L, Keller C, Schoch G, Meyers JD. Ganciclovir prophylaxis to prevent cytomegalovirus disease after allogeneic marrow transplant. *Ann Intern Med.* 1993;118(3):173–178.

63. Winston DJ, Ho WG, Bartoni K, et al. Ganciclovir prophylaxis of cytomegalovirus infection and disease in allogeneic bone marrow transplant recipients. Results of a placebo-controlled, double-blind trial. *Ann Intern Med.* 1993;118(3):179–184.

64. Boeckh M, Boivin G. Quantitation of cytomegalovirus: methodologic aspects and clinical applications. *Clin Microbiol Rev.* 1998;11(3):533–554.

65. Mattes FM, Hainsworth EG, Geretti AM, et al. A randomized, controlled trial comparing ganciclovir to ganciclovir plus foscarnet (each at half dose) for preemptive therapy of cytomegalovirus infection in transplant recipients. *J Infect Dis.* 2004;189(8):1355–1361.

66. Chawla JS, Ghobadi A, Mosley 3rd J, et al. Oral valganciclovir versus ganciclovir as delayed pre-emptive therapy for patients after allogeneic hematopoietic stem cell transplant: a pilot trial (04-0274) and review of the literature. *Transpl Infect Dis.* 2012;14(3):259–267.

67. Ichihara H, Nakamae H, Hirose A, et al. Immunoglobulin prophylaxis against cytomegalovirus infection in patients at high risk of infection following allogeneic hematopoietic cell transplantation. *Transplant Proc.* 2011;43(10):3927–3932.

68. Platzbecker U, Bandt D, Thiede C, et al. Successful preemptive cidofovir treatment for CMV antigenemia after dose-reduced conditioning and allogeneic blood stem cell transplantation. *Transplantation.* 2001;71(7):880–885.

69. Ljungman P, Deliliers GL, Platzbecker U, et al. Cidofovir for cytomegalovirus infection and disease in allogeneic stem cell transplant recipients. The infectious diseases working party of the European group for blood and marrow transplantation. *Blood.* 2001;97(2):388–392.

70. Tan SK, Waggoner JJ, Pinsky BA. Cytomegalovirus load at treatment initiation is predictive of time to resolution of viremia and duration of therapy in hematopoietic cell transplant recipients. *J Clin Virol.* 2015;69:179–183.

71. Peggs KS, Verfuerth S, Pizzey A, Chow SL, Thomson K, Mackinnon S. Cytomegalovirus-specific T cell immunotherapy promotes restoration of durable functional antiviral immunity following allogeneic stem cell transplantation. *Clin Infect Dis.* 2009;49(12):1851–1860.

72. Hassan Z, Remberger M, Svenberg P, et al. Hemorrhagic cystitis: a retrospective single-center survey. *Clin Transplant.* 2007;21(5):659–667.

73. Yamamoto R, Kusumi E, Kami M, et al. Late hemorrhagic cystitis after reduced-intensity hematopoietic stem cell transplantation (RIST). *Bone Marrow Transplant.* 2003;32(11):1089–1095.

74. Leung AY, Suen CK, Lie AK, Liang RH, Yuen KY, Kwong YL. Quantification of polyoma BK viruria in hemorrhagic cystitis complicating bone marrow transplantation. *Blood.* 2001;98(6):1971–1978.

75. Azzi A, Cesaro S, Laszlo D, et al. Human polyomavirus BK (BKV) load and haemorrhagic cystitis in bone marrow transplantation patients. *J Clin Virol.* 1999;14(2):79–86.

76. Bedi A, Miller CB, Hanson JL, et al. Association of BK virus with failure of prophylaxis against hemorrhagic cystitis following bone marrow transplantation. *J Clin Oncol.* 1995;13(5):1103–1109.

77. Dosin G, Aoun F, El Rassy E, et al. Viral-induced hemorrhagic cystitis after allogeneic hematopoietic stem cell transplant. *Clin Lymphoma Myeloma Leuk.* 2017;17(7):438–442.

78. Yaghobi R, Ramzi M, Dehghani S. The role of different risk factors in clinical presentation of hemorrhagic cystitis in hematopoietic stem cell transplant recipients. *Transplant Proc.* 2009;41(7):2900–2902.

79. Tsuboi K, Kishi K, Ohmachi K, et al. Multivariate analysis of risk factors for hemorrhagic cystitis after hematopoietic stem cell transplantation. *Bone Marrow Transplant.* 2003;32(9):903–907.

80. Miller AN, Glode A, Hogan KR, et al. Efficacy and safety of ciprofloxacin for prophylaxis of polyomavirus BK virus-associated hemorrhagic cystitis in allogeneic hematopoietic stem cell transplantatin recipients. *Biol Blood Marrow Transplant.* 2011;17(8):1176–1181.

81. Vu D, Shah T, Ansari J, Naraghi R, Min D. Efficacy of intravenous immunoglobulin in the treatment of persistent BK viremia and BK virus nephropathy in renal transplant recipients. *Transplant Proc.* 2015;47(2):394–398.

82. Philippe M, Ranchon F, Gilis L, et al. Cidofovir in the treatment of BK virus-associated hemorrhagic cystitis after allogeneic hematopoietic stem cell transplantation. *Biol Blood Marrow Transplant.* 2016;22(4):723–730.

83. Lee S-S, Ahn J-S, Jung S-H, et al. Treatment of BK virus-associated hemorrhagic cystitis with low-dose intravenous cidofovir in patients undergoing allogeneic hematopoietic cell transplantation. *Korean J Intern Med.* 2015;30(2):212–218.

84. Sakurada M, Kondo T, Umeda M, Kawabata H, Yamashita K, Takaori-Kondo A. Successful treatment with intravesical cidofovir for virus-associated hemorrhagic cystitis after allogeneic hematopoietic stem cell transplantation: a case report and a review of the literature. *J Infect Chemother.* 2016;22(7):495–500.

85. Park YH, Lim JH, Yi HG, Lee MH, Kim CS. BK virus-hemorrhagic cystitis following allogeneic stem cell transplantation: clinical characteristics and utility of Leflunomide treatment. *Turkish J Hematol.* 2016;33(3):223–230.

86. Tzannou I, Papadopoulou A, Naik S, et al. Off-the-Shelf virus-specific T cells to treat BK virus, human herpesvirus 6, cytomegalovirus, Epstein-Barr virus, and adenovirus infections after allogeneic hematopoietic stem-cell transplantation. *J Clin Oncol.* 2017;35(31):3547–3557.

87. Yamanishi KMY, Pellett PE. Human Herpesvirus 6 and 7. In: 6th ed. Knipe DM, Howley P, eds. *Fields Virology.* Vol. 2. Philadelphia: Wolters Kluwer Health; 2013:2058.

88. Zerr DM, Meier AS, Selke SS, et al. A population-based study of primary human herpesvirus 6 infection. *N Engl J Med.* 2005;352(8):768–776.

89. Pellett PE, Ablashi DV, Ambros PF, et al. Chromosomally integrated human herpesvirus 6: questions and answers. *Rev Med Virol.* 2012;22(3):144–155.

90. Sedlak RH, Hill JA, Nguyen T, et al. Detection of human herpesvirus 6B (HHV-6B) reactivation in hematopoietic cell transplant recipients with inherited chromosomally integrated HHV-6A by droplet digital PCR. *J Clin Microbiol.* 2016;54(5):1223–1227.

91. Colombier MA, Amorim S, Salmona M, Thieblemont C, Legoff J, Lafaurie M. HHV-6 reactivation as a cause of fever in autologous hematopoietic stem cell transplant recipients. *J Infect.* 2017;75(2):155–159.

92. Blennow O, Fjaertoft G, Winiarski J, Ljungman P, Mattsson J, Remberger M. Varicella-zoster reactivation after allogeneic stem cell transplantation without routine prophylaxis—the incidence remains high. *Biol Blood Marrow Transplant.* 2014;20(10):1646–1649.

93. Kamber C, Zimmerli S, Suter-Riniker F, et al. Varicella zoster virus reactivation after autologous SCT is a frequent event and associated with favorable outcome in myeloma patients. *Bone Marrow Transplant.* 2015;50(4):573–578.

94. Arvin AM. Varicella-zoster virus: pathogenesis, immunity, and clinical management in hematopoietic cell transplant recipients. *Biol Blood Marrow Transplant.* 2000;6(3):219–230.

95. Seo HM, Kim YS, Bang CH, et al. Antiviral prophylaxis for preventing herpes zoster in hematopoietic stem cell transplant recipients: a systematic review and meta-analysis. *Antivir Res.* 2017;140:106–115.

96. Marin MGD, Chaves SS. Prevention of varicella: recommendations of the Advisory Committee on Immunization Practices (ACIP). *MMWR Recomm Rep.* 2007;56(RR-4):1. https://www.cdc.gov/mmwr/preview/mmwrhtml/rr5604a1.htm. 2007.

97. Wade JC, Newton B, Flournoy N, Meyers JD. Oral acyclovir for prevention of herpes simplex virus reactiva-

tion after marrow transplantation. *Ann Intern Med.* 1984;100(6):823–828.

98. Saral R, Burns WH, Laskin OL, Santos GW, Lietman PS. Acyclovir prophylaxis of herpes-simplex-virus infections. *N Engl J Med.* 1981;305(2):63–67.

99. Dignani MC, Mykietiuk A, Michelet M, et al. Valacyclovir prophylaxis for the prevention of Herpes simplex virus reactivation in recipients of progenitor cells transplantation. *Bone Marrow Transplant.* 2002;29(3):263–267.

100. El-Haddad D, El Chaer F, Vanichanan J, et al. Brincidofovir (CMX-001) for refractory and resistant CMV and HSV infections in immunocompromised cancer patients: a single-center experience. *Antivir Res.* 2016;134:58–62.

101. Piret J, Boivin G. Antiviral drug resistance in herpesviruses other than cytomegalovirus. *Rev Med Virol.* 2014;24(3):186–218.

102. van Esser JW, van der Holt B, Meijer E, et al. Epstein-Barr virus (EBV) reactivation is a frequent event after allogeneic stem cell transplantation (SCT) and quantitatively predicts EBV-lymphoproliferative disease following T-cell–depleted SCT. *Blood.* 2001;98(4):972–978.

103. Nash RA, Dansey R, Storek J, et al. Epstein-Barr virus-associated posttransplantation lymphoproliferative disorder after high-dose immunosuppressive therapy and autologous CD34-selected hematopoietic stem cell transplantation for severe autoimmune diseases. *Biol Blood Marrow Transplant.* 2003;9(9):583–591.

104. Rasche L, Kapp M, Einsele H, Mielke S. EBV-induced post transplant lymphoproliferative disorders: a persisting challenge in allogeneic hematopoetic SCT. *Bone Marrow Transplant.* 2014;49(2):163–167.

105. van Esser JW, Niesters HG, van der Holt B, et al. Prevention of Epstein-Barr virus-lymphoproliferative disease by molecular monitoring and preemptive rituximab in high-risk patients after allogeneic stem cell transplantation. *Blood.* 2002;99(12):4364–4369.

106. Leen AM, Christin A, Myers GD, et al. Cytotoxic T lymphocyte therapy with donor T cells prevents and treats adenovirus and Epstein-Barr virus infections after haploidentical and matched unrelated stem cell transplantation. *Blood.* 2009;114(19):4283–4292.

107. Dignan FL, Clark A, Aitken C, et al. BCSH/BSBMT/UK clinical virology network guideline: diagnosis and management of common respiratory viral infections in patients undergoing treatment for haematological malignancies or stem cell transplantation. *Br J Haematol.* 2016;173(3):380–393.

108. Abbas S, Raybould JE, Sastry S, de la Cruz O. Respiratory viruses in transplant recipients: more than just a cold. Clinical syndromes and infection prevention principles. *Int J Infect Dis.* 2017;62:86–93.

109. Chemaly RF, Shah DP, Boeckh MJ. Management of respiratory viral infections in hematopoietic cell transplant recipients and patients with hematologic malignancies. *Clin Infect Dis.* 2014;59(suppl 5):S344–S351.

110. Shah JN, Chemaly RF. Management of RSV infections in adult recipients of hematopoietic stem cell transplantation. *Blood.* 2011;117(10):2755–2763.

111. Shah DP, Ghantoji SS, Shah JN, et al. Impact of aerosolized ribavirin on mortality in 280 allogeneic haematopoietic stem cell transplant recipients with respiratory syncytial virus infections. *J Antimicrob Chemother.* 2013;68(8):1872–1880.

112. Grimley MPG, Prasad VK, et al. *Treatment of Adenovirus (AdV) Infection in Allogeneic Hematopoietic Cell Transplant (HCT) Patients (Pts) with Brincidofovir: 24-week Interim Results from the AdVise Trial. ID Week.* New Orleans, LA: Infectious Diseases Society of America; 2016:2339:abstract.

113. Suyani E, Aki Z, Guzel O, Altindal S, Senol E, Sucak G. H1N1 infection in a cohort of hematopoietic stem cell transplant recipients: prompt antiviral therapy might be life saving. *Transpl Infect Dis.* 2011;13(2):208–212.

114. Derouin F, Pelloux H. Prevention of toxoplasmosis in transplant patients. *Clin Microbiol Infect.* 2008;14(12):1089–1101.

115. Foot AB, Garin YJ, Ribaud P, Devergie A, Derouin F, Gluckman E. Prophylaxis of toxoplasmosis infection with pyrimethamine/sulfadoxine (Fansidar) in bone marrow transplant recipients. *Bone Marrow Transplant.* 1994;14(2):241–245.

116. Tuncer HH, Rana N, Milani C, Darko A, Al-Homsi SA. Gastrointestinal and hepatic complications of hematopoietic stem cell transplantation. *World J Gastroenterology WJG.* 2012;18(16):1851–1860.

117. Lucena CM, Torres A, Rovira M, et al. Pulmonary complications in hematopoietic SCT: a prospective study. *Bone Marrow Transplant.* 2014;49(10):1293–1299.

118. Panoskaltsis-Mortari A, Griese M, Madtes DK, et al. An official American Thoracic Society research statement: noninfectious lung injury after hematopoietic stem cell transplantation: idiopathic pneumonia syndrome. *Am J Respir Crit Care Med.* 2011;183(9):1262–1279.

119. Strasser SI, Myerson D, Spurgeon CL, et al. Hepatitis C virus infection and bone marrow transplantation: a cohort study with 10-year follow-up. *Hepatology.* 1999;29(6):1893–1899.

120. Ruutu T, Eriksson B, Remes K, et al. Ursodeoxycholic acid for the prevention of hepatic complications in allogeneic stem cell transplantation. *Blood.* 2002;100(6):1977–1983.

121. Hogan WJ, Maris M, Storer B, et al. Hepatic injury after nonmyeloablative conditioning followed by allogeneic hematopoietic cell transplantation: a study of 193 patients. *Blood.* 2004;103(1):78–84.

122. McDonald GB. Hepatobiliary complications of hematopoietic cell transplant, 40 years on. *Hepatol Baltim Md.* 2010;51(4):1450–1460.

123. Cox GJ, Matsui SM, Lo RS, et al. Etiology and outcome of diarrhea after marrow transplantation: a prospective study. *Gastroenterology.* 1994;107(5):1398–1407.

124. Claas EC, Burnham CA, Mazzulli T, Templeton K, Topin F. Performance of the xTAG(R) gastrointestinal pathogen panel, a multiplex molecular assay for simultaneous detection of bacterial, viral, and parasitic

causes of infectious gastroenteritis. *J Microbiol Biotechnol.* 2013;23(7):1041–1045.

125. Avery KRFJ *Infectious Diseases in Transplantation.* http://wwwblackwellpublishingcom/content/hricikastprimercom/chapters/c04pdf.

126. Green M, Covington S, Taranto S, et al. Donor-derived transmission events in 2013: a report of the organ procurement transplant network ad hoc disease transmission advisory committee. *Transplantation.* 2015;99(2):282–287.

127. Fishman JA. Infection in organ transplantation. *Am J Transplant.* 2017;17(4):856–879.

128. Seem DL, Lee I, Umscheid CA, Kuehnert MJ. PHS guideline for reducing human immunodeficiency virus, hepatitis B virus, and hepatitis C virus transmission through organ transplantation. *Public Health Rep.* 2013;128(4):247–343.

129. Frieden TRKR https://www.cdc.gov/oid/docs/ID-Framework.pdf.

130. Ariza-Heredia EJ, Gulbis AM, Stolar KR, et al. Vaccination guidelines after hematopoietic stem cell transplantation: practitioners' knowledge, attitudes, and gap between guidelines and clinical practice. *Transplant Infect Dis.* 2014;16(6):878–886.

131. Aucouturier P, Barra A, Intrator L, et al. Long lasting IgG subclass and antibacterial polysaccharide antibody deficiency after allogeneic bone marrow transplantation. *Blood.* 1987;70(3):779–785.

132. Ljungman P, Cordonnier C, Einsele H, et al. Vaccination of hematopoietic cell transplant recipients. *Bone Marrow Transplant.* 2009;44(8):521–526.

133. Einsele H, Ehninger G, Hebart H, et al. Polymerase chain reaction monitoring reduces the incidence of cytomegalovirus disease and the duration and side effects of antiviral therapy after bone marrow transplantation. *Blood.* 1995;86(7):2815–2820.

134. Boeckh M, Bowden RA, Gooley T, Myerson D, Corey L. Successful modification of a pp65 antigenemia-based early treatment strategy for prevention of cytomegalovirus disease in allogeneic marrow transplant recipients. *Blood.* 1999;93(5):1781–1782.

135. Allain J-P, Hewitt PE, Tedder RS, Williamson LM. For the anti Hssg. Evidence that anti-HBc but not HBV DNA testing may prevent some HBV transmission by transfusion. *Br J Haematol.* 1999;107(1):186–195.

136. Ison MG, Hager J, Blumberg E, et al. Donor-derived disease transmission events in the United States: data reviewed by the OPTN/UNOS Disease Transmission Advisory Committee. *Am J Transpl.* 2009;9(8):1929–1935.

137. Tomblyn M, Chiller T, Einsele H, et al. Guidelines for preventing infectious complications among hematopoietic cell transplantation recipients: a global perspective. *Biol Blood Marrow Transplant.* 2009;15(10):1143–1238.

138. Tomblyn M, Chiller T, Einsele H, et al. Guidelines for preventing infectious complications among hematopoietic cell transplant recipients: a global perspective. *Pref Bone Marrow Transplant.* 2009;44(8):453–455.

Hematopoietic Stem Cell Transplantation for Hematologic Malignancies in HIV-Positive Patients

LIANA NIKOLAENKO, MD • AMRITA KRISHNAN, MD

INTRODUCTION

The introduction of combination antiretroviral therapy (cART) in the 1990s has improved the survival of patients with human immunodeficiency virus-1 (HIV-1) infection worldwide.[1-3] However, HIV-1–infected patients are at higher risk for developing AIDS-related lymphoma, such as non-Hodgkin lymphoma (NHL), as well as other hematologic malignancies, including Hodgkin lymphoma, multiple myeloma, and leukemia. The incidence of lymphomas in HIV-infected patients has decreased with widespread use of cART.[4,5] In turn, the treatment strategies have changed for HIV-1–infected patients with hematologic malignancies with the implementation of aggressive induction chemotherapy improving overall survival (OS) for patients with AIDS-related lymphomas.[6] For example, the complete remission (CR) rate in the era of pre-CART and post-CART implementation improved from 47% to 61%, as did 2-year progression-free survival (PFS) from 43% to 65% and 2-year OS from 24% to 57%. The most significant improvements were seen between the years of 2005 and 2010, with CR 65%, 2-year PFS of 76%, and 2-year OS of 67%.[7]

High-dose therapy followed by autologous stem cell transplantation (ASCT) is a well-established treatment option in the relapsed setting for NHL and classical Hodgkin lymphoma (cHL) as well as a consolidation treatment for multiple myeloma and allogeneic stem cell transplant (allo-SCT) similarly for acute leukemia in HIV-negative patients. Recent studies have shown that combination of cART and ASCT in HIV-infected patients on cART with relapsed lymphoma is a feasible treatment option and that outcomes are similar to those in HIV-negative patients.[8] Similarly, case series have reported favorable outcomes for allo-SCT for HIV-positive patients with hematologic malignancies.[9] Thus we now have ample data to demonstrate that HIV-1 infection is not a contraindication to stem cell transplantation and may be performed with similar outcomes to the HIV-negative population.

cART suppresses replication of HIV allowing for immune reconstitution and T-cell recovery; however, HIV-1 can persist in its latent form in the resting CD4+ cells and macrophages that contain an integrated copy of the viral DNA in the host genome. Discontinuation of cART ultimately leads to rebound rises in HIV-1 viral load with subsequent replication and immunodeficiency.[10] Hence cART is unlikely able to eradicate the virus and HIV-1 reservoir. High-dose therapy as part of conditioning regimen for stem cell transplantation with myelodepletion and elimination of host lymphoid cells did not result in cure of HIV-1 infection, but an intriguing possibility is the potential to cure HIV-1 infection by using stem cell transplantation with HIV-resistant stem cells.[11,12] Options for this include allogeneic stem cell transplantation using an HIV-1–resistant stem cell source such as CCR5-delta 32 homozygous donors or genetically modified CCR5-resistant autologous or allogeneic stem cells.

Since the introduction of cART, there have been substantial developments and improvement in treatment options for patients with HIV-1 infection affected by hematologic malignancies. In this chapter we will review the current treatment approach to HIV-associated hematologic malignancies, the role of ASCT and allogeneic transplant in HIV-positive patients, and the recent advances in treatment strategies that are evolving for the goal of an HIV/AIDS cure.

EPIDEMIOLOGY OF HIV-ASSOCIATED LYMPHOMA

HIV-Associated Lymphoma

Although survival of HIV-infected patients has improved with the implementation of cART, the cancer incidence and associated mortality rates remain substantial.[13] HIV infection is associated with an increased risk of NHL, especially B-cell lymphomas.[14] The reported incidence of systemic NHL in Europe was 463 per 100,000 person-years not on cART and 205 per 100,000 person-years patients on antiviral treatment, The United States reported a crude annual percent change from −15.7% (1996–2003) to −5.5% (2003–10) for NHL and −4.0% for HL (1996–2010).[4,15] NHL is considered an AIDS-defining illness and comprises 53% of all AIDS-defining malignancies and is the most common cause of cancer-related deaths in HIV-infected individuals in the United States. As aforementioned, the incidence of NHL declined in the era of cART, but the incidence of cHL continued to increase during 1996–2006.[16,17]

Lymphomas in the HIV setting tend to be aggressive in clinical presentation, with advanced-stage disease and extranodal sites of disease being common. Standard treatment for B-cell NHL is a combination of immunochemotherapy with rituximab in combination with multidrug chemotherapy, such as CHOP (cyclophosphamide, doxorubicin, vincristine, and prednisone). Initial studies, however, reported inferior outcomes in HIV-positive patients treated with rituximab combination chemotherapy due to high infectious complications.[18] The AIDS Malignancy Consortium in a randomized phase 3 study evaluating the addition of rituximab to CHOP in HIV-associated NHL showed a higher risk of treatment-related death than CHOP alone, 14% versus 2%, P = .035 However, subsequent studies reported the feasibility and survival benefit of combination immunochemotherapy, such as infusional EPOCH (etoposide, vincristine, doxorubicin, cyclophosphamide, and prednisone) with rituximab showing complete response (CR) of 73% and mortality rate of 9.8% due to opportunistic infections. Two-year PFS and OS were 66% and 70%, respectively.[19] However, although it became an accepted paradigm to use standard dose chemotherapy such as the described regimens in the treatment of HIV-associated NHL and cHL, the use of high-dose chemotherapy was initially considered not feasible.

ASCT IN HIV PATIENTS

The initial reticence for the use of high-dose therapy in HIV-1 patients was due to earlier poor outcomes of ASCT in HIV-positive patients in the pre-cART era. A case report of a 40-year-old male with HIV-1 infection and relapsed NHL treated with high-dose conditioning BEAM (BCNU [carmustine], etoposide, arabinofuranosyl

cytidine [cytarabine], and melphalan) and ASCT described a complicated posttransplant course with multiple opportunistic infections including cytomegalovirus viremia, mycobacterium pneumonia, and cryptosporidiosis, underscoring the risk conferred by AIDS-related immune dysfunction after stem cell transplantation. However, the report also demonstrated the feasibility of mobilizing stem cells and successful engraftment in the bone marrow despite active viral replication.[20]

A later French study in the early era of cART described autologous transplantation in eight patients with AIDS and refractory or relapsed lymphoma, who had undetectable HIV-1 plasma levels while on cART. The patients received conditioning regimens consisting either of radiation plus chemotherapy or chemotherapy alone. Four of eight patients were alive, and in complete remission at the time of reporting, three died of lymphoma within 3 months after ASCT and one died of an opportunistic infection.[21] This laid the foundation that high-dose therapy was feasible and could lead to control of the lymphoma in HIV-positive patients.

An EBMT retrospective case-control study comparing 53 HIV-1–infected lymphoma patients (66% NHL and 34% HL) with 53 HIV-1–negative controls matched for histology, non–age-adjusted international prognostic index, and disease status at the time of transplant demonstrated the minimum effect of HIV-1 infection on the outcome. OS was 61.5% for HIV-1–positive patients and 70% for controls (P=not significant). There was a trend toward delayed platelet engraftment in the HIV-1 cohort. A nonstatistically significant difference in nonrelapse mortality was reported in the HIV-1–infected cohort (8% vs. 2%), primarily due to the higher rate of bacterial infections.[8] This study provided evidence that ASCT led to similar outcomes and survival for patients with HIV lymphoma as compared with patients without HIV-1 infection with no significant difference in PFS or OS per histology or disease status before ASCT.

Another EBMT retrospective multicenter study with 68 patients from 20 institutions reported outcomes with ASCT in high-risk patients in first CR (n = 16), with relapsed disease (n = 44), or chemorefractory disease (n = 8). Relapse or progression after ASCT occurred in 29.5% of patients, and treatment-related mortality was 7.5%, mainly due to bacterial infections. At a median follow-up of 32 months, PFS was 56%, and analysis of prognostic factors demonstrated that histology, other than diffuse large B cell lymphoma, the use of more than two regimens, and not achieving CR at the time of transplant were significantly associated with a higher risk of post-ASCT relapse.[22] The study included patients with chemotherapy refractory disease, which is a challenging-to-treat group of patients irrespective of the HIV status but demonstrated feasibility of the procedure.

The multicenter phase II study (BMT CTN0803/AMC 071) evaluated ASCT for HIV-infected patients with chemotherapy-sensitive relapsed or refractory HL or NHL. This trial was important as it had a standard conditioning regimen and also was designed to see if the single institution outcomes could be replicated in a multicenter trial. Forty-three patients were enrolled of which 40 underwent ASCT. The conditioning regimen was with BEAM chemotherapy for all patients. At the time of enrollment, the HIV viral load was undetectable (<50 copies/mL) in 80% of the patients, and median CD4 count was 249/μL (range 39–797). One-year and 2-year OS probabilities were 87.3% and 82%, respectively, with 2-year PFS probability of 79.8%, and the estimated risk of 1-year treatment-related mortality (TRM) was 5.2%.[23] This study clearly demonstrated favorable outcomes in this patient population using ASCT for treatment of aggressive HIV lymphoma and was consistent with the previously published European results.

The challenges and caveats of managing HIV-positive patients in the peritransplant setting were well described by the City of Hope group. Their initial experience included 20 patients with chemotherapy-sensitive relapsed HL or NHL. The patients were required to have HIV-1 viral levels in plasma <10,000 gc/mL on cART. The majority of patients received high-dose conditioning chemotherapy consisting of CBV (cyclophosphamide, BCNU [carmustine], etoposide). Engraftment times were similar to those of HIV-1–negative patients, except for one patient who had delayed engraftment until day 23. This patient engrafted after the discontinuation of the zidovudine component of the cART. Attempts were made to continue cART throughout the transplant period; however, 11 of 20 patients were unable to tolerate oral antiviral medications because of nausea or mucositis. PFS and OS were superior to the French series [85% and 85%, respectively] likely due to the inclusion of only chemosensitive patients.[24] The cohort was expanded to 29 patients to evaluate a long-term outcome in a matched-case-control study. During a median follow-up of 41 months, the PFS remained high at 78%, and 2-year disease-free survival (DFS) and OS were also similar [75% DFS and OS 75% in HIV-1–infected group versus 56% (P = not significant) and 75%, respectively in the HIV-negative group]. The

nonrelapse-related mortality was also similar between the groups, 11% (95%, CI 4%–28%) in HIV-1–positive patients versus 4% (95% CI 1%–25%) in HIV-negative controls. Infectious complications were different between the groups with more opportunistic infections seen in the HIV-positive patients without impacting OS.[25] The results of this study provided further evidence that HIV status does not affect the long-term outcome of ASCT for NHL.

The Italian Cooperative Group on AIDS and Tumors reported results of their long-term follow-up study of 50 patients with HIV-1 infection and relapsed/refractory NHL or HL. This study was important as it followed up patients from diagnosis and underscored the challenges of getting patients to ASCT. Forty-six patients were already on cART, and 4 started cART at the time of enrollment or stem cell mobilization. HIV-1 plasma RNA level at study entry ranged from 204 to 750,000 gc/mL. Thirteen patients were withdrawn before stem cell collection due to death (n = 2), disease progression (n = 10), or patient refusal (n = 1). Of the remaining 37 patients, 31 adequately mobilized CD34 + cells. Four patients had early disease progression after stem cell mobilization and were unable to undergo ASCT. Twenty-seven of the initial 50 patients underwent ASCT after BEAM conditioning regimen. All patients engrafted at a median time of 10 days after ASCT. Three-year PFS for these patients was 76.3%. Multivariate analysis of prognostic factors for survival showed that marrow involvement, performance status <2, and CD4 count <100 cells/μL were significantly associated with worse outcome.[26] The group reported updated long-term follow-up on the 26 evaluable patients who reached CR after ASCT in which 24 of 26 patients remained alive at the time of the report. Two patients had relapse of the lymphoma, and five patients developed a second malignancy. At a median follow-up of 6 years, OS and PFS were 91% and 36%, respectively, once again confirming a long-term efficacy of ASCT for HIV lymphoma.[27]

The body of evidence suggests that the ASCT is a feasible, safe, and effective treatment option or treatment of HIV lymphoma. However, the ultimate effectiveness of lymphoma treatment is the control of HIV infection before, during, and after ASCT.

ALLOGENEIC STEM CELL TRANSPLANTATION IN HIV PATIENTS

Allo-SCT provides a curative option for treatment of hematologic malignancies by eliminating residual malignant cells via the graft-versus-tumor effect from the donor T cells in addition to the myeloablative chemotherapy. The greatest challenge in the setting of allo-SCT in the HIV-positive patients is the need for chronic immunosuppression for graft-versus-host disease (GVHD) prophylaxis or treatment. In the era of cART, survival of HIV-infected patients after allogeneic stem cell transplantation has improved, providing this treatment option available for high-risk hematologic malignancies in this population.[9]

In 1996 the first case of allo-SCT was performed in an HIV-positive patient with chronic myeloid leukemia (CML) while receiving cART therapy during stem cell transplant. The patient was conditioned with busulfan and cyclophosphamide followed by HLA-matched sibling donor bone marrow stem cell infusion. The patient engrafted by day 17 and had undetectable levels of HIV viral load through day 100. His posttransplant course was complicated by grade III/IV oral GVHD, which improved with prolonged cyclosporine taper. Reactivation of HIV was noted about 4 months after allo-SCT, with suggested uncertain compliance and suboptimal HIV therapy. At the time of the report, 3 years after allo-SCT, the patient remained in remission from CML despite poorly controlled HIV infection.[28]

Subsequent reports of successful allo-SCT for high-risk hematologic disorders in HIV-infected patients on cART were published.[29] Additionally, a first case of unrelated cord blood stem cell transplantation (HSCT-cb) in an HIV-positive patient for Philadelphia-positive acute lymphocytic leukemia after achieving remission with two cycles of induction chemotherapy while continued on cART was published. The patient had no available HLA-matched related or unrelated donors and was transplanted with HSCT-cb mismatched at HLA-B and HLA-DR. The conditioning regimen included 12 Gy total-body irradiation and 120 mg/kg cyclophosphamide. The GVHD prophylaxis consisted of cyclosporine and methotrexate. Owing to possible immunosuppression, cART was discontinued on day +28, and because the patient remained pancytopenic, she received a second HSCT-cb with one locus mismatch at HLA-DR after conditioning with fludarabine of 40 mg/m². She engrafted by day +27 of the second HSCT-cb with full-donor chimerism. HIV RNA levels increased to 3×10^6 copies/mL on day +27, which became undetectable by day +195 after resuming cART on day +38. The CD4 count remained above 300/μL from day +170 without evidence of bacterial or fungal infections. The patient had grade I acute GVHD which resolved without additional immunosuppressants. The patient remained free of leukemia at the time of report at 15 months after the transplant.[30] HSCT-cb procedure can be challenging due to prolonged engraftment associated with the treatment,[31] and in immunocompromised patients due to HIV infection, persistent immunosuppression also necessitates discontinuation of cART, placing patients at further risk of infections and TRM. Double umbilical cord stem cell transplantation is more frequently used now to decrease the rates of graft failures.[32–34] This was an important case in which Tomonari et al. were able to demonstrate a successful treatment of leukemia in the HIV-positive patient with an alternative stem cell source when a matched sibling and unrelated donor were not available. The case, however, clearly identified challenges with HSCT-cb in the HIV-positive patient of poor initial engraftment with one umbilical cord blood unit and the need for discontinuation of cART with rebound HIV reactivation during prolonged myelosuppression.

cART MANAGEMENT DURING HSCT

Owing to significant interactions between cART and conditioning regimen, it is important to have a high awareness of the potential drug-drug interactions. Some cART medications might be strong CYP3A4 inducers and should be discontinued before starting a conditioning regimen. One example of inducers are ritonavir-boosted protease inhibitors, which should be discontinued and substituted with another agent, such as raltegravir. Although less of an issue, as this drug is uncommon in modern regimens, zidovudine leads to myelosuppression and therefore should be avoided during stem cell transplantation to allow for successful engraftment. Antiretrovirals with a long half-life, such as efavirenz and efavirenz-containing combinations, can remain in the system after discontinuation and lead to single drug exposure and induction of resistance. It is therefore recommended to stop efavirenz 2 weeks before discontinuation of other cART and starting conditioning. Immunosuppressive regimens for GVHD prophylaxis and concomitant use of cART also have significant interactions. Owing to inhibition of CYP3A4, ritonavir can increase both tacrolimus and sirolimus serum levels. On the other hand, induction of CYP3A4 with nonnucleoside reverse transcriptase inhibitors (NNRTIs), such as efavirenz and nevirapine, may decrease the levels of tacrolimus and sirolimus. Another important consideration is the presence of significant interactions between -azole antifungals, cART, conditioning regimens, and GVHD prophylaxis. The echinocandins (anidulafungin, caspofungin, and micafungin) and amphotericin B are thus preferred antifungal prophylaxis during the peritransplant period. Substitution with enfurviritide, which is administered intravenously, can be considered in patients who are unable to maintain oral intake during stem cell transplantation. Even though there is no standard cART schedule that is used in the peri-HCT setting, careful planning can allow a regimen to be continued through the transplant.

HIV RESERVOIR

It is apparent that the autologous transplant can lead to changes in HIV reservoir and alteration of immune responses but will not eliminate the reservoir. Assessment of HIV antigens and antibodies, HIV-specific CD4 T-cell responses, and HIV RNA and DNA in plasma peripheral blood mononuclear cells (PBMCs) provides valuable insight into behavior of the virus and function of the immune system in response to chemotherapy and stem cell transplantation. A multicenter, cross-sectional study lead by Cillo et al. evaluated 10 patients after ASCT on cART. Low-level plasma viremia was detected in 9 of 10 patients, and total HIV-1 DNA was noted in all 10 patients, indicating persistence of HIV and inability of cytoablative therapy to eliminate the HIV reservoir.[12]

The stem cell transplantation from an unrelated HLA-matched donor lacking functional CCR5 receptor, a surface chemokine receptor on immune cells used by HIV-1 for entry into the host cells, was successfully performed on Timothy Ray Brown, an HIV patient with acute myeloid leukemia, "the Berlin patient". Twenty months at the time of report after allo-SCT, the patient had undetectable levels of HIV viral load and was leukemia free.[35,36] Hence the concept of HIV eradication with CCR5-modified stem cells is currently under investigation.

Genetic approaches targeting CCR5 in autologous cells have been explored. In a small pilot study, four patients received gene-modified peripheral blood–derived [CD34(+)] hematopoietic progenitor cells expressing three RNA-based anti-HIV moieties (tat/rev short hairpin RNA, trans-activation response element decoy, and CCR5 ribozyme). In vitro analysis of these gene-modified cells showed no differences in their hematopoietic potential compared with nontransduced cells. Patients received both gene-modified and unmanipulated hematopoietic progenitor cells. Transfected cells were successfully engrafted in

all four patients by day 11 without any unexpected infusion-related toxicities. They were able to demonstrate stable vector expression in human blood cells after transplantation of autologous gene-modified hematopoietic progenitor cells though at very low and likely nontherapeutic levels. These results support the development of a therapeutic strategy implementing an RNA-based cell therapy platform for treatment of HIV.[37] Further process improvement needs to be done in regard to increasing levels of gene marking to the point that true resistance to at least CCR5 virus could be conferred.

An alternative allogeneic approach is the use of HSCT-cb that has been screened for innate HIV-1 resistance. It is estimated that there are as many as 400,000 cord blood units worldwide. There are a small number of cord blood units with the identified CCR5-Δ32/Δ32 mutation, which could serve as an alternative donor source to matched unrelated donor transplants for AIDS-related hematologic malignancies.[38] However, appropriate engraftment requires at least two matched cord blood units, and the statistical probability of finding a suitable match within such a cord blood bank is limiting.[39,40] The delayed immune recovery after conventional HSCT-cb could be challenging in already immunocompromised patients, but emerging evidence shows the feasibility of this approach. Duarte et al. presented a patient with aggressive HIV lymphoma, progressing after 5 lines of therapy including ASCT, who underwent an allo-SCT with four of six HLA-matched CCR5 Δ32 homozygous cord blood cells (StemCyte, Covina, CA), supported with purified CD34 + cells from a haploidentical sibling. cART was continued during the transplant, and the patient was monitored for HIV infection.[38] Other studies included chimerism analysis, CCR5 genotyping and viral tropism, viral isolation and sequence, viral reservoir analysis, immune activation and proliferation, and ex vivo cell infectivity assays. After HCT-cb, plasma HIV DNA load was undetectable by ultrasensitive analyses. The patient achieved full cord blood chimerism, producing CCR5 Δ32 homozygous CD4+ T cells, which became resistant to HIV infection by the patient's viral isolate and laboratory-adapted HIV-1 strains.

GENE THERAPY FOR TREATMENT OF HIV-1

Anti-HIV gene therapy has been classified into three groups targeting different pathways of the viral life cycle and replication: Class I targets genes that affect either chemokine receptors or reverse transcriptase and integrase, which ultimately leads to inhibition of early stages of viral replication and integration; and class II targets expression of HIV proteins involved in replication such as ribosomes and transdominant negative mutants of Rev (tdRev). Class II therapy requires much higher inhibitory activity than class I genes to stimulate T-cell regeneration and decrease viral load. The third class of gene therapy targets viral assembly and release of the virus. Therapeutic success of the gene therapy depends on accumulation of genetically selected cells after transduction and infusion into the patient.[41] Mathematical analysis developed by van Laer et al. predicts that a significant therapeutic benefit can be derived from class I where antiviral gene product would inhibit viral replication before integration into human DNA.[41]

The first allo-SCT with stems cells that were genetically programmed to inhibit viral replication was conducted by Kang et al. The donor CD34 + cells were transduced with genetically altered tdRev, which would subsequently decrease viral replication by inhibiting wild-type Rev. The patient tolerated the procedure well and remained free of leukemia and maintained an undetectable HIV viral load. The therapeutic and control gene transfer vectors remained detectable at low levels more than 2 years after transplantation.[29]

RNA-based gene therapy involves the use of small interfering RNA (siRNA), which can produce a sequence-specific downregulation of the HIV-1 replication by targeting its receptors or coreceptor. The inhibition of HIV replication can be achieved by either transfection of preformed siRNAs or endogenous expression of siRNA via use of polymerase (pol) II or pol III. A combination of pol II and pol III promoters can express two different siRNAs, hence increasing the efficacy in targeting HIV-1 replication.[42]

Encouraging clinical trials of the gene therapy using hematopoietic stem cells offer substantial advantages against HIV-1 infection if genetically modified stem cells engraft with and retain the ability to produce HIV-1 resistance. Mitsuyasu et al. conducted a randomized, phase II double-blind study in 74 patients with HIV infection receiving a *tat-vpr* specific anti-HIV ribozyme (OZ1) or placebo delivered in autologous CD34 + hematopoietic progenitor cells. The patients were monitored over 100 weeks after stem cell infusion.

There were no reported OZ1-related adverse events. HIV-1 viral load was lower, and CD4+ lymphocyte counts were higher in the treatment group versus placebo group, although nonstatistically significant.[43,44]

In summary, current advances in the gene therapy and both autologous and allogeneic stem cell transplantation have shown the safety and feasibility of the anti-HIV-targeted approach.

CONCLUSIONS

Patients with HIV-1 infection remain at high risk for developing hematologic malignancies, and since the introduction of cART, there have been substantial advances in the treatment options available for patients with HIV-1 infection and hematologic malignancies. HIV-positive patients are now offered standard chemoimmunotherapy as induction therapy of hematologic malignancies. Moreover, in the setting of relapsed lymphoma, trials with applying high-dose therapy followed by ASCT have proven to be successful without increased risk of opportunistic infection or death, providing improved survival outcomes for this population. Allogeneic stem cell transplantation reports also demonstrated feasibility of the treatment for acute leukemia in HIV-positive patients with particular attention paid to the management of cART during the peritransplant period due to drug-drug interactions with chemotherapy and GVHD prophylaxis. Management of HIV-positive patients undergoing transplant may require consultation with an infectious disease specialist to assist with the choice of cART during stem cell transplant. When well coordinated, stem cell transplant can offer curative options for HIV-positive patients with hematologic malignancies. Hence the HIV-1 infection is not a contraindication for standard treatment of hematologic malignancies, including stem cell transplantation. Table 26.1 summarizes treatments that have been used to treat patients with HIV-associated lymphoma, including chemotherapy, stem cell transplant, and gene therapy. More exciting are the new developments in the field of HIV-1 treatment with the use of stem cell transplant and gene therapy, where ongoing research for potential curative strategies for HIV-1 infection continues.

TABLE 26.1

Treatment of HIV-Associated Hematologic Malignancies, Including Chemotherapy, Stem Cell Transplant, and Gene Therapy

References	Type of Therapy	n	Regimen	Response	Survival	Comments
Sparano et al. *Blood*. 2010	Induction chemotherapy	48 patients in concurrent rituximab plus chemotherapy group and 53 patients in sequential group (rituximab given after completion of all chemotherapy)	R-EPOCH	CR 73% in concurrent versus 55% in sequential group	2-year PFS 64% in concurrent and 60% in sequential arms 2-year OS 63% in concurrent and 66% in sequential arms	9.8% mortality rate in concurrent versus 7.3% in sequential group due to OI
Diez-Martin et al. *Blood*. 2009, EBMT	ASCT	53 HIV patients and 53 HIV-negative matched controls	TBI and ASCT	Patients in CR before ASCT had improved PFS in both groups	PFS 61% HIV+ versus 56% for controls, OS was 61.5% in both groups at 30-month median follow-up	
Alvarnas et al. *Blood*. 2016, BMT CTN0803/AMC071	ASCT, phase 2, multicenter	43 patients enrolled, 40 received ASCT	BEAM and ASCT		2-year probability PFS 79.8%, 2-yr OS 82%	1-yr TRM 5.2%
DiGiusto et al. *Sci Transl Med*. 2010	Gene therapy, Pilot study CCR5 gene-modified autologous CD34+ cells transplant	4 patients with HIV NHL eligible for ASCT	BCNU/VP16/Cytoxan	Successful gene modification, vector transfer, and engraftment after transplant		
Kang et al. *Blood*. 2002	Gene therapy, allogeneic transplant	1 patient with HIV and treatment-related AML, eligible for allogeneic transplant	Cyclophosphamide/fludarabine conditioning	Leukemia-free and undetectable viral load	At 2 years, therapeutic and control gene transfer vectors remained detectable	

ASCT, autologous stem cell transplantation; *BEAM, BCNU*, etoposide, cytarabine, and melphalan; *CR*, complete remission; *OI*, opportunistic infection; *OS*, overall survival; *PFS*, progression-free survival; *R-EPOCH*, rituximab, etoposide, vincristine, doxorubicin, cyclophosphamide, and prednisone; *TBI*, total-body irradiation; *TMR*, treatment-related mortality.

REFERENCES

1. Detels R, Munoz A, McFarlane G, et al. Effectiveness of potent antiretroviral therapy on time to AIDS and death in men with known HIV infection duration. Multicenter AIDS Cohort Study Investigators. *JAMA*. 1998;280:1497–1503.
2. Bartlett JA, DeMasi R, Quinn J, Moxham C, Rousseau F. Overview of the effectiveness of triple combination therapy in antiretroviral-naive HIV-1 infected adults. *AIDS*. 2001;15:1369–1377.
3. Sterne JA, Hernan MA, Ledergerber B, et al. Long-term effectiveness of potent antiretroviral therapy in preventing AIDS and death: a prospective cohort study. *Lancet*. 2005;366:378–384.
4. Robbins HA, Shiels MS, Pfeiffer RM, Engels EA. Epidemiologic contributions to recent cancer trends among HIV-infected people in the United States. *AIDS*. 2014;28:881–890.

5. Sutton L, Guenel P, Tanguy ML, et al. Acute myeloid leukaemia in human immunodeficiency virus-infected adults: epidemiology, treatment feasibility and outcome. *Br J Haematol.* 2001;112:900–908.

6. Olszewski AJ, Fallah J, Castillo JJ. Human immunodeficiency virus-associated lymphomas in the antiretroviral therapy era: analysis of the National Cancer Data Base. *Cancer.* 2016;122:2689–2697.

7. Barta SK, Samuel MS, Xue X, et al. Changes in the influence of lymphoma- and HIV-specific factors on outcomes in AIDS-related non-Hodgkin lymphoma. *Ann Oncol.* 2015;26:958–966.

8. Diez-Martin JL, Balsalobre P, Re A, et al. Comparable survival between HIV+ and HIV- non-Hodgkin and Hodgkin lymphoma patients undergoing autologous peripheral blood stem cell transplantation. *Blood.* 2009;113:6011–6014.

9. Hutter G, Zaia JA. Allogeneic haematopoietic stem cell transplantation in patients with human immunodeficiency virus: the experiences of more than 25 years. *Clin Exp Immunol.* 2011;163:284–295.

10. Lori F, Foli A, Lisziewicz J. Structured treatment interruptions as a potential alternative therapeutic regimen for HIV-infected patients: a review of recent clinical data and future prospects. *J Antimicrob Chemother.* 2002;50:155–160.

11. Zaia JA, Forman SJ. Transplantation in HIV-infected subjects: is cure possible? *Hematol Am Soc Hematol Educ Program.* 2013;2013:389–393.

12. Cillo AR, Krishnan A, Mitsuyasu RT, et al. Plasma viremia and cellular HIV-1 DNA persist despite autologous hematopoietic stem cell transplantation for HIV-related lymphoma. *J Acquir Immune Defic Syndr.* 2013;63:438–441.

13. Wolf T, Brodt HR, Fichtlscherer S, et al. Changing incidence and prognostic factors of survival in AIDS-related non-Hodgkin's lymphoma in the era of highly active antiretroviral therapy (HAART). *Leuk Lymphoma.* 2005;46:207–215.

14. Bonnet F, Lewden C, May T, et al. Malignancy-related causes of death in human immunodeficiency virus-infected patients in the era of highly active antiretroviral therapy. *Cancer.* 2004;101:317–324.

15. Bohlius J, Schmidlin K, Costagliola D, et al. Incidence and risk factors of HIV-related non-Hodgkin's lymphoma in the era of combination antiretroviral therapy: a European multicohort study. *Antivir Ther.* 2009;14:1065–1074.

16. Simard EP, Pfeiffer RM, Engels EA. Spectrum of cancer risk late after AIDS onset in the United States. *Arch Intern Med.* 2010;170:1337–1345.

17. Biggar RJ, Jaffe ES, Goedert JJ, Chaturvedi A, Pfeiffer R, Engels EA. Hodgkin lymphoma and immunodeficiency in persons with HIV/AIDS. *Blood.* 2006;108:3786–3791.

18. Kaplan LD, Lee JY, Ambinder RF, et al. Rituximab does not improve clinical outcome in a randomized phase 3 trial of CHOP with or without rituximab in patients with HIV-associated non-Hodgkin lymphoma: AIDS-Malignancies Consortium Trial 010. *Blood.* 2005;106:1538–1543.

19. Sparano JA, Lee JY, Kaplan LD, et al. Rituximab plus concurrent infusional EPOCH chemotherapy is highly effective in HIV-associated B-cell non-Hodgkin lymphoma. *Blood.* 2010;115:3008–3016.

20. Gabarre J, Leblond V, Sutton L, et al. Autologous bone marrow transplantation in relapsed HIV-related non-Hodgkin's lymphoma. *Bone Marrow Transpl.* 1996;18:1195–1197.

21. Gabarre J, Azar N, Autran B, Katlama C, Leblond V. High-dose therapy and autologous haematopoietic stem-cell transplantation for HIV-1-associated lymphoma. *Lancet.* 2000;355:1071–1072.

22. Balsalobre P, Diez-Martin JL, Re A, et al. Autologous stem-cell transplantation in patients with HIV-related lymphoma. *J Clin Oncol.* 2009;27:2192–2198.

23. Alvarnas JC, Le Rademacher J, Wang Y, et al. Autologous hematopoietic cell transplantation for HIV-related lymphoma: results of the BMT CTN 0803/AMC 071 trial. *Blood.* 2016;128:1050–1058.

24. Krishnan A, Molina A, Zaia J, et al. Durable remissions with autologous stem cell transplantation for high-risk HIV-associated lymphomas. *Blood.* 2005;105:874–878.

25. Krishnan A, Palmer JM, Zaia JA, Tsai NC, Alvarnas J, Forman SJ. HIV status does not affect the outcome of autologous stem cell transplantation (ASCT) for non-Hodgkin lymphoma (NHL). *Biol Blood Marrow Transpl.* 2010;16:1302–1308.

26. Re A, Michieli M, Casari S, et al. High-dose therapy and autologous peripheral blood stem cell transplantation as salvage treatment for AIDS-related lymphoma: long-term results of the Italian Cooperative Group on AIDS and Tumors (GICAT) study with analysis of prognostic factors. *Blood.* 2009;114:1306–1313.

27. Zanet E, Durante C, Rupolo M, et al. Post-transplantation long-term events in a cohort of HIV-positive patients affected by relapsed/refractory lymphoma. *J Clin Oncol.* 2015;33(Suppl S):7031.

28. Schlegel P, Beatty P, Halvorsen R, McCune J. Successful allogeneic bone marrow transplant in an HIV-1-positive man with chronic myelogenous leukemia. *J Acquir Immune Defic Syndr.* 2000;24:289–290.

29. Kang EM, de Witte M, Malech H, et al. Nonmyeloablative conditioning followed by transplantation of genetically modified HLA-matched peripheral blood progenitor cells for hematologic malignancies in patients with acquired immunodeficiency syndrome. *Blood.* 2002;99:698–701.

30. Tomonari A, Takahashi S, Shimohakamada Y, et al. Unrelated cord blood transplantation for a human immunodeficiency virus-1-seropositive patient with acute lymphoblastic leukemia. *Bone Marrow Transpl.* 2005;36:261–262.

31. Marks DI, Woo KA, Zhong X, et al. Unrelated umbilical cord blood transplant for adult acute lymphoblastic leukemia in first and second complete remission: a comparison with allografts from adult unrelated donors. *Haematologica.* 2014;99:322–328.

32. Cutler C, Stevenson K, Kim HT, et al. Double umbilical cord blood transplantation with reduced intensity conditioning and sirolimus-based GVHD prophylaxis. *Bone Marrow Transpl.* 2011;46:659–667.

33. Barker JN, Weisdorf DJ, DeFor TE, et al. Transplantation of 2 partially HLA-matched umbilical cord blood units to enhance engraftment in adults with hematologic malignancy. *Blood.* 2005;105:1343–1347.

34. Ballen KK, Spitzer TR, Yeap BY, et al. Double unrelated reduced-intensity umbilical cord blood transplantation in adults. *Biol Blood Marrow Transpl.* 2007;13:82–89.

35. Hutter G, Nowak D, Mossner M, et al. Long-term control of HIV by CCR5 Delta32/Delta32 stem-cell transplantation. *N Engl J Med.* 2009;360:692–698.

36. Allers K, Hutter G, Hofmann J, et al. Evidence for the cure of HIV infection by CCR5Delta32/Delta32 stem cell transplantation. *Blood.* 2011;117:2791–2799.

37. DiGiusto DL, Krishnan A, Li L, et al. RNA-based gene therapy for HIV with lentiviral vector–modified CD34(+) cells in patients undergoing transplantation for AIDS-related lymphoma. *Sci Transl Med.* 2010;2:36ra43.

38. Duarte RF, Salgado M, Sanchez-Ortega I, et al. CCR5 Delta32 homozygous cord blood allogeneic transplantation in a patient with HIV: a case report. *Lancet HIV.* 2015;2:e236–e242.

39. Gonzalez G, Park S, Chen D, Armitage S, Shpall E, Behringer R. Identification and frequency of CCR5Delta32/Delta32 HIV-resistant cord blood units from Houston area hospitals. *HIV Med.* 2011;12:481–486.

40. Alarifi M, Al-Amro F, Alalwan A, et al. The prevalence of CCR5-Delta32 mutation in a cohort of Saudi stem cell donors. *HLA.* 2017;90:292–294.

41. von Laer D, Baum C, Protzer U. Antiviral gene therapy. *Handb Exp Pharmacol.* 2009:265–297.

42. Anderson J, Li MJ, Palmer B, et al. Safety and efficacy of a lentiviral vector containing three anti-HIV genes-CCR5 ribozyme, tat-rev siRNA, and TAR decoy-in SCID-hu mouse-derived T cells. *Mol Ther.* 2007;15:1182–1188.

43. Mitsuyasu RT, Merigan TC, Carr A, et al. Phase 2 gene therapy trial of an anti-HIV ribozyme in autologous CD34+ cells. *Nat Med.* 2009;15:285–292.

44. Mitsuyasu RT, Zack JA, Macpherson JL, Symonds GP. Phase I/II clinical trials using gene-modified adult hematopoietic stem cells for HIV: lessons learnt. *Stem Cells Int.* 2011;2011:393698.

CHAPTER 27

Symptom Control and Palliative Care in Hematopoietic Stem Cell Transplantation

SOLA KIM, MD • NHU-NHU NGUYEN, MD • ALI HAIDER, MD

INTRODUCTION

Patients' with hematologic malignancies undergoing hematopoietic stem cell transplantation (HSCT) or simply stem cell transplantation (SCT) often experience adverse physical and psychosocial symptoms which can impact their quality of life (QOL).[1–4] Studies have reported several biomedical, psychological, and social variables that can be associated with the intensity of these symptoms.[5,6] It is imperative to screen high-risk individuals for such factors with the provision of additional psychological interventions before initiating transplantation.[5] The severity of physical symptoms is dependent on multiple factors such as the type of transplant, type and dose of chemotherapy and radiation therapy used during conditioning, the degree of cytopenias and associated infections, and other organ dysfunction such as liver and kidneys.[5] In our opinion, there are certain symptoms that are relatively common such as pain, nausea and vomiting, diarrhea, mucositis, and delirium.

Graft-versus-host disease (GVHD) is a complication of SCT with high morbidity and mortality and is a frequent reason for SCT failure.[7] Because it affects multiple organ systems, a multidisciplinary approach is often recommended which should include the provision of supportive care. We aim to provide a brief overview of the management of symptoms related to acute and chronic GVHD. Mucositis due to SCT is common and often poorly controlled which can lead to frequent emergency room visits and hospital admissions, increased reliance on total parenteral nutrition (TPN), and a 3.9-fold rise in rate of mortality.[8] The discussion will be focused on the prevention and treatment aspects. This chapter will provide a comprehensive overview of nausea and vomiting related to SCT. In the end, we will discuss delirium which is usually underdiagnosed, and inadequate treatment can lead to patient and caregiver distress.

There is a small but significant body of literature examining the benefits of early integration of palliative care with standard transplant care leading to improvement in physical and psychosocial well-being.[3,9,10] Our chapter will cover a brief overview of the recent literature.

QOL MEASURES

The most common QOL measures used in transplant care include MD Anderson Symptom Inventory (MDASI)[11,12] and the Functional Assessment of Cancer Therapy-Bone Marrow Transplant Scale (FACT-BMT).[13] MDASI is a validated multisymptom patient-reported outcome measure for clinical and research purposes used to assess the severity of symptoms experienced by patients with cancer and the interference of daily living. It consists of 13 symptoms based on a 0–10 scale (0 = symptom not present and 10 = symptom as bad as you can imagine) which can be applied broadly across cancer types and treatments. Specific to bone marrow transplant patients, the FACT-BMT combines the Functional Assessment of Cancer Therapy and the Bone Marrow Transplantation Subscale. It is a 47-item questionnaire that can be used to assess five areas of well-being (physical, social/family, emotional, functional, and doctor-patient relationship) using a 0–4 scale (0 = not at all and 4 = very much).[13] Edmonton Symptom Assessment Scale (ESAS) can also be used to measure physical and psychological symptoms.[14] ESAS is a validated tool to assess patient rating of pain, fatigue, nausea, anxiety, depression, drowsiness, appetite, feeling of well-being, shortness of breath, and sleep. The patient will be asked to grade the severity of their symptoms from "no symptom" with a 0 to "worst symptom" with 10 in the last 24 hours. ESAS has high test-retest reliability of >0.8 and has been validated in many clinical settings including cancer population.[15]

Hematopoietic Cell Transplantation for Malignant Conditions. https://doi.org/10.1016/B978-0-323-56802-9.00027-4

GRAFT-VERSUS-HOST DISEASE

GVHD is a complication of SCT with high morbidity and mortality and is an important reason for SCT failure.[7] Definitions and underlying pathophysiology of the common symptoms are discussed in Chapter 22. In this section, we will briefly discuss the management of acute and chronic symptoms related to GVHD.

The rash is a most common manifestation of acute GVHD, affecting 81% of patients, followed by gastrointestinal (54%) and liver dysfunctions (50%).[16] Skin is frequently the first organ involved, and common sites early on include palms and soles, upper back, lateral neck, cheeks, and the external ear.[17] Treatment includes immunosuppressive agents such as steroids and psoralen plus ultraviolet A irradiation or extracorporeal photophoresis for limited skin disease.[18] Gastrointestinal involvement can be diffuse with the comparable diagnostic yield at the rectal, sigmoid, gastric, and duodenal biopsy sites.[7] The symptoms may include nausea, vomiting, anorexia, abdominal pain, and diarrhea; if symptoms are severe, rectal bleeding can occur as well.[19] Pain and nausea are discussed separately in this chapter. Abdominal pain related to GVHD can be treated with anticholinergic medications such as dicyclomine or glycopyrrolate.[6] It is important to consider infectious causes of diarrhea, with *Salmonella, Shigella, Campylobacter, Cryptosporidium,* and *Clostridium difficile* being common culprits along with viral etiologies. Extensive GVHD involving the gastrointestinal tract can result in up to 10 L of diarrhea in a day. Therefore, it is important to manage metabolic derangements, dehydration, and nutrition. Loperamide and octreotide can be given to help patients with diarrhea after infectious causes are ruled out.[6] Jaundice from hyperbilirubinemia is commonly seen, especially in the early stages of hepatic involvement. Ursodeoxycholic acid has been shown to decrease the frequency of jaundice, lower acute GVHD incidence, and improve survival.[20,21]

Symptoms commonly seen in chronic GVHD are related to increased dryness. Sicca symptoms experienced in chronic GVHD can be palliated by artificial tears, moisture-chamber eyewear, gas-permeable scleral lens, or in more severe cases, plugging or ligation of the tear ducts.[22] Patients with xerostomia may find relief from medications, which increase the salivary flow such as cevimeline.[23] Oral involvement may respond to therapy with topical steroid wash. Genitalia involvement is more common in chronic GVHD and includes vaginal GVHD, which manifests as ulcerated and thickened mucosa and narrowed introitus with scar tissue. Treatment includes topical immunosuppressive medications such as cyclosporine and vaginal dilators, and

in severe disease, surgical lysis is used.[24] Myositis, fasciitis, contractures, and joint stiffness are also seen in the chronic disease.[19] Deep tissue massage, frequent weight-bearing exercise, and physical activity help with these symptoms.[22] Other chronic gastrointestinal manifestations include esophageal webs and strictures. Lung disease includes bronchiolitis obliterans, cryptogenic organizing pneumonia, and restrictive lung disease.[22]

MUCOSITIS

Incidence and Risk Factors

Oral mucositis due to SCT is common and experienced by 76% of patients undergoing this procedure. Almost 42% of patients have described mucositis as the most significant adverse effect of SCT.[25] In one study, 84% of patients with mucositis thought symptoms were more severe than expected, with 65% reporting poor or no control of symptoms. Patients who are at increased risk of mucositis after HCT include those who receive total-body irradiation, have a body mass index ≥ 25, do not receive multivitamins before transplantation, and those with the methylenetetrahydrofolate reductase 677TT genotype.[26] Mucositis can result in many complications for the patient and can stress resources leading to more frequent emergency room visits and hospital admissions, increased reliance on TPN, and a 3.9-fold rise in mortality.[8]

There are several grading scales that can assist with the clinical diagnosis of mucositis. The World Health Organization scale[27] was developed before the National Cancer Institute Common Terminology Criteria for Adverse Events scale, which uses clinical and functional components to determine the grades (Table 27.1).[8]

Clinical Presentation and Course

Injury occurs at the start of chemotherapy or radiation and becomes evident a few days later. Cellular apoptosis occurs, which leads to the syndrome. Patients may experience a burning sensation on the oral mucosa with erythema and removable white plaques.[28] Desquamation and epithelial sloughing occur, with symptoms peaking at 1 week, eventually leading to ulceration and severe pain.[29] Certain areas of the oral mucosa are prone to mechanical injury from normal activity. Cytokines and interleukins released after chemotherapy and radiotherapy may cause increased vascularity in those areas. Bacterial, viral, and fungal infections may arise and can be complicated by bacteremia, especially in the setting of neutropenia.[30] The most common infection seen with mucositis is candidiasis.[31] This is followed by a herpes simplex virus 1 (HSV-1) infection, most commonly due to reactivation of HSV-1.[32] Mucositis is

TABLE 27.1
Oral Mucositis Grading Scales

Grades	WHO Scale	NCI-CTCAE Scale
Grade 1	Oral soreness, erythema	Painless ulcers, erythema, or mild pain in the absence of lesions; interventions not required
Grade 2	Erythema, ulcers; patient can swallow solid food	Painful erythema, edema, or ulcers, but eating or swallowing possible; modified diet indicated
Grade 3	Ulcers with extensive erythema; patient cannot swallow food	Painful erythema, edema, or ulcers, interfering with oral intake, requiring intravenous hydration
Grade 4	Mucositis to the extent that alimentation is not possible	Severe ulceration or requiring parenteral or enteral nutritional support or prophylactic intubation
Grade 5	NA	Death related to toxicity

NCI-CTCAE, National Cancer Institute Common Terminology Criteria for Adverse Events; *WHO*, World Health Organization; *NA*, Not Applicable.

known to be self-limited, and lesions are usually healed by 2 weeks after chemotherapy administration.[29]

Prevention

The guidelines for prevention of mucositis include good oral hygiene, with the addition of some useful interventions if needed. Good oral hygiene includes use of a soft toothbrush on a regular basis, consulting dental care before and after treatments, drinking plenty of liquids, regular flossing, abstaining from tobacco and alcohol as well as acidic foods, use of mouth lubricants such as artificial saliva or jellies, performing baking soda mouth rinses, and good denture care. Interventions for prevention include oral cryotherapy for patients receiving bolus 5-fluorouracil chemotherapy or high-dose melphalan or bolus doses of methotrexate. Recombinant keratinocyte growth factor-1 known as palifermin could be given to patients with hematologic malignancies receiving high-dose chemotherapy and total-body irradiation, followed by SCT.[33] Low-level laser therapy can be given to patients receiving SCT conditioned with high-dose chemotherapy and head and neck cancer patients receiving radiotherapy.[28]

Of note, chlorhexidine and sucralfate mouthwashes are not recommended for prevention.

Treatment

Treatment for established oral mucositis is usually aimed at symptom control. This consists of mouth protectants, analgesia, and treatment of infection in addition to good oral hygiene. Mouth protectants include baking soda rinses, and denture cares as discussed previously are important to maintain.[28] For mucositis with mild pain, patients can try bland rinses with normal saline and sodium bicarbonate.[8] If the pain is moderate, topical analgesia mouthwash options including preparations comprising of the previous ingredients in combinations with lidocaine, hydrocortisone, and diphenhydramine known as magic or miracle mouthwashes are used.[8] Doxepin, xyloxylin, and morphine sulfate mouthwashes are also available options. Of note, these mouthwashes require frequent swish and swallow use several times per day. For more severe pain with mucositis, systemic opioids are considered. Patients are usually started on oral opioids such as morphine, keeping in mind that due to severe pain, the oral route may not be feasible. If so, clinicians can consider a fentanyl patch or parenteral opioid administration.[28] For infections, certain populations can be considered for infection prophylaxis. Neutropenic patients often receive hematopoietic growth factors. Treatment with bortezomib is linked with reactivation of HSV-1, so antiviral prophylaxis is recommended.[8] For patients with established candida infections, nystatin swish and swallow, clotrimazole, or fluconazole can be given. For HSV infections, acyclovir or valacyclovir can be given while cultures are collected. Practice guidelines are available for review with the Infectious Diseases Society of America. Refractory or systemic infections require the use of parenteral medications and consultation with an infectious disease specialist.[34]

NAUSEA AND VOMITING

Nausea is an unpleasant, subjective sensation with an involuntary urge to vomit. The act of vomiting is defined as the forceful expulsion of stomach contents through the mouth which may or may not be associated with nausea. Two organ systems play a major role in nausea: (1) gastrointestinal tract and (2) brain. Specific areas involved are the gastrointestinal lining, chemoreceptor trigger zone (CTZ), vestibular apparatus, and cerebral cortex. Stimulation of one or more of these areas emanate from the vomiting center culminating in the neuromuscular reflex in the final common pathway (Fig. 27.1).[35]

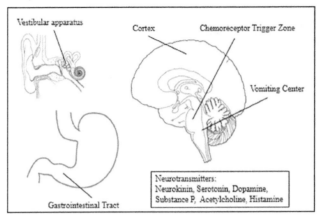

FIG. 27.1 Pathophysiology of nausea and vomiting.

The CTZ is directly accessible to emetogenic substances. Contraction or distension of the gut mucosa or chemoreceptors including serotonin can activate visceral afferents in the gastrointestinal tract which in turn can stimulate the vomiting center directly or via the chemoreceptor zone. Pathways from both peripheral and central nervous system are involved using various neurotransmitters such as serotonin (5-hydroxytryptophan 3), dopamine (D2), substance P (natural killer-1), acetylcholine (muscarinic), and histamine (histaminic).[36] The etiology of nausea in the SCT patient can be difficult to uncover. Therefore a thorough assessment must be performed to document the onset, intensity, duration, frequency, aggravating and relieving factors, relation to food, bowel patterns, and use of current antiemetics' and their success.

Well-performed physical examination and diagnostic studies can also provide insight into the diagnosis and guidance of treatment plans. Physical examination findings such as signs of significant dehydration (decreased urine output, skin tenting, and dry mucous membranes), severe abdominal pain/distension, or abnormal funduscopic examination can help guide the need for further laboratory and diagnostic imaging studies.[37]

Management of nausea depends on the etiology as each requires different interventions to control symptoms adequately. Eleven M's of emesis etiology and management are summarized in (Table 27.2).[38] Supportive therapy should be used in fluid hydration, electrolyte correction, and avoidance of triggers.

Chemotherapy-Induced Nausea

One of the most frequent side effects of chemotherapy is nausea and vomiting which can interfere with compliance and primarily affect the QOL. Three types of chemotherapy-induced nausea and vomiting (CIMV) exist.[39] Symptoms can be acute which occurs within 24 h after chemotherapy administration or delayed which occurs after 24 h of chemotherapy administration and can last up to 4 days or more. Most commonly happens with cisplatin but may be associated with cyclophosphamide, anthracyclines, and carboplatin. Anticipatory nausea is a conditioned response to a prior episode of CIMV. It typically occurs 3–4 h after the treatment. It is usually a learned response which is not regulated by neurotransmitters.

The National Cancer Institute developed a grading system and criteria to describe nausea severity which is as follows[40]:

1. Grade 1: loss of appetite but without alteration in eating habits, and 1–2 episodes of vomiting (separated by 5 minutes) in 24 hours;
2. Grade 2: decreased oral intake without significant weight loss, malnutrition, or dehydration, 3–5 episodes (separated by 5 min in 24 h);
3. Grade 3: inadequate oral caloric or fluid intake, artificial feeding (tube feeds) or TPN indicated for hospitalization, and >6 episodes of vomiting (separated by 5 min) in 24 h;
4. Grade 4: life-threatening, emergent medical attention is required;
5. Grade 5: death.

Treatment is driven by etiology and should focus on correction of the underlying issue. However, the cause of nausea is often multifactorial and will require a unique treatment plan for each patient. Pharmacological therapy should start with a single agent, preferably target the neurotransmitter thought to be

TABLE 27.2
"M's" of Etiology and Management of Nausea/Vomiting

Etiology	Pathophysiology	Therapy
METASTASES		
Cerebral	Increased ICP, direct effect on CMZ	Steroids, mannitol, anti-DA/Histamine
Liver	Toxin accumulation	Anti-DA/Histamine
Meningeal irritation	Increased ICP	Steroids
Movement	Vestibular stimulation	Anti-Ach
Mentation (ex. anxiety)	Cortical activity	Anxiolytics
MEDICATIONS		
Opioids	CTZ, vestibular effects, GIT	Anti-DA/histamine, anti-Ach, prokinetic agents, simulant cathartics
Chemotherapy	CMZ, GIT	Anti-5HT/DA, steroids
Others (ex, nonsteroidal anti-inflammatory drugs)	CMZ	Anti-DA/histamine
MUCOSAL IRRITATION		
Nonsteroidal anti-inflammatory drugs	GIT, gastritis	Cytoprotective agents
Hyperacidity, gastroesophageal reflux	GIT, gastritis, duodenitis	Antacids
MECHANICAL OBSTRUCTION		
Intraluminal	Constipation, obstipation	Manage constipation
Extraluminal	Tumor, fibrotic stricture	Reversible: Surgery Irreversible: fluid management, steroids, inhibit secretions with Octreotide, scopolamine
MOTILITY		
Opioids, ileus, other medications	GIT, central nervous system	Prokinetic agents, stimulate laxatives
METABOLIC		
Hypercalcemia, hyponatremia, hepatic/renal failure	CMZ	Anti-DA/histamine, rehydration, steroids
MICROBES		
Local irritation esophagitis, gastritis (Candida, Helicobacter pylori, herpes, CMV)	GIT	Antibacterial, antivirals, antifungals, antacids
Systemic sepsis	CMZ	Anti-DA/Histamine, antibacterial, antiviral, antifungal
MYOCARDIAL		
Ischemia, congestive heart failure	Vagal stimulation, cortical, CMZ	Oxygen, opioids, Anti-DA/Histamine, anxiolytics

Anti-5HT, serotonin antagonist; *Anti-Ach*, acetylcholine antagonist; *Anti-DA*, dopamine antagonist; *CMZ*, chemoreceptor zone; *GIT*, gastrointestinal tract; *ICP*, intracranial pressure.

involved. A detailed description of antiemetics has been consolidated in (Table 27.3) and includes name, dose, indication, and adverse effects.[41,42] It is recommended that one antiemetic should be maximized before another agent with a different mechanism of action.[43] Sequential titration of treatment should then be continued to reach adequate symptom control and improve QOL.[44]

TABLE 27.3
Antiemetic Drugs

Name	Dosage	Main Indication	Adverse Effects	Additional Comments
DOPAMINE−2 RECEPTOR ANTAGONIST				
Haloperidol	1–2 mg BID, IV, PO, SC		Diarrhea, sedating	Less EPS
Chlorpromazine	25–50 mg PO, rectal, IM q8-12h PRN		Anticholinergic effects, sedating	Anticholinergic effects
Prochlorperazine	5–20 mg PO, PR, IM, IV q4H PRN or scheduled	Opioid induced	Dry mouth, drowsiness, blurred vision	
Metoclopramide (prokinetic)	5–10 mg PO, IM, SC, IV 3–4 times/day, 30 min before meals and at bedtime	Opioid induced, gastroparesis, pseudo-obstruction	Gynecomastia, galactorrhea, amenorrhea	Increased risk of perforation of bowel obstruction
SEROTONIN (5-HT₃) RECEPTOR ANTAGONIST				
Ondansetron	4–16 mg PO, IV, SL q8H PRN	CINV	Headache, constipation, QT prolongation, fatigue, dizziness	
Granisetron	2 mg PO up to 1 h before chemotherapy and 12h later Alternate dosing for IV and TD	CINV		
Palonosetron	0.25 mg IV or 0.5 mg po daily	CINV		
HISTAMINE ANTAGONISTS (ANTIHISTAMINES)				
Diphenhydramine	25–50 mg PO, IV, SC q 6–8h PRN	Intestinal obstruction, ICP, vestibular	Sedation, dizziness, confusion, dry mouth	Anticholinergic properties
Hydroxyzine	25 mg PO, IV q6-8H PRN			
Promethazine	12.5 mg PO, PR, IV q4H PRN			
SUBSTANCE P/NEUROKININ ANTAGONIST **USED IN COMBINATION WITH CORTICOSTEROID AND A 5−HT ANTAGONIST FOR CINV**				
Aprepitant	125 mg PO 1h before chemotherapy on day 1, 80 mg PO q am on days 2 and 3	CIMV	Dizziness Anorexia Diarrhea	New class of antiemetics
Fosaprepitant	150 mg IV 50 to 60 minutes prior to chemotherapy on day 1 only	CIMV	Fatigue Diarrhea Infusion site pain	New class of antiemetics
ACETYLCHOLINE ANTAGONISTS (ANTICHOLINERGICS)				
Hyoscine	0.2–0.4 mg q4H SL, SC,TD	Intestinal obstruction, colic, secretions	Dry mouth, blurry vision, urinary retention	Contraindicated in dementia, delirium, glaucoma
Scopolamine	one patch q3days PRN			
CANNABINOIDS				
Dronabinol	2.5 mg PO q8-12H and titrate		Ataxia, depression, sedation	Appetite stimulant
Nabilone	1–2 mg twice daily started 1–3h before chemotherapy			

TABLE 27.3
Antiemetic Drugs—cont'd

Name	Dosage	Main Indication	Adverse Effects	Additional Comments
OTHERS				
Glucocorticoid, Dexamethasone	0.5-8 mg PO, IV, IM, SC daily to q6H	CINV	Infection, gastritis, gastric bleed, myopathy, salt, water retention	Slow taper to avoid adre-nocorticoid insufficiency or withdrawal
Benzodiazepine, Lorazepam	1–4 mg PO, SC, IV q6-8H		Sedation, confusion	Avoid use with other CNS depressants
Synthetic analog of somatostatin, octreotide	100ug SC q8H for 48 hours or 10ug/hour by continuous SC, IV infusion and titrate	Cancer-related bowel obstruction	GI side effects	Palliative
Neuroleptic, olanzapine	2.5 mg PO	Nausea refractory to standard therapy	Sedation, weight gain, somnolence	Atypical antipsychotic

EPS, extrapyramidal symptoms; *IV*, intravenously; *PO*, oral; *PR*, per rectum; *SC*, subcutaneously; *SL*, sublingual; *TD*, transdermal.

PAIN

One early source of discomfort for recipients of stem cell transplant is the adverse reactions that can arise from an infusion of progenitor cells. Several uncomfortable reactions can occur, notably gastrointestinal effects (nausea, vomiting, and abdominal pain), as well as allergic symptoms (bronchospasm and swelling) and dysfunction of the renal and cardiovascular systems. Much of this is thought to be attributable to the effects of the cryoprotectant dimethyl sulphoxide and cellular debris.[45] Pain from mucositis, a very frequent morbidity in SCT, and pain from GVHD are discussed elsewhere in this chapter. Some medications that are given to facilitate SCT are known to cause neuropathic pain, such as chemotherapeutic and immunosuppressant agents. Calcineurin inhibitors that are given for GVHD prophylaxis can cause neuropathic pain.[46] Generalized bone pain due to bone marrow necrosis can occur after administration of granulocyte colony-stimulating factor.[47] Hemorrhagic cystitis is a common and painful symptom after SCT, which is frequently caused by chemotherapy regimens and viral infections.[48] Other iatrogenic causes of pain include neuropathies related to chemotherapy or immunosuppressive drugs. Later sources of discomfort include pain due to complications. For instance, there may be bone marrow expansion related to the engraftment, infections such as neutropenic colitis, or viruses such as HSV and cytomegalovirus (CMV).[49] Pain due to

chronic GVHD is common and often occurs at multiple sites. In addition, high rates of bone loss causing bone pain are seen in SCT patients who had received high-dose cytoreductive chemotherapy and could be exacerbated by exposure to glucocorticoids.[50]

Mechanisms of Pain

It is important to characterize pain before the appropriate therapy is selected. It is important to consider the temporal account of pain, such as acute (weeks to months), chronic (more than 3 months), or breakthrough (a brief augmented intensity). Pain can be characterized by mechanisms, such as nociceptive (the result of tissue injury and divided as somatic and visceral), neuropathic pain (due to neuronal injury), or a combination of both.[51]

Pain Assessment

Before starting patients on pain regimens, careful history taking is necessary. A patient's nonmedical and medical history should be evaluated through interviewing and examination. This should include screening for chemical coping, addiction or abuse history by using tools such as the Cut-down, Annoyed, Guilty, Eye-opener[52] questionnaire for alcoholism, and appropriate psychiatric history. In addition, many patients may have emotional or spiritual pain, contributing to their overall pain, therefore; psychosocial and spiritual distress must be recognized and treated, preferably by working with a multidisciplinary team.[51] Patients with high psychosocial distress, such as those who report depressed mood or high anxiety, are more likely to have increased pain expression.[53] It is also important to consider whether patients have ever received opioids before. Patients may be opioid-naive, thus requiring lower initial dosing. Patients may have responded different ways to different opioids in the past. This is influenced by genetic factors and due to different opioids acting on different receptors.[28] It should be stressed that the patient's cognition should be regularly assessed to prevent opioid-induced neurotoxicity (OIN) which is a spectrum of symptoms that include

myoclonus, excessive sedation, and delirium that some patients may experience while on opioids.[28,54] The severity of pain is important to assess. An example of an analytical tool for the cancer patient is the ESAS (Table 27.4) which is meant to ask the patient directly how they rate the severity of common symptoms, from 0 being the absence of that symptom to 10 being the worse possible severity of that symptom.[14] Other commonly used scales include MDASI[11,12] and the FACT-BMT.[13]

Selecting a Pain Regimen

In considering pain regimens for SCT patients, there are limitations in route of administration as patients

---

TABLE 27.4
Edmonton Symptom Assessment Scale

Please circle the number that best describes how you feel within the past 24 hours:

No pain	0	1	2	3	4	5	6	7	8	9	10	Worst possible pain
No fatigue	0	1	2	3	4	5	6	7	8	9	10	Worst possible fatigue
No nausea	0	1	2	3	4	5	6	7	8	9	10	Worst possible nausea
Not depressed	0	1	2	3	4	5	6	7	8	9	10	Worst possible depression
No anxiety	0	1	2	3	4	5	6	7	8	9	10	Worst possible anxiety
Not drowsy	0	1	2	3	4	5	6	7	8	9	10	Worst possible drowsiness
Best appetite	0	1	2	3	4	5	6	7	8	9	10	Worst possible appetite
Best feeling of well-being	0	1	2	3	4	5	6	7	8	9	10	Worst possible feeling of well being
No shortness of breath	0	1	2	3	4	5	6	7	8	9	10	Worst possible shortness of breath
Best sleep	0	1	2	3	4	5	6	7	8	9	10	Worst possible sleep

Bruera, E., Kuehn, N., Miller, M. J., Selmser, P., & Macmillan, K. (1991). The Edmonton Symptom Assessment System (ESAS): a simple method for the assessment of palliative care patients. *J Palliat Care*, 7(2), 6–9.
Permission obtained from Eduardo Bruera, MD

may have inflammation, infections, or GVHD complications that affect mucosal surfaces and the skin. SCT patients often have thrombocytopenia, which makes the subcutaneous route unwarranted.[6] Analgesics such as nonsteroidal anti-inflammatory drugs and acetaminophen are discouraged in SCT patients due to effects on renal, gastrointestinal, and hepatic function. Thus knowledge of opioids is important in the management of pain in SCT patients.[49] The patient's biochemical profile should be kept in mind when choosing a pain regimen. The opioids that are more commonly seen in OIN are those opioids with active metabolites. This includes morphine, codeine, meperidine, and hydromorphone. Fentanyl and methadone do not have active metabolites, and patients are less likely to experience OIN while on these medications.[55] It is also important to keep in mind that opioids must be chosen discriminately based on the patients' circumstances. Patients with renal failure, who are elderly, and have infections or dehydration could experience increased metabolite accumulation, thus increased neurotoxicity and other side effects.[55] It can be helpful to use a scoring system such as the Memorial Delirium Assessment Scale (MDAS), a ten-point tool for the screening of the severity of delirium.[56] Patients with hepatic dysfunction are also at risk of experiencing side effects of opioid medications and are another population that poses a challenge in pain management. Owing to decreased clearance of medications in these patients, it is recommended that there is a reduced initial dose and that there are longer periods between doses.[57]

Weak opioids include tramadol, codeine, and hydrocodone, whereas strong opioids include morphine, oxycodone, oxymorphone, hydromorphone, fentanyl, and methadone.[51] Morphine serves as a standard of comparison for opioid analgesics (Table 27.5).[28] There are equianalgesic conversion tables available for common dose conversions (Table 27.6).[28] For opioid-naive patients, longer acting regimens can be considered later on based on the amount of initial opioid use. To sustain satisfactory opioid levels throughout the day, most patients should have extended-release opioids in combination with immediate-release opioids for breakthrough pain. Pain regimens should initially have conservative dosing which should be titrated over several days to attain the best pain relief. Intermediate-release opioids should be dosed at 10% of the 24-hour dose.[28] For opioid maintenance, it is imperative to continually reevaluate the patient's disease status, medication side effects, and psychosocial parameters in addition to the analgesic effect.[51] Opioid dose titration may be necessary when the pain has not been adequately controlled. Dose reduction may be necessary if there are toxicities and side effects seen on the current pain regimen such as over-sedation and intractable nausea.[28] Opioid rotation may be necessary for patients with inadequate pain control despite multiple titrations and in patients who develop OIN.[51] A brief overview of strong opioids is provided in (Table 27.7).[28]

DELIRIUM

Delirium is defined as an acute fluctuating disturbance in attention, awareness, and cognition including disorganized thinking, memory impairment, disorientation, or perceptual disturbance.[58] Interestingly, a prospective study found that 50% of patients in the peritransplant period and up to 90% of patients during the final days

TABLE 27.5
Types of Opioids Based on Their Strength

OPIOID STRENGTH	
Weak Opioids	**Strong Opioids**
Codeine	Morphine
Hydrocodone	Oxycodone
Tramadol	Oxymorphone
	Hydromorphone
	Methadone
	Fentanyl

TABLE 27.6
Conversion Factors to Calculate Morphine Equianalgesic Daily Dose (MEDD)

Type of Opioid and Route	Conversion factor to calculate Morphine Equianalgesic Daily Dose (MEDD)
Morphine (Oral)	1
Hydrocodone (Oral)	1.5
Oxycodone (Oral)	1.5
Hydromorphone (Oral)	5
Oxymorphone (Oral)	3
Morphine (Intravenous)	2.5
Hydromorphone (Intravenous)	10-12
Fentanyl patch microgram/hour	2.5 (requires experience)

Published in The MD Anderson Supportive and Palliative Care Handbook, Fifth Edition Permission Obtained from Eduardo Bruera, MD

TABLE 27.7
Overview of Strong Opioids

Opioid	Onset (minutes)	Peak effect (hours)	Duration (hours)	Initial scheduled dose	Available Oral/TD Formulation	Comments
Hydrocodone/ Acetaminophen Hydrocodone ER	PO: 30 PO: 60	1-1.5 5	IR: 4 LA: 12	5/325 mg PO q4h 10mg PO q12h	Tablet, Liquid, Tablet	Co-ingestion with alcohol increases peak concentration
Morphine	PO: 30	0.5-1	IR: 3-6 LA: 12	LA: 15 mg po q12h, IR: 7.5mg po q 4 hrs prn	Tablet, cap, liquid	Kadian® can be given via PEG tube (16Fr or larger)
Oxycodone	PO: 10-15	0.5-1	IR: 3-6 LA: 12	LA:10 mg PO q12h IR: 2.5-5mg PO q 4 h prn	Tablet, Liquid	Long-acting formulation reformulated to minimize drug abuse
Hydromorphone	PO: 15-30	0.5-1	IR: 3-5 LA: 24	LA: 8mg po once daily IR: 1-2 mg po q4h	Tablet, Liquid	ER Hydromorphone available in 8mg, 12mg, 16mg, 32mg
Methadone	PO: 30-60	1-7.5	Variable	PO: 2.5 mg po q12h	Tablet, Liquid	Multiple drug interactions, monitor electrolytes, QTc
Oxymorphone	PO: 10-15	0.5	8 (IR) 12 (ER)	ER: 10 mg PO q12h IR: 5mg PO q 6-8h prn	Tablet	Co-ingestion with alcohol and food increases peak concentration
Fentanyl Transdermal	TD: variable Typically takes >5 hrs	24-48	72	12mcg patch Q 72 hrs	patch	Adjust dose after three days. May take up to 2 applications to reach steady state

Abbreviation: ER: Extended Release; PO: Per Oral; mg: Milligram; mcg: Microgram; hrs: Hours; IR: prn: Pro Re Nata (as necessary); Immediate Release; LA: Long Acting; TD: Transdermal
Published in The MD Anderson Supportive and Palliative Care Handbook, Fifth Edition Permission Obtained from Eduardo Bruera, MD

of life will experience delirium.[59,60] Delirium remains underdiagnosed which may result in mismanagement and distress to both patient and caregiver.

Three subtypes of delirium exist which are classified according to motor or arousal disturbances. Hypoactive delirium includes somnolence and confusion and may be difficult to differentiate between sedative effects of opioids and depression.[61] Hyperactive delirium is characterized by restlessness, agitation, hallucinations, delusions, and hyperalgesia and may be mistaken for psychosis or extrapyramidal side effects of medications.[28] Mixed delirium is a combination of symptoms that alternate between hyperactive and hypoactive delirium. In the general cancer population, mixed delirium remains most common;[5] however, studies have shown hypoactive delirium predominance in HSCT populations.[62]

The cause of delirium in cancer patients is often multifactorial. Medication side effects (specifically opioids, anticholinergics, benzodiazepines) are a common cause of delirium, especially in the setting of dehydration and renal failure. Other common reasons include organ dysfunction (hepatic, renal), infection, electrolyte disturbances, dehydration, chemotherapy or radiation therapy, CNS involvement of malignancy, drug withdrawal or intoxication, or nutritional deficiencies.[63] It is important to note that less than 50% of cases will result in an etiology;[64] however, this should not deter the clinician in evaluating for a reversible cause and treat if indicated.

The best practice is to maintain a high level of suspicion for delirium in cancer patients. Several screening tools exist to aid in the diagnosis of delirium including MDAS,[65,66] Confusion Assessment Method,[67] and Delirium Rating Scale.[68] These should be used in all patients, along with clinical observations from nurses or caregivers, to facilitate early diagnosis.

TABLE 27.8
Overview of Treatment of Delirium

Medication	Class	Dose, Route	Adverse Effects	Additional Comments
Haloperidol	Typical Antipsychotic	0.5-2 mg every 2-12 h PO, IV, IM, SC	Extrapyramidal syndrome, prolonged QTc	First line Oral bioavailability is approximately 60-70% May add Lorazepam for agitated patients.
Chlorpromazine	Typical Antipsychotic	12.5-50mg every 4-6 h PO, IV, IM, SC, PR	Sedation, Hypotension	More sedating and anticholinergic when compared to haloperidol
Olanzapine	Atypical Antipsychotic	2.5-5 mg every 12-24 h PO	Extrapyramidal syndrome, prolonged QTc, Hyperglycemia, Weight gain, Hyperlipidemia	
Risperidone	Atypical Antipsychotic	0.25-1 mg every 12-24 h PO	Extrapyramidal syndrome, prolonged QTc, Weight gain	
Quetiapine	Atypical Antipsychotic	12.5-100 mg every 12-24 h PO	Extrapyramidal syndrome, prolonged QTc, Weight gain	
Lorazepam	Benzodiazepine	0.5-3mg q2-12 h PO, IV	Sedative, Respiratory depression	Can have paradoxical effect causing worsening delirium

Abbreviation: PO – Per Oral; IV: Intravenous; IM: Intramuscular; SC: Subcutaneous; PR: Per Rectum
Published in The MD Anderson Supportive and Palliative Care Handbook, Fifth Edition Permission Obtained from Eduardo Bruera, MD

Management of delirium relies on treating the underlying cause, which proves to be difficult in cancer patients as etiology can be broad and complex. Nonpharmacological therapy can assist with symptoms and include daily orientation, early mobilization, maintaining a safe and familiar environment, and use of hearing or visual aids if indicated.[69]

Pharmacologic treatment should be considered for uncontrolled symptoms of delirium. Neuroleptics and benzodiazepines are the mainstays of therapy. Specifically, haloperidol is the first-line therapy for delirium for terminally ill cancer patients, followed by chlorpromazine as an acceptable choice.[66,70] Atypical antipsychotics such as olanzapine, quetiapine, and risperidone can also be used as an alternative and may be equally as effective in some patients[71] (Table 27.8).[28,66,72] Benzodiazepines are typically reserved for cases where delirium is present in the setting of alcohol withdrawal or contraindications to neuroleptic use.

Palliative sedation should be considered in cases of refractory delirium and life expectancy less than 2 weeks.[73,74] Indications and goals should be thoroughly discussed with both the patient and family reinforcing that treatment aims to control symptoms and not shorten life; this should be documented in the medical chart. Midazolam is the drug of choice due to the rapid onset of action, short half-life, and dose-dependent sedative effect. Start with a loading dose of 2.5–5 mg and continuous infusion at 1 mg/h, titrating by 0.5–1 mg/h increments every 30 minutes according to clinical response[75] with tools such as the Richmond Agitation–Sedation Scale.[76] In the terminally ill patient, delirium is a poor prognostic sign. Symptoms of delirium may be distressing for caregivers, and adequate education should be provided.

DIARRHEA

Patients with hematopoietic malignancies are at high risk for diarrhea (approximately 66% of patients), especially in the first 3 months after SCT. Patients who are undergoing allogeneic SCT are more significantly affected than autologous SCT recipients.[77] Evaluation begins with a careful history including duration, frequency, quantity, quality, associated symptoms, and subsequent correction of volume depletion and metabolic abnormalities.

Infectious etiologies are common in SCT populations given their immunocompromised state, including bacterial (*Salmonella, Shigella, Yersinia, Clostridium difficile*), viral (adenovirus, rotavirus, and CMV), and fungal agents.[78] In SCT patients the most commonly reported bacterial cause is *Clostridium difficile* infection (CDI) as sequelae of antibiotic therapy causing intestinal microbiome shifts.[79] CDI is critical to evaluate as there is increasing antibiotic resistance, toxin production, and the emergence of virulent strain NAP-1/027 all correlating with severity of the disease.[80]

Noninfectious etiologies include regimens for hematopoietic stem cell transplant, with or without total-body irradiation, which are highly mucotoxic agents and can affect the entire alimentary tract.[81] A common and significant cause of diarrhea in this specific patient population includes acute gastrointestinal GVHD associated with allogeneic bone marrow transplantation. Gastrointestinal GVHD can affect any segment of the intestinal tract, along with skin and liver. Specifically, intestinal GVHD causes profuse watery diarrhea with or without hematochezia, nausea, emesis, and abdominal discomfort which start approximately 3 weeks after SCT.[82] Gastrointestinal GVHD is distinguished from other causes of gastroenteritis (infectious, protocol induced) including the presence of hyperbilirubinemia and maculopapular rash at palms, soles, and trunk. Endoscopy may be required to assist in establishing an accurate and early diagnosis.[83] The mainstay of treatment relies on glucocorticoids and supportive therapy (aggressive fluid and electrolyte replacement, nutrition). Development of gastrointestinal GVHD is associated with higher morbidity and mortality (please see Graft-Versus-Host Disease section for further details).

After infectious etiologies are ruled out, symptom management for patients with high-volume diarrhea (>10 L/day) may find relief with loperamide (maximum dose of 16 mg daily). Unfortunately, severe gastrointestinal GVHD will result in poor absorption, and octreotide proves to be beneficial (200–600 μg daily subcutaneous or intravenous bolus or continues infusion with a maximum dose of 900 μg daily).[84]

PALLIATIVE CARE IN HEMATOPOIETIC CELL TRANSPLANTATION

SCT is often a curative therapy for patients with hematological malignancies.[85] In the United States, SCT is mostly offered in an inpatient setting and requires prolonged hospitalization, usually 3–4 weeks.[86] It is not uncommon that patients often experience high physical and psychosocial symptoms which can lead to decrease in QOL.[1-4] Posttraumatic stress disorder (PTSD) and depression are relatively common in SCT survivors. For those patients who do not survive, death is often a consequence of prolonged hospitalization due to organ failure, cytopenias leading to infections, and GVHD.[87]

There is a small but significant body of literature examining the benefits of early integration of palliative care with standard transplant care leading to improvement in physical and psychosocial well-being. In a recent nonblinded randomized clinical trial among 160 patients undergoing autologous/allogeneic SCT, El-Jawahri et al. found that patients who received twice-weekly inpatient palliative care interventions reported a smaller decrease in QOL at 2 weeks after transplantation versus those who received standard care.[9] Also, patients in the intervention arm reported lower anxiety, less increase in depression, and less increase in overall symptom burden.[9] Patients reported higher QOL and less depression at 3 months after transplantation.[9] Also, in a separate 6-month follow-up study on the same cohort, authors reported lower depression symptoms on the Hospital Anxiety and Depression Scale and lower PTSD symptoms but no difference in QOL and anxiety.[10] Authors also reported that symptom burden and anxiety symptoms partially mediated the effect of the intervention on patients with PTSD and depression at 6 months after transplantation.[10] Therefore, it is reasonable to consider referral to interdisciplinary palliative care team for symptom management and psychological support during the early transplant phase. This approach has potential to improve depression and PTSD symptoms in survivors.

According to American Society of Clinical Oncology clinical practice guidelines,[88] patients with advanced cancer and/or high symptom burden should be considered for a referral to interdisciplinary palliative care team early in their disease trajectory concurrent with active cancer treatment. A potential barrier to palliative care referral in patients with hematological malignancies undergoing SCT can be its prognostic uncertainty.[89] Nevertheless, patients with high symptom burden will likely benefit from early palliative care interventions. More research is needed to find an optimal model of integration of early palliative care in transplant care for symptom management, complex decision-making, and survivorship care.[90] At this point, there are no consensus guidelines or recommendations on the appropriate timings of palliative care integration.

REFERENCES

1. Pidala J, Anasetti C, Jim H. Health-related quality of life following haematopoietic cell transplantation: patient education, evaluation and intervention. *Br J Haematol.* 2010;148(3):373–385.
2. Jim HS, Quinn GP, Gwede CK, et al. Patient education in allogeneic hematopoietic cell transplant: what patients wish they had known about quality of life. *Bone Marrow Transplant.* 2014;49(2):299–303.
3. El-Jawahri AR, Traeger LN, Kuzmuk K, et al. Quality of life and mood of patients and family caregivers during hospitalization for hematopoietic stem cell transplantation. *Cancer.* 2015;121(6):951–959.
4. El-Jawahri AR, Vandusen HB, Traeger LN, et al. Quality of life and mood predict posttraumatic stress disorder after hematopoietic stem cell transplantation. *Cancer.* 2016;122(5):806–812.
5. Schulz-Kindermann F, Hennings U, Ramm G, Zander AR, Hasenbring M. The role of biomedical and psychosocial factors for the prediction of pain and distress in patients undergoing high-dose therapy and BMT/PBSCT. *Bone Marrow Transplant.* 2002;29(4):341–351.
6. Roeland E, Mitchell W, Elia G, et al. Symptom control in stem cell transplantation: a multidisciplinary palliative care team approach. part 1: physical symptoms. *J Support Oncol.* 2010;8(3):100–116.
7. Aslanian H, Chander B, Robert M, et al. Prospective evaluation of acute graft-versus-host disease. *Dig Dis Sci.* 2012;57(3):720–725.
8. Bensinger W, Schubert M, Ang KK, et al. NCCN Task Force Report. prevention and management of mucositis in cancer care. *J Natl Compr Canc Netw.* 2008;6(suppl 1):S1–S21; quiz S22–24.
9. El-Jawahri A, LeBlanc T, VanDusen H, et al. Effect of inpatient palliative care on quality of life 2 Weeks after hematopoietic stem cell transplantation: a randomized clinical trial. *Jama.* 2016;316(20):2094–2103.
10. El-Jawahri A, Traeger L, Greer JA, et al. Effect of inpatient palliative care during hematopoietic stem-cell transplant on psychological distress 6 Months after transplant: results of a randomized clinical trial. *J Clin Oncol.* 2017: Jco2017732800.
11. Cleeland CS, Mendoza TR, Wang XS, et al. Assessing symptom distress in cancer patients: the M.D. Anderson Symptom Inventory. *Cancer.* 2000;89(7):1634–1646.
12. Shah N, Shi Q, Williams LA, et al. Higher stem cell dose infusion after intensive chemotherapy does not improve symptom burden in older patients with multiple myeloma and amyloidosis. *Biol Blood Marrow Transpl.* 2016;22(2):226–231.
13. McQuellon RP, Russell GB, Cella DF, et al. Quality of life measurement in bone marrow transplantation: development of the Functional Assessment of Cancer Therapy-Bone Marrow Transplant (FACT-BMT) scale. *Bone Marrow Transpl.* 1997;19(4):357–368.
14. Bruera E, Kuehn N, Miller MJ, Selmser P, Macmillan K. The Edmonton Symptom Assessment System (ESAS): a simple method for the assessment of palliative care patients. *J Palliat Care.* 1991;7(2):6–9.
15. Richardson LA, Jones GW. A review of the reliability and validity of the Edmonton symptom assessment system. *Curr Oncol.* 2009;16(1):55.
16. Martin PJ, Schoch G, Fisher L, et al. A retrospective analysis of therapy for acute graft-versus-host disease: initial treatment. *Blood.* 1990;76(8):1464–1472.
17. Villarreal CD, Alanis JC, Perez JC, Candiani JO. Cutaneous graft-versus-host disease after hematopoietic stem cell transplant - a review. *An Bras Dermatol.* 2016;91(3):336–343.
18. Penas PF, Zaman S. Many faces of graft-versus-host disease. *Australas J Dermatol.* 2010;51(1):1–10; quiz 11.
19. Ferrara JL, Levine JE, Reddy P, Holler E. Graft-versus-host disease. *Lancet.* 2009;373(9674):1550–1561.
20. Ruutu T, Eriksson B, Remes K, et al. Ursodeoxycholic acid for the prevention of hepatic complications in allogeneic stem cell transplantation. *Blood.* 2002;100(6):1977–1983.
21. Ruutu T, Juvonen E, Remberger M, et al. Improved survival with ursodeoxycholic acid prophylaxis in allogeneic stem cell transplantation: long-term follow-up of a randomized study. *Biol Blood Marrow Transpl.* 2014;20(1):135–138.
22. Flowers ME, Martin PJ. How we treat chronic graft-versus-host disease. *Blood.* 2015;125(4):606–615.
23. Carpenter PA, Schubert MM, Flowers ME. Cevimeline reduced mouth dryness and increased salivary flow in patients with xerostomia complicating chronic graft-versus-host disease. *Biol Blood Marrow Transpl.* 2006;12(7):792–794.
24. Spiryda LB, Laufer MR, Soiffer RJ, Antin JA. Graft-versus-host disease of the vulva and/or vagina: diagnosis and treatment. *Biol Blood Marrow Transpl.* 2003;9(12):760–765.
25. Bellm LA, Epstein JB, Rose-Ped A, Martin P, Fuchs HJ. Patient reports of complications of bone marrow transplantation. *Support Care Cancer.* 2000;8(1):33–39.
26. Robien K, Schubert MM, Bruemmer B, Lloid ME, Potter JD, Ulrich CM. Predictors of oral mucositis in patients receiving hematopoietic cell transplants for chronic myelogenous leukemia. *J Clin Oncol.* 2004;22(7):1268–1275.
27. Sonis ST, Elting LS, Keefe D, et al. Perspectives on cancer therapy-induced mucosal injury: pathogenesis, measurement, epidemiology, and consequences for patients. *Cancer.* 2004;100(suppl 9):1995–2025.
28. Bruera EE A. *The MD Anderson Symptom Control and Palliative Care Handbook.* Houston, TX: University of Health Science Center at Houston; 2015.
29. Epstein JB, Schubert MM. Oropharyngeal mucositis in cancer therapy. Review of pathogenesis, diagnosis, and management. *Oncol Willist Park.* 2003;17(12):1767–1779; discussion 1779-1782, 1791-1762.
30. Stiff P. Mucositis associated with stem cell transplantation: current status and innovative approaches to management. *Bone Marrow Transpl.* 2001;27(suppl 2):S3–S11.

31. Dreizen S, Bodey GP, Valdivieso M. Chemotherapy-associated oral infections in adults with solid tumors. *Oral Surg Oral Med Oral Pathol.* 1983;55(2):113–120.

32. Redding SW. Role of herpes simplex virus reactivation in chemotherapy-induced oral mucositis. *NCI Monogr.* 1990;(9):103–105.

33. Keefe DM, Schubert MM, Elting LS, et al. Updated clinical practice guidelines for the prevention and treatment of mucositis. *Cancer.* 2007;109(5):820–831.

34. Freifeld AG, Bow EJ, Sepkowitz KA, et al. Clinical practice guideline for the use of antimicrobial agents in neutropenic patients with cancer: 2010 Update by the Infectious Diseases Society of America. *Clin Infect Dis.* 2011;52(4):427–431.

35. Gralla RJ, Osoba D, Kris MG, et al. Recommendations for the use of antiemetics: evidence-based, clinical practice guidelines. American Society of Clinical Oncology. *J Clin Oncol.* 1999;17(9):2971–2994.

36. Hesketh PJ. Chemotherapy-induced nausea and vomiting. *N Engl J Med.* 2008;358(23):2482–2494.

37. Anderson 3rd WD, Strayer SM. Evaluation of nausea and vomiting: a case-based approach. *Am Fam Physician.* 2013;88(6):371–379.

38. Lingen MW, Abt E, Agrawal N, et al. Evidence-based clinical practice guideline for the evaluation of potentially malignant disorders in the oral cavity: a report of the American Dental Association. *J Am Dent Assoc.* 2017;148(10):712–727.e710.

39. Adel N. Overview of chemotherapy-induced nausea and vomiting and evidence-based therapies. *Am J Manag Care.* 2017;23(suppl 14):S259–S265.

40. Berger MJ, Ettinger DS, Aston J, et al. NCCN guidelines insights: antiemesis, Version 2.2017. *J Natl Compr Canc Netw.* 2017;15(7):883–893.

41. Hesketh PJ. Defining the emetogenicity of cancer chemotherapy regimens: relevance to clinical practice. *Oncologist.* 1999;4(3):191–196.

42. Navari RM, Aapro M. Antiemetic prophylaxis for chemotherapy-induced nausea and vomiting. *N Engl J Med.* 2016;374(14):1356–1367.

43. Janelsins MC, Tejani MA, Kamen C, Peoples AR, Mustian KM, Morrow GR. Current pharmacotherapy for chemotherapy-induced nausea and vomiting in cancer patients. *Expert Opin Pharmacother.* 2013;14(6):757–766.

44. Ballatori E, Roila F. Impact of nausea and vomiting on quality of life in cancer patients during chemotherapy. *Health Qual Life Outcomes.* 2003;1:46.

45. Ferrucci PF, Martinoni A, Cocorocchio E, et al. Evaluation of acute toxicities associated with autologous peripheral blood progenitor cell reinfusion in patients undergoing high-dose chemotherapy. *Bone Marrow Transpl.* 2000;25(2):173–177.

46. Fujii N, Ikeda K, Koyama M, et al. Calcineurin inhibitor-induced irreversible neuropathic pain after allogeneic hematopoietic stem cell transplantation. *Int J Hematol.* 2006;83(5):459–461.

47. Katayama Y, Deguchi S, Shinagawa K, et al. Bone marrow necrosis in a patient with acute myeloblastic leukemia during administration of G-CSF and rapid hematologic recovery after allotransplantation of peripheral blood stem cells. *Am J Hematol.* 1998;57(3):238–240.

48. Lunde LE, Dasaraju S, Cao Q, et al. Hemorrhagic cystitis after allogeneic hematopoietic cell transplantation: risk factors, graft source and survival. *Bone Marrow Transpl.* 2015;50(11):1432–1437.

49. Niscola P, Romani C, Scaramucci L, et al. Pain syndromes in the setting of haematopoietic stem cell transplantation for haematological malignancies. *Bone Marrow Transpl.* 2008;41(9):757–764.

50. Schulte C, Beelen DW, Schaefer UW, Mann K. Bone loss in long-term survivors after transplantation of hematopoietic stem cells: a prospective study. *Osteoporos Int.* 2000;11(4):344–353.

51. Dalal S, Tanco KC, Bruera E. State of art of managing pain in patients with cancer. *Cancer J.* 2013;19(5):379–389.

52. Mayfield D, McLeod G, Hall P. The CAGE questionnaire: validation of a new alcoholism screening instrument. *Am J Psychiat.* 1974;131(10):1121–1123.

53. Strasser F, Walker P, Bruera E. Palliative pain management: when both pain and suffering hurt. *J Palliat Care.* 2005;21(2):69–79.

54. Mercadante S. Opioid rotation for cancer pain: rationale and clinical aspects. *Cancer.* 1999;86(9):1856–1866.

55. Gallagher R. Opioid-induced neurotoxicity. *Can Fam Physician.* 2007;53(3):426–427.

56. Breitbart W, Rosenfeld B, Roth A, Smith MJ, Cohen K, Passik S. The memorial delirium assessment scale. *J Pain Symptom Management.* 1997;13(3):128–137.

57. Soleimanpour H, Safari S, Shahsavari Nia K, Sanaie S, Alavian SM. Opioid drugs in patients with liver disease: a systematic review. *Hepat Mon.* 2016;16(4):e32636.

58. Association AP. *Diagnostic and Statistical Manual of Mental Disorders.* 5th ed. Arlington, VA: DSM-5; 2013.

59. Fann JR, Roth-Roemer S, Burington BE, Katon WJ, Syrjala KL. Delirium in patients undergoing hematopoietic stem cell transplantation. *Cancer.* 2002;95(9):1971–1981.

60. Hosie A, Davidson PM, Agar M, Sanderson CR, Phillips J. Delirium prevalence, incidence, and implications for screening in specialist palliative care inpatient settings: a systematic review. *Palliat Med.* 2013;27(6):486–498.

61. Kiely DK, Jones RN, Bergmann MA, Marcantonio ER. Association between psychomotor activity delirium subtypes and mortality among newly admitted post-acute facility patients. *J Gerontol Ser A Biol Sci Med Sci.* 2007;62(2):174–179.

62. Beglinger LJ, Duff K, Van Der Heiden S, Parrott K, Langbehn D, Gingrich R. Incidence of delirium and associated mortality in hematopoietic stem cell transplantation patients. *Biol Blood Marrow Transpl.* 2006;12(9):928–935.

63. Morita T, Tei Y, Tsunoda J, Inoue S, Chihara S. Underlying pathologies and their associations with clinical features in terminal delirium of cancer patients. *J Pain Symptom Management.* 2001;22(6):997–1006.

64. Bruera E, Miller L, McCallion J, Macmillan K, Krefting L, Hanson J. Cognitive failure in patients with terminal cancer: a prospective study. *J Pain Symptom Management.* 1992;7(4):192–195.

65. Lawlor PG, Nekolaichuk C, Gagnon B, Mancini IL, Pereira JL, Bruera ED. Clinical utility, factor analysis, and further validation of the memorial delirium assessment scale in patients with advanced cancer: assessing delirium in advanced cancer. *Cancer.* 2000;88(12):2859–2867.

66. Breitbart W, Marotta R, Platt MM, et al. A double-blind trial of haloperidol, chlorpromazine, and lorazepam in the treatment of delirium in hospitalized AIDS patients. *Am J Psychiat.* 1996;153(2):231–237.

67. Inouye SK, van Dyck CH, Alessi CA, Balkin S, Siegal AP, Horwitz RI. Clarifying confusion: the confusion assessment method. A new method for detection of delirium. *Ann Intern Med.* 1990;113(12):941–948.

68. Trzepacz PT. The Delirium Rating Scale. Its use in consultation-liaison research. *Psychosomatics.* 1999;40(3):193–204.

69. Inouye SK, Bogardus Jr ST, Charpentier PA, et al. A multicomponent intervention to prevent delirium in hospitalized older patients. *N Engl J Med.* 1999;340(9):669–676.

70. Jackson KC, Lipman AG. Drug therapy for delirium in terminally ill patients. *Cochrane Database Syst Rev.* 2004;(2):Cd004770.

71. Grassi L, Caraceni A, Mitchell AJ, et al. Management of delirium in palliative care: a review. *Curr Psychiat Rep.* 2015;17(3):550.

72. Breitbart W, Alici Y. Agitation and delirium at the end of life: "We couldn't manage him". *Jama.* 2008;300(24):2898–2910.e2891.

73. Lo B, Rubenfeld G. Palliative sedation in dying patients: "we turn to it when everything else hasn't worked". *Jama.* 2005;294(14):1810–1816.

74. Dean MM, Cellarius V, Henry B, Oneschuk D. Librach Canadian Society of palliative care physicians taskforce SL. Framework for continuous palliative sedation therapy in Canada. *J Palliat Med.* 2012;15(8):870–879.

75. Bush SH, Tierney S, Lawlor PG. Clinical assessment and management of delirium in the palliative care setting. *Drugs.* 2017.

76. Sessler CN, Gosnell MS, Grap MJ, et al. The Richmond Agitation-Sedation Scale: validity and reliability in adult intensive care unit patients. *Am J Respir Crit Care Med.* 2002;166(10):1338–1344.

77. van Kraaij MG, Dekker AW, Verdonck LF, et al. Infectious gastro-enteritis: an uncommon cause of diarrhoea in adult allogeneic and autologous stem cell transplant recipients. *Bone Marrow Transpl.* 2000;26(3):299–303.

78. Yuen KY, Woo PC, Liang RH, et al. Clinical significance of alimentary tract microbes in bone marrow transplant recipients. *Diagn Microbiol Infect Dis.* 1998;30(2):75–81.

79. Yolken RH, Bishop CA, Townsend TR, et al. Infectious gastroenteritis in bone-marrow-transplant recipients. *N Engl J Med.* 1982;306(17):1010–1012.

80. Shallis RM, Terry CM, Lim SH. Changes in intestinal microbiota and their effects on allogeneic stem cell transplantation. *Am J Hematol.* 2017.

81. Bowen JM, Wardill HR. Advances in the understanding and management of mucositis during stem cell transplantation. *Curr Opin Support Palliat Care.* 2017;11(4):341–346.

82. Naymagon S, Naymagon L, Wong SY, et al. Acute graft-versus-host disease of the gut: considerations for the gastroenterologist. *Nat Rev Gastroenterol Hepatol.* 2017.

83. Cruz-Correa M, Poonawala A, Abraham SC, et al. Endoscopic findings predict the histologic diagnosis in gastrointestinal graft-versus-host disease. *Endoscopy.* 2002;34(10):808–813.

84. Ippoliti C, Champlin R, Bugazia N, et al. Use of octreotide in the symptomatic management of diarrhea induced by graft-versus-host disease in patients with hematologic malignancies. *J Clin Oncol.* 1997;15(11):3350–3354.

85. Braamse AM, Gerrits MM, van Meijel B, et al. Predictors of health-related quality of life in patients treated with auto- and allo-SCT for hematological malignancies. *Bone Marrow Transpl.* 2012;47(6):757–769.

86. Majhail NS, Mau LW, Chitphakdithai P, et al. National survey of hematopoietic cell transplantation center personnel, infrastructure, and models of care delivery. *Biol Blood Marrow Transpl.* 2015;21(7):1308–1314.

87. D'Souza A, Lee S, Zhu X, Pasquini M. Current use and trends in hematopoietic cell transplantation in the United States. *Biol Blood Marrow Transpl.* 2017;23(9):1417–1421.

88. Ferrell BR, Temel JS, Temin S, et al. Integration of palliative care into standard Oncology care: American Society of clinical Oncology clinical practice guideline update. *J Clin Oncol.* 2017;35(1):96–112.

89. LeBlanc TW, El-Jawahri A. When and why should patients with hematologic malignancies see a palliative care specialist? *Hematol Am Soc Hematol Educ Program.* 2015;2015:471–478.

90. El-Jawahri A, Temel JS. Palliative care integration in hematopoietic stem-cell transplantation: the need for additional research. *J Oncol Pract.* 2017;13(9):578–579.

CHAPTER 28

Principles and Applications of Cellular Therapy in the Setting of Hematopoietic Cell Transplant

MALIHA KHAN, MD • RABBIA SIDDIQI, MB, BS • ELIZABETH J. SHPALL, MD • AMANDA OLSON, MD

IMMUNOLOGIC STATUS AND RECONSTITUTION AFTER HEMATOPOIETIC CELL TRANSPLANT

Hematopoietic cell transplant (HCT) is widely performed for patients with hematological and other diseases and is often the only potentially curative treatment option available to these patients. Unfortunately, restoration of normal immune function after HCT is significantly delayed and may never be fully achieved.[1] Impaired adaptive immune response in the posttransplant period limits the success rate of HCT and carries serious risks to the patient, including infection, malignant relapse, secondary cancers, and decreased response to tumor vaccines.

Host immunosuppression in the pretransplant phase results from preparative conditioning regimens involving cytotoxic and/or radiation-induced injury to both mucosal barriers and hematopoietic tissues. Myeloablative regimens are associated with myeloid suppression and persistent lymphodepletion, which may be seen in recipients of both myeloablative and nonmyeloablative conditioning.[2] The resultant tissue damage is responsible for a "cytokine storm", i.e., widespread release of proinflammatory mediators including IL-6, IL-1, and tumor necrosis factor (TNF)-α that activate the host innate immune system.[3] Interaction between host antigen-presenting cells (APCs) and donor T lymphocytes stimulate the latter to differentiate and assume T-effector function, triggering acute graft-versus-host disease (GVHD).[4] T-helper cells further produce IL-2 and other cytokines that potentiate host APC activity via an increase in costimulatory signaling (CD40–CD40L interaction). CD8+ cytotoxic lymphocytes (CTLs)

mediate host tissue destruction, including damage to hematopoietic niches in the bone marrow[5] and thymus.[6,7] As a result, the graft-versus-host response contributes to a more severe and prolonged immune depletion.

Transplant-related factors, such as stem cell source, appear to influence the severity and duration of immune suppression. Immune reconstitution is often delayed for patients undergoing allogenic versus autologous transplant, those with unrelated versus related donors (possibly because of minor histocompatibility (MHC) antigen mismatch) and for those receiving T-cell depleted versus T-cell replete grafts.[8-11] Furthermore, recipients of umbilical cord blood (UCB) grafts experience prolonged lymphopenia compared to patients receiving bone marrow or peripheral blood-derived stem cells.[12-15] Immunosuppression with antithymocyte globulin (ATG) has also been associated with slower immune recovery after HCT, predisposing patients to infectious complications.[16]

Numerical recovery of innate immune cells occurs within weeks of HCT; neutrophils, NK cells, and monocytes reach normal counts by 2–4 weeks after transplantation; however, neutrophil function may remain suboptimal for an extended period.[2,17,18] Adaptive immunity recovers over a longer timeframe, taking months to years for B and T lymphocyte numbers to normalize.[2] B cell counts return to normal levels within 1–2 years of transplant, although full recovery may be delayed in the presence of GVHD.[19-21] Despite rising numbers of B lymphocytes, humoral immunity post-HCT is still deficient due to a lack of memory B cells, persistently low levels of certain immunoglobulin subsets,[22-24] and diminished

Hematopoietic Cell Transplantation for Malignant Conditions. https://doi.org/10.1016/B978-0-323-56802-9.00028-6

somatic hypermutation.[25] HCT-induced depression of CD4[+] function also contributes to humoral immune incompetence.[26,27] Immunization of the donor before transplant (e.g., with *H. influenza b* and tetanus toxoid vaccines) can extend important immune protection to the recipient posttransplant.[28,29]

CD8[+] T lymphocytes transiently rise to supranormal levels by approximately 6 months after transplantation, whereas low CD4[+] counts persist for over a year.[30] T-cell regeneration can occur through either homeostatic peripheral expansion (HPE) of memory/effector cells, which is a thymus-independent process, or through a lengthier thymus-dependent pathway which enables diversification of the T-cell repertoire.[31,32] In the months after HCT, CD8[+] T cell numbers recover rapidly after clonal HPE, giving increased CD8/CD4 ratios.[33–36] Increased post-HCT IL-7 (and possibly IL-15) levels, and antigen presentation drive homeostatic proliferation of T lymphocytes.[37–39] Thymus-dependent regeneration of T cells is limited in post-HCT immune recovery because of age-related decrease in thymic function and thymic damage resulting from conditioning regimens and GVHD.[30,40–42] As a consequence of this lack of thymopoiesis, which is more pronounced in older patients, the T-cell repertoire remains skewed and oligoclonal, and may never reach former levels of receptor diversity.[43–45] Thymic-dependent CD4[+] recovery is therefore severely deficient, resulting in a lack of critical stimulatory signals from CD4[+] T helper (Th) cells which further compromises the ability of CD8[+] T cells and B cells to mount an effective response.[46] Dendritic cells, which serve both the innate and adaptive arms of the immune system, take up to 1 year after transplant to recover.[47]

Cellular therapies administered in the pretransplant or posttransplant period focus on three key areas: (1) restoring normal immune function and reducing infection-related morbidity and mortality; (2) controlling GVHD; and (3) enhancing the graft versus tumor effect in the setting of malignant disease. Although deficits in lymphoid recovery present a challenge to generation of long-term antitumor immunity, adoptive T cell therapy is particularly well-suited to capitalize on the post-HCT inflammatory milieu[48] and HPE of cytotoxic cells in malignant diseases.[49,50] Novel strategies using adoptive transfer of T cells to prevent or fight against viral infections, as well as to generate antitumor immunity, are closely associated with the lympho-depleted status of the host.[51] Finally, natural killer (NK) cells are an important focus of immunomodulatory therapies, in addition to being among the earliest cell types to recover from HCT, they demonstrate effective cytolytic activity against leukemia cells,[52] support engraftment,[53] and suppress development of GVHD[54,55] (Fig. 28.1).

ROLE OF CELLULAR THERAPY IN REDUCING INFECTIOUS POST-HCT MORBIDITY AND MORTALITY

Infectious complications are a major cause of posttransplant morbidity and mortality with 20%–30% deaths in HCT recipients being directly attributable to infection.[56,57] Risk of infection is related to graft T cell depletion, donor/recipient HLA mismatch, donor immune status, use of intensive immunosuppressive drugs and severe acute or extensive chronic GVHD.[2,58–61] In the preengraftment phase (first month of transplant), the breakdown of innate immune defenses predisposes patients to bacterial and fungal infections, whereas in the engraftment (first 100 days of transplant) and postengraftment phases, opportunistic viral infections and reactivations of cytomegalovirus (CMV) and Epstein-Barr virus (EBV) predominate.[62,63] Persistent cellular and humoral immune defects also render patients susceptible to infections with encapsulated bacteria (including *S. pneumoniae* and *H. influenzae*) and varicella zoster virus (VZV) reactivation months after transplant.[64] Table 28.1 shows the time course of common infections in the peri-transplant period.

In the post-HCT setting, the most clinically relevant viral infections are CMV, EBV, human herpes virus 6 (HHV-6), polyoma viruses 'BK and 'JC virus, and adenovirus (AdV). Pharmacological antiviral prophylaxis and treatment, although useful, are often suboptimal because of toxicity, limited viral sensitivity and potential for drug resistant infection.[65–67] Vaccination strategies are also ineffective due to significant functional B and T cell deficits post-HCT.[68–71] As T lymphocytes mediate the immune response to viral infection, cellular immunotherapy involving infusion of virus-specific CTLs has been pursued.[72] Adoptive transfer of lymphocytes from the donor to HCT recipient, however, carries the risk of dose-limiting GVHD.[73,74] This understanding has led to development of approaches involving selective isolation of CMV-specific (and later EBV) T cells from the donor and expansion of these cells by means of ex vivo culture prior to infusion.[75–77] Although other biological and cellular therapeutic strategies such as infusion of T-cell precursors and administration of thymopoiesis-stimulating cytokines have been investigated, the generation and ex vivo expansion of virus-specific CTLs has been the most successful therapy to date.[78,79]

Principles of Generating Virus-Specific T Lymphocytes (VSTs)

In one of the pioneering works, Riddell et al. (1992) provided proof of principle that CMV-specific CD8[+]

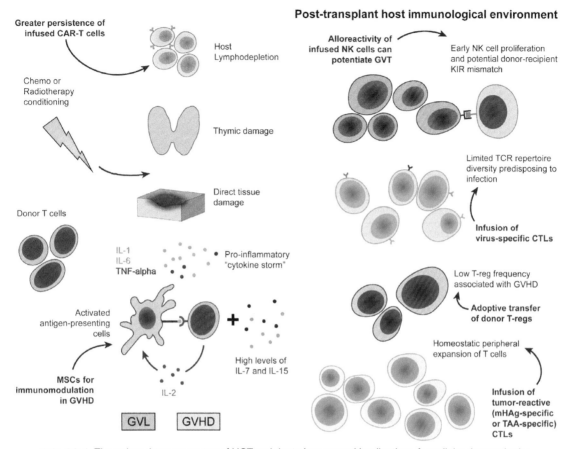

Post-transplant host immunological environment

FIG. 28.1 The unique immune status of HCT recipients has several implications for cellular therapy in the early posttransplant period, as shown here (blue arrows). High levels of circulating cytokines as well as lymphodepletion of the host result in a precarious balance between graft-versus-tumor and graft-versus-host effects. Infusion of mesenchymal stem cells (MSCs) and Tregs may be a potential approach to ameliorate GVHD. In addition, the posttransplant period may be optimal for the infusion of NK cells, CAR-T cells, and tumor-specific T cells, as high IL-7 and homeostatic peripheral expansion offers greater in vivo proliferation. Finally adoptive transfer of virus-specific lymphocytes can extend immune protection to the immunodeficient host. *CAR*, chimeric antigen receptor; *CTL*, cytotoxic lymphocyte; *GVHD*, graft-versus-host disease; *GVL*, graft-versus-leukemia; *GVT*, graft-versus-tumor; *HCT*, hematopoietic cell transplant; *mHAg*, minor histocompatibility antigens; *NK*, natural killer; *TAA*, tumor-associated antigen; *TCR*, T-cell receptor; *TNF*, tumor necrosis factor.

T cells isolated from a donor, expanded in vitro and adoptively transferred to HCT recipients could restore CMV-specific immunity.[77] Essentially adoptive therapy with VSTs comprises of isolation of the virus-specific lymphocytes, depletion of alloreactive cells, and clonal expansion of virus-specific cells to reach clinically relevant doses (Fig. 28.2).

One method to generate VSTs is to directly isolate T cells from donor blood, using rapid selection strategies and eliminating the need for ex vivo culture. The successful application of this method was thought to depend on high numbers of relevant virus-specific cells in donor peripheral blood, which is not a limiting factor in the case of CMV and EBV infections.[80] Rather, in practice even relatively low numbers of adenovirus-specific CTLs infused were shown to be clinically effective, likely because of in vivo proliferation in the host.[81–84] Rapid generation strategies to derive VSTs from donor blood products are based on either interferon-gamma (IFN-γ)

TABLE 28.1
Common Viral, Bacterial, and Fungal Causes of Infection in the HCT Setting

	Preengraftment Phase (Within 30 days of Transplant)	Early Posttransplant Phase (31–100 days of Transplant)	Late Posttransplant (>100 days of Transplant)
Immune factors predisposing to infection	Neutropenia, mucosal, and skin barrier breakdown	Impaired cellular and humoral immunity; limited T-cell diversity	Impaired cellular and humoral immunity; gradual B- and T-cell recovery
Viral	HSV; respiratory and enteric seasonal	CMV, VZV, HHV-6, EBV, adenovirus	VZV
Bacterial	Gram-negative and gram-positive organisms; viridans group streptococci and staphylococci	Gram-positive organisms	Encapsulated bacteria
Fungal	Aspergillus; Candida	Aspergillus; Pneumocystis	

CMV, cytomegalovirus; *EBV*, Epstein-Barr virus; *HHV6*, human herpes virus 6; *HSV*, herpes simplex virus; *VZV*, varicella zoster virus.

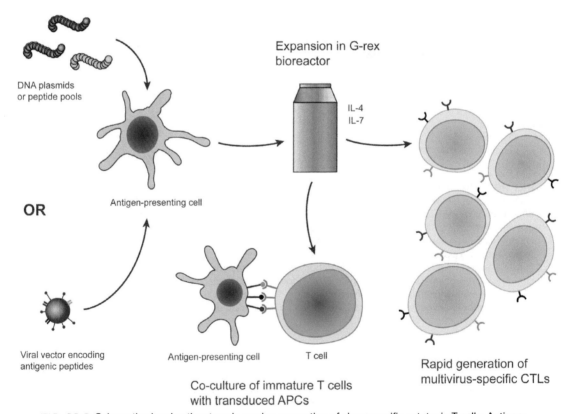

FIG. 28.2 Schematic showing the steps in ex vivo generation of virus-specific cytotoxic T cells. Antigen-presenting cells can be induced to express the viral antigen or antigens of interest through either transduction with viral vectors (commonly adenovirus) or DNA plasmids. The transduced antigen-presenting cells are then cultured with naive T cells in G-rex expansion bioreactors to yield large numbers of single virus or multivirus specific T cells, which can then be infused into transplant recipients to provide antiviral immunity. *APC*, antigen-presenting cell; *CTL*, cytotoxic lymphocyte.

capture, or peptide/MHC multimer labeling.[85,86] The latter approach selects only CD8[+] cells. It is unclear how the lack of coinfused CD4[+] helper T cells affects clinical responses, as these cells have a role in maintaining CD8[+] cytotoxic functionality and long-term immunity, yet are also associated with higher risk of alloreactivity.[77,85,87-89]

Another, lengthier method of generating virus-specific T cells is coculture of T cells with in vitro-stimulated antigen-presenting cells. This can be done by transducing donor-derived dendritic cells with viral vectors expressing immunodominant peptides, e.g., the CMVpp65 transgene, or using EBV-transformed B cells to stimulate expansion of specific antiviral T cells.[90,91] This approach further allows generation of multi-virus specific T cells. Alternatively, DNA plasmids or peptide pools can be used to pulse dendritic cells, bypassing the use of viral vectors and their associated safety and regulatory hurdles.

Clinical Use of VSTs

Early trials show that multivirus-specific CTLs targeting CMV, EBV, adenovirus and VZV are a safe and clinically effective means of antiviral prophylaxis as well as treatment of viral reactivation in post-HCT patients (summarized in Table 28.2).[92-95] A rapid protocol which reduces culture time to 10–12 days was developed in which transfection of dendritic cells with plasmids was followed by G-rex, gas-permeable rapid expansion, culture expansion to generate VSTs.[96] Using this protocol, CTLs specific for five viruses: CMV, EBV, Adv, BKV and HHV-6 were given to patients post-HCT and effective long-term antiviral protection was observed.[91,97]

For HCT recipients who have pathogen-naïve or UCB donors, generation of donor VSTs is not possible. For those patients, infusion of virus-specific cells derived from third party donors (HLA matched at loci dependent on viral target) is an option. Use of 'off the shelf' CTL lines from third party donors has produced partial or complete antiviral responses in recipients, with one study showing a correlation between outcomes and degree of donor-recipient HLA match.[98-100] Phase 1/2 trials of third party VSTs in post-SCT patients have shown this approach to be safe and effective with successful viral clearance after infusion of single- and multi-virus specific T lymphocytes.[101,102] Although in vitro experience suggest that expanded VSTs have the potential to cross-react with allogenic HLA antigens and produce GVHD, significant alloreactivity has not been reported in clinical studies.[82,103-106]

ROLE OF CELLULAR THERAPY IN CONTROLLING GRAFT-VERSUS-HOST DISEASE

Graft-versus-host disease is result of donor T cell alloreactivity. Despite the use of routine pharmacological immunosuppression as prophylaxis, GVHD complicates up to 40%–60% of allogeneic HCT cases.[107,108] The incidence of acute GVHD is higher in cases with donor-recipient HLA mismatch,[109] and in matched unrelated donor transplant recipients relative to matched related donor recipients.[108] The primary treatment for acute GVHD is corticosteroids; however, approximately half of patients are resistant to steroid therapy.[110,111] GVHD is mediated by donor T cells, coinfused with stem cell graft or derived from post-HCT donor lymphocyte infusions (DLI), and is a result of an altered interplay of inflammatory cytokines and certain T cell subsets.[112,113] Correspondingly, CD8[+] cytotoxic T cell depletion (TCD) of the graft, through ex vivo physical or immunologic separation techniques, or in vivo administration of anti-thymocyte globulin (ATG), was developed to prevent the occurrence of GVHD after HCT.[114,115] Unfortunately, although TCD reduces GVHD, any potential survival benefit appears to be offset by an increased risk of graft failure,[116] opportunistic infections due to delayed immune reconstitution,[117] and disease relapse.[109,118-124] Thus, the goal of immunomodulatory therapies in GVHD remains to restore balance between effector and regulatory immune functions, selective enrichment/depletion of T cell subsets, and genetic manipulation of T cells which may alleviate or prevent graft-versus-host (GVH) complications.[125,126] Given the close association of graft-versus-host and graft-versus-tumor mechanisms, strategies modifying the post-HCT immune status of the host are aimed at maximally preserving the beneficial graft-versus-tumor effect in malignant diseases.

Several approaches have been developed to selectively deplete GVHD-causing alloreactive donor lymphocytes, to preferentially infuse the host with immunoregulatory T cells, and to promote specific subpopulations that provide antiviral and antitumor immune function.

Depletion of αβ (Alpha-Beta) T Cells

T-cell receptor (TCR) αβ cells are implicated in the pathophysiology behind GVHD,[127,128] whereas increased numbers of γδ cells in the context of HLA-mismatched SCT are associated with improved survival. Thus, approaches to specifically eliminate αβ T cells have been developed with the aim of reducing GVHD

TABLE 28.2
Clinical Studies Involving Multivirus-Specific CTL Infusion in HCT Patients

Virus	References	Patients	Method of VST Generation	Outcome	Finding
EBV and AdV	Leen et al.[93]	N = 13 (12 on study, 1 compassionate); pediatric allo-HCT patients at high risk for viral infection, 2 with active AdV	CTLs activated by EBV-associated lymphoblastoid cells and monocytes transduced with adenoviral vector	None developed EBV or AdV disease; both AdV patients had complete clearance; no GVHD reported	Safety and efficacy of VST as antiviral prophylaxis in partially matched or unrelated HCT recipients
CMV and EBV	Dong et al.[259]	N = 3 pediatric allo-HCT patients with active CMV or EBV	CTLs activated by DC pulsed with antigenic viral peptides	Clearance in 2/2 CMV patients; none developed CMV or EBV infection	Therapeutic and preventive efficacy
EBV, CMV, and AdV	Gerdemann et al.[91]	N = 10 allo-HCT patients with active CMV, EBV, and/or AdV	CTLs activated by DC nucleofected with viral antigen-encoding DNA plasmids	CR in 3/4 EBV, CR in 4/5 CMV, CR in 4/5 AdV; no significant alloreactivity	Safety and efficacy of VSTs in treatment of post-HCT infections
EBV, CMV, and AdV	Leen et al.[98]	N = 50 allo-HCT patients with severe refractory infection	Third-party CTLs activated by EBV-associated lymphoblastoid cells and monocytes transduced with adenoviral vector	Cumulative overall response at 6 weeks of infusion: 74.0% (CMV, 73.9%; EBV, 66.7%; AdV, 77.8%)	Safety, efficacy, and feasibility of banked third-party VSTs in treatment of post-HCT infections
EBV, CMV, AdV, BKV, and HHV6	Papadopoulou et al.[97]	N = 11 allo-HCT patients, 8 with active infection, and 3 at risk	CTLs activated by DC pulsed with synthetic antigenic viral peptides	Overall response rate 94%, at 12 weeks of infusion; 1 patient had grade 2 GVHD	Safety and sustained long-term efficacy of VSTs in prophylaxis and treatment of post-HCT infections
EBV, CMV, AdV, and VZV	Ma et al.[95]	N = 10 allo-HCT patients at risk of viral infection	CTLs activated by MoDC transduced with viral vector or vaccine	5 patients had CMV reactivation, no other viral reactivation; 3 patients had grades 2–4 GVHD	Safety and efficacy of additional VZV-specific CTLs as prophylaxis

AdV, adenovirus; *CMV*, cytomegalovirus; *CTL*, cytotoxic lymphocyte; *DC*, dendritic cell; *EBV*, Epstein-Barr virus; *GVHD*, graft-versus-host disease; *HHV6*, human herpes virus 6; *MoDC*, monocyte-derived dendritic cell; *VST*, virus-specific T lymphocyte; *VZV*, varicella zoster virus.

complications.[129,130] Twenty-three children with non-malignant disorders who received αβ TCD haploidentical stem cell grafts, without any posttransplant GVHD prophylaxis, exhibited sustained engraftment, rapid immune reconstitution and low incidence of GVHD (3 patients experienced grade 1–2 aGVHD of the skin).[131] In 34 patients with high-risk acute leukemia, who received αβ T-cell–depleted haploidentical HCT, grade 3–4 aGVHD and cGVHD each occurred only in 2 patients.[132]

Depletion of Antigen-Naïve T Cells

T lymphocytes may be classified into antigen-experienced 'T-memory' and 'T-naïve' cells based on antigen exposure and antigen-induced activation. Naïve T cells have high expression of homing molecules, enabling these cells to home to secondary lymphoid organs and proliferate into antigen-reactive cells.[133,134] This may explain why graft-versus-host responses are mediated chiefly by T-naïve (CD44^{low}CCR7^{high}CD45RA) cells, rather than T-memory (CD44^{high}CCR7$^{high/low}$CD45RA) cells.[135] Selective depletion of T-naïve but not the T-memory cell subset before DLI can be a rational strategy for GVHD prophylaxis.[136,137] In murine models of GVHD, T-memory cell recipients were more immunetolerant than T-naïve cell recipients. Antiviral immunity and graft-versus-leukemia effect were relatively preserved in the former.[138,139]

Infusion of 'Suicide Gene'-Transduced Donor Lymphocytes

A novel strategy, which is now progressing beyond early phase clinical trials, involves genetic modification of donor lymphocytes to express a 'suicide gene' which can be activated to induce cell apoptosis at the earliest manifestation of GVHD. In one approach, donor T cells are transduced with the herpes simplex virus-thymidine kinase (HSV-TK) gene. In the event of GVHD, gancicyclovir can be administered, which is activated by thymidine kinase and results in cell death via inhibition of DNA polymerase. This approach was deemed safe in a phase 1/2 multicenter study, with prompt resolution in all 10 patients who developed aGVHD.[140] Interestingly, an improvement in antiviral immunity was seen in this study as well as in a subsequent study, possibly because of enhanced thymic recovery in the absence of aGVHD.[141]

Although this work demonstrated the practical feasibility of this strategy, the use of gancicyclovir is not ideal, since it is commonly used to prevent or treat CMV reactivation in post-SCT patients. Alternatively, another group engineered T cells to express an inducible caspase 9 protein which is modified to abrogate its endogenous mechanism of activation and to instead bind a dimerizing agent, AP1903. This dimerization of caspase 9 protein with exogenously administered AP1903 triggers apoptotic cell death. These modified T cells were successful in expanding in vivo in HCT patients and in eliminating alloreactive cells while sparing virus-reactive T cells.[142–144]

Infusion of Donor-Derived T-Regulatory Cells (Tregs)

Regulatory T cells (Tregs), a subpopulation of T cells defined as $CD4^+$, $CD25^+$ and $FOXP3^+$ are important modulators of the immune response that suppress autoreactive lymphocytes and maintain self-tolerance.[145] The level of Tregs after HCT is negatively correlated with the incidence of acute and chronic GVHD.[146–148] Low frequency of Tregs in peripheral blood is associated with more frequent[149] and more severe acute GVHD.[150,151] Some studies[151,152] have found a similar association between peripheral Treg counts and chronic

GVHD, but others have negated it.[153–155] Infusion of donor-derived Tregs has been investigated as a preventive and/or therapeutic approach in the development of acute GVHD.

As naïve Tregs are found in low frequencies in peripheral blood (PB) (representing 5%–10% of $CD4^+$ cells in PB), obtaining sufficient numbers of donor Tregs for infusion may be a challenge.[156] Tregs are isolated based on flow cytometry: positive selection for CD4 and CD25 followed by negative selection for CD127, and expanded ex vivo prior to infusion. In a first-in-human phase 1 study of UCB-derived Tregs infused in 23 post-SCT patients, the strategy was found to be safe to administer, although efficacy in preventing aGVHD could not be determined in this trial.[157] Promising results were reported by DiIanni et al., who administered donor-derived Tregs to 28 patients along with no other posttransplant prophylaxis for GVHD–only 2 of these patients developed grade 2–4 GVHD, and the incidence of CMV reactivation was lower than in controls.[158] Similar results were obtained when Tregs were coinfused with conventional T cells in a 2:1 ratio.[159]

Although these small-scale studies offer encouragement about the prophylactic use of Tregs for post-SCT GVHD, there remain several barriers to the widespread clinical adoption of this strategy. The first is the problem of ex vivo expansion of Tregs, which is a lengthy process and requires specialized expertise. In addition, instability of the expanded cellular product, with loss of FOXP3 expression, and relative anergy of Tregs are a limitation.[160] At present, Tregs survive about 14 days in vivo; improvement in the persistence of these cells would greatly expand the scope for Treg immunotherapy.[161]

Another approach is to foster in vivo expansion of Tregs by the administration of ultra-low doses of IL-2, which is required by T-cells for proliferation.[162,163] A phase 2 single-arm study demonstrated its safe application, none of the 16 patients receiving ultra-low dose IL-2 as prophylaxis developed grades 2–4 aGVHD, and there was successful expansion of Tregs in vivo, with preservation of antiviral and antileukemic activity.[164] In the treatment of steroid-refractory cGVHD with low-dose IL-2, objective responses occurred in 61% of 35 patients, although no complete response was seen. IL-2 infusion in this case was further associated with specific rises in peripheral blood Treg and NK frequencies, and in the Treg:conventional $CD4^+$ T cell ratio.[165]

Given the selective inhibitory effect of Tregs on alloreactive donor cells and their favorable impact on immune reconstitution,[166] strategies to harness Tregs constitute an attractive area of research. The optimal timing (prophylactic vs. after development of GVHD) and dosage of Treg infusion is yet to be determined. Another issue that remains to be addressed is how to broaden the clinical feasibility and applicability of these approaches beyond the investigational setting.

Photodepletion of Alloreactive T Cells

Donor T cells can be cultured in the presence of host antigen-presenting cells, to activate alloreactive donor cells, but not tumor- or pathogen-reactive cells. The activated alloreactive cells have preferential retention of photoactive compounds such as TH9402, and these cells can then be selectively eliminated.[167] Results from early clinical studies suggest that this may be an efficient means of T-cell depletion that contributes to lower rates of GVHD and improved survival in the case of haploidentical SCT.[168,169]

Infusion of Mesenchymal Stem Cells (MSCs)

Mesenchymal stem cells (MSCs) have been investigated for their possible role in preventing and resolving graft-versus-host reactions that occur after HCT. MSCs are progenitor cells found in low frequencies in a variety of tissues, and have potential for multilineage differentiation. Based on recent findings relating to MSC biology, these cells are thought to possess local and systemic immunomodulatory functions, and have a role in tissue regeneration and repair. In vitro, MSCs suppress T cell proliferation and in vivo mouse models, they have been found to home to GVHD-injured organs and the thymus thus supporting a therapeutic role for these cells in GVHD.[170,171] By improving thymic function, post-transplant administration of MSCs may reduce the incidence and severity of acute and chronic GVHD.[172,173] Additionally, infusion of MSCs is not associated with the risk of inducing allogenic lymphocyte responses, making them suitable for use in the HCT setting.

The first evidence for clinical success of MSCs is a report of a pediatric patient with grade 4 acute GVHD that was refractory to multiple lines of treatment, but resolved completely after infusion of an MSC dose 2×10^6/kg.[174] Since then many studies have investigated MSCs for the treatment and prophylaxis of acute and chronic GVHD. In a multicenter study of the European Group for Blood and Marrow Transplantation, 39 out of 55 patients with steroid-resistant grades 2–4 aGVHD responded to infusion of third-party MSCs.[175] The overall response rate was 71%, and no infusion-related toxicities were noted. Similar responses were noted in subsequent patient series.[176,177] A prospective controlled study for aGVHD confirmed that outcomes of MSC-treated patients were significantly superior

compared to controls (odds ratio, 75% vs. 42%), and that there was a lower incidence of chronic GVHD in the former group.[172] However, other prospective trials have contradicted this finding,[178,179] suggesting that response to MSCs differ significantly according to different target organs and patient populations, in addition to variations of trial design and dosing schedule. Additionally, there is a lack of consensus over the optimal tissue of origin, methods of isolation and cell surface phenotype of MSCs most suitable for the treatment and prevention of GVHD.[180]

Studies of MSC as GVHD prophylaxis have been controversial, with some reporting a reduced incidence of aGVHD in post HCT patients, and others finding no effect.[181-184]

ROLE OF CELLULAR THERAPY IN PROMOTING ENGRAFTMENT AND POTENTIATING GRAFT-VERSUS-TUMOR (GVT) EFFECT

HCT remains a treatment goal for many patients with various refractory and aggressive hematological malignancies. However, despite improvements in HLA haplotype matching and pre-transplant conditioning regimens, a significant proportion of alloHCT patients experience disease relapse,[185] posing a significant clinical challenge.

Much of the survival benefit of HCT is a consequence of the GVT or GVL effect, an immunologic response mediated by donor T cells opposing tumor cells. This response requires presentation of tumor-specific antigens by host antigen-presenting cells (APCs), utilizing appropriate costimulatory signaling and stimulation by specific cytokines, importantly interferon-gamma. Tumor cells acquire several strategies to evade immune response, including: downregulation of costimulatory and HLA class 1 molecules, induction of coinhibitory signaling molecules, production of inhibitory cytokines, and induction of regulatory T cells and suppressor cells in the tumor microenvironment.

This understanding has provided the rationale and impetus to reinforce GVL through various novel strategies that seek to modulate cellular and cytokine mediators of tumor immune evasion. Specifically, it has become clear that attempts to enhance engraftment, expansion and long-term persistence of T cells are critical to achieving durable responses after HCT. In fact, the presence of tumor-specific CTLs and NK cells correlates with remission in acute leukemias and other malignancies.[186-190] Unfortunately, the T cell mechanisms that mediate GVL and GVHD are closely interrelated such that adoptive transfer of immune cells to an

HCT recipient is often complicated by the alloreactive potential of donor cells.[191] Thus, although aspects of the post-HCT inflammatory milieu, particularly high levels of IL-15[192,193] favor the in vivo expansion of adoptively transferred unmodified or modified lymphocytes, they can also potentiate unwanted GVHD effects.

Unmodified Donor Lymphocyte Infusion (DLI)

Unmodified donor lymphocyte infusion (DLI) given to HCT recipients with the goal of alleviating malignant disease relapse, is one of the best examples of adoptive cellular therapy using alloreactive donor T cells. The first use of DLI was in overt relapse after transplant, but this technique may be also be used as a preventive strategy in high-risk patients (e.g., those receiving TCD grafts), who develop falling donor chimerism or minimal residual disease.

Responses to DLI in relapsed leukemia vary with underlying disease and lymphocyte dose, with a different dose-response curve for each disease.[194] Studies have reported on the safety and efficacy of DLI (with or without interferon-alpha) in a variety of patient populations and malignancies with post-SCT relapse.[194–200] Chronic myeloid leukemia (CML) is the most responsive to DLI, with 70%–80% cytogenetic remissions. Multiple myeloma, myelodysplastic syndrome and myeloproliferative disease are less responsive, and acute leukemias particularly ALL, are minimally responsive.[201]

In addition, prophylactic/preemptive DLI has been shown to be effective in reducing risk of relapse.[202] Striking (>80%) responses have been achieved in CML patients with cytogenetic or molecular relapse.[203,204] Nevertheless, the use of DLI is associated with a concomitant increased risk of exacerbating or provoking GVHD, prompting strategies to select T cell subsets that mediate GVL but not GVHD. Finally, until formal guidelines are published on the use of donor cellular products as adjuncts to SCT, the potential antitumor benefit of these strategies must be carefully weighed against the risks of potential GVHD and marrow hypoplasia.

Adoptive Transfer of Tumor-specific Cytotoxic T Lymphocytes

After HCT in hematological malignancies, GVL-producing donor T cells are directed against two types of tissue-specific antigens: minor histocompatibility antigens (mHAgs), and tumor-associated antigens (TAAs).

Some mHAgs are expressed on hematopoietic and certain other tissues, but not on GVHD-affected organs. Donor-recipient differences in these mHAgs are responsible for eliciting T-cell-mediated GVL responses;

therefore adoptive transfer of mHAg-reactive CTLs can potentially produce antitumor immunity.[205] In a report of 3 patients with myeloid malignancies who received DLI with donor-recipient mismatch of the mHAg HA-1/2, all patients achieved complete remission after generation of HA-1/2-reactive CD8+ CTLs.[206] A further Phase1/2 feasibility study showed moderate to high cytotoxic activity of leukemia-reactive CTLs in vitro.[207] Of 8 relapsed patients receiving 1–7 manufactured CTL lines, 2 had CR, 2 had stable disease and 4 had no response. Adoptive transfer of CTLs in leukemia patients has achieved in vivo persistence of up to 21 days. However, 3/7 MHC-matched alloSCT patients who were infused with CTLs, exhibited pulmonary toxicity that correlated with the level of mHAg expression in lung tissue.[208]

Tumor-associated antigens are proteins that are overexpressed in malignant cells, such as Wilms tumor gene 1 (WT-1), gp100 and others (see Table 28.3). The most widely studied, WT-1, is overexpressed in more than 70% patients with hematologic malignancies, and in AML, elevated WT-1 levels are associated with poor response to chemotherapy, increased risk of relapse, and shorter disease-free survival.[209,210] Moreover, the presence and levels of TAA-specific CTLs have independently been correlated with likelihood and durability of remission in acute and chronic leukemias.[189,211] Chapuis et al. showed that adoptively transferred WT-1 specific CTLs had selective antileukemic activity, long-term persistence in vivo, and were successful in reducing disease burden and risk of relapse post-HCT.[212]

Adoptive Transfer of γδ (Gamma-Delta) T Cells

T-cell receptor (TCR) γδ T lymphocytes comprise 1%–10% of the circulating T-cell population.[213] These cells are stimulated via γδ TCR and NKG2D receptor activation, and are capable of strong cytotoxic responses as well as secretion of cytokines such as IFN-γ and TNF-α.[214,215] Importantly, unlike αβ T cells, γδ cells participate in MHC-independent killing and consequently do not mediate GVHD effects. In HCT patients who received αβ and CD19+ cell depleted grafts, increased numbers of γδ cells were observed and these increased frequencies were associated with longer disease-free survival.[216] Similar findings were noted in a longer prospective follow-up of 153 AML/ALL patients who underwent mismatched related HCT and received partially T-cell depleted grafts.[128] In this study, patients who had high levels of γδ T cells had significantly greater 5-year leukemia-free survival and overall survival than those with

TABLE 28.3
Tumor Related Antigens that May Be Potential Targets for Adoptively Transferred Tumor-Reactive CTLs

Antigen	References	Malignancy	Notable Toxicity
WT-1	Chapuis et al.[212]; Provasi et al.[260]	Hematological	
gp100	Johnson et al.[261]	Melanoma	Melanocyte toxicity; uveitis, hearing loss
MART-1	Morgan et al.[262]	Melanoma	
Cancer-testis antigens: NY-ESO-1 and LAGE-1	Rapoport et al.[263]; Robbins et al.[264]; Robbins et al.[265]	Multiple myeloma, synovial sarcoma, melanoma	
MAGE-A3	Linette et al.[266]	Myeloma, melanoma	Cardiovascular, neurological
CEA	Parkhurst et al.[267]	Colorectal carcinoma	Colitis
Other TAAs: proteinase 3, human neutrophil elastase			
Patient-specific neoantigens, e.g., ERBB2IP (erbb2 interacting protein) mutation	Tran et al. [268]	Cholangiocarcinoma, colorectal carcinoma	
Tumor-specific mutated antigens, e.g., BCR-ABL and BRAF$_{v600E}$ mutations	Somasundaram et al.[269]		
Overexpressed self-proteins associated with driver mutations, e.g., c–erbB2	Conrad et al.[270]	Breast carcinoma	
Minor histocompatibility antigens (mHAg)	Warren et al.[208]; Marijt et al.[206]; Marijt et al.[207]		

CEA, carcinoembryonic antigen; *gp100*, glycoprotein 100; *MART-1*, melanoma antigen recognized by T cells 1; *MAGE-A3*, melanoma-associated antigen A3; *TAA*, tumor-associated antigen; *WT-1*, Wilms tumor 1.

normal or decreased γδ levels (54.4% vs. 19.1%, and 70.8% vs. 19.6% respectively).

Given these data, several studies have evaluated γδ T cells for immune therapy in patients with hematological malignancies and found it to be a safe and feasible approach.[217–219] Airoldi et al. demonstrated efficient in vivo cytotoxicity of a subset of γδ T cells against leukemic blasts in patients who received TCD HCT.[220]

Owing to the low frequency of γδ T cells in peripheral blood, adoptive transfer strategies require in vitro activation and expansion of isolated donor γδ cells prior to infusion. Aminobisphosphonates, such as zoledronic acid, have been used to expand these cells and shown some clinical success.[217,221,222] Further clinical trials of adoptive γδ T cell transfer are needed to validate this approach in post-HCT patients, and to determine the optimal timing (prophylactic or postrelapse) and source (peripheral blood or tissue) of γδ cells that

have prolonged in vivo persistence and adequate homing to tumor niches.

Chimeric Antigen Receptor (CAR)-Transduced T Cell Therapy

CAR-T cell therapy involves genetic modification of autologous T cells to express an antigen receptor that allows immune recognition of tumor molecules, for example, CD19 in B-cell malignancies.[223–225] The CAR construct comprises a single chain monoclonal antibody directed against tumor-specific antigen which is coupled via an extracellular hinge domain and transmembrane domain to a cytoplasmic signaling domain, generally the CD3 zeta chain.[226] The advantage of CAR-T cells is their MHC-unrestricted mode of action as it bypasses key tumor escape mechanisms, namely the downregulation of HLA class 1 and costimulatory molecules[227,228] and impairments in antigen presentation (Fig. 28.3).

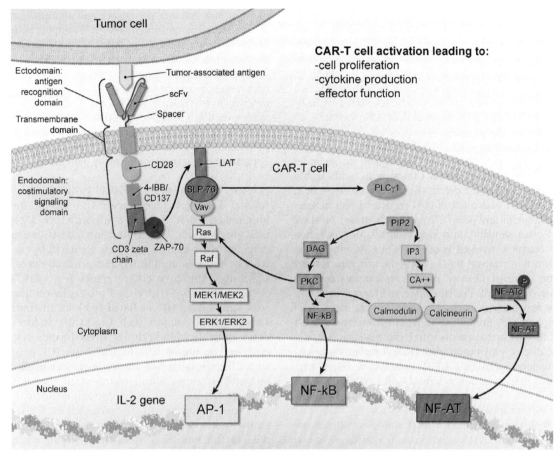

FIG. 28.3 Structure and mechanism of third-generation CAR-modified T cells. The CAR consists of a single-chain monoclonal antibody (scFv) linked via a transmembrane domain to an intracellular signaling domain. Recognition of tumor-associated antigens by the scFv activates T-cell signaling pathways downstream of ZAP-70. Upregulation of IL-2 gene enhances T effector function and cytokine production, leading to T-cell–mediated killing of tumor cells. *CAR*, chimeric antigen receptor; *MEK*, MAPK/ERK kinase; *ERK*, extracellular signal-regulated kinase; *IL-2*, interleukin-2; *AP-1*, activator protein-1; *NF-AT*, nuclear factor of activated T-cells; *DAG*, diacylglycerol; *PKC*, protein kinase C; *PLC*, phospholipase C; *PIP2*, phosphatidylinositol 4,5-bisphosphate 2; *IP3*, inositol triphosphate.

Development and optimization of CAR-T cell strategies

Strategies to develop and infuse tumor-targeted CAR-T cells incorporate principles of gene transfer as well as of standard adoptive cellular therapy. Autologous or donor-derived T cells are obtained from a peripheral blood draw, and then transduced with the CAR using either gamma lentiviral or retroviral vectors, or through transposon systems, e.g., the Sleeping Beauty (SB) system.[229] An advantage of the latter is its larger gene transfer capacity and possibly lower cost. However, longer culture times of SB-transduced cells may be unsuitable for acute and highly aggressive leukemias.[230]

CAR-transduced cells are expanded ex vivo with CD3-or CD28-expressing beads and supplemental cytokines.[231] Bead-manufactured T cells reportedly have greater in vivo proliferative potential than older methods of culture and expansion.[232]

A major problem with first-generation CAR-modified T cells was lack of in vivo persistence and expansion; responses to CAR-T cells appear to related more to in vivo cell proliferation than the infused dose. Addition of costimulatory domains such as CD28 and 4-1BB to the CAR construct,[233] as well as specific cytokines (e.g., IL-15) have been successful in improving survival and antileukemic efficacy of these cells in vivo.[234,235]

In theory, the development of CAR-T cells is subject to several procedure-related safety concerns, most importantly insertional mutagenesis or induction of a T-cell lymphoproliferative syndrome.[236] However, long-term follow-up results indicate no such practical risks.[237,238] The potential risk of alloreactivity in the setting of CAR-T cell transfer peri-transplant, can be countered with the transduction of suicide genes in the CAR construct.

Clinical results with CAR-T cells

CD19-targeted CAR-T cells for B-cell malignancies have been tested in several clinical trials, with significant responses noted overall. The best results have been seen in ALL, with a CR of 90% reported in 30 blinatumomab-refractory post-HCT patients.[239] Based on these and other similarly promising results, CAR-T cell therapy has now received Food and Drug Administration approval in relapsed B-ALL, being the first gene therapy to be approved. Of note, durable remissions have been achieved with CAR-T cell therapy even in aggressive refractory malignancies, such as relapsed diffuse large B-cell lymphoma.[240] Brudno, et al. reported results of CAR-T cell therapy in 20 patients with B cell malignancies who had disease progression after HCT: 8 patients achieved remissions, including 6 CR.[241] A systematic review concluded that use of donor-derived CAR T cells after SCT is highly effective in relapse prophylaxis, minimal residual disease clearance and salvage from relapse.[242]

Toxicities reported for CAR T therapy represent on-target effects of CD19 targeting, such as cytokine release syndrome (CRS), tumor lysis syndrome and B-cell aplasia. CRS is characterized by high levels of IL-6 and IFN-gamma, but in most cases is manageable with the IL-6 inhibitor, tocilizumab (approved for this indication), or the chimeric anti-IL-6 monoclonal antibody, siltuximab. In refractory or severe cases, corticosteroids can also be used to control the inflammatory response, albeit at the cost of impaired antitumor efficacy of T cells. Neurological toxicity, termed as CAR-T cell related encephalopathy syndrome, is the second most common adverse event after CRS, and is characterized by a toxic encephalopathic state involving mental status changes, seizures, raised intracranial pressure and cerebral edema. Rarely, immune overactivation can result in fulminant hemophagocytic lymphohistiocytosis. Recently guidelines on the assessment, grading and management of CAR-T cell toxicities have been published by a multi-institutional team of experts.[243]

Outlook for CAR-T cell therapy

CAR-T cell therapy is a very promising cellular therapy for malignant disorders, and has unique potential in the transplant setting as the lymphodepleted status of the host may enhance persistence and antitumor activity of adoptively transferred cells.[51,244] Adoptive transfer of CAR-transduced T cells in post-HCT patients may be used in place of conventional DLI, as prophylactic or preemptive therapy in minimal residual disease-positive nonrelapse disease, or may be restricted to patients who experience overt relapse. In addition, CAR-T cell therapy may be used as a bridge to transplant. Given the limited responses to current reinduction regimens, even transient remissions induced by CAR-T cells may increase the opportunity for transplant for many patients.

Adoptive Transfer of Natural Killer (NK) Cells

Natural killer (NK) cells are CD3⁻ CD56⁺ innate immune cells that make up a minority (5%–15%) of total lymphocytes. NK cell function is MHC-independent and NK cytotoxic activity is regulated by careful balance between inhibitory and activating receptor signaling. Inhibitory NK receptors (e.g., KIR and NKG2A) recognize HLA class 1 molecules on normal cells, suppressing NK-mediated cytolysis. In contrast, activating NK receptors such as NKG2D, induce cell death when they bind cellular 'stress' ligands that are expressed on tumor cells. In TCD haploSCT, patients with KIR mismatch had a lower incidence of disease relapse.[54] It is therefore hypothesized that donor-recipient NK alloreactivity (due to KIR mismatch) can enhance GVT effects with low potential for GVHD.[245] Furthermore, despite imperfect functionality of NK cells in the immediate post-HCT period, NK cells recover within a month of transplant, and recovery of these cells is correlated with reduced risk of relapse and improved survival.[246] The HCT setting is ideal for adoptive NK strategies in malignant diseases, since in vivo NK proliferation is greatly enhanced in the lymphodepleted IL-15-high host status postconditioning therapy.[247]

NK cells can be positively selected from donor blood by performing a CD3 depletion procedure followed by CD56 enrichment–CD3⁻ CD56⁺ NK cells with a median purity of 95% can be obtained this way.[248–250] The selected NK cells can then be activated and expanded in vitro with the addition of IL-2 and IL-15.[247] Alternately, autologous or genetically modified 'feeder' cells may be used, shortening culture time and improving upon NK cell yield.[251]

Multiple clinical trials have established the safety of administering NK infusion to patients peritransplant or posttransplant.[249,252–256] Regarding the efficacy of this approach in preventing or treating disease relapse, there has been conflicting data. Although a few studies showed improved progression-free and overall survival for NK-infused post-SCT patients than non-NK treated,[257,258] prospective randomized controlled studies are lacking to conclusively demonstrate clinical benefit of NK infusion.

REFERENCES

1. Bosch M, Khan FM, Storek J. Immune reconstitution after hematopoietic cell transplant. *Curr Opin Hematol.* 2012;19(4):324–335.
2. Mackall C, Fry T, Gress R, et al. Background to hematopoietic cell transplant, including post transplant immune recovery. *Bone Marrow Transpl.* 2009;44(8):457–462.
3. Levine JE. Implications of TNF-alpha in the pathogenesis and management of GVHD.. *Int J Hematol.* 2011;93(5):571–577.
4. Ferrara JL, Levine JE, Reddy P, Holler E. Graft-versus-host disease. *Lancet.* 2009;373(9674):1550–1561.
5. Shono Y, Ueha S, Wang Y, et al. Bone marrow graft-versus-host disease: early destruction of hematopoietic niche after MHC-mismatched hematopoietic stem cell transplantation. *Blood.* 2010;115(26):5401–5411.
6. Krenger W, Rossi S, Hollander GA. Apoptosis of thymocytes during acute graft-versus-host disease is independent of glucocorticoids. *Transplantation.* 2000;69(10):2190–2193.
7. Krenger W, Hollander GA. The immunopathology of thymic GVHD. *Semin Immunopathol.* 2008;30(4):439–456.
8. Small TN, Papadopoulos EB, Boulad F, et al. Comparison of immune reconstitution after unrelated and related T-cell-depleted bone marrow transplantation: effect of patient age and donor leukocyte infusions. *Blood.* 1999;93(2):467–480.
9. Barker JN, Hough RE, van Burik JA, et al. Serious infections after unrelated donor transplantation in 136 children: impact of stem cell source. *Biol Blood Marrow Transpl.* 2005;11(5):362–370.
10. Rizzieri DA, Koh LP, Long GD, et al. Partially matched, nonmyeloablative allogeneic transplantation: clinical outcomes and immune reconstitution. *J Clin Oncol.* 2007;25(6):690–697.
11. Fallen PR, McGreavey L, Madrigal JA, et al. Factors affecting reconstitution of the T cell compartment in allogeneic haematopoietic cell transplant recipients. *Bone Marrow Transpl.* 2003;32(10):1001–1014.
12. Komanduri KV, St John LS, de Lima M, et al. Delayed immune reconstitution after cord blood transplantation is characterized by impaired thymopoiesis and late memory T-cell skewing. *Blood.* 2007;110(13):4543–4551.
13. Hamza NS, Lisgaris M, Yadavalli G, et al. Kinetics of myeloid and lymphocyte recovery and infectious complications after unrelated umbilical cord blood versus HLA-matched unrelated donor allogeneic transplantation in adults. *Br J Haematol.* 2004;124(4):488–498.
14. Inoue H, Yasuda Y, Hattori K, et al. The kinetics of immune reconstitution after cord blood transplantation and selected CD34+ stem cell transplantation in children: comparison with bone marrow transplantation. *Int J Hematol.* 2003;77(4):399–407.
15. Klein AK, Patel DD, Gooding ME, et al. T-Cell recovery in adults and children following umbilical cord blood transplantation. *Biol Blood Marrow Transpl.* 2001;7(8):454–466.
16. Sauter C, Abboud M, Jia X, et al. Serious infection risk and immune recovery after double-unit cord blood transplantation without antithymocyte globulin. *Biol Blood Marrow Transpl.* 2011;17(10):1460–1471.
17. Jacobs R, Stoll M, Stratmann G, Leo R, Link H, Schmidt RE. CD16- CD56+ natural killer cells after bone marrow transplantation. *Blood.* 1992;79(12):3239–3244.
18. Zimmerli W, Zarth A, Gratwohl A, Speck B. Neutrophil function and pyogenic infections in bone marrow transplant recipients. *Blood.* 1991;77(2):393–399.
19. Storek J, Wells D, Dawson MA, Storer B, Maloney DG. Factors influencing B lymphopoiesis after allogeneic hematopoietic cell transplant. *Blood.* 2001;98(2):489–491.
20. Storek J, Dawson MA, Storer B, et al. Immune reconstitution after allogeneic marrow transplantation compared with blood stem cell transplantation. *Blood.* 2001;97(11):3380–3389.
21. Park BG, Park CJ, Jang S, et al. Reconstitution of lymphocyte subpopulations after hematopoietic stem cell transplantation: comparison of hematologic malignancies and donor types in event-free patients. *Leuk Res.* 2015;39(12):1334–1341.
22. Avigan D, Pirofski LA, Lazarus HM. Vaccination against infectious disease following hematopoietic stem cell transplantation. *Biol Blood Marrow Transpl.* 2001;7(3):171–183.
23. Suzuki I, Milner EC, Glas AM, et al. Immunoglobulin heavy chain variable region gene usage in bone marrow transplant recipients: lack of somatic mutation indicates a maturational arrest. *Blood.* 1996;87(5):1873–1880.
24. Storek J, Witherspoon RP, Storb R. Reconstitution of membrane IgD- (mIgD-) B cells after marrow transplantation lags behind the reconstitution of mIgD+ B cells. *Blood.* 1997;89(1):350–351.
25. Glas AM, van Montfort EH, Storek J, et al. B-cell-autonomous somatic mutation deficit following bone marrow transplant. *Blood.* 2000;96(3):1064–1069.
26. Li F, Jin F, Freitas A, Szabo P, Weksler ME. Impaired regeneration of the peripheral B cell repertoire from bone marrow following lymphopenia in old mice. *Eur J Immunol.* 2001;31(2):500–505.
27. Storek J. B-cell immunity after allogeneic hematopoietic cell transplant. *Cytotherapy.* 2002;4(5):423–424.
28. Molrine DC, Guinan EC, Antin JH, et al. Donor immunization with Haemophilus influenzae type b (HIB)-conjugate vaccine in allogeneic bone marrow transplantation. *Blood.* 1996;87(7):3012–3018.

29. Storek J, Dawson MA, Lim LC, et al. Efficacy of donor vaccination before hematopoietic cell transplant and recipient vaccination both before and early after transplantation. *Bone Marrow Transpl.* 2004;33(3):337–346.

30. Hakim FT, Cepeda R, Kaimei S, et al. Constraints on CD4 recovery postchemotherapy in adults: thymic insufficiency and apoptotic decline of expanded peripheral CD4 cells. *Blood.* 1997;90(9):3789–3798.

31. Mackall CL, Gress RE. Pathways of T-cell regeneration in mice and humans: implications for bone marrow transplantation and immunotherapy. *Immunol Rev.* 1997;157:61–72.

32. Hakim FT, Memon SA, Cepeda R, et al. Age-dependent incidence, time course, and consequences of thymic renewal in adults. *J Clin Invest.* 2005;115(4):930–939.

33. Fagnoni FF, Lozza L, Zibera C, et al. T-cell dynamics after high-dose chemotherapy in adults: elucidation of the elusive CD8+ subset reveals multiple homeostatic T-cell compartments with distinct implications for immune competence. *Immunology.* 2002;106(1):27–37.

34. Heitger A, Neu N, Kern H, et al. Essential role of the thymus to reconstitute naive (CD45RA+) T-helper cells after human allogeneic bone marrow transplantation. *Blood.* 1997;90(2):850–857.

35. Godthelp BC, van Tol MJ, Vossen JM, van Den Elsen PJ. T-Cell immune reconstitution in pediatric leukemia patients after allogeneic bone marrow transplantation with T-cell-depleted or unmanipulated grafts: evaluation of overall and antigen-specific T-cell repertoires. *Blood.* 1999;94(12):4358–4369.

36. Mackall CL, Fleisher TA, Brown MR, et al. Distinctions between CD8+ and CD4+ T-cell regenerative pathways result in prolonged T-cell subset imbalance after intensive chemotherapy. *Blood.* 1997;89(10):3700–3707.

37. Guimond M, Veenstra RG, Grindler DJ, et al. Interleukin 7 signaling in dendritic cells regulates the homeostatic proliferation and niche size of CD4+ T cells. *Nat Immunol.* 2009;10(2):149–157.

38. Bolotin E, Annett G, Parkman R, Weinberg K. Serum levels of IL-7 in bone marrow transplant recipients: relationship to clinical characteristics and lymphocyte count. *Bone Marrow Transpl.* 1999;23(8):783–788.

39. Schluns KS, Williams K, Ma A, Zheng XX, Lefrancois L. Cutting edge: requirement for IL-15 in the generation of primary and memory antigen-specific CD8 T cells. *J Immunol.* 2002;168(10):4827–4831.

40. Nordoy T, Kolstad A, Endresen P, et al. Persistent changes in the immune system 4-10 years after ABMT. *Bone Marrow Transpl.* 1999;24(8):873–878.

41. Clave E, Busson M, Douay C, et al. Acute graft-versus-host disease transiently impairs thymic output in young patients after allogeneic hematopoietic stem cell transplantation. *Blood.* 2009;113(25):6477–6484.

42. Roux E, Helg C, Dumont-Girard F, Chapuis B, Jeannet M, Roosnek E. Analysis of T-cell repopulation after allogeneic bone marrow transplantation: significant differences between recipients of T-cell depleted and unmanipulated grafts. *Blood.* 1996;87(9):3984–3992.

43. Sfikakis PP, Gourgoulis GM, Moulopoulos LA, Kouvatseas G, Theofilopoulos AN, Dimopoulos MA. Age-related thymic activity in adults following chemotherapy-induced lymphopenia. *Eur J Clin Invest.* 2005;35(6):380–387.

44. Mackall CL, Fleisher TA, Brown MR, et al. Lymphocyte depletion during treatment with intensive chemotherapy for cancer. *Blood.* 1994;84(7):2221–2228.

45. Williams KM, Mella H, Lucas PJ, Williams JA, Telford W, Gress RE. Single cell analysis of complex thymus stromal cell populations: rapid thymic epithelia preparation characterizes radiation injury. *Clin Transl Sci.* 2009;2(4):279–285.

46. Janssen EM, Lemmens EE, Wolfe T, Christen U, von Herrath MG, Schoenberger SP. CD4+ T cells are required for secondary expansion and memory in CD8+ T lymphocytes. *Nature.* 2003;421(6925):852–856.

47. Chklovskaia E, Nowbakht P, Nissen C, Gratwohl A, Bargetzi M, Wodnar-Filipowicz A. Reconstitution of dendritic and natural killer-cell subsets after allogeneic stem cell transplantation: effects of endogenous flt3 ligand. *Blood.* 2004;103(10):3860–3868.

48. Rapoport AP, Stadtmauer EA, Aqui N, et al. Rapid immune recovery and graft-versus-host disease-like engraftment syndrome following adoptive transfer of costimulated autologous T cells. *Clin Cancer Res.* 2009;15(13):4499–4507.

49. Surh CD, Sprent J. Homeostasis of naive and memory T cells. *Immunity.* 2008;29(6):848–862.

50. Dummer W, Niethammer AG, Baccala R, et al. T cell homeostatic proliferation elicits effective antitumor autoimmunity. *J Clin Invest.* 2002;110(2):185–192.

51. Laport GG, Levine BL, Stadtmauer EA, et al. Adoptive transfer of costimulated T cells induces lymphocytosis in patients with relapsed/refractory non-Hodgkin lymphoma following CD34+-selected hematopoietic cell transplant. *Blood.* 2003;102(6):2004–2013.

52. Asai O, Longo DL, Tian ZG, et al. Suppression of graft-versus-host disease and amplification of graft-versus-tumor effects by activated natural killer cells after allogeneic bone marrow transplantation. *J Clin Invest.* 1998;101(9):1835–1842.

53. Bornhauser M, Thiede C, Brendel C, et al. Stable engraftment after megadose blood stem cell transplantation across the HLA barrier: the case for natural killer cells as graft-facilitating cells. *Transplantation.* 1999;68(1):87–88.

54. Ruggeri L, Capanni M, Urbani E, et al. Effectiveness of donor natural killer cell alloreactivity in mismatched hematopoietic transplants. *Science.* 2002;295(5562):2097–2100.

55. Olson JA, Leveson-Gower DB, Gill S, Baker J, Beilhack A, Negrin RS. NK cells mediate reduction of GVHD by inhibiting activated, alloreactive T cells while retaining GVT effects. *Blood.* 2010;115(21):4293–4301.

56. Schuster MG, Cleveland AA, Dubberke ER, et al. Infections in hematopoietic cell transplant recipients: results from the organ transplant infection project, a multicenter, prospective, cohort study. *Open Forum Infect Dis.* 2017;4(2). ofx050.

57. Gratwohl A, Brand R, Frassoni F, et al. Cause of death after allogeneic haematopoietic stem cell transplantation (HSCT) in early leukaemias: an EBMT analysis of lethal infectious complications and changes over calendar time. *Bone Marrow Transpl.* 2005;36(9):757–769.

58. Sundin M, Le Blanc K, Ringden O, et al. The role of HLA mismatch, splenectomy and recipient Epstein-Barr virus seronegativity as risk factors in post-transplant lymphoproliferative disorder following allogeneic hematopoietic stem cell transplantation. *Haematologica.* 2006;91(8):1059–1067.

59. Hakki M, Riddell SR, Storek J, et al. Immune reconstitution to cytomegalovirus after allogeneic hematopoietic stem cell transplantation: impact of host factors, drug therapy, and subclinical reactivation. *Blood.* 2003;102(8):3060–3067.

60. Brunstein CG, Weisdorf DJ, DeFor T, et al. Marked increased risk of Epstein-Barr virus-related complications with the addition of antithymocyte globulin to a nonmyeloablative conditioning prior to unrelated umbilical cord blood transplantation. *Blood.* 2006;108(8):2874–2880.

61. Curtis RE, Travis LB, Rowlings PA, et al. Risk of lymphoproliferative disorders after bone marrow transplantation: a multi-institutional study. *Blood.* 1999;94(7):2208–2216.

62. Ogonek J, Kralj Juric M, Ghimire S, et al. Immune reconstitution after allogeneic hematopoietic stem cell transplantation. *Front Immunol.* 2016;7:507.

63. D'Orsogna LJ, Wright MP, Krueger RG, et al. Allogeneic hematopoietic stem cell transplantation recipients have defects of both switched and igm memory B cells. *Biol Blood Marrow Transpl.* 2009;15(7):795–803.

64. Mehta RS, Rezvani K. Immune reconstitution post allogeneic transplant and the impact of immune recovery on the risk of infection. *Virulence.* 2016;7(8): 901–916.

65. Biron KK. Antiviral drugs for cytomegalovirus diseases. *Antivir Res.* 2006;71(2–3):154–163.

66. Boeckh M. Current antiviral strategies for controlling cytomegalovirus in hematopoietic stem cell transplant recipients: prevention and therapy. *Transpl Infect Dis.* 1999;1(3):165–178.

67. Boeckh M, Zaia JA, Jung D, Skettino S, Chauncey TR, Bowden RA. A study of the pharmacokinetics, antiviral activity, and tolerability of oral ganciclovir for CMV prophylaxis in marrow transplantation. *Biol Blood Marrow Transpl.* 1998;4(1):13–19.

68. Kumar D, Chen MH, Welsh B, et al. A randomized, double-blind trial of pneumococcal vaccination in adult allogeneic stem cell transplant donors and recipients. *Clin Infect Dis.* 2007;45(12):1576–1582.

69. Avanzini MA, Carra AM, Maccario R, et al. Immunization with Haemophilus influenzae type b conjugate vaccine in children given bone marrow transplantation: comparison with healthy age-matched controls. *J Clin Immunol.* 1998;18(3):193–201.

70. Yager EJ, Ahmed M, Lanzer K, Randall TD, Woodland DL, Blackman MA. Age-associated decline in T cell repertoire diversity leads to holes in the repertoire and impaired immunity to influenza virus. *J Exp Med.* 2008;205(3):711–723.

71. Kroon FP, van Dissel JT, de Jong JC, van Furth R. Antibody response to influenza, tetanus and pneumococcal vaccines in HIV-seropositive individuals in relation to the number of CD4+ lymphocytes. *AIDS.* 1994;8(4):469–476.

72. Reusser P, Riddell SR, Meyers JD, Greenberg PD. Cytotoxic T-lymphocyte response to cytomegalovirus after human allogeneic bone marrow transplantation: pattern of recovery and correlation with cytomegalovirus infection and disease. *Blood.* 1991;78(5):1373–1380.

73. Roddie C, Peggs KS. Donor lymphocyte infusion following allogeneic hematopoietic stem cell transplantation. *Expert Opin Biol Ther.* 2011;11(4):473–487.

74. Anasetti C, Beatty PG, Storb R, et al. Effect of HLA incompatibility on graft-versus-host disease, relapse, and survival after marrow transplantation for patients with leukemia or lymphoma. *Hum Immunol.* 1990;29(2):79–91.

75. Heslop HE, Brenner MK, Rooney CM. Donor T cells to treat EBV-associated lymphoma. *N Engl J Med.* 1994;331(10):679–680.

76. Heslop HE, Slobod KS, Pule MA, et al. Long-term outcome of EBV-specific T-cell infusions to prevent or treat EBV-related lymphoproliferative disease in transplant recipients. *Blood.* 2010;115(5):925–935.

77. Riddell SR, Watanabe KS, Goodrich JM, Li CR, Agha ME, Greenberg PD. Restoration of viral immunity in immunodeficient humans by the adoptive transfer of T cell clones. *Science.* 1992;257(5067):238–241.

78. Zakrzewski JL, Kochman AA, Lu SX, et al. Adoptive transfer of T-cell precursors enhances T-cell reconstitution after allogeneic hematopoietic stem cell transplantation. *Nat Med.* 2006;12(9):1039–1047.

79. Barrett AJ, Bollard CM. The coming of age of adoptive T-cell therapy for viral infection after stem cell transplantation. *Ann Transl Med.* 2015;3(5):62.

80. Icheva V, Kayser S, Wolff D, et al. Adoptive transfer of epstein-barr virus (EBV) nuclear antigen 1-specific t cells as treatment for EBV reactivation and lymphoproliferative disorders after allogeneic stem-cell transplantation. *J Clin Oncol.* 2013;31(1): 39–48.

81. Feucht J, Opherk K, Lang P, et al. Adoptive T-cell therapy with hexon-specific Th1 cells as a treatment of refractory adenovirus infection after HSCT. *Blood.* 2015;125(12):1986–1994.

82. Feuchtinger T, Matthes-Martin S, Richard C, et al. Safe adoptive transfer of virus-specific T-cell immunity for the treatment of systemic adenovirus infection after allogeneic stem cell transplantation. *Br J Haematol.* 2006;134(1):64–76.

83. Moosmann A, Bigalke I, Tischer J, et al. Effective and long-term control of EBV PTLD after transfer of peptide-selected T cells. *Blood.* 2010;115(14):2960–2970.

84. Qasim W, Gilmour K, Zhan H, et al. Interferon-gamma capture T cell therapy for persistent Adenoviraemia following allogeneic haematopoietic stem cell transplantation. *Br J Haematol.* 2013;161(3):449–452.

85. Feuchtinger T, Opherk K, Bethge WA, et al. Adoptive transfer of pp65-specific T cells for the treatment of chemorefractory cytomegalovirus disease or reactivation after haploidentical and matched unrelated stem cell transplantation. *Blood.* 2010;116(20):4360–4367.

86. Odendahl M, Grigoleit GU, Bonig H, et al. Clinical-scale isolation of 'minimally manipulated' cytomegalovirus-specific donor lymphocytes for the treatment of refractory cytomegalovirus disease. *Cytotherapy.* 2014;16(9):1245–1256.

87. Walter EA, Greenberg PD, Gilbert MJ, et al. Reconstitution of cellular immunity against cytomegalovirus in recipients of allogeneic bone marrow by transfer of T-cell clones from the donor. *N Engl J Med.* 1995;333(16):1038–1044.

88. Landais E, Morice A, Long HM, et al. EBV-specific CD4+ T cell clones exhibit vigorous allogeneic responses. *J Immunol.* 2006;177(3):1427–1433.

89. Martins SL, St John LS, Champlin RE, et al. Functional assessment and specific depletion of alloreactive human T cells using flow cytometry. *Blood.* 2004;104(12):3429–3436.

90. Meij P, Jedema I, Zandvliet ML, et al. Effective treatment of refractory CMV reactivation after allogeneic stem cell transplantation with in vitro-generated CMV pp65-specific CD8+ T-cell lines. *J Immunother.* 2012;35(8):621–628.

91. Gerdemann U, Katari UL, Papadopoulou A, et al. Safety and clinical efficacy of rapidly-generated trivirus-directed T cells as treatment for adenovirus, EBV, and CMV infections after allogeneic hematopoietic stem cell transplant. *Mol Ther.* 2013;21(11):2113–2121.

92. Leen AM, Myers GD, Sili U, et al. Monoculture-derived T lymphocytes specific for multiple viruses expand and produce clinically relevant effects in immunocompromised individuals. *Nat Med.* 2006;12(10):1160–1166.

93. Leen AM, Christin A, Myers GD, et al. Cytotoxic T lymphocyte therapy with donor T cells prevents and treats adenovirus and Epstein-Barr virus infections after haploidentical and matched unrelated stem cell transplantation. *Blood.* 2009;114(19):4283–4292.

94. Micklethwaite KP, Clancy L, Sandher U, et al. Prophylactic infusion of cytomegalovirus-specific cytotoxic T lymphocytes stimulated with Ad5f35pp65 gene-modified dendritic cells after allogeneic hemopoietic stem cell transplantation. *Blood.* 2008;112(10):3974–3981.

95. Ma CK, Blyth E, Clancy L, et al. Addition of varicella zoster virus-specific T cells to cytomegalovirus, Epstein-Barr virus and adenovirus tri-specific T cells as adoptive immunotherapy in patients undergoing allogeneic hematopoietic stem cell transplantation. *Cytotherapy.* 2015;17(10):1406–1420.

96. Gerdemann U, Keirnan JM, Katari UL, et al. Rapidly generated multivirus-specific cytotoxic T lymphocytes for the prophylaxis and treatment of viral infections. *Mol Ther.* 2012;20(8):1622–1632.

97. Papadopoulou A, Gerdemann U, Katari UL, et al. Activity of broad-spectrum T cells as treatment for AdV, EBV, CMV, BKV, and HHV6 infections after HSCT. *Sci Transl Med.* 2014;6(242). 242ra83.

98. Leen AM, Bollard CM, Mendizabal AM, et al. Multicenter study of banked third-party virus-specific T cells to treat severe viral infections after hematopoietic stem cell transplantation. *Blood.* 2013;121(26):5113–5123.

99. Haque T, Taylor C, Wilkie GM, et al. Complete regression of posttransplant lymphoproliferative disease using partially HLA-matched Epstein Barr virus-specific cytotoxic T cells. *Transplantation.* 2001;72(8):1399–1402.

100. Barker JN, Doubrovina E, Sauter C, et al. Successful treatment of EBV-associated posttransplantation lymphoma after cord blood transplantation using third-party EBV-specific cytotoxic T lymphocytes. *Blood.* 2010;116(23):5045–5049.

101. Qian C, Campidelli A, Wang Y, et al. Curative or pre-emptive adenovirus-specific T cell transfer from matched unrelated or third party haploidentical donors after HSCT, including UCB transplantations: a successful phase I/II multicenter clinical trial. *J Hematol Oncol.* 2017;10(1):102.

102. Tzannou I, Papadopoulou A, Naik S, et al. Off-the-Shelf virus-specific T cells to treat 'BK virus, human herpesvirus 6, cytomegalovirus, epstein-barr virus, and adenovirus infections after allogeneic hematopoietic stem-cell transplantation. *J Clin Oncol.* 2017. JCO2017730655.

103. Morice A, Charreau B, Neveu B, et al. Cross-reactivity of herpesvirus-specific CD8 T cell lines toward allogeneic class I MHC molecules. *PLoS One.* 2010;5(8):e12120.

104. D'Orsogna LJ, Roelen DL, Doxiadis II, Claas FH. Alloreactivity from human viral specific memory T-cells. *Transpl Immunol.* 2010;23(4):149–155.

105. Amir AL, D'Orsogna LJ, Roelen DL, et al. Allo-HLA reactivity of virus-specific memory T cells is common. *Blood.* 2010;115(15):3146–3157.

106. Melenhorst JJ, Leen AM, Bollard CM, et al. Allogeneic virus-specific T cells with HLA alloreactivity do not produce GVHD in human subjects. *Blood.* 2010;116(22):4700–4702.

107. Choi SW, Reddy P. Current and emerging strategies for the prevention of graft-versus-host disease. *Nat Rev Clin Oncol.* 2014;11(9):536–547.

108. Jagasia M, Arora M, Flowers ME, et al. Risk factors for acute GVHD and survival after hematopoietic cell transplant. *Blood.* 2012;119(1):296–307.

109. Ash RC, Horowitz MM, Gale RP, et al. Bone marrow transplantation from related donors other than HLA-identical siblings: effect of T cell depletion. *Bone Marrow Transpl.* 1991;7(6):443–452.

110. Martin PJ, Rizzo JD, Wingard JR, et al. First- and second-line systemic treatment of acute graft-versus-host disease: recommendations of the American Society of Blood and Marrow Transplantation. *Biol Blood Marrow Transpl.* 2012;18(8):1150–1163.

111. MacMillan ML, Weisdorf DJ, Wagner JE, et al. Response of 443 patients to steroids as primary therapy for acute graft-versus-host disease: comparison of grading systems. *Biol Blood Marrow Transpl.* 2002;8(7):387–394.

112. Kernan NA, Collins NH, Juliano L, Cartagena T, Dupont B, O'Reilly RJ. Clonable T lymphocytes in T cell-depleted bone marrow transplants correlate with development of graft-v-host disease. *Blood.* 1986;68(3):770–773.

113. Korngold R, Sprent J. Lethal graft-versus-host disease after bone marrow transplantation across minor histocompatibility barriers in mice. Prevention by removing mature T cells from marrow. *J Exp Med.* 1978;148(6):1687–1698.

114. Ho VT, Soiffer RJ. The history and future of T-cell depletion as graft-versus-host disease prophylaxis for allogeneic hematopoietic stem cell transplantation. *Blood.* 2001;98(12):3192–3204.

115. Giralt S, Hester J, Huh Y, et al. CD8-depleted donor lymphocyte infusion as treatment for relapsed chronic myelogenous leukemia after allogeneic bone marrow transplantation. *Blood.* 1995;86(11):4337–4343.

116. Patterson J, Prentice HG, Brenner MK, et al. Graft rejection following HLA matched T-lymphocyte depleted bone marrow transplantation. *Br J Haematol.* 1986;63(2):221–230.

117. Zutter MM, Martin PJ, Sale GE, et al. Epstein-Barr virus lymphoproliferation after bone marrow transplantation. *Blood.* 1988;72(2):520–529.

118. Goldman JM, Gale RP, Horowitz MM, et al. Bone marrow transplantation for chronic myelogenous leukemia in chronic phase. Increased risk for relapse associated with T-cell depletion. *Ann Intern Med.* 1988;108(6):806–814.

119. Wagner JE, Thompson JS, Carter SL, Kernan NA, Unrelated Donor Marrow Transplantation T. Effect of graft-versus-host disease prophylaxis on 3-year disease-free survival in recipients of unrelated donor bone marrow (T-cell Depletion Trial): a multi-centre, randomised phase II-III trial. *Lancet.* 2005;366(9487):733–741.

120. Apperley JF, Jones L, Hale G, et al. Bone marrow transplantation for patients with chronic myeloid leukaemia: T-cell depletion with Campath-1 reduces the incidence of graft-versus-host disease but may increase the risk of leukaemic relapse. *Bone Marrow Transpl.* 1986;1(1):53–66.

121. Pavletic SZ, Carter SL, Kernan NA, et al. Influence of T-cell depletion on chronic graft-versus-host disease: results of a multicenter randomized trial in unrelated marrow donor transplantation. *Blood.* 2005;106(9):3308–3313.

122. Mitsuyasu RT, Champlin RE, Gale RP, et al. Treatment of donor bone marrow with monoclonal anti-T-cell antibody and complement for the prevention of graft-versus-host disease. A prospective, randomized, double-blind trial. *Ann Intern Med.* 1986;105(1):20–26.

123. Theurich S, Fischmann H, Shimabukuro-Vornhagen A, et al. Polyclonal anti-thymocyte globulins for the prophylaxis of graft-versus-host disease after allogeneic stem cell or bone marrow transplantation in adults. *Cochrane Database Syst Rev.* 2012;(9):CD009159.

124. Marmont AM, Horowitz MM, Gale RP, et al. T-cell depletion of HLA-identical transplants in leukemia. *Blood.* 1991;78(8):2120–2130.

125. Yi T, Chen Y, Wang L, et al. Reciprocal differentiation and tissue-specific pathogenesis of Th1, Th2, and Th17 cells in graft-versus-host disease. *Blood.* 2009;114(14):3101–3112.

126. Haase D, Starke M, Puan KJ, Lai TS, Rotzschke O. Immune modulation of inflammatory conditions: regulatory T cells for treatment of GvHD. *Immunol Res.* 2012;53(1–3):200–212.

127. Blazar BR, Murphy WJ, Abedi M. Advances in graft-versus-host disease biology and therapy. *Nat Rev Immunol.* 2012;12(6):443–458.

128. Godder KT, Henslee-Downey PJ, Mehta J, et al. Long term disease-free survival in acute leukemia patients recovering with increased gammadelta T cells after partially mismatched related donor bone marrow transplantation. *Bone Marrow Transpl.* 2007;39(12):751–757.

129. Schumm M, Lang P, Bethge W, et al. Depletion of T-cell receptor alpha/beta and CD19 positive cells from apheresis products with the CliniMACS device. *Cytotherapy.* 2013;15(10):1253–1258.

130. Li Pira G, Malaspina D, Girolami E, et al. Selective depletion of alphabeta T cells and B cells for human leukocyte antigen-haploidentical hematopoietic stem cell transplantation. A three-year follow-up of procedure efficiency. *Biol Blood Marrow Transpl.* 2016;22(11):2056–2064.

131. Bertaina A, Merli P, Rutella S, et al. HLA-haploidentical stem cell transplantation after removal of alphabeta+ T and B cells in children with nonmalignant disorders. *Blood.* 2014;124(5):822–826.

132. Kaynar L, Demir K, Turak EE, et al. TcR alphabeta-depleted haploidentical transplantation results in adult acute leukemia patients. *Hematology.* 2017;22(3):136–144.

133. Bradley LM, Watson SR, Swain SL. Entry of naive CD4 T cells into peripheral lymph nodes requires L-selectin. *J Exp Med.* 1994;180(6):2401–2406.

134. Croft M, Bradley LM, Swain SL. Naive versus memory CD4 T cell response to antigen. Memory cells are less dependent on accessory cell costimulation and can respond to many antigen-presenting cell types including resting B cells. *J Immunol.* 1994;152(6):2675–2685.

135. Anderson BE, McNiff J, Yan J, et al. Memory CD4+ T cells do not induce graft-versus-host disease. *J Clin Invest.* 2003;112(1):101–108.

136. Bleakley M, Heimfeld S, Jones LA, et al. Engineering human peripheral blood stem cell grafts that are depleted of naive T cells and retain functional pathogen-specific memory T cells. *Biol Blood Marrow Transpl.* 2014;20(5):705–716.

137. Huang W, Chao NJ. Memory T cells: a helpful guard for allogeneic hematopoietic stem cell transplantation without causing graft-versus-host disease. *Hematol Oncol Stem Cell Ther.* 2017.

138. Chen BJ, Cui X, Sempowski GD, Liu C, Chao NJ. Transfer of allogeneic CD62L- memory T cells without graft-versus-host disease. *Blood.* 2004;103(4):1534–1541.

139. Chen BJ, Deoliveira D, Cui X, et al. Inability of memory T cells to induce graft-versus-host disease is a result of an abortive alloresponse. *Blood.* 2007;109(7):3115–3123.

140. Ciceri F, Bonini C, Stanghellini MT, et al. Infusion of suicide-gene-engineered donor lymphocytes after family haploidentical haemopoietic stem-cell transplantation for leukaemia (the TK007 trial): a non-randomised phase I-II study. *Lancet Oncol.* 2009;10(5):489–500.

141. Vago L, Oliveira G, Bondanza A, et al. T-cell suicide gene therapy prompts thymic renewal in adults after hematopoietic stem cell transplantation. *Blood.* 2012;120(9):1820–1830.

142. Zhou X, Di Stasi A, Tey SK, et al. Long-term outcome after haploidentical stem cell transplant and infusion of T cells expressing the inducible caspase 9 safety transgene. *Blood.* 2014;123(25):3895–3905.

143. Zhou X, Dotti G, Krance RA, et al. Inducible caspase-9 suicide gene controls adverse effects from alloreplete T cells after haploidentical stem cell transplantation. *Blood.* 2015;125(26):4103–4113.

144. Di Stasi A, Tey SK, Dotti G, et al. Inducible apoptosis as a safety switch for adoptive cell therapy. *N Engl J Med.* 2011;365(18):1673–1683.

145. Hori S, Nomura T, Sakaguchi S. Control of regulatory T cell development by the transcription factor Foxp3. *Science.* 2003;299(5609):1057–1061.

146. Rieger K, Loddenkemper C, Maul J, et al. Mucosal FOXP3+ regulatory T cells are numerically deficient in acute and chronic GvHD. *Blood.* 2006;107(4):1717–1723.

147. Taylor PA, Lees CJ, Blazar BR. The infusion of ex vivo activated and expanded CD4(+)CD25(+) immune regulatory cells inhibits graft-versus-host disease lethality. *Blood.* 2002;99(10):3493–3499.

148. Rezvani K, Mielke S, Ahmadzadeh M, et al. High donor FOXP3-positive regulatory T-cell (Treg) content is associated with a low risk of GVHD following HLA-matched allogeneic SCT. *Blood.* 2006;108(4):1291–1297.

149. Magenau JM, Qin X, Tawara I, et al. Frequency of CD4(+)CD25(hi)FOXP3(+) regulatory T cells has diagnostic and prognostic value as a biomarker for acute graft-versus-host-disease. *Biol Blood Marrow Transpl.* 2010;16(7):907–914.

150. Bremm M, Huenecke S, Lehrnbecher T, et al. Advanced flowcytometric analysis of regulatory T cells: CD127 downregulation early post stem cell transplantation and altered Treg/CD3(+)CD4(+)-ratio in severe GvHD or relapse. *J Immunol Methods.* 2011;373(1–2):36–44.

151. Li Q, Zhai Z, Xu X, et al. Decrease of CD4(+)CD25(+) regulatory T cells and TGF-beta at early immune reconstitution is associated to the onset and severity of graft-versus-host disease following allogeneic haematogenesis stem cell transplantation. *Leuk Res.* 2010;34(9):1158–1168.

152. McIver Z, Melenhorst JJ, Wu C, et al. Donor lymphocyte count and thymic activity predict lymphocyte recovery and outcomes after matched-sibling hematopoietic stem cell transplant. *Haematologica.* 2013;98(3):346–352.

153. Watanabe N, Narita M, Furukawa T, et al. Kinetics of pDCs, mDCs, gammadeltaT cells and regulatory T cells in association with graft versus host disease after hematopoietic stem cell transplantation. *Int J Lab Hematol.* 2011;33(4):378–390.

154. Schneider M, Munder M, Karakhanova S, Ho AD, Goerner M. The initial phase of graft-versus-host disease is associated with a decrease of CD4+CD25+ regulatory T cells in the peripheral blood of patients after allogeneic stem cell transplantation. *Clin Lab Haematol.* 2006;28(6):382–390.

155. Ukena SN, Grosse J, Mischak-Weissinger E, et al. Acute but not chronic graft-versus-host disease is associated with a reduction of circulating CD4(+)CD25(high)CD127(low/-) regulatory T cells. *Ann Hematol.* 2011;90(2):213–218.

156. Baecher-Allan C, Brown JA, Freeman GJ, Hafler DA. CD4+CD25high regulatory cells in human peripheral blood. *J Immunol.* 2001;167(3):1245–1253.

157. Brunstein CG, Miller JS, Cao Q, et al. Infusion of ex vivo expanded T regulatory cells in adults transplanted with umbilical cord blood: safety profile and detection kinetics. *Blood.* 2011;117(3):1061–1070.

158. Di Ianni M, Falzetti F, Carotti A, et al. Immunoselection and clinical use of T regulatory cells in HLA-haploidentical stem cell transplantation. *Best Pract Res Clin Haematol.* 2011;24(3):459–466.

159. Martelli MF, Di Ianni M, Ruggeri L, et al. HLA-haploidentical transplantation with regulatory and conventional T-cell adoptive immunotherapy prevents acute leukemia relapse. *Blood.* 2014;124(4):638–644.

160. Ramlal R, Hildebrandt GC. Advances in the use of regulatory T-cells for the prevention and therapy of graft-vs.-host disease. *Biomedicines.* 2017;5(2).

161. Brunstein CG, Miller JS, McKenna DH, et al. Umbilical cord blood-derived T regulatory cells to prevent GVHD: kinetics, toxicity profile, and clinical effect. *Blood.* 2016;127(8):1044–1051.

162. Ito S, Bollard CM, Carlsten M, et al. Ultra-low dose interleukin-2 promotes immune-modulating function of regulatory T cells and natural killer cells in healthy volunteers. *Mol Ther.* 2014;22(7):1388–1395.

163. Zhao XY, Zhao XS, Wang YT, et al. Prophylactic use of low-dose interleukin-2 and the clinical outcomes of hematopoietic stem cell transplantation: a randomized study. *Oncoimmunology.* 2016;5(12):e1250992.

164. Kennedy-Nasser AA, Ku S, Castillo-Caro P, et al. Ultra low-dose IL-2 for GVHD prophylaxis after allogeneic hematopoietic stem cell transplantation mediates expansion of regulatory T cells without diminishing antiviral and antileukemic activity. *Clin Cancer Res.* 2014;20(8):2215–2225.

165. Koreth J, Kim HT, Jones KT, et al. Efficacy, durability, and response predictors of low-dose interleukin-2 therapy for chronic graft-versus-host disease. *Blood.* 2016;128(1):130–137.

166. Edinger M, Hoffmann P, Ermann J, et al. CD4+CD25+ regulatory T cells preserve graft-versus-tumor activity while inhibiting graft-versus-host disease after bone marrow transplantation. *Nat Med.* 2003;9(9):1144–1150.

167. Mielke S, Nunes R, Rezvani K, et al. A clinical-scale selective allodepletion approach for the treatment of HLA-mismatched and matched donor-recipient pairs using expanded T lymphocytes as antigen-presenting cells and a TH9402-based photodepletion technique. *Blood.* 2008;111(8):4392–4402.

168. McIver ZA, Melenhorst JJ, Grim A, et al. Immune reconstitution in recipients of photodepleted HLA-identical sibling donor stem cell transplantations: T cell subset frequencies predict outcome. *Biol Blood Marrow Transpl.* 2011;17(12):1846–1854.

169. Roy D-C, Lachance S, Roy J, et al. Donor lymphocytes depleted of alloreactive T-cells (ATIR101) improve event-free survival (GRFS) and overall survival in a T-cell depleted haploidentical HSCT: phase 2 trial in patients with AML and ALL. *Blood.* 2016;128(22):1226.

170. Joo SY, Cho KA, Jung YJ, et al. Bioimaging for the monitoring of the in vivo distribution of infused mesenchymal stem cells in a mouse model of the graft-versus-host reaction. *Cell Biol Int.* 2011;35(4):417–421.

171. Hu KX, Wang MH, Fan C, Wang L, Guo M, Ai HS. CM-DiI labeled mesenchymal stem cells homed to thymus inducing immune recovery of mice after haploidentical bone marrow transplantation. *Int Immunopharmacol.* 2011;11(9):1265–1270.

172. Zhao K, Lou R, Huang F, et al. Immunomodulation effects of mesenchymal stem cells on acute graft-versus-host disease after hematopoietic stem cell transplantation. *Biol Blood Marrow Transpl.* 2015;21(1):97–104.

173. Munneke JM, Spruit MJ, Cornelissen AS, van Hoeven V, Voermans C, Hazenberg MD. The potential of mesenchymal stem cells as treatment for severe steroid-refractory acute graft-versus-host disease: a critical review of the literature. *Transplantation.* 2016;100(11):2309–2314.

174. Le Blanc K, Rasmusson I, Sundberg B, et al. Treatment of severe acute graft-versus-host disease with third party haploidentical mesenchymal stem cells. *Lancet.* 2004;363(9419):1439–1441.

175. Le Blanc K, Frassoni F, Ball L, et al. Mesenchymal stem cells for treatment of steroid-resistant, severe, acute graft-versus-host disease: a phase II study. *Lancet.* 2008;371(9624):1579–1586.

176. Ball LM, Bernardo ME, Roelofs H, et al. Multiple infusions of mesenchymal stem cells induce sustained remission in children with steroid-refractory, grade III-IV acute graft-versus-host disease. *Br J Haematol.* 2013;163(4):501–509.

177. Kurtzberg J, Prockop S, Teira P, et al. Allogeneic human mesenchymal stem cell therapy (remestemcel-L, Prochymal) as a rescue agent for severe refractory acute graft-versus-host disease in pediatric patients. *Biol Blood Marrow Transpl.* 2014;20(2):229–235.

178. Galipeau J. The mesenchymal stem cells dilemma–does a negative phase III trial of random donor mesenchymal stem cells in steroid-resistant graft-versus-host disease represent a death knell or a bump in the road? *Cytotherapy.* 2013;15(1):2–8.

179. von Dalowski F, Kramer M, Wermke M, et al. Mesenchymal stem cells for treatment of acute steroid-refractory graft versus host disease: clinical responses and long-term outcome. *Stem Cells.* 2016;34(2):357–366.

180. Yin F, Battiwalla M, Ito S, et al. Bone marrow mesenchymal stem cells to treat tissue damage in allogeneic stem cell transplant recipients: correlation of biological markers with clinical responses. *Stem Cells.* 2014;32(5):1278–1288.

181. Kuzmina LA, Petinati NA, Parovichnikova EN, et al. Multipotent mesenchymal stem cells for the prophylaxis of acute graft-versus-host disease-A phase II study. *Stem Cells Int.* 2012;2012:968213.

182. Baron F, Lechanteur C, Willems E, et al. Cotransplantation of mesenchymal stem cells might prevent death from graft-versus-host disease (GVHD) without abrogating graft-versus-tumor effects after HLA-mismatched allogeneic transplantation following nonmyeloablative conditioning. *Biol Blood Marrow Transpl.* 2010;16(6):838–847.

183. Lee SH, Lee MW, Yoo KH, et al. Co-transplantation of third-party umbilical cord blood-derived MSCs promotes engraftment in children undergoing unrelated umbilical cord blood transplantation. *Bone Marrow Transpl.* 2013;48(8):1040–1045.

184. Lazarus HM, Koc ON, Devine SM, et al. Cotransplantation of HLA-identical sibling culture-expanded mesenchymal stem cells and hematopoietic stem cells in hematologic malignancy patients. *Biol Blood Marrow Transpl.* 2005;11(5):389–398.

185. Miller JS, Warren EH, van den Brink MR, et al. NCI first international workshop on the biology, prevention, and treatment of relapse after allogeneic hematopoietic stem cell transplantation: report from the committee on the biology underlying recurrence of malignant disease following allogeneic HSCT: graft-versus-tumor/leukemia reaction. *Biol Blood Marrow Transpl.* 2010;16(5):565–586.

186. Reid GS, Shan X, Coughlin CM, et al. Interferon-gamma-dependent infiltration of human T cells into neuroblastoma tumors in vivo. *Clin Cancer Res.* 2009;15(21):6602–6608.

187. Lowdell MW, Craston R, Samuel D, et al. Evidence that continued remission in patients treated for acute leukaemia is dependent upon autologous natural killer cells. *Br J Haematol.* 2002;117(4):821–827.

188. Barbaric D, Corthals SL, Jastaniah WA, et al. Detection of WT1-specific T cells in paediatric acute lymphoblastic leukaemia patients in first remission. *Br J Haematol.* 2008;141(2):271–273.

189. Montagna D, Maccario R, Locatelli F, et al. Emergence of antitumor cytolytic T cells is associated with maintenance of hematologic remission in children with acute myeloid leukemia. *Blood.* 2006;108(12):3843–3850.

190. Berghuis D, Santos SJ, Baelde HJ, et al. Pro-inflammatory chemokine-chemokine receptor interactions within the Ewing sarcoma microenvironment determine CD8(+) T-lymphocyte infiltration and affect tumour progression. *J Pathol.* 2011;223(3):347–357.

191. Yegin ZA, Ozkurt ZN, Aki SZ, Sucak GT. Donor lymphocyte infusion for leukemia relapse after hematopoietic stem cell transplantation. *Transfus Apher Sci.* 2010;42(3):239–245.

192. Kumaki S, Minegishi M, Fujie H, et al. Prolonged secretion of IL-15 in patients with severe forms of acute graft-versus-host disease after allogeneic bone marrow transplantation in children. *Int J Hematol.* 1998;67(3):307–312.

193. Chik KW, Li K, Pong H, Shing MM, Li CK, Yuen PM. Elevated serum interleukin-15 level in acute graft-versus-host disease after hematopoietic cell transplant. *J Pediatr Hematol Oncol.* 2003;25(12):960–964.

194. Huang XJ, Liu DH, Liu KY, Xu LP, Chen H, Han W. Donor lymphocyte infusion for the treatment of leukemia relapse after HLA-mismatched/haploidentical T-cell-replete hematopoietic stem cell transplantation. *Haematologica.* 2007;92(3):414–417.

195. Zeidan AM, Forde PM, Symons H, et al. HLA-haploidentical donor lymphocyte infusions for patients with relapsed hematologic malignancies after related HLA-haploidentical bone marrow transplantation. *Biol Blood Marrow Transpl.* 2014;20(3):314–318.

196. Ghiso A, Raiola AM, Gualandi F, et al. DLI after haploidentical BMT with post-transplant CY. *Bone Marrow Transpl.* 2015;50(1):56–61.

197. Huff CA, Fuchs EJ, Smith BD, et al. Graft-versus-host reactions and the effectiveness of donor lymphocyte infusions. *Biol Blood Marrow Transpl.* 2006;12(4):414–421.

198. Michallet AS, Nicolini F, Furst S, et al. Outcome and long-term follow-up of alloreactive donor lymphocyte infusions given for relapse after myeloablative allogeneic hematopoietic stem cell transplantations (HSCT). *Bone Marrow Transpl.* 2005;35(6):601–608.

199. Kolb HJ, Schattenberg A, Goldman JM, et al. Graft-versus-leukemia effect of donor lymphocyte transfusions in marrow grafted patients. *Blood.* 1995;86(5):2041–2050.

200. Collins Jr RH, Shpilberg O, Drobyski WR, et al. Donor leukocyte infusions in 140 patients with relapsed malignancy after allogeneic bone marrow transplantation. *J Clin Oncol.* 1997;15(2):433–444.

201. Kolb HJ. Hematopoietic stem cell transplantation and cellular therapy. *HLA.* 2017;89(5):267–277.

202. Wang Y, Liu DH, Xu LP, et al. Prevention of relapse using granulocyte CSF-primed PBPCs following HLA-mismatched/haploidentical, T-cell-replete hematopoietic SCT in patients with advanced-stage acute leukemia: a retrospective risk-factor analysis. *Bone Marrow Transpl.* 2012;47(8):1099–1104.

203. Liga M, Triantafyllou E, Tiniakou M, et al. High alloreactivity of low-dose prophylactic donor lymphocyte infusion in patients with acute leukemia undergoing allogeneic hematopoietic cell transplant with an alemtuzumab-containing conditioning regimen. *Biol Blood Marrow Transpl.* 2013;19(1):75–81.

204. Montero A, Savani BN, Shenoy A, et al. T-cell depleted peripheral blood stem cell allotransplantation with T-cell add-back for patients with hematological malignancies: effect of chronic GVHD on outcome. *Biol Blood Marrow Transpl.* 2006;12(12):1318–1325.

205. Bleakley M, Riddell SR. Exploiting T cells specific for human minor histocompatibility antigens for therapy of leukemia. *Immunol Cell Biol.* 2011;89(3):396–407.

206. Marijt WA, Heemskerk MH, Kloosterboer FM, et al. Hematopoiesis-restricted minor histocompatibility antigens HA-1- or HA-2-specific T cells can induce complete remissions of relapsed leukemia. *Proc Natl Acad Sci USA.* 2003;100(5):2742–2747.

207. Marijt E, Wafelman A, van der Hoorn M, et al. Phase I/II feasibility study evaluating the generation of leukemia-reactive cytotoxic T lymphocyte lines for treatment of patients with relapsed leukemia after allogeneic stem cell transplantation. *Haematologica.* 2007;92(1):72–80.

208. Warren EH, Fujii N, Akatsuka Y, et al. Therapy of relapsed leukemia after allogeneic hematopoietic cell transplant with T cells specific for minor histocompatibility antigens. *Blood.* 2010;115(19):3869–3878.

209. Schwarzinger I, Valent P, Koller U, et al. Prognostic significance of surface marker expression on blasts of patients with de novo acute myeloblastic leukemia. *J Clin Oncol.* 1990;8(3):423–430.

210. Tyler EM, Jungbluth AA, O'Reilly RJ, Koehne G. WT1-specific T-cell responses in high-risk multiple myeloma patients undergoing allogeneic T cell-depleted hematopoietic stem cell transplantation and donor lymphocyte infusions. *Blood.* 2013;121(2):308–317.

211. Wang ZD, Li D, Huang XJ. Graft-versus-leukemia effects of Wilms' tumor 1 protein-specific cytotoxic T lymphocytes in patients with chronic myeloid leukemia after allogeneic hematopoietic stem cell transplantation. *Chin Med J Engl.* 2010;123(7):912–916.

212. Chapuis AG, Ragnarsson GB, Nguyen HN, et al. Transferred WT1-reactive CD8+ T cells can mediate antileukemic activity and persist in post-transplant patients. *Sci Transl Med.* 2013;5(174). 174ra27.

213. Bonneville M, O'Brien RL, Born WK. Gammadelta T cell effector functions: a blend of innate programming and acquired plasticity. *Nat Rev Immunol.* 2010;10(7):467–478.

214. Hayday AC. Gammadelta T cells and the lymphoid stress-surveillance response. *Immunity.* 2009;31(2):184–196.

215. Jameson J, Havran WL. Skin gammadelta T-cell functions in homeostasis and wound healing. *Immunol Rev.* 2007;215:114–122.

216. Lamb Jr LS, Henslee-Downey PJ, Parrish RS, et al. Increased frequency of TCR gamma delta + T cells in disease-free survivors following T cell-depleted, partially mismatched, related donor bone marrow transplantation for leukemia. *J Hematother.* 1996;5(5):503–509.

217. Wilhelm M, Kunzmann V, Eckstein S, et al. Gammadelta T cells for immune therapy of patients with lymphoid malignancies. *Blood.* 2003;102(1):200–206.

218. Kunzmann V, Smetak M, Kimmel B, et al. Tumor-promoting versus tumor-antagonizing roles of gammadelta T cells in cancer immunotherapy: results from a prospective phase I/II trial. *J Immunother.* 2012;35(2):205–213.

219. Abe Y, Muto M, Nieda M, et al. Clinical and immunological evaluation of zoledronate-activated Vgamma9gammadelta T-cell-based immunotherapy for patients with multiple myeloma. *Exp Hematol.* 2009;37(8):956–968.

220. Airoldi I, Bertaina A, Prigione I, et al. Gammadelta T-cell reconstitution after HLA-haploidentical hematopoietic transplantation depleted of TCR-alphabeta+/CD19+ lymphocytes. *Blood.* 2015;125(15):2349–2358.

221. Fisher JP, Heuijerjans J, Yan M, Gustafsson K, Anderson J. Gammadelta T cells for cancer immunotherapy: a systematic review of clinical trials. *Oncoimmunology.* 2014;3(1):e27572.

222. Gomes AQ, Martins DS, Silva-Santos B. Targeting gammadelta T lymphocytes for cancer immunotherapy: from novel mechanistic insight to clinical application. *Cancer Res.* 2010;70(24):10024–10027.

223. Brentjens RJ, Curran KJ. Novel cellular therapies for leukemia: CAR-modified T cells targeted to the CD19 antigen. *Hematol Am Soc Hematol Educ Program.* 2012;2012:143–151.

224. Lipowska-Bhalla G, Gilham DE, Hawkins RE, Rothwell DG. Targeted immunotherapy of cancer with CAR T cells: achievements and challenges. *Cancer Immunol Immunother.* 2012;61(7):953–962.

225. Jena B, Dotti G, Cooper LJ. Redirecting T-cell specificity by introducing a tumor-specific chimeric antigen receptor. *Blood.* 2010;116(7):1035–1044.

226. Eshhar Z, Waks T, Gross G, Schindler DG. Specific activation and targeting of cytotoxic lymphocytes through chimeric single chains consisting of antibody-binding domains and the gamma or zeta subunits of the immunoglobulin and T-cell receptors. *Proc Natl Acad Sci USA.* 1993;90(2):720–724.

227. Hirano N, Takahashi T, Takahashi T, et al. Expression of costimulatory molecules in human leukemias. *Leukemia.* 1996;10(7):1168–1176.

228. Brouwer RE, van der Heiden P, Schreuder GM, et al. Loss or downregulation of HLA class I expression at the allelic level in acute leukemia is infrequent but functionally relevant, and can be restored by interferon. *Hum Immunol.* 2002;63(3):200–210.

229. Singh H, Figliola MJ, Dawson MJ, et al. Manufacture of clinical-grade CD19-specific T cells stably expressing chimeric antigen receptor using Sleeping Beauty system and artificial antigen presenting cells. *PLoS One.* 2013;8(5):e64138.

230. Maus MV, Grupp SA, Porter DL, June CH. Antibody-modified T cells: CARs take the front seat for hematologic malignancies. *Blood.* 2014;123(17):2625–2635.

231. Kalamasz D, Long SA, Taniguchi R, Buckner JH, Berenson RJ, Bonyhadi M. Optimization of human T-cell expansion ex vivo using magnetic beads conjugated with anti-CD3 and Anti-CD28 antibodies. *J Immunother.* 2004;27(5):405–418.

232. Barrett DM, Singh N, Liu X, et al. Relation of clinical culture method to T-cell memory status and efficacy in xenograft models of adoptive immunotherapy. *Cytotherapy.* 2014;16(5):619–630.

233. Savoldo B, Ramos CA, Liu E, et al. CD28 costimulation improves expansion and persistence of chimeric antigen receptor-modified T cells in lymphoma patients. *J Clin Invest.* 2011;121(5):1822–1826.

234. Hoyos V, Savoldo B, Quintarelli C, et al. Engineering CD19-specific T lymphocytes with interleukin-15 and a suicide gene to enhance their anti-lymphoma/leukemia effects and safety. *Leukemia.* 2010;24(6):1160–1170.

235. Kochenderfer JN, Somerville RPT, Lu T, et al. Lymphoma remissions caused by anti-CD19 chimeric antigen receptor T cells are associated with high serum Interleukin-15 levels. *J Clin Oncol.* 2017;35(16):1803–1813.

236. Hackett PB, Largaespada DA, Switzer KC, Cooper LJ. Evaluating risks of insertional mutagenesis by DNA transposons in gene therapy. *Transl Res.* 2013;161(4):265–283.

237. Muul LM, Tuschong LM, Soenen SL, et al. Persistence and expression of the adenosine deaminase gene for 12 years and immune reaction to gene transfer components: long-term results of the first clinical gene therapy trial. *Blood.* 2003;101(7):2563–2569.

238. Scholler J, Brady TL, Binder-Scholl G, et al. Decade-long safety and function of retroviral-modified chimeric antigen receptor T cells. *Sci Transl Med.* 2012;4(132). 132ra53.

239. Maude SL, Frey N, Shaw PA, et al. Chimeric antigen receptor T cells for sustained remissions in leukemia. *N Engl J Med.* 2014;371(16):1507–1517.

240. Kochenderfer JN, Somerville RPT, Lu T, et al. Long-duration complete remissions of diffuse large B cell lymphoma after anti-CD19 chimeric antigen receptor T cell therapy. *Mol Ther.* 2017.

241. Brudno JN, Somerville RP, Shi V, et al. Allogeneic T cells that express an anti-CD19 chimeric antigen receptor induce remissions of B-cell malignancies that progress after allogeneic hematopoietic stem-cell transplantation without causing graft-versus-host disease. *J Clin Oncol.* 2016;34(10):1112–1121.

242. Anwer F, Shaukat AA, Zahid U, et al. Donor origin CAR T cells: graft versus malignancy effect without GVHD, a systematic review. *Immunotherapy.* 2017;9(2):123–130.

243. Neelapu SS, Tummala S, Kebriaei P, et al. Chimeric antigen receptor T-cell therapy - assessment and management of toxicities. *Nat Rev Clin Oncol.* 2017.

244. Dudley ME, Wunderlich JR, Robbins PF, et al. Cancer regression and autoimmunity in patients after clonal repopulation with antitumor lymphocytes. *Science.* 2002;298(5594):850–854.

245. Bennett M. Biology and genetics of hybrid resistance. *Adv Immunol.* 1987;41:333–445.

246. Savani BN, Mielke S, Adams S, et al. Rapid natural killer cell recovery determines outcome after T-cell-depleted HLA-identical stem cell transplantation in patients with myeloid leukemias but not with acute lymphoblastic leukemia. *Leukemia.* 2007;21(10):2145–2152.

247. Miller JS, Soignier Y, Panoskaltsis-Mortari A, et al. Successful adoptive transfer and in vivo expansion of human haploidentical NK cells in patients with cancer. *Blood.* 2005;105(8):3051–3057.

248. Koehl U, Sorensen J, Esser R, et al. IL-2 activated NK cell immunotherapy of three children after haploidentical stem cell transplantation. *Blood Cells Mol Dis.* 2004;33(3):261–266.

249. Brehm C, Huenecke S, Quaiser A, et al. IL-2 stimulated but not unstimulated NK cells induce selective disappearance of peripheral blood cells: concomitant results to a phase I/II study. *PLoS One.* 2011;6(11):e27351.

250. Stern M, Passweg JR, Meyer-Monard S, et al. Pre-emptive immunotherapy with purified natural killer cells after haploidentical SCT: a prospective phase II study in two centers. *Bone Marrow Transpl.* 2013;48(3):433–438.

251. Becker PS, Suck G, Nowakowska P, et al. Selection and expansion of natural killer cells for NK cell-based immunotherapy. *Cancer Immunol Immunother.* 2016;65(4):477–484.

252. Passweg JR, Tichelli A, Meyer-Monard S, et al. Purified donor NK-lymphocyte infusion to consolidate engraftment after haploidentical stem cell transplantation. *Leukemia.* 2004;18(11):1835–1838.

253. Koehl U, Esser R, Zimmermann S, et al. Ex vivo expansion of highly purified NK cells for immunotherapy after haploidentical stem cell transplantation in children. *Klin Padiatr.* 2005;217(6):345–350.

254. Shi J, Tricot G, Szmania S, et al. Infusion of haplo-identical killer immunoglobulin-like receptor ligand mismatched NK cells for relapsed myeloma in the setting of autologous stem cell transplantation. *Br J Haematol.* 2008;143(5):641–653.

255. Yoon SR, Lee YS, Yang SH, et al. Generation of donor natural killer cells from CD34(+) progenitor cells and subsequent infusion after HLA-mismatched allogeneic hematopoietic cell transplant: a feasibility study. *Bone Marrow Transpl.* 2010;45(6):1038–1046.

256. Rizzieri DA, Storms R, Chen DF, et al. Natural killer cell-enriched donor lymphocyte infusions from A 3-6/6 HLA matched family member following nonmyeloablative allogeneic stem cell transplantation. *Biol Blood Marrow Transpl.* 2010;16(8):1107–1114.

257. Choi I, Yoon SR, Park SY, et al. Donor-derived natural killer cells infused after human leukocyte antigen-haploidentical hematopoietic cell transplant: a dose-escalation study. *Biol Blood Marrow Transpl.* 2014;20(5):696–704.

258. Killig M, Friedrichs B, Meisig J, et al. Tracking in vivo dynamics of NK cells transferred in patients undergoing stem cell transplantation. *Eur J Immunol.* 2014;44(9):2822–2834.

259. Dong L, Gao ZY, Chang LJ, et al. Adoptive transfer of cytomegalovirus/Epstein-Barr virus-specific immune effector cells for therapeutic and preventive/preemptive treatment of pediatric allogeneic cell transplant recipients. *J Pediatr Hematol Oncol.* 2010;32(1):e31–e37.

260. Provasi E, Genovese P, Lombardo A, et al. Editing T cell specificity towards leukemia by zinc finger nucleases and lentiviral gene transfer. *Nat Med.* 2012;18(5):807–815.

261. Johnson LA, Morgan RA, Dudley ME, et al. Gene therapy with human and mouse T-cell receptors mediates cancer regression and targets normal tissues expressing cognate antigen. *Blood.* 2009;114(3):535–546.

262. Morgan RA, Dudley ME, Wunderlich JR, et al. Cancer regression in patients after transfer of genetically engineered lymphocytes. *Science.* 2006;314(5796):126–129.

263. Rapoport AP, Stadtmauer EA, Binder-Scholl GK, et al. NY-ESO-1-specific TCR-engineered T cells mediate sustained antigen-specific antitumor effects in myeloma. *Nat Med.* 2015;21(8):914–921.

264. Robbins PF, Morgan RA, Feldman SA, et al. Tumor regression in patients with metastatic synovial cell sarcoma and melanoma using genetically engineered lymphocytes reactive with NY-ESO-1. *J Clin Oncol.* 2011;29(7):917–924.

265. Robbins PF, Kassim SH, Tran TL, et al. A pilot trial using lymphocytes genetically engineered with an NY-ESO-1-reactive T-cell receptor: long-term follow-up and correlates with response. *Clin Cancer Res.* 2015;21(5):1019–1027.

266. Linette GP, Stadtmauer EA, Maus MV, et al. Cardiovascular toxicity and titin cross-reactivity of affinity-enhanced T cells in myeloma and melanoma. *Blood.* 2013;122(6):863–871.

267. Parkhurst MR, Yang JC, Langan RC, et al. T cells targeting carcinoembryonic antigen can mediate regression of metastatic colorectal cancer but induce severe transient colitis. *Mol Ther.* 2011;19(3):620–626.

268. Tran E, Turcotte S, Gros A, et al. Cancer immunotherapy based on mutation-specific CD4+ T cells in a patient with epithelial cancer. *Science.* 2014;344(6184):641–645.

269. Somasundaram R, Swoboda R, Caputo L, et al. Human leukocyte antigen-A2-restricted CTL responses to mutated BRAF peptides in melanoma patients. *Cancer Res.* 2006;66(6):3287–3293.

270. Conrad H, Gebhard K, Kronig H, et al. CTLs directed against HER2 specifically cross-react with HER3 and HER4. *J Immunol.* 2008;180(12):8135–8145.

Index

Note: Page numbers followed by "f" indicate figures and "t" indicate tables.

Printed and bound by CPI Group (UK) Ltd, Croydon, CR0 4YY

03/10/2024

01040300-0013